small animal
internal medicine

The National Veterinary Medical Series for Independent Study

small animal internal medicine

Darcy H. Shaw, D.V.M., M.V.Sc.
Diplomate ACVIM (Internal Medicine)
Associate Professor
Department of Companion Animals
University of Prince Edward Island
Charlottetown, Prince Edward Island, Canada

Sherri L. Ihle, D.V.M., M.S.
Diplomate ACVIM (Internal Medicine)
Associate Professor
Department of Companion Animals
University of Prince Edward Island
Charlottetown, Prince Edward Island, Canada

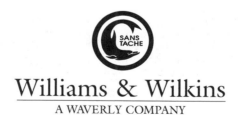

Williams & Wilkins
A WAVERLY COMPANY

BALTIMORE • PHILADELPHIA • LONDON • PARIS • BANGKOK
BUENOS AIRES • HONG KONG • MUNICH • SYDNEY • TOKYO • WROCLAW

1997

WILLIAMS & WILKINS

Editor: Elizabeth A. Nieginski
Manager, Development Editing: Julie Scardiglia
Marketing Manager: Diane M. Harnish
Development Editors: Melanie Cann, Lynne Stockton
Managing Editor: Darrin Kiessling
Editorial Assistant: Lisa Kiesel
Production Coordinator: Cindy Park
Series Editor, Clinical Sciences: Brian Hill, D.V.M.
Typesetter: Maryland Composition Co., Inc.
Printer: Mack Printing
Digitized Illustrations: Maryland Composition Co., Inc.
Binder: Mack Printing

Copyright © 1997 Williams & Wilkins

351 West Camden Street
Baltimore, Maryland 21201-2436 USA

Rose Tree Corporate Center
1400 North Providence Road
Building II, Suite 5025
Media, Pennsylvania 19063-2043 USA

Accurate indications, adverse reactions, and dosage schedules for drugs are provided in this book, but it is possible that they may change. The reader is urged to review the package information data of the manufacturers of the medications mentioned.

Printed in the United States of America

First Edition,

Library of Congress Cataloging-in-Publication Data

Shaw, Darcy H.
    Small animal internal medicine / Darcy H. Shaw, Sherri L. Ihle.—
1st ed.
      p.   cm — (The national veterinary medical series for independent study)
    Includes index.
    ISBN 0-683-07670-1
    1. Dogs—Diseases.   2. Cats—Diseases.   3. Veterinary internal medicine.   I. Ihle, Sherri L.   II. Title.   III. Series.
SF991.S53   1997
636.7'0896—dc21
                                              97-3958
                                              CIP

The publishers have made every effort to trace the copyright holders for borrowed material. If they have inadvertently overlooked any, they will be pleased to make the necessary arrangements at the first opportunity.

To purchase additional copies of this book, call our customer service department at **(800) 638-0672** or fax orders to **(800) 447-8438.** For other book services, including chapter reprints and large quantity sales, ask for the Special Sales department.

Canadian customers should call **(800) 665-1148,** or fax **(800) 665-0103.** For all other calls originating outside of the United States, please call **(410) 528-4223** or fax us at **(410) 528-8550.**

Visit Williams & Wilkins on the Internet: **http://www.wwilkins.com** or contact our customer service department at **custserv@wwilkins.com.** Williams & Wilkins customer service representatives are available from 8:30 am to 6:00 pm, EST, Monday through Friday, for telephone access.

97 98 99 00
1 2 3 4 5 6 7 8 9 10

Dedication

To Tao, Ted, Wally, Henry, and Norm, truly wonderful cats who have enriched my life immensely with their antics, eccentricities, and unconditional affection.

To all of my canine and feline patients who through my mistakes and successes have taught me so much about medicine and life.

To my past students who have kept me honest and enthused.

To my wife, Shelly Burton, who is my best friend and who makes it all worthwhile.

D. H. S.

Contents

Preface

The objectives of *NVMS Small Animal Internal Medicine* are to provide students with a concise, well-organized, and up-to-date overview of the discipline and to offer the opportunity to test comprehension of the material. In our effort to be concise and emphasize the key points regarding clinical signs, diagnosis, and treatment, information relating to pathophysiologic mechanisms and detailed treatment strategies is decidedly brief. Consequently, other textbooks and scientific publications should be sought for this information.

The main audience for *NVMS Small Animal Internal Medicine* is third- and fourth-year veterinary students, but interns, residents, and private practitioners will also find the book useful. *NVMS Small Animal Internal Medicine* is organized into three general sections. The first section, Chapters 1 through 38, deals with clinical problems and their causes. The next section, Chapters 39 through 50, covers diseases associated with organ systems. A self-assessment section containing a 100-question multiple choice examination concludes the book.

We are confident that readers will find this a current, accurate, and complete overview of small animal internal medicine and will be challenged by the self-assessment activities. A companion volume, *NVMS Small Animal Internal Medicine Case Management Test Booklet*, is also available to readers who wish to practice working through cases similar to those encountered in clinical practice and on national board examinations.

Darcy H. Shaw
Sherri L. Ihle

Acknowledgments

The authors would like to thank Williams & Wilkins for providing us with the opportunity to write this book, and Melanie Cann, our development editor, for her patience, timely prodding, and editorial contributions. We would also like to thank Lisa Kiesel and Lynne Stockton for their editorial contributions.

PART I

CLINICAL PROBLEMS

Chapter 1

Halitosis

I. DEFINITION. Halitosis is offensive or foul-smelling breath.

II. CAUSES of halitosis are listed in Table 1-1.

  A. In many cases, necrotic tissue, bacterial proliferation in retained food particles, or both are responsible for the odor.

  B. Consumption of a foul-smelling substance can cause transient halitosis.

III. CLINICAL FINDINGS vary with the underlying disease.

  A. Drooling may be seen with any of the oral or pharyngeal disorders listed in Table 1-1.

  B. Oral pain may indicate periodontal disease, neoplasia, or inflammation.

  C. Dysphagia in the presence of normal food prehension may indicate pharyngeal or esophageal disease.

IV. DIAGNOSTIC APPROACHES

  A. History and physical examination, including a full **oral examination,** will usually narrow the list of differential diagnoses.

  B. Viral serology or **biopsy** may be useful if oral ulceration or a mass is found.

TABLE 1-1. Causes of Halitosis

Oral disease
Dental tartar or periodontal disease
Neoplasia
Granuloma
Stomatitis or pharyngitis
Food retention
Esophageal disease
Neuromuscular disease with retention of food
Neoplasia
Granuloma
Miscellaneous causes
Gastritis (rare)

C. **Complete blood count (CBC), serum biochemical profile,** and **urinalysis** may help rule out systemic diseases that may cause oral lesions.

D. **Observation of the animal eating,** to assess food prehension and swallowing, may be helpful in the absence of dental tartar, oral ulceration, or oral masses (see Chapter 2).

V. **TREATMENT** is aimed at the primary disease.

Chapter 2

Dysphagia and Regurgitation

I. DEFINITION

A. **Dysphagia** is difficulty in prehending or swallowing food.

B. **Regurgitation** is the passive expulsion of undigested food from the esophagus.

II. CAUSES

A. **Dysphagia.** The causes of dysphagia are listed in Table 2-1.

B. **Regurgitation.** The causes of regurgitation are listed in Table 2-2.

III. CLINICAL FINDINGS

A. **Dysphagia.** A dysphagic animal may attempt to eat but is either unable to prehend the food, chew the food, or move the food to or beyond the pharyngeal region. The extent to which the animal is able to proceed with food consumption is determined by the site and type of disease. The clinical findings vary according to the underlying disorder.

   1. **Drooling** may result from an inability or reluctance to swallow.

   2. **Pain**

      a. **Oral pain** may occur with oral or pharyngeal trauma or foreign bodies.

      b. **Oral pain** accompanied by **halitosis** may occur with periodontitis, stomatitis or pharyngitis, neoplasia, or granuloma.

   3. **Neurologic abnormalities**

      a. A **"dropped jaw"** will be found with trigeminal nerve dysfunction.

      b. **Facial muscle pain** or **atrophy** may occur with facial myositis.

      c. The presence of **other neurologic abnormalities** (e.g., **weakness, abnormal mentation, ataxia**) suggests the presence of a central nervous system (CNS) disorder or a neuromuscular disease.

B. **Regurgitation.** Food prehension, mastication, tongue movement, and pharyngeal motility are usually normal, but esophageal structure or function is abnormal. The ejected material is often tubular in shape and alkaline.

IV. DIAGNOSTIC APPROACHES.
If differentiation between dysphagia and regurgitation is not possible from the history, watching the animal eat and drink may be helpful.

A. **Dysphagia** (see Table 2-1). A thorough neurologic and oral examination should be performed on all dogs and cats with dysphagia.

   1. If **neurologic abnormalities** are present, useful tests include a cerebrospinal fluid (CSF) tap, electrodiagnostic tests, and nerve or muscle biopsy.

   2. If **oral lesions** are present, a biopsy or further dental evaluation may be needed.

TABLE 2-1. Causes of and Diagnostic Tests for Dysphagia

Cause	Diagnostic Test
Neuromuscular disease	
Oral	
Myositis	Serum creatine kinase, electromyography, biopsy
Trigeminal nerve dysfunction	Physical examination, biopsy
Neuromuscular trauma	. . .
Pharyngeal	
Cricopharyngeal achalasia	Contrast radiographs with fluoroscopy
Myasthenia gravis	Acetylcholine receptor antibody titer
Myositis	Serum creatine kinase, electromyography, biopsy
Rabies	Histopathologic studies
Idiopathic	. . .
Obstructive disease	
Tumor	Biopsy
Granuloma	Biopsy
Foreign bodies	Oral examination, radiography
Sialocoele	Oral examination
Infectious and inflammatory disease	
Periodontitis	Oral examination
Stomatitis or pharyngitis	Oral examination, biopsy
Abscess (tooth root, retrobulbar)	Oral examination, radiography
Osteomyelitis	Radiography, biopsy, culture
Miscellaneous causes	
Trauma (e.g., fracture, laceration, hematoma)	Oral examination, radiography
Temporomandibular joint problems	Physical examination, radiography

TABLE 2-2. Causes of Regurgitation

Esophageal obstruction
  Foreign body
  Granuloma
  Periesophageal mass or fibrosis
  Persistent right aortic arch (PRAA) and other vascular ring anomalies
  Stricture
Megaesophagus
  Idiopathic megaesophagus
    Congenital
    Acquired
  Secondary megaesophagus
Miscellaneous causes
  Esophagitis
  Esophageal diverticulum
  Esophageal fistula
  Hiatal hernia

3. If **no abnormalities** are found, then contrast radiographs with fluoroscopy may delineate a pharyngeal or upper esophageal sphincter problem.

B. **Regurgitation** must be differentiated from vomiting (see Chapter 3). Diagnostic approaches to esophageal disease are discussed in Chapter 41 II A 4.

V. TREATMENT

A. **Dysphagia.** Treatment is aimed at the primary disorder. Parenteral fluid administration may be necessary.

B. **Regurgitation.** Treatment is aimed at the primary disorder. Retention of ingesta in the esophagus should be minimized by elevating the food and water supply and feeding the animal multiple small meals, consisting of a food of optimal consistency (the optimal consistency varies with the individual).

Chapter 3

Vomiting

I. DEFINITION

A. **Vomiting** is a reflex act characterized by forceful expulsion of gastric or small intestinal contents from the stomach, coordinated by the vomiting center in the medulla.

1. The vomiting center can be stimulated directly by drugs and toxins (endogenous and exogenous).

2. It can be triggered by afferent nerves from the viscera (especially the abdominal viscera), the chemoreceptor trigger zone, the vestibular apparatus, or the cerebrum.

B. **Hematemesis** is the vomiting of blood.

II. CAUSES of vomiting are summarized in Tables 3-1 through 3-4.

A. Vomiting soon after eating is most commonly due to overeating, dietary indiscretion, or gastritis.

B. Vomiting more than 8 hours after eating is more suggestive of gastric outflow obstruction or a motility disorder.

III. CLINICAL FINDINGS

A. Vomiting is usually preceded by nausea (evidenced by **hypersalivation, frequent swallowing,** and **restlessness**) and **anxiety** and is accompanied by repeated contractions of the diaphragm and abdomen. The ejected material may be digested or undigested and often contains bile.

B. Clinical findings that may accompany vomiting vary according to the cause of the vomiting (see Tables 3-1 through 3-4).

TABLE 3-1. Causes of Acute Vomiting without Systemic Signs of Illness

Cause	Common Concurrent Clinical Findings
Change in diet	Diarrhea
Dietary intolerance	Diarrhea
Dietary indiscretion	Diarrhea
Gastric foreign body	Abdominal discomfort
Motion sickness	Usually none
Medication	Variable, depending on the medication
Parasitic infection	Diarrhea
Psychogenic	Usually none
Early stage of a more chronic or serious disorder	Variable

TABLE 3-2. Causes of Acute Vomiting with Systemic Signs of Illness

Cause	Possible Concurrent Clinical Findings
Extra-gastrointestinal disorders	
Central nervous system (CNS) disease	Abnormal mentation, neurologic deficits
Diabetic ketoacidosis	Polyuria, polydipsia, anorexia, depression, dehydration, weight loss, polyphagia
Hepatic disease	Anorexia, diarrhea, icterus, ascites, neurologic abnormalities
Hypercalcemia	Weakness, anorexia, polyuria, polydipsia
Hypoadrenocorticism	Anorexia, diarrhea, dehydration, weakness, bradycardia
Hypocalcemia	Anorexia, muscle twitches, tetany
Hypokalemia	Weakness, polyuria
Pancreatitis	Anorexia, cranial abdominal discomfort, fever, dehydration, diarrhea, icterus
Peritonitis	Anorexia, depression, dehydration, abdominal pain, shock
Prostatitis	Anorexia, fever, hematuria, palpable prostatomegaly, prostatic pain
Pyometra	Anorexia, polyuria, polydipsia, vaginal discharge, depression, fever
Renal disease	Anorexia, depression, weight loss, polyuria or oliguria
Sepsis	Anorexia, fever, depression, dehydration
Urinary obstruction	Anorexia, abdominal discomfort
Vestibular disease	Head tilt, nystagmus
Primary gastrointestinal disorders	
Gastric dilatation	Anorexia, cranial abdominal distention
Gastric dilatation/volvulus (GDV)	Cranial abdominal distention, nonproductive retching, shock
Gastritis or enteritis	Anorexia, diarrhea, dehydration
Hemorrhagic gastroenteritis (HGE)	Hematemesis, hemorrhagic diarrhea, dehydration
Intestinal volvulus	Abdominal pain, shock
Neoplasia	Variable, depending on the type and site of neoplasia
Obstipation	Anorexia; dehydration; palpable, distended, firm colon
Obstruction (gastric or intestinal)	Diarrhea, abdominal discomfort, dehydration, shock
Parasitic infection	Diarrhea
Ulcers	Hematemesis, melena, abdominal discomfort, pale mucous membranes
Viral infection	Diarrhea, fever
Early stage of a more chronic disorder	Variable
Miscellaneous causes	
Diaphragmatic hernia	Anorexia, respiratory distress, history of trauma
Hyperthermia	Hyperthermia, depression, shock
Medications	Variable, depending on the medication
Toxins	Variable, depending on the toxin

TABLE 3-3. Causes of Chronic or Intermittent Vomiting

Cause	Possible Concurrent Clinical Findings
Extra-gastrointestinal disorders	
Diabetes mellitus	Polyuria, polydipsia, weight loss, polyphagia
Heartworm disease (cats)	Anorexia, coughing, dyspnea
Hepatic disease	Anorexia, diarrhea, icterus, ascites
Hyperthyroidism (cats)	Polyuria, polydipsia, polyphagia, weight loss, diarrhea, hyperactivity, palpable cervical mass
Hypoadrenocorticism	Anorexia, diarrhea, weight loss, weakness, bradycardia
Hypocalcemia	Anorexia, muscle twitching, tetany
Pancreatitis	Anorexia, cranial abdominal discomfort, fever, diarrhea
Renal disease	Anorexia, depression, polyuria and polydipsia or oliguria, weight loss
Primary gastrointestinal disorders	
Colitis	Large bowel diarrhea
Chronic inflammatory gastritis	Anorexia, weight loss, diarrhea
Enterogastric reflux (bilious vomiting syndrome)	Usually none
Fungal infection	Anorexia, fever, diarrhea, lymphadenopathy, other organ involvement
Idiopathic gastric hypomotility	Anorexia
Inflammatory bowel disease	Anorexia, diarrhea, weight loss
Irritable bowel syndrome	Diarrhea
Neoplasia	Variable, depending on the type and site of neoplasia
Obstruction	
Gastric antral mucosal hypertrophy	Usually none
Pyloric stenosis	Usually none
Upper intestinal (partial)	Diarrhea, anorexia, weight loss
Parasitic infection	Diarrhea
Ulcers (usually secondary to another disorder)	Anorexia, hematemesis, melena, abdominal discomfort, pale mucous membranes, other signs specific to the underlying disease
Miscellaneous causes	
Diaphragmatic hernia	Anorexia, history of trauma
Abdominal neoplasia	Variable, depending on the type and site of neoplasia

TABLE 3-4. Causes of Hematemesis

Cause	Possible Concurrent Clinical Findings
Gastrointestinal disorders	
Gastritis or enteritis	Anorexia, diarrhea, dehydration
Hemorrhagic gastroenteritis (HGE)	Depression, hemorrhagic diarrhea, dehydration
Neoplasia	Variable, depending on the type and site of neoplasia
Ulcers (usually secondary to another disorder)	Anorexia, melena, abdominal discomfort, pale mucous membranes, other signs specific to the underlying disorder
Other causes	
Coagulopathy	Petechiae, ecchymoses, other types of hemorrhage
Swallowed blood from hemoptysis	Cough, hemoptysis, tachypnea
Swallowed blood from oral hemorrhage	Oral lesions

IV. DIAGNOSTIC APPROACHES

A. Acute vomiting without systemic signs of illness

1. The diagnosis is often one of exclusion based on the **history** and the **physical examination.** A lack of response to conservative medical therapy indicates a need for additional testing.

2. Ascariasis is detected by fecal examination or response to treatment with pyrantel pamoate.

B. Acute vomiting with systemic signs of illness or chronic intermittent vomiting

1. **Complete blood count (CBC)**
   a. **Leukocytosis** may be seen with pancreatitis, peritonitis, pyometra, sepsis, or severe gastrointestinal (GI) inflammation.
   b. **An increased hematocrit but normal serum protein concentration** in a dog with hematemesis and bloody diarrhea is highly suggestive of hemorrhagic gastroenteritis (HGE).
   c. **Nonregenerative anemia** may be seen with chronic disease, peracute or chronic blood loss, or malnutrition.
   d. **Regenerative anemia** may be seen with subacute gastric hemorrhage.
   e. **Eosinophilia** may be seen with some parasitic infections, eosinophilic gastroenteritis, or hypoadrenocorticism.

2. **Serum biochemical profile**
   a. **Hypochloremic metabolic alkalosis** suggests loss of gastric acid because of gastric or upper duodenal vomiting.
   b. **Hyper- or hypocalcemia** may be the cause of the vomiting.
   c. **Hypoproteinemia** may result from blood loss, severe inflammation, or hepatic failure (hypoalbuminemia).
   d. **Hyperglycemia** is consistent with diabetes mellitus if concurrent glucosuria is present.
   e. **Increased serum hepatic enzyme concentrations** may be seen with hepatic disease.
   f. **Hypoalbuminemia** may be seen with hepatic failure, severe inflammatory disease, or severe GI hemorrhage.

g. Hypoglycemia may be seen with hypoadrenocorticism, pancreatitis, hepatic failure, and sepsis.

h. Hyperkalemia, hyponatremia, and **hypochloremia** may be seen with hypoadrenocorticism.

i. Increased serum amylase and **lipase concentrations** are suggestive of pancreatitis.

j. Azotemia with concurrent **isosthenuria** is most consistent with renal failure but can also be seen with acute hypoadrenocorticism.

k. Hyperbilirubinemia may be seen with hepatic disease or biliary obstruction caused by pancreatitis.

3. Urinalysis

a. Glucosuria is consistent with diabetes mellitus if hyperglycemia is also present. **Concurrent ketonuria** suggests diabetic ketoacidosis.

b. Isosthenuria may be seen with diabetes mellitus, hepatic failure, hypercalcemia, hypoadrenocorticism, hypokalemia, pyometra, and renal failure.

4. Fecal flotation may reveal parasitic infection.

5. Radiology

a. Survey radiographs

(1) Hepatomegaly or microhepatica may be seen with hepatic disease.

(2) Loss of cranial abdominal detail may be seen with pancreatitis.

(3) A generalized loss of abdominal detail may be seen with ascites (e.g., hepatic failure) or peritonitis.

(4) A large, fluid-filled tubular structure (i.e., an enlarged uterus) may be seen in the caudal abdomen with pyometra.

(5) Renomegaly or small kidneys may be seen with renal disease.

(6) Radiographic findings suggestive of gastric disease are discussed in Chapter 41 III A 5 a (1).

(7) A mass, lymphadenopathy, or other organomegaly may also be diagnostic.

b. Contrast radiographs (with fluoroscopy if possible) may be helpful [see Chapter 41 III A 5 a (2)].

6. An **adrenocorticotrophic hormone (ACTH) stimulation test** is indicated if the history, clinical findings, or laboratory results suggest hyperadrenocorticism.

7. Serum bile acid concentrations should be assessed if the history, clinical findings, or laboratory results suggest hepatic failure.

8. Ultrasound

a. A gastric foreign body, mass lesion, or gastric wall thickening may be visible.

b. Ultrasound can better assess any mass or change in organ size seen on survey radiographs.

9. Endoscopic evaluation (see Chapter 41 III A 5 c) may help with the diagnosis.

10. Exploratory laparotomy

a. Full-thickness gastrointestinal biopsies and biopsies of multiple organs can be obtained.

b. Surgery may be diagnostic as well as therapeutic in some situations (e.g., foreign bodies, neoplasms, obstructive lesions, peritonitis).

C. **Hematemesis** is usually an indication for a diagnostic evaluation.

1. History. The owner should be questioned about any current medications or the presence of a cough.

2. Physical examination

a. The mouth and nose should be examined for hemorrhage.

b. The skin should be evaluated for any masses (i.e., possible mast cell tumors).

3. Laboratory tests can be assessed to rule out extra-GI causes of GI ulceration or hemorrhage (see Chapter 41 III B 4) if no abnormalities are found on physical examination. Useful tests include the following:

   a. **CBC**
   b. **Serum biochemical profile**
   c. **Urinalysis**
   d. **Clotting tests** [i.e., activated clotting time or prothrombin time (PT) and partial thromboplastin time (PTT)]

   4. **Upper GI endoscopy** should be performed if laboratory test results are within normal limits. Endoscopy may be used to look for erosions or ulcers and to obtain biopsies for histopathology.

V. TREATMENT

A. **Acute vomiting without systemic signs of illness.** Food and water should be withheld for at least 12 hours to rest the GI tract, progressing to small amounts of water for 12–24 hours and later small meals of a bland, low-fat diet (e.g., cottage cheese or boiled meat mixed with rice or potatoes).

B. **Acute vomiting with systemic signs of illness**

   1. The primary disorder should be treated.

   2. Food and water should be withheld for at least 12–24 hours to rest the GI tract. Parenteral fluids are often needed during this time to correct or prevent dehydration and to correct electrolyte imbalances.

   3. Antiemetics (e.g., chlorpromazine, prochlorperazine, metoclopramide) can be considered if vomiting is excessive; however, it should be remembered that these agents do not resolve the main problem. Metoclopramide is contraindicated in the presence of an obstruction. Phenothiazines are contraindicated in animals with severe seizure disorders.

C. **Chronic intermittent vomiting**

   1. The primary disorder should be treated.

   2. Parenteral fluid administration is not often needed but should be instituted if dehydration or electrolyte imbalances are present.

D. **Hematemesis**

   1. Food and water should be withheld and parenteral fluid administered to correct and maintain hydration and to correct any electrolyte imbalances.

   2. A transfusion may also be needed if the hemorrhage is severe.

   3. Because gastrointestinal ulceration is the most common cause of hematemesis, treatment with sucralfate and a histamine-2 (H_2) antagonist may be instituted while awaiting the results of diagnostic tests.

Chapter 4

Diarrhea

I. DEFINITIONS

A. **Diarrhea** is excess water in the feces.

1. **Secretory** diarrhea results from increased intestinal secretion of fluid.

2. **Osmotic** diarrhea results from increased luminal osmotic pressure and subsequent water retention.

3. **Exudative** diarrhea results from exudation of fluid and cells because of increased permeability.

B. **Steatorrhea** is excess fat in the feces.

II. CLINICAL SYNDROMES THAT MAY BE ASSOCIATED WITH DIARRHEA

A. **Malassimilation** is a syndrome, not a disease, that can result from maldigestion, malabsorption, or a combination of these two.

1. **Maldigestion** can result from digestive enzyme deficiency, bile acid deficiency, conditions that alter the activity of enzymes or bile acids, primary small intestinal disorders, bacterial overgrowth, and pancreatic duct obstruction. Exocrine pancreatic insufficiency (EPI), discussed in Chapter 42 II B 4, is the most common cause of maldigestion in dogs; bile acid deficiency is very rare. Diarrhea, weight loss, and sometimes steatorrhea are seen.

2. **Malabsorption** involves loss of mucosal cells (e.g., villous atrophy), problems with movement of absorbed nutrients from mucosal cells to capillaries and lymphatics (e.g., lymphocytic–plasmacytic enteritis) or problems with intestinal circulation because of venous or lymphatic obstruction (e.g., lymphangiectasia). Fat malabsorption may occur first because multiple steps are involved in fat digestion and a large portion of the intestine is needed for normal absorption. Protein and carbohydrate malabsorption occur with more severe generalized small intestinal disease. Diarrhea and weight loss are common.

B. **Protein-losing enteropathy (PLE)** is a syndrome, not a specific disease, caused by obstruction, infection, toxins, inflammation, and neoplasia. Inflammatory bowel disease, lymphosarcoma, and lymphangiectasia are the most common causes. Both albumin and globulins are lost (panhypoproteinemia), in contrast to the solitary hypoalbuminemia seen with protein-losing nephropathy and hepatic failure.

III. CAUSES of diarrhea are summarized in Tables 4-1 through 4-4.

IV. CLINICAL FINDINGS vary with the underlying disorder (see Tables 4-1 through 4-4).
The typical clinical findings associated with **small bowel diarrhea** are differentiated from those of **large bowel diarrhea** in Table 4-5.

TABLE 4-1. Causes of Acute Diarrhea without Systemic Signs of Illness

Cause	Possible Concurrent Clinical Findings
Change in diet	Vomiting
Dietary intolerance	Vomiting
Dietary indiscretion	Vomiting
Parasitic infection	Vomiting
Early stage of a more chronic or serious disorder	Variable

TABLE 4-2. Causes of Acute Small Bowel Diarrhea with Systemic Signs of Illness

Cause	Possible Concurrent Clinical Findings
Extra-gastrointestinal disorders	
Hepatic disease	Anorexia, vomiting, icterus, ascites
Hyperthyroidism (primarily cats)	Polyphagia, polyuria, polydipsia, weight loss, tachycardia, palpable cervical mass
Hypoadrenocorticism	Anorexia, vomiting, weakness, bradycardia
Pancreatitis	Anorexia, vomiting, fever, cranial abdominal discomfort
Renal disease	Anorexia, vomiting, polyuria or oliguria, weight loss
Right-sided heart failure	Anorexia, vomiting, ascites, pleural effusion
Primary gastrointestinal disorders	
Dietary indiscretion	Vomiting
Hemorrhagic gastroenteritis (HGE)	Anorexia, hematemesis, depression, shock
Infection	
Bacterial	Anorexia, vomiting, fever, depression
Fungal	Anorexia, vomiting, fever, depression, lymphadenopathy, other organ involvement
Rickettsial	Anorexia, vomiting, diarrhea, fever, lymphadenopathy, petechiae, lameness
Viral	Anorexia, vomiting, depression
Inflammatory bowel disease	Anorexia, vomiting, weight loss
Irritable bowel syndrome	Vomiting
Neoplasia	Variable, depending on the type and site of neoplasia
Obstruction	
Foreign body	Anorexia, vomiting, intestinal "mass," or bunched intestines, abdominal pain, shock
Intussusception	Anorexia, vomiting, tubular abdominal "mass," abdominal pain, shock
Parasitic infection	Vomiting, weight loss
Ulcers (duodenal)	Anorexia, vomiting, abdominal discomfort, other signs specific to the underlying cause
Other causes	
Toxins	Variable, depending on the toxin

TABLE 4-3. Causes of Chronic or Intermittent Small Bowel Diarrhea

Cause	Possible Concurrent Clinical Findings
Extra-gastrointestinal disorders	
Exocrine pancreatic insufficiency (EPI)	Weight loss, steatorrhea, polyphagia
Hepatic disease	Anorexia, vomiting, icterus (less common), ascites
Hyperthyroidism (primarily cats)	Polyphagia, polyuria, polydipsia, weight loss, tachycardia, palpable cervical mass
Hypoadrenocorticism	Anorexia, vomiting, weakness, bradycardia
Pancreatitis (chronic)	Anorexia, vomiting, cranial abdominal discomfort
Renal disease	Anorexia, vomiting, weight loss, polyuria, polydipsia
Primary gastrointestinal disorders	
Dietary intolerance	Vomiting
Infection	
Bacterial	Anorexia, fever
Fungal	Anorexia, fever, lymphadenopathy, other organ involvement
Viral (cats)	Anorexia, fever, pale mucous membranes, depression, weight loss
Inflammatory bowel disease	Anorexia, vomiting, weight loss
Irritable bowel syndrome	Vomiting
Lymphangiectasia	Anorexia, vomiting, weight loss, abdominal fluid
Neoplasia	Variable, depending on the type and site of neoplasia
Obstruction	
Partial mechanical obstruction	Anorexia, vomiting, weight loss
Physiologic obstruction	Variable, depending on the underlying cause
Parasitic infection	Vomiting, weight loss
Small intestinal bacterial overgrowth	Anorexia, vomiting, weight loss
Villous atrophy	Anorexia or polyphagia, weight loss

TABLE 4-4. Causes of Chronic or Intermittent Large Bowel Diarrhea

Dietary intolerance
Infection
   Algal
   Bacterial
   Fungal
   Parasitic
   Viral (cats)
Inflammatory colitis
Neoplasia
Obstruction
   Cecocolic intussusception or cecal inversion
   Foreign body
   Stricture
Stress colitis or irritable colon

TABLE 4-5. Comparison of Clinical Findings in Small Bowel Diarrhea and Large Bowel Diarrhea

	Small Bowel	**Large Bowel**
Volume	Usually increased	Usually decreased because of increased frequency
Frequency of defecation	Normal or slightly increased	Increased
Steatorrhea	May be present	Absent
Mucus	Rare	Usually present
Melena	May be present	Absent
Frank blood	Rare	May be present
Tenesmus	Absent	Usually present
Weight loss	May be present	Rare
Vomiting	May be present	May be present
Appetite	Usually normal or decreased	Usually normal
Borborygmus	May be present	Absent

V. **DIAGNOSTIC APPROACHES.** The diagnostic approach varies depending on the severity and chronicity of the problem and whether the diarrhea is large bowel or small bowel in origin.

A. **Acute diarrhea without systemic signs of illness**

   1. The diagnosis is often a diagnosis of exclusion based on the **history** and **physical examination.** Lack of response to conservative medical therapy indicates a need for additional testing.

   2. Parasitic infection may be diagnosed by a fecal flotation, direct fecal examination, or by response to treatment with fenbendazole.

B. **Acute small bowel diarrhea with systemic signs of illness or chronic or intermittent small bowel diarrhea**

   1. **Complete blood count (CBC)**
      a. An **increased hematocrit with normal serum total solids** will occur with hemorrhagic gastroenteritis (HGE).
      b. **Lymphopenia** may occur with stress or lymphangiectasia.
      c. **Leukopenia** may be seen with parvoviral infection or sepsis.
      d. **Leukocytosis** may be seen with severe intestinal inflammation or perforation.
      e. **Nonregenerative anemia** can be seen with peracute or chronic hemorrhagic diarrhea, chronic disease, or malnutrition.
      f. **Regenerative anemia** can be seen with subacute intestinal hemorrhage caused by ulceration, inflammation, or neoplasia.
      g. **Eosinophilia** can be seen with some parasitic and fungal infections and eosinophilic enteritis.

   2. **Serum biochemical profile**
      a. **Electrolyte abnormalities,** especially **hypokalemia, hyponatremia,** and **hypochloremia,** may be seen with many disorders involving diarrhea.
      b. **Hyperkalemia** with **concurrent hyponatremia** and **hypochloremia** is suggestive of hypoadrenocorticism but can also occur with renal disease and primary gastrointestinal disorders.
      c. **Panhypoproteinemia** is typically seen in patients with PLE or severe blood loss, although globulin concentrations may be normal or increased if concurrent inflammation is seen.
      d. **Hypoalbuminemia** alone may be seen with hepatic failure.

   e. **Increased serum hepatic enzyme concentrations** may be seen with hepatic disease or hepatic congestion secondary to right-sided heart failure.
   f. **Increased serum amylase** and **lipase concentrations** are suggestive of pancreatitis.
   g. **Azotemia** with concurrent **isosthenuria** is most consistent with renal failure but can also be seen with acute hypoadrenocorticism.
   h. **Hypercalcemia** is commonly associated with lymphosarcoma.
   i. **Hypoglycemia** may occur with hypoadrenocorticism, pancreatitis, sepsis, hepatic failure, or as a result of inadequate food intake or malassimilation in young animals.
   j. **Hyperbilirubinemia** may be seen with hepatic disease or biliary obstruction due to pancreatitis.

3. **Urinalysis** is needed to rule out proteinuria as a cause of hypoproteinemia or hypoalbuminemia. Isosthenuria may be seen with renal disease, hepatic failure, hypoadrenocorticism, and hyperthyroidism.

4. **Fecal examination** [see Chapter 41 IV A 5 a (4)] may be of value.

5. **Radiology**
   a. **Survey radiographs**
      (1) Hepatomegaly or microhepatica may be seen with hepatic disease.
      (2) Loss of cranial abdominal detail may be seen with pancreatitis.
      (3) A generalized loss of abdominal detail may be seen with ascites (e.g., as a result of hepatic failure or severe hypoproteinemia), peritonitis, or cachexia.
      (4) Renomegaly or small kidneys may be seen with renal disease.
      (5) Cardiomegaly or pleural effusion may be seen with right-sided heart failure.
      (6) Radiographic findings suggestive of small intestinal disease are discussed in Chapter 41 IV A 5 b (1).
      (7) Finding a mass, lymphadenopathy, or other type of organomegaly may also help lead to the diagnosis.
   b. **Contrast radiographs** may be helpful [see Chapter 41 IV A 5 b (2)].

6. An **adrenocorticotropic (ACTH) stimulation test** should be run if the history, clinical findings, or laboratory results suggest hyperadrenocorticism.

7. **Serum bile concentrations** should be assessed if hepatic failure is suspected.

8. **Serum thyroxine concentration** should be assessed for all middle-aged to older cats with small bowel diarrhea and systemic signs of illness.

9. **Serologies** for **feline leukemia virus (FeLV)** and **feline immunodeficiency virus (FIV)** should be considered in cats with chronic diarrhea.

10. **Tests for malassimilation** are discussed in Chapter 41 IV A 5 a (5).

11. **Ultrasound.** Ultrasonographic findings suggestive of small intestinal disease are discussed in Chapter 41 IV A 5 c. In addition, ultrasound can better assess any mass or change in organ size (e.g., liver or kidneys) seen on survey radiographs. Ultrasound may also be useful if abdominal fluid obscures radiographic detail. Other relevant findings include:
    a. Pancreatic enlargement or a small amount of cranial abdominal fluid, which may indicate pancreatitis
    b. Pericardial fluid or right-sided heart enlargement, which may suggest heart failure

12. **Endoscopic evaluation** (see Chapter 41 IV A 5 d) may help with the diagnosis.

13. **Exploratory laparotomy**
    a. Full-thickness gastrointestinal biopsies and biopsies of multiple organs can be obtained.
    b. Surgery may be diagnostic as well as therapeutic if the diarrhea is caused by foreign bodies, neoplasms, obstructive lesions, or peritonitis.

C. **Chronic or intermittent large bowel diarrhea**

1. **CBC**
   a. **Leukocytosis** may be seen with inflammation or infection.
   b. **Nonregenerative anemia** can be seen with chronic hemorrhage or chronic disease.
   c. **Eosinophilia** can be seen with some parasitic and fungal infections and with eosinophilic colitis.

2. **Multiple fecal examinations** for parasites should be performed. Deworming with fenbendazole should also be considered before pursuing more costly or invasive diagnostic tests.

3. A **rectal scraping** for cytologic evaluation may reveal inflammatory cells, bacterial pathogens, or *Histoplasma* organisms.

4. A **serum biochemical profile** and **urinalysis** are usually unremarkable in dogs or cats with large bowel diarrhea.

5. **Radiology**
   a. **Survey radiographs** are usually unremarkable in dogs or cats with large bowel diarrhea but may reveal a radiodense foreign body or regional lymphadenopathy.
   b. **Contrast radiographs.** A **barium enema** may be considered if flexible colonoscopy is not feasible. A barium enema study can localize lesions of the transverse or ascending colon but does not allow definitive diagnosis; a biopsy is still required.

6. **Proctoscopy** may allow visualization of intraluminal masses (i.e., neoplasia or granuloma), erosions or ulcers (i.e., inflammation or neoplasia), hyperemia or an irregular mucosa (i.e., inflammation or neoplasia), a foreign body, parasites, stricture, or polyps of the descending colon. In some inflammatory conditions and submucosal diseases, the mucosa may appear grossly normal; therefore, multiple biopsies should be taken even if the mucosa is grossly normal.

7. **Flexible colonoscopy** allows visualization of the entire colon and should be considered if previous diagnostic tests do not yield a diagnosis.

VI. TREATMENT

A. **Acute diarrhea without systemic signs of illness**

1. Food should be withheld for at least 12–48 hours to rest the gastrointestinal (GI) tract. Water can be given ad libitum if there is not concurrent vomiting. If the diarrhea lessens or resolves, then small meals of a bland, low-fat diet (e.g., cottage cheese, boiled meat mixed with rice or potatoes) can be fed.

2. Deworming with pyrantel pamoate (small bowel diarrhea) or fenbendazole (large bowel diarrhea) should be strongly considered, especially in young animals.

3. Antidiarrheals (e.g., bismuth subsalicylate, diphenoxylate, loperamide) are usually not needed and do not resolve the main problem. Bismuth subsalicylate may be effective for symptomatic control of mild to moderate diarrhea, but one of the opiates may be needed for severe cases. These agents should be used with caution in cats.

B. **Acute small bowel diarrhea with systemic signs of illness.** The primary disorder should be treated. Food should be withheld for at least 12–48 hours to rest the GI tract. Antibiotics are indicated if the animal is febrile, neutropenic, or septic. Parenteral fluids should be administered if the animal is dehydrated or vomiting, is systemically ill, or to correct electrolyte imbalances. Electrolytes may be given orally if there is not vomiting and the clinical signs are not severe. Dextrose supplementation may be necessary for young, anorexic animals that have inadequate hepatic glucose reserves, or for animals with sepsis.

C. **Chronic or intermittent small bowel diarrhea** may respond to treatment of the primary disorder with no additional treatment. Parenteral fluids may be needed if concurrent anorexia, dehydration, or electrolyte imbalances are present.

D. **Chronic large bowel diarrhea.** The primary disorder should be treated. Supportive treatment for acute diarrhea without systemic signs (see VI A) may be helpful.

Chapter 5

Melena and Hematochezia

I. DEFINITIONS

A. **Melena** is black, tarry feces resulting from the presence of digested blood. If blood is swallowed or if upper gastrointestinal (GI) hemorrhage occurs, the hemoglobin from the blood is oxidized and degraded as it passes through the intestinal tract. Thus, melena usually is an indication of upper GI hemorrhage. Melena is rare in cats.

B. **Hematochezia** denotes fresh blood on the feces. Hematochezia is usually an indicator of large bowel or perianal disease. It can occasionally be seen with upper GI hemorrhage if the hemorrhage is rapid, massive, or intestinal transit time is decreased.

II. CAUSES of melena and hematochezia are listed in Tables 5-1 and 5-2, respectively.

III. CLINICAL FINDINGS. Pale mucous membranes may result from anemia, and weakness or collapse may result from severe hemorrhage. Other associated clinical findings vary according to the underlying disorder (see Tables 5-1 and 5-2).

IV. DIAGNOSTIC APPROACHES

A. Melena

1. **History** and **physical examination** should help rule out swallowed blood from hemoptysis, epistaxis, or oral lesions.

2. A **fecal occult blood test** can be used to differentiate true melena from feces colored black by a meat diet, iron supplementation, or some medications (e.g., bismuth, salicylates). A meat-free diet should be fed for 2–3 days prior to testing so that blood in the ingested meat does not influence the test results.

3. **Coagulation tests** and a **platelet count** should be evaluated to rule out a clotting disorder as the cause of the hemorrhage.

4. A **complete blood count (CBC), serum biochemical profile,** and **urinalysis** should be performed to rule out extra-GI causes of GI hemorrhage. A microcytic, hypochromic anemia may be seen with chronic blood loss.

5. **Fecal examinations** for parasites should be performed.

6. **Endoscopy** and **biopsies** are the optimal way to diagnose and determine the inciting cause of esophageal, gastric, or upper duodenal erosions or ulcers.

7. A **scintigraphic study** using technetium-labeled erythrocytes may be considered if the above tests fail to identify the source and cause of the bleeding.

B. Hematochezia

1. **Perianal** and digital **rectal examination** will identify any abnormalities of the caudal rectum, anus, or anal sacs.

TABLE 5-1. Causes of Melena

Cause	Possible Concurrent Clinical Findings
Swallowed blood	
Nasal disease	Epistaxis, nasal discharge, sneezing
Oropharyngeal hemorrhage	Oral or pharyngeal erosion, ulceration, or mass
Pulmonary or airway disease	Cough, hemoptysis, tachypnea
Extra-gastrointestinal disorders	
Coagulopathies	Petechiae, ecchymoses, other types of hemorrhage
Hepatic disease	Anorexia, weight loss, vomiting, diarrhea, icterus, ascites
Neurologic disease	Neurologic deficits, abnormal mentation
Pancreatitis	Anorexia, vomiting, fever, cranial abdominal discomfort
Shock	Depressed mentation, weak pulses, pale mucous membranes, hypothermia, tachycardia, tachypnea, reduced urine output
Uremia	Anorexia, vomiting, weight loss, polyuria, polydipsia, oral ulceration
Vasculitis	
Rocky Mountain spotted fever	Anorexia, fever, lymphadenopathy, petechiae, lameness
Primary gastrointestinal disorders	
Esophagitis	Anorexia, regurgitation, odynophagia
Inflammatory gastritis and enteritis	Anorexia, vomiting, diarrhea
Ischemia	Anorexia, abdominal pain, fever, depression, shock
Medications	Variable, depending on the medication
Neoplasia	Variable, depending on the type and site of neoplasia
Parasitic infection (severe)	Diarrhea, vomiting, weight loss
Ulcers (usually secondary to another disorder)	Vomiting, diarrhea, abdominal discomfort, other signs specific to the underlying disorder

2. **Clotting function tests** should be evaluated if there are no clinical signs other than hematochezia.

3. If the perianal area and clotting are normal, then the diagnostic approaches for large bowel diarrhea should be followed (see Chapter 4 V C).

V. TREATMENT

A. **Melena.** The primary disease should be treated.

1. **Parenteral fluid therapy,** a **transfusion,** or both may be necessary if hemorrhaging is severe.

2. Because ulceration is the most common cause of significant upper GI hemorrhage, treatment with **sucralfate** and **histamine-2 (H_2) antagonists** is often also instituted while pursuing a definitive diagnosis.

TABLE 5-2. Causes of Hematochezia

Cause	Possible Concurrent Clinical Findings
Extra-gastrointestinal disorders	
Anal sac infection	Dyschezia, perianal swelling or erythema
Coagulopathy	Petechiae, ecchymoses, other types of hemorrhage
Primary gastrointestinal disorders	
Dietary intolerance	Vomiting, diarrhea
Foreign body	Anorexia, vomiting, diarrhea, dyschezia, constipation
Hemorrhagic gastroenteritis (HGE)	Anorexia, vomiting, hematemesis, diarrhea, depression
Inflammatory colitis	Inappetance, diarrhea, vomiting
Intussusception	Anorexia, diarrhea, vomiting, abdominal discomfort
Neoplasia	Variable, depending on the type and site of neoplasia
Parasitic infection	Diarrhea
Parvovirus infection	Anorexia, vomiting, diarrhea, depression
Polyps	Usually none

3. The use of **antibiotics** in dogs and cats with melena is controversial. These agents should be considered if a secondary bacteremia is suspected (i.e., as a result of bacteria from the GI tract entering the bloodstream through breaks in the mucosa).

B. **Hematochezia.** The primary disease should be treated.

Chapter 6

Tenesmus and Dyschezia

I. **DEFINITIONS**

A. **Tenesmus** is straining to defecate or urinate.

B. **Dyschezia** denotes pain or difficulty in defecation.

II. **CAUSES** (Table 6-1). Dyschezia and tenesmus due to large bowel or perianal disease are often seen together.

III. **CLINICAL FINDINGS** vary with the underlying disorder (see Table 6-1). Large bowel diarrhea is often seen in conjunction with tenesmus or dyschezia.

IV. **DIAGNOSTIC APPROACHES**

A. **Tenesmus**

1. The **history** will help differentiate between straining during urination and straining during defecation. The diagnostic approach to dysuria is discussed in Chapter 32.
2. The **physical examination,** including **abdominal palpation** and a **rectal examination,** should allow identification of constipation (i.e., a colon distended with firm feces), anal sac enlargement or pain, a rectal mass or stricture, a caudal abdominal mass, a pelvic fracture, perianal fistulas, or a perineal hernia.
3. If the physical examination is unremarkable, then the large bowel should be evaluated as for large bowel diarrhea (see Chapter 4 V C).

B. **Dyschezia**

1. As with tenesmus, **physical examination** usually reveals the cause of the dyschezia (see IV A 2). Dyschezia is more common with rectal, anal, and perianal disease.
2. If the cause is still unclear following physical examination, then the large bowel should be evaluated as for large bowel diarrhea.

TABLE 6-1. Causes of Tenesmus and Dyschezia

Cause	Possible Concurrent Clinical Findings
Anal sac abscess	Perianal swelling, erythema, pain, fever, ruptured anal sac
Anal sac neoplasia	Palpable mass, systemic signs of hypercalcemia
Caudal abdominal mass	Depression, palpable mass
Pelvic fracture	History of trauma, pain on palpation, lameness
Perianal fistulas	Pain, visible fistulas
Perineal hernia	Perineal swelling, palpable hernia
Urethral obstruction or urogenital disease (tenesmus only)	Dysuria, hematuria, depression
Colorectal disease	Variable

V. **TREATMENT.** The primary disease should be treated.

A. **Loperamide** or **diphenoxylate** may be used to decrease the symptoms until the primary disease can be controlled if the tenesmus is the result of colorectal disease.

B. **Propantheline** or **dicyclomine** can also be considered for short-term symptomatic treatment of severe tenesmus.

Chapter 7

Constipation and Obstipation

I. **DEFINITIONS**

A. **Constipation** is difficult or infrequent defecation with retention of feces in the colon.

B. **Obstipation** is severe constipation in which the retained feces have become so firm that defecation is no longer possible.

II. **CAUSES** of constipation and obstipation are summarized in Table 7-1.

III. **CLINICAL FINDINGS**

A. There is often a history of **tenesmus, pain,** and the passage of **no feces** or **hard, dry feces. Diarrhea** will sometimes be seen as liquid feces pass around the impacted fecal material.

B. **Anorexia, vomiting, lethargy,** and **weight loss** may occur if the constipation is severe or prolonged.

C. A delay in transit of feces through the colon will result in increased water resorption and drying and hardening of the feces. If the problem goes untreated, **dehydration** and **electrolyte imbalances** may be seen.

D. Specific **associated clinical findings** are summarized in Table 7-1.

IV. **DIAGNOSTIC APPROACHES**

A. **History** and **physical examination,** including **neurologic** and **rectal examination,** will allow identification of dietary, environmental, iatrogenic (i.e., medication-induced), neuromuscular, and some painful or obstructive disorders. An enlarged colon filled with firm feces is usually palpable.

B. **Abdominal radiographs** and possibly **ultrasound** can identify an extraluminal cause of obstruction or the presence of a radiodense foreign body if the history and physical examination reveal only a feces-filled colon.

C. A **complete blood count (CBC)** may identify any secondary systemic inflammation.

D. A **serum biochemical profile** may identify a systemic disorder causing colonic weakness.

E. **Thyroid testing** [see Chapter 44 III A 3 a (3)] should be done if other signs of hypothyroidism are present.

F. **Proctoscopy** or **colonoscopy** and **biopsies** should be considered after general treatment of the constipation if less invasive tests fail to reveal the cause.

TABLE 7-1. Causes of Constipation and Obstipation

Cause	Possible Concurrent Clinical Findings
Dietary causes	
Foreign material	History of access to foreign material, dyschezia, hematochezia
Insufficient fiber	None
Colonic weakness	
Neuromuscular disease	
Bilateral pelvic nerve damage	History of trauma
Dysautonomia	Mydriasis, regurgitation
Lumbosacral disease	Pain, hindlimb weakness
Systemic disorders	
Dehydration	Tacky mucous membranes
Hypercalcemia	Anorexia, vomiting, polyuria, polydipsia, weakness
Hypokalemia	Weakness
Hypothyroidism	Lethargy, bilaterally symmetrical alopecia
Prolonged severe colonic distention	Variable
Obstructive disease	
Intraluminal or intramural obstruction	
Diverticulum	Palpable diverticulum on rectal examination
Foreign body	Pain, hematochezia
Granuloma	Hematochezia
Neoplasia	Hematochezia, weight loss, diarrhea
Perineal hernia	Perineal swelling, palpable hernia on rectal examination
Stricture	Dyschezia
Extraluminal obstruction	
Granuloma	Dyschezia, other signs specific to the type and site of the granuloma
Neoplasia	Anorexia, weight loss, other signs specific to the type and site of neoplasia
Pelvic fracture	History of trauma, pain, crepitus or displacement on palpation, lameness
Prostatic disease	Palpable prostatomegaly and pain, hematuria, dysuria, fever
Pseudocoprostasis	None
Sublumbar lymphadenopathy	Variable, depending on the cause of the lymphadenopathy

(continued)

TABLE 7-1. *(continued)*

Cause	Possible Concurrent Clinical Findings
Pain	
Anal sac abscess	Perianal swelling, pain, fever, erythema, ruptured anal sac
Anal or rectal mass	Hematochezia, dyschezia, palpable mass
Anal or rectal stricture	Dyschezia
Rectal or anal inflammation	Hematochezia, dyschezia
Pelvic fracture	History of trauma, pain, crepitus, or displacement on palpation, lameness
Perianal fistula	Visible tracts
Spinal cord disease or injury	Neurologic deficits
Miscellaneous causes	
Hospitalization	None
Dirty litter box	None
Idiopathic megacolon	None
Medication	Variable

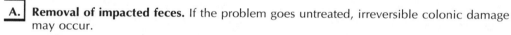

V. TREATMENT

A. **Removal of impacted feces.** If the problem goes untreated, irreversible colonic damage may occur.

1. **Oral therapy** may be effective for mild constipation. A **high-fiber diet** and oral **osmotic** or **emollient laxatives** can be prescribed and the animal reevaluated in 48 hours.

2. **Enemas** may be required if the constipation is severe or if oral therapy fails. Warm water or retention enemas should be given. Multiple enemas given over several days may be required.

3. **Manual evacuation** of the feces under general anesthesia is needed if enemas are ineffective.

B. **Supportive treatment**

1. **Fluid therapy** may be needed if the animal is dehydrated or has electrolyte imbalances.

2. **Antibiotic therapy** may be needed if fever or leukocytosis is present or if the obstipation is severe and has compromised the integrity of the colonic mucosa.

C. **Definitive therapy.** The primary disorder should be treated.

Chapter 8

Acute Abdominal Distress

I. **DEFINITION.** Acute abdominal distress (acute abdomen) is the sudden onset of severe abdominal pain, distention, inflammation, or infection.

II. **CAUSES** are summarized in Table 8-1.

A. An abdominal organ, the peritoneum, or both may be involved in the disease process.

B. Pain referred from the spine may also appear as abdominal pain.

III. **CLINICAL FINDINGS.** **Secondary shock** or **sepsis** may occur. Other clinical findings vary with the underlying disorder (see Table 8-1).

IV. **DIAGNOSTIC APPROACHES**

A. A **physical examination** will often identify organomegaly (e.g., gastric distention, hepatomegaly), an abdominal mass, abdominal pain, bunched intestines (e.g., probable linear foreign body), a tubular abdominal mass (i.e., probable intussusception), or the presence of abdominal fluid.

B. A **complete blood count (CBC)** may show a leukocytosis (e.g., infection, inflammation) or an anemia (e.g., gastrointestinal or intraabdominal hemorrhage).

C. A **serum biochemical profile** will identify any concurrent electrolyte imbalances and may show increased serum hepatic enzyme concentrations, azotemia (as a result of dehydration or renal disease), panhypoproteinemia (as a result of intestinal disease or severe glomerular disease), or increased amylase and lipase levels (a sign of possible pancreatitis).

D. A **urinalysis** may show hematuria or leukuria, findings that may indicate urinary tract disease, prostatic disease, trauma, or sepsis.

E. **Abdominal radiographs** and **ultrasound** may show abdominal fluid, organomegaly, gastric or intestinal distention, a radiodense foreign body, a mass, displaced abdominal structures, or pneumoperitoneum.

F. An **abdominocentesis** should be performed if abdominal fluid is present. The fluid should be analyzed (see Chapter 10).

G. A **radiographic contrast study** of the upper gastrointestinal (GI) tract should be considered if a GI obstruction is suspected.

H. An **exploratory laparotomy** may be needed in some cases.

TABLE 8-1. Causes of Acute Abdominal Distress in Dogs and Cats

Cause	Possible Concurrent Clinical Findings
Abdominal hemorrhage (trauma, neoplasia)	History of trauma, pale mucous membranes
Bladder rupture	History of trauma or dysuria
Gastric dilatation	Abdominal distention, vomiting
Gastric dilatation–volvulus (GDV)	Abdominal distention, nonproductive retching, shock
Hepatitis or cholangitis	Anorexia, vomiting, diarrhea, icterus, ascites
Intestinal inflammation	Anorexia, vomiting, diarrhea
Intestinal obstruction	Anorexia, vomiting, diarrhea, distended bowel loops, shock
Intussusception	Anorexia, vomiting, diarrhea, tubular abdominal "mass," shock
Neoplasia	Variable, depending on the type and site of neoplasia
Peritonitis	
Nonseptic	
Iatrogenic (e.g., surgical sponge)	Anorexia, vomiting
Pancreatitis	Anorexia, vomiting, diarrhea, cranial abdominal pain, fever
Septic	
Abscess	Variable, depending on the type and site of the abscess
Biliary rupture	History of hepatobiliary disease, icterus
Gastrointestinal perforation	Anorexia, vomiting, hematemesis, diarrhea, melena, abdominal discomfort
Prostatitis or prostatic abscess	Palpable prostatomegaly and pain, fever, vomiting, hematuria, dysuria, tenesmus
Pyometra	Anorexia, vomiting, polyuria, polydipsia, abdominal distention
Referred spinal pain	Neurologic deficits
Splenic torsion	Splenomegaly, shock
Testicular torsion	Testicular enlargement
Urethral obstruction	History of dysuria; anorexia; enlarged, turgid bladder; vomiting

V. TREATMENT

A. Stabilization

1. **Intravenous fluids** and a **rapid-acting glucocorticoid** should be administered as needed for shock and to correct any electrolyte abnormalities.

2. **Parenteral antibiotic therapy** should be instituted if infection or sepsis is suspected.

B. Definitive therapy. The primary disease should be treated. For example, if a foreign body, gastric dilatation–volvulus (GDV), mass, obstruction, or pneumoperitoneum is found, an exploratory laparotomy should be performed as soon as possible after initial stabilization.

VI. PROGNOSIS.
The prognosis is guarded with septic peritonitis or severe obstruction and ischemia.

Chapter 9

Jaundice

I. DEFINITIONS

A. **Jaundice** is yellow discoloration of body tissues, caused by hyperbilirubinemia.

B. **Icterus** is a term often used interchangeably with jaundice.

II. CAUSES

A. **General mechanisms.** There are three mechanisms of jaundice:

1. **Prehepatic icterus** occurs as a result of **increased bilirubin presented to the liver** (e.g., as a result of hemolysis).

2. **Hepatic icterus** occurs as a result of **decreased uptake, conjugation,** and **secretion of bilirubin by the liver** (e.g., as a result of hepatic dysfunction)..

3. **Posthepatic icterus** occurs as a result of decreased **bile outflow** (e.g., as a result of bile duct obstruction).

B. **Specific causes** of jaundice are listed in Tables 9-1 and 9-2.

III. CLINICAL FINDINGS vary with the underlying disorder (see Tables 9-1 and 9-2).

A. **Discoloration of the sclera, mucous membranes,** and **skin.** As the serum bilirubin concentration increases, scleral icterus, icteric mucous membranes, and then icteric skin is seen. Clinical icterus persists for several days following resolution of the hyperbilirubinemia because of staining of the tissues.

1. Plasma icterus cannot be detected until serum bilirubin concentrations exceed 1.5 mg/dl (25 μmol/L).

2. Tissue icterus is not visible until serum bilirubin concentrations exceed 2.0–3.0 mg/dl (34–50 μmol/L).

B. **Pale mucous membranes** and **weakness** may be seen with **hemolytic disease.**

C. **Dark urine** may result from hyperbilirubinuria (from hyperbilirubinemia) or hemoglobinuria (from intravascular hemolysis).

D. **Pale gray feces** (i.e., acholic feces) may be present if complete posthepatic biliary obstruction is present or biliary rupture has occurred.

IV. DIAGNOSTIC APPROACHES. Regardless of the cause of the jaundice, renal, neurologic, and additional hepatic damage can occur with hyperbilirubinemia; therefore, diagnosis and treatment should be prompt.

A. **Complete blood count (CBC)**

TABLE 9-1. Causes of Jaundice in Dogs

Cause	Possible Concurrent Clinical Findings
Prehepatic causes	
Hemolysis	
Babesiosis	Anorexia, pale mucous membranes, discolored urine, fever, collapse
Dirofilariasis	Anorexia, lethargy, cough, ascites
Hemobartonellosis	Pale mucous membranes, fever
Heinz body anemia	Pale mucous membranes
Immune-mediated hemolytic anemia	Pale mucous membranes, lethargy, fever
Septicemia	Anorexia, fever, lethargy
Resorption of a large hematoma	History of hematoma
Hepatic causes	
Acute hepatitis	Anorexia, vomiting, diarrhea, lethargy, neurologic abnormalities
Chronic hepatitis	Anorexia, weight loss, vomiting, diarrhea, lethargy, ascites
Cirrhosis	Anorexia, weight loss, vomiting, diarrhea, lethargy, ascites
Copper storage disease	Anorexia, vomiting, diarrhea, lethargy
Leptospirosis	Anorexia, vomiting, diarrhea, fever, polyuria or oliguria
Medications	Variable
Necrosis	Anorexia, vomiting, diarrhea, lethargy, abnormal mentation
Neoplasia	Anorexia, lethargy, vomiting, diarrhea
Sepsis	Anorexia, fever, lethargy
Posthepatic causes	
Choleliths	Anorexia, abdominal discomfort, vomiting
Neoplasia	Anorexia, vomiting
Pancreatitis	Anorexia, vomiting, fever, cranial abdominal discomfort, diarrhea

1. **Anemia** (i.e., nonregenerative with acute disease, regenerative with subacute or chronic disease), **spherocytosis, autoagglutination, reddish** or **icteric plasma,** or a **leukocytosis** may be seen with hemolysis. A normal hematocrit will rule out prehepatic icterus.

2. A **normocytic normochromic nonregenerative anemia** may be seen with chronic hepatic disease.

3. A **leukocytosis with a marked shift toward immaturity** may be seen with sepsis.

B. Serum biochemical profile

1. The **serum bilirubin concentration** is always increased with jaundice.
   a. Theoretically:
      (1) With prehepatic icterus, most of the increase in bilirubin will result from an increase in unconjugated (i.e., indirect) bilirubin levels.
      (2) With hepatic icterus, both conjugated and unconjugated bilirubin levels are increased.

TABLE 9-2. Causes of Jaundice in Cats

Cause	Possible Concurrent Clinical Findings
Prehepatic causes	
Hemolysis	
Cytauxozoonosis	Pale mucous membranes, fever, dyspnea
Heinz body anemia	Pale mucous membranes
Hemobartonellosis	Anorexia, lethargy, fever
Medication	Variable
Hepatic causes	
Cholangitis or cholangiohepatitis	Anorexia, vomiting, diarrhea, lethargy, fever
Feline infectious peritonitis (FIP)	Anorexia, fever, lethargy, other signs specific to the organs involved
Histoplasmosis	Anorexia, fever, lethargy, vomiting, diarrhea, lymphadenopathy
Idiopathic feline hepatic lipidosis	Anorexia, vomiting
Medications	Variable
Neoplasia	Anorexia, lethargy, vomiting, diarrhea
Sepsis	Anorexia, fever, lethargy
Posthepatic causes	
Choleliths	Anorexia, vomiting, abdominal discomfort, fever
Neoplasia	Anorexia vomiting, lethargy
Pancreatitis	Anorexia, fever, vomiting, cranial abdominal discomfort

      (3) With posthepatic icterus, mainly conjugated bilirubin levels are increased.

  b. Clinically, however, these guidelines rarely hold true.

      (1) If mainly unconjugated bilirubin is increased, then a prehepatic cause for the icterus should be strongly suspected.

      (2) Often both forms of bilirubin are increased with all three types of icterus.

2. Hypoglycemia, hypoalbuminemia, hypocholesterolemia, and a **decreased serum blood urea nitrogen (BUN) concentration** are suggestive of chronic hepatic disease.

3. Serum alanine aminotransferase (SALT), serum aspartate aminotransferase (SAST) and **serum alkaline phosphatase (SAP)** may be increased with hepatic and posthepatic disorders.

4. Serum amylase and **lipase concentrations** may be increased with pancreatitis.

C. Urinalysis

1. Greater than 2+ bilirubin in canine urine and any bilirubin in feline urine is consistent with hyperbilirubinemia.

2. Hemoglobinuria may be seen with some forms of immune-mediated hemolytic anemia.

3. An **absence of urobilinogen** in the urine of a jaundiced dog or cat suggests a complete bile duct obstruction, but urobilinogen is also influenced by other factors.

4. Urate crystals may be seen in dogs or cats with chronic hepatic dysfunction.

5. Dilute or **isosthenuric urine** may be seen in animals with severe hepatic disease.

D. **Other blood tests** to be considered if hemolysis is found include a **Coomb's test, antinu-**

clear antibody (ANA) test, lupus erythematosus (LE) preparation, and tests for blood parasites.

E. Abdominal radiographs and ultrasonograms should be evaluated in dogs or cats with hepatic or posthepatic icterus.

F. A serum thyroxine concentration (in cats) and hepatic biopsy should also be obtained if hepatic disease is found.

V. TREATMENT

A. Prehepatic icterus. The primary disease should be treated. Supportive measures include transfusion [if the anemia is causing clinical signs (e.g., weakness, tachypnea)] and intravenous fluid therapy (if the animal is not drinking, the hyperbilirubinemia is severe, or there are electrolyte imbalances).

B. Hepatic icterus. The primary disease should be treated. Intravenous fluid therapy is often needed to correct dehydration, hypokalemia, and hypoglycemia and to maintain hydration.

C. Posthepatic icterus

1. Biliary obstruction usually requires prompt surgical treatment. An exception is obstruction caused by pancreatitis, which will sometimes resolve with medical treatment of the pancreatitis.

2. Prior to surgery the animal should be rehydrated and electrolyte imbalances corrected.

Chapter 10

Abdominal Distention and Ascites

I. **DEFINITIONS. Ascites** refers to the accumulation of fluid in the abdominal cavity. The fluid may be a transudate or exudate (Table 10-1) and may contain bile, blood, chyle, or urine.

II. **CAUSES**

A. Causes of abdominal distention are listed in Table 10-2.

B. Causes of ascites are listed in Table 10-3. Portal hypertension, hypoproteinemia, inflammation, trauma, sodium and water retention, coagulopathies, and lymphatic obstruction or trauma can all contribute to ascites formation.

III. **CLINICAL FINDINGS** vary with the cause (see Tables 10-2 and 10-3).

IV. **DIAGNOSTIC APPROACHES**

A. **History** and **physical examination** will often provide enough information to differentiate abdominal fluid accumulation from other causes of abdominal distention.

B. **Abdominal radiographs** may be necessary to better define the cause of the distention. Fluid may impart a "ground glass" appearance to the abdomen or may completely obscure most abdominal structures.

C. **Specific diagnostic approaches** depend on the findings.
1. **Abdominal weakness**
   a. An **adrenocorticotropic (ACTH) stimulation test** or a **low-dose dexamethasone suppression test** should be considered [see Chapter 44 V C 3 b (4)] if other signs of hyperadrenocorticism are present or if the serum alkaline phosphatase (SAP) level is increased.
   b. **Electromyography** and **muscle biopsy** should be considered (see Chapter 47 VI B,

TABLE 10-1. Fluid Characteristics

	Transudate	Modified Transudate	Exudate
Specific gravity	<1.018	1.018–1.025	>1.025
Protein (g/dl)	<2.5	2.5–6.0	>2.5
Cells	<1000–2500 nucleated cells/mm^3	<7000 cells/mm^3	>7000 cells/mm^3

TABLE 10-2. Causes of Abdominal Distention

Cause	Possible Concurrent Clinical Findings
Abdominal muscle weakness	
Hyperadrenocorticism	Polyuria and polydipsia, hepatomegaly, bilaterally symmetrical truncal alopecia
Malnutrition	Cachexia, weakness
Myopathy	Pain, muscle atrophy
Ascites	See Table 10-3
Mass	
Granuloma	Variable, depending on the site and size of the granuloma
Neoplasia	Variable, depending on the type and site of neoplasia
Obesity	Generalized obesity
Organomegaly	
Gastric dilatation	Anorexia, vomiting
Hepatomegaly	Anorexia, icterus, abdominal discomfort, vomiting, diarrhea
Renomegaly	Anorexia, abdominal discomfort, hematuria, polyuria and polydipsia
Splenomegaly	None
Uterine enlargement	
Pregnancy	Mammary development
Pyometra	Anorexia, vomiting, polyuria and polydipsia
Pneumoperitoneum	
Ruptured hollow viscus	Shock, anorexia, fever, vomiting
Penetrating wound	Shock, fever
Postoperative	History of surgery

C) if other signs of a myopathy are present or if serum creatine kinase is increased.

2. **Abdominal effusion**
   a. **Abdominal ultrasound** can help identify masses, abscesses, organomegaly, or alterations in organ shape.
   b. **Abdominocentesis.** Analysis of the fluid should be performed to better characterize the fluid.
      (1) **Transudate**
         (a) **Hypoalbuminemia** [suggestive of hepatic failure, protein-losing enteropathy (PLE), or protein-losing nephropathy (PLN)] or **increased serum hepatic enzyme concentrations** (portal hypertension) may be seen.
         (b) **Serum bile acid concentrations** can identify hepatic dysfunction.
         (c) **Exploratory laparotomy** may be considered to determine the cause of the ascites if ultrasound and the serum test results are unremarkable.
      (2) **Modified transudate**
         (a) **Thoracic radiographs** and **echocardiography** are useful for detecting pericardial or right-sided heart disease or a cardiac neoplasm.
         (b) **Tests for microfilaria** and **adult heartworm antigen** should be performed if there are radiographic changes consistent with dirofilariasis or if the animal lives in an endemic heartworm area.
         (c) **Serum hepatic enzyme concentrations** may increase with disease that causes hepatic portal hypertension or with passive congestion associated with heart failure.

TABLE 10-3. Causes of Ascites

Cause	Possible Concurrent Clinical Findings
Transudate	
Hypoproteinemia	
Hepatic failure	Anorexia, vomiting, diarrhea, abnormal mentation, icterus
Protein-losing enteropathy (PLE)	Anorexia, vomiting, diarrhea, weight loss
Protein-losing nephropathy (PLN)	Anorexia, vomiting, weight loss, polyuria and polydipsia
Neoplasia	Variable, depending on the type and site of neoplasia
Lymphatic obstruction	Variable, depending on the cause of the obstruction
Prehepatic and hepatic portal hypertension	Anorexia, vomiting, icterus
Modified transudate	
Neoplasia	Variable, depending on the type and site of neoplasia
Lymphatic obstruction	Variable, depending on the cause of the obstruction
Right-sided heart failure	Anorexia, lethargy, tachypnea, dyspnea
Pericardial effusion	Anorexia, lethargy, collapse
Posthepatic portal hypertension	
Right-sided heart failure	Anorexia, lethargy, tachypnea, dyspnea
Pericardial effusion	Anorexia, lethargy, collapse
Cardiac neoplasia	Anorexia, lethargy, weight loss, collapse
Dirofilariasis	Anorexia, lethargy, exercise intolerance, weight loss
Compression of the caudal vena cava	Variable, depending on the cause of the compression
Exudate	
Purulent	
Gastrointestinal perforation	Shock, abdominal pain, vomiting, diarrhea
Penetrating wound	Shock, abdominal pain
Abscess	Variable, depending on the type and site of the abscess
Ruptured pyometra	Shock, abdominal pain, vomiting, history of polyuria and polydipsia
Sepsis	Anorexia, fever, lethargy
Volvulus	Shock, abdominal discomfort, vomiting
Hemorrhagic	
Coagulopathy	Petechiae, ecchymoses, hemorrhage, pale mucous membranes
Trauma	Abdominal discomfort, pale mucous membranes, history of trauma
Hemangiosarcoma	Pale mucous membranes, lethargy, collapse, abdominal discomfort
Neoplasia eroding a vessel	Variable, depending on the type and site of neoplasia

(continued)

TABLE 10-3. *(continued)*

Cause	Possible Concurrent Clinical Findings
Chylous*	
Lymphatic obstruction	
Cardiomyopathy	Anorexia, exercise intolerance, cough, tachypnea, dyspnea, weight loss
Cirrhosis	Anorexia, vomiting, diarrhea, lethargy, icterus
Hereditary	None
Infection	Anorexia, fever, abdominal discomfort
Intestinal obstruction	Anorexia, abdominal discomfort, vomiting, diarrhea, weight loss, shock
Lymphangiectasia	Anorexia, vomiting, diarrhea, weight loss
Neoplasia	Variable, depending on the type and site of neoplasia
Pancreatitis	Anorexia, vomiting, abdominal discomfort, fever, diarrhea
Trauma	Pain
Pseudochylous	
Chronic inflammation	Anorexia, vomiting, diarrhea, weight loss
Neoplasia	Variable, depending on the type and site of neoplasia
Other	
Bile peritonitis	Anorexia, abdominal discomfort, icterus, shock
Diaphragmatic hernia	Variable, depending on the organ displacement
Feline infectious peritonitis (FIP)	Anorexia, fever, other signs specific to the involved organs
Hepatopathy (chronic)	Anorexia, vomiting, diarrhea, icterus
Neoplasia	Variable, depending on the type and site of neoplasia
Pancreatitis	Anorexia, vomiting, abdominal discomfort, fever, diarrhea
Steatitis	Anorexia, abdominal discomfort, fever
Urine peritonitis	Anorexia, vomiting, abdominal discomfort, history of oliguria or trauma

* Triglyceride content greater than 100 g/dl; clears with ether.

      (d) Serum bile acid concentrations may also be helpful in identifying hepatic disease.
      (e) Radiographic contrast studies of the caudal vena cava should be considered to look for an obstructive lesion if radiographs, ultrasound, and a serum biochemical profile are unremarkable.
   (3) Exudate
      (a) Purulent exudate. The presence of a septic purulent exudate is an indication for prompt exploratory laparotomy.
      (b) Hemorrhagic exudate
         (i) Clotting tests should be performed to rule out a coagulopathy if there is no history of trauma.
         (ii) Exploratory laparotomy should be considered if clotting is normal.
      (c) Chylous exudate
         (i) Thoracic radiographs and **echocardiography** should be used to assess cardiac function if clinical signs of cardiac failure are present.

(ii) **Serum biochemical profile**
—Hypoglycemia, hypoalbuminemia, hypocholesterolemia, and a decreased blood urea nitrogen (BUN) concentration are suggestive of hepatic dysfunction and possible cirrhosis.

—Increased serum amylase and lipase concentrations are suggestive of pancreatitis.

(iii) **Exploratory laparotomy** should be considered if there is no history of trauma and the results of other diagnostic tests are unremarkable.

(d) **Pseudochylous exudate. Exploratory laparotomy** is the usual method of determining the cause of pseudochylous ascites.

(e) **Other**

(i) **Exploratory laparotomy** is indicated promptly if bile or urine is present, and when clinical findings and others tests are not diagnostic.

(ii) **Radiographs** and **ultrasound** will usually reveal a diaphragmatic hernia, if that is the cause of the distention.

(iii) **Serum biochemical profile**
—Increased serum hepatic enzyme concentrations are suggestive of a hepatopathy.

—Increased serum amylase and lipase concentrations are suggestive of pancreatitis.

—If a yellow, high-protein, sterile exudate is found in a cat, feline infectious peritonitis (FIP) should be suspected (see Chapter 49 V F).

3. **Mass.** A **biopsy** should be obtained, using a percutaneous or surgical approach, depending on the location and size of the mass.

4. **Organomegaly**
   a. **Gastric dilatation** (see Chapter 41 III B 3)
   b. **Hepatomegaly** [see Chapter 42 I A 4 d (1) (a) (i)]
   c. **Renomegaly** (see Chapter 43 I B 2 a)
   d. **Splenomegaly** (see Chapter 48 V B)
   e. **Uterine enlargement.** Concurrent **clinical findings** and results of abdominal **ultrasound** will allow differentiation of pyometra and pregnancy.

5. **Pneumoperitoneum. Exploratory laparotomy** is indicated promptly, unless the pneumoperitoneum is seen within 10 days following surgery.

V. TREATMENT

A. The primary disorder should be treated.

B. Diuretics are only useful with some causes of ascites. In other situations, they may actually be deleterious.

C. If ascites is so severe that the respiratory capacity is seriously hindered, then some of the fluid should be slowly drained. Rapid drainage of a large amount of fluid may result in hypovolemia and collapse.

Chapter 11

Weight Loss

I. DEFINITIONS

A. **Weight loss** occurs when energy use or loss is greater than energy intake. Weight loss is often considered significant if more than 10% of the body weight is lost.

B. **Emaciation** is more severe, usually defined as the loss of more than 20% of the body weight, at which point the dorsal vertebral processes and other bony prominences are quite noticeable.

C. **Cachexia** denotes weight loss that is so extreme that weakness and depression are also seen.

II. CAUSES of weight loss are summarized in Table 11-1.

III. CLINICAL FINDINGS. The clinical findings vary according to the cause of the weight loss (see Table 11-1). Particularly helpful in narrowing the list of differential diagnoses are the presence or absence of:

A. Anorexia (see Chapter 13)

B. Polyphagia (see Chapter 15)

C. Fever (see Chapter 16)

D. Concurrent gastrointestinal (GI) signs (see Chapters 2–4, Chapter 41)

IV. DIAGNOSTIC APPROACHES

A. **General measures**

1. The **patient history** should help rule out dietary causes of weight loss.

2. A **complete blood count (CBC)** may reveal:
   a. **Leukocytosis** (suggestive of infection or inflammation)
   b. **Anemia** (suggestive of chronic blood loss or chronic disease)
   c. **Eosinophilia** (suggestive of parasitic infection, eosinophilic inflammation, hypoadrenocorticism)

3. A **serum biochemical profile** may reveal:
   a. **Hypoproteinemia** [suggestive of protein-losing enteropathy (PLE), protein-losing nephropathy (PLN), or hepatic failure]
   b. **Hyperbilirubinemia** (suggestive of hepatic disease or bile duct obstruction)
   c. **Increased serum hepatic enzyme concentrations** (suggestive of hepatic disease)
   d. **Azotemia** (suggestive of renal disease)
   e. **Hyperglycemia** (suggestive of diabetes mellitus)

4. **Urinalysis** may reveal:

TABLE 11-1. Causes of Weight Loss

Cause	Possible Concurrent Clinical Findings
Anorexia	Variable
Dietary causes	
Underfeeding	Ravenous appetite
Poor-quality food	Poor haircoat, dry skin
Dysphagia	Variable
Increased nutrient loss	
Blood loss (chronic)	Variable, depending on the site of blood loss (e.g., melena, hematuria)
Burns	Eschars, history of thermal injury
Diabetes mellitus	Polyphagia, polyuria, polydipsia, cataracts (dogs)
Effusions	Abdominal distention, dyspnea
Neoplasia	Variable, depending on the type and site of neoplasia
Protein-losing enteropathy (PLE)	Polyphagia or inappetence, diarrhea, vomiting
Protein-losing nephropathy (PLN)	Anorexia, polyuria, polydipsia
Pyoderma (severe)	Skin lesions, fever, lethargy
Increased nutrient use	
Cold environment	None
Exercise	None
Fever	Variable, depending on the cause of the fever
Hyperthyroidism	Polyphagia, polyuria, polydipsia, vomiting, diarrhea, tachycardia, palpable cervical mass
Lactation	Mammary development
Pregnancy	Abdominal enlargement, mammary development
Neoplasia	Variable, depending on the type and site of neoplasia
Malassimilation	
Bile salt deficiency	Steatorrhea
Cardiac failure	Exercise intolerance, weakness, increased capillary refill time, auscultable murmur or crackles, arrhythmia
Exocrine pancreatic insufficiency	Steatorrhea, diarrhea, polyphagia
Hepatic failure	Anorexia, vomiting, diarrhea, icterus, ascites
Hypoadrenocorticism	Anorexia, vomiting, diarrhea, weakness, bradycardia
Neoplasia	Variable, depending on the type and site of neoplasia
Renal failure	Anorexia, vomiting, polyuria, polydipsia
Small intestinal disease	Anorexia, vomiting, diarrhea
Pseudoanorexia	
Dental disease	Drooling, halitosis, dental tartar
Masseter myositis	Muscle atrophy, pain on opening the mouth
Temporomandibular joint problem	Pain on opening the mouth, crepitus
Regurgitation	Variable, depending on the cause of the dysphagia
Vomiting	Variable, depending on the cause of the vomiting

   a. **Proteinuria** (suggestive of PLN)
   b. **Glucosuria** (suggestive of diabetes mellitus, renal glucosuria)
5. A **fecal sample** should be assessed for parasites and cytologic abnormalities.

B. **Specific tests** for the evaluation of dogs or cats with anorexia, dysphagia, regurgitation, or vomiting are discussed in Chapters 2, 3, and 13.

C. **Other tests**

1. **Serum thyroxine concentration** should be assessed in a middle-aged or older cat with weight loss if the previously described tests fail to yield a diagnosis.

2. **Serologic tests** for feline leukemia virus (FeLV), feline immunodeficiency virus (FIV), rickettsial disease, heartworm disease, and others may be useful depending on concurrent clinical signs.

3. **Serum trypsin-like immunoreactivity (STLI)** should be assessed in a dog with weight loss if other test results are normal, especially if diarrhea or polyphagia is also present.

4. **Radiographs** may be useful.
   a. **Thoracic radiographs** may reveal cardiac disease or occult neoplasia.
   b. **Abdominal radiographs** and possibly ultrasound may show lymphadenopathy (e.g., inflammation, neoplasia), a mass (e.g., neoplasia, granuloma), an increase or decrease in organ size (e.g., liver, kidney, uterus), or the presence of abdominal effusion.

5. **Serum bile acid concentrations** (fasting and postprandial), **tests of intestinal absorption** [see Chapter 41 IV A 5 a (5)], or an **adrenocorticotropic hormone (ACTH) stimulation test** [see Chapter 44 V A 3 a (2) (d)] may be helpful based on concurrent clinical signs and other test results.

6. **Endoscopy** or an **exploratory laparotomy** should be considered to obtain intestinal **biopsies** for histopathology if noninvasive tests fail to yield a diagnosis. This is especially helpful if diarrhea is present, although significant intestinal disease and malassimilation can occur even in the absence of diarrhea.

V. **TREATMENT.** The primary disease should be treated. Enteral or parenteral feeding may be helpful as an interim treatment if anorexia is the primary cause of the weight loss.

Chapter 12
Weight Gain

I. **DEFINITION. Obesity** is usually defined as an increase in body fat to a level where the body weight is at least 15% greater than the ideal.

II. **CAUSES** (Table 12-1)

A. Overeating and overfeeding are the most common causes of obesity. Weight gain occurs if caloric intake is increased or if energy use is decreased.

B. Organomegaly, ascites, and peripheral edema may also cause weight gain.

III. **CLINICAL FINDINGS** vary with the cause of weight gain (see Table 12-1).

A. **Obesity**

1. **Increased appetite (polyphagia)** is suggestive of simple overeating, boredom, or an endocrinopathy (i.e., hyperadrenocorticism, acromegaly). Some medications (e.g., glucocorticoids, phenobarbital) may also cause polyphagia.

2. **Normal** or **decreased appetite** concurrent with weight gain is suggestive of overfeeding or an endocrinopathy (i.e., hypothyroidism, hypogonadism, hyperinsulinism).

B. **Ascites** (see Chapter 10)

C. **Peripheral edema** (see Chapter 17)

D. **Organomegaly** (see Chapter 10)

IV. **DIAGNOSTIC APPROACHES**

A. **Obesity**

1. **History** and **physical examination** can usually differentiate excess body fat from other causes of weight gain. Details about the animal's diet and environment may help identify overfeeding or overeating as the cause of obesity.

2. **Laboratory studies.** If excess caloric intake does not seem to be a problem, a **complete blood count (CBC), serum biochemical profile,** and **urinalysis** should be assessed for the presence of:
   a. Hyperglycemia (suggestive of acromegaly)
   b. Hypoglycemia (suggestive of hyperinsulinism)
   c. Hypercholesterolemia (suggestive of hypothyroidism)
   d. Increased serum alkaline phosphatase (SAP) concentration (suggestive of hyperadrenocorticism)
   e. Other abnormalities

3. **Other tests** that may be indicated include:
   a. Thyroid function tests (see Chapter 44)

TABLE 12-1. Causes of Weight Gain

Cause	Possible Concurrent Clinical Findings
Ascites or fluid accumulation	
Ascites	Abdominal distention, other signs specific to the cause of the ascites
Peripheral edema	Variable, depending on the cause of the edema
Obesity or increased body fat	
Dietary	
Overfeeding	None
Overeating	
Boredom	None
Medications	Variable, depending on the medication
Endocrinopathies	
Acromegaly	Increased interdental spaces, polyuria, polydipsia, polyphagia
Hyperadrenocorticism	Abdominal distention, polyuria, polydipsia, polyphagia, bilaterally symmetrical truncal alopecia
Hypogonadism	Truncal alopecia
Hypothyroidism	Bilaterally symmetrical truncal alopecia, lethargy
Hyperinsulinism	Weakness, seizures
Organomegaly	
Gastric dilatation	Anorexia, vomiting
Hepatomegaly	Anorexia, icterus, abdominal discomfort, vomiting, diarrhea
Renomegaly	Anorexia, abdominal discomfort, hematuria, polyuria and polydipsia
Splenomegaly	None
Uterine enlargement	
Pregnancy	Mammary development
Pyometra	Anorexia, vomiting, polyuria and polydipsia

    b. An adrenocorticotropic hormone (ACTH) stimulation test or low-dose dexamethasone suppression test (see Chapter 44)
    c. Computed tomography (CT) scans
    d. Serum insulin concentrations

B. **Ascites** and **organomegaly.** Diagnostic approaches are given in Chapter 10.

C. **Peripheral edema.** Diagnostic approaches are given in Chapter 17.

V. **TREATMENT**

A. The underlying disorder should be treated.

B. A weight reduction plan based on reduced caloric intake and increased energy expenditure should be instituted if simple obesity is the cause of the weight gain. The prognosis for simple obesity is good with treatment. If obesity persists, however, the animal may be at increased risk for diabetes mellitus, dystocia, exercise intolerance, hepatic lipidosis, intervertebral disk disease, joint disease, and pancreatitis.

Chapter 13

Anorexia

I. DEFINITIONS

A. **Anorexia** is the loss of appetite. True anorexia must be differentiated from pseudoanorexia.

B. **Pseudoanorexia** is a condition in which the animal wants to eat but is unwilling or unable to do so, usually because of pain or neuromuscular dysfunction.

II. CAUSES of anorexia are listed in Table 13-1. Because hormones, the nervous system, and metabolic substances all play a role in appetite and satiety, many diseases and environmental factors can disrupt normal hunger and feeding.

III. CLINICAL FINDINGS vary with the underlying disorder (see Table 13-1).

IV. DIAGNOSTIC APPROACHES

A. **History** and **observation** of the animal should be used to rule out environmental or psychological causes of anorexia.

1. If the animal is interested in food, the oral and pharyngeal region should be carefully examined and the cranial nerve (CN) reflexes assessed.

2. If the animal is not interested in food, a **complete blood count (CBC), serum biochemical profile,** and **urinalysis** should be evaluated for evidence of infection, inflammation, electrolyte imbalances, or organ dysfunction.

B. **Radiographs** and **ultrasound** may reveal a mass, organ displacement, a decrease or increase in organ size, or a change in organ shape or architecture.

C. **Other tests** that may be indicated include:

1. **Adrenocorticotropic hormone (ACTH) stimulation test,** to rule out hypoadrenocorticism

2. **Serum bile acid concentrations,** to rule out hepatic dysfunction

3. **Radiographic contrast studies,** to rule out esophageal disease, partial gastrointestinal obstruction or mass

4. **Exploratory laparotomy**

5. **Computed tomography (CT),** to rule out a brain mass

V. TREATMENT. The primary disorder should be treated.

A. **Parenteral fluid therapy** may be needed to correct dehydration (if present), maintain hydration, or correct electrolyte abnormalities.

TABLE 13-1. Causes of Anorexia

Cause	Possible Concurrent Clinical Findings
Pseudoanorexia	
Oral disease	Pain, drooling, halitosis
Neurologic dysfunction	Dropped jaw, facial asymmetry, cranial nerve (CN) deficits (CN 5, 7, 9, 10, 12)
Retrobulbar abscess	Pain on opening the mouth, unilateral exophthalmus
Mandibular or maxillary fracture	Pain, hemorrhage, crepitus, history of trauma
Myositis	Pain, muscle swelling or atrophy
Blindness	Lack of menace, inability to negotiate a maze of unfamiliar surroundings
Esophageal disease	Regurgitation
True anorexia	
Primary anorexia	
Hypothalamic disease	Depression, seizures, hyperthermia
Intracranial disease	Abnormal behavior, seizures, neurologic deficits
Anosomia	Variable, depending on the cause of the anosomia
Psychological	None, possibly a history of change in environment
Secondary anorexia	
Pain	Variable
Fever	Variable, depending on the cause of the fever
Neoplasia	Variable, depending on the type and site of neoplasia
Infection	Variable, depending on the type and site of infection
Inflammatory disease	Variable, depending on the type and site of inflammation
Renal disease	Polyuria, polydipsia, vomiting, weight loss
Hepatic disease	Vomiting, diarrhea, icterus, abnormal behavior, ascites
Hypoadrenocorticism	Vomiting, diarrhea, weakness, bradycardia
Gastrointestinal (GI) disease	Vomiting, diarrhea, weight loss
Cardiac failure	Exercise intolerance, cough, dyspnea
Hypercalcemia	Vomiting, polyuria, polydipsia, weakness

B. **Nutritional support** should be considered if the anorexia persists for more than 5–7 days.

1. **Warmed food** and foods with a **strong odor** should be offered.

2. **Benzodiazepines, cyproheptadine,** and **stanozolol** may stimulate appetite in some patients.

3. A **nasogastric, gastrostomy,** or **enterostomy tube** for feeding may be placed if other attempts at feeding are unsuccessful and response to treatment of the primary disease is likely to be delayed. Parenteral nutrition can also be considered in such patients.

Chapter 14

Polyuria and Polydipsia

I. DEFINITIONS

A. **Polyuria** is urine production greater than 1.5 times the normal amount of 25–35 ml/kg/day.

B. **Polydipsia** is water consumption 1.5 times the normal amount of 50–70 ml/kg/day.

II. CAUSES of polyuria and polydipsia are summarized in Table 14-1.

III. CLINICAL FINDINGS

A. **History** and **predisposition**

1. **Species** and **breed**
   a. In basenjis, mixed-breed dogs, Norwegian elkhounds, schnauzers, Scottish terriers, and Shetland sheepdogs, renal glucosuria or a Fanconi-like syndrome has been recognized.
   b. In cats, renal failure, diabetes mellitus, and hyperthyroidism are the most common disorders causing polyuria and polydipsia.

2. **Age** and **sex**
   a. In younger animals, congenital kidney disease and portosystemic shunts are more common.
   b. In middle-aged to older animals, diabetes mellitus, chronic renal failure, hyperadrenocorticism, hyperthyroidism, and neoplasia are more common.
   c. In the polyuric female dog or cat, pyometra should be considered especially if there is a history of recent estrus.

B. **Concurrent clinical signs** are summarized in Table 14-1.

IV. DIAGNOSTIC APPROACHES

A. **Urinalysis** should be one of the first tests performed, both to help document the presence of polyuria and polydipsia and to help establish a definitive diagnosis.

1. **Specific gravity**
   a. If the urine specific gravity is > 1.025 in a nonglucosuric, nondehydrated dog, or > 1.030 in a nonglucosuric, nondehydrated cat, either the pet is not polyuric and polydipsic or large amounts of solutes are present in the urine.
   b. A urine specific gravity of 1.001–1.007 is most consistent with the presence of hepatic disease, hyperadrenocorticism, hypoadrenocorticism, pyometra, central diabetes insipidus, congenital nephrogenic diabetes insipidus, or psychogenic polydipsia.
   c. A urine specific gravity of 1.008–1.029 is most consistent with diabetes mellitus, renal glycosuria, primary renal failure, pyelonephritis, hypercalcemia, hypoka-

TABLE 14-1. Causes of Polyuria and Polydipsia

Cause	Possible Concurrent Clinical Findings
Iatrogenic causes	
Low-protein diet	None
Medication	Variable, depending on the medication
Metabolic causes	
Central diabetes insipidus	None
Diabetes mellitus	Polyphagia, weight loss, cataracts
Escherichia coli infection	Variable, depending on the site of infection
Hepatic disease	Anorexia, vomiting, diarrhea; icterus, behavior change, ascites
Hyperadrenocorticism	Polyphagia, abdominal distention, bilaterally symmetrical truncal alopecia
Hypercalcemia	Anorexia, vomiting, weakness, other signs specific to the cause of the hypercalcemia
Hyperthyroidism	Polyphagia, weight loss, vomiting, diarrhea, tachycardia, palpable cervical mass
Hypoadrenocorticism	Anorexia, vomiting, diarrhea, weakness, bradycardia
Hypokalemia	Anorexia, weakness, other signs specific to the cause of the hypokalemia
Nephrogenic diabetes insipidus	
Congenital	None
Secondary to other disorders	Variable, depending on the primary disorder
Polycythemia	Reddish mucous membranes; weakness, vomiting, diarrhea, seizures
Pyelonephritis	Anorexia, fever, vomiting, weight loss, pain on palpation of the kidneys
Pyometra	Anorexia, vomiting, fever, vaginal discharge, abdominal enlargement
Renal failure	Anorexia, vomiting, weight loss, increase or decrease in renal size
Renal glucosuria	Weight loss
Miscellaneous causes	
Psychogenic polydipsia	History of change in environment

lemia, liver disease, hyperadrenocorticism, hypoadrenocorticism, hyperthyroidism, or polycythemia.

2. **Glucosuria** will be seen with diabetes mellitus or renal glucosuria.

3. **Bacteriuria** and **pyuria** may suggest pyelonephritis or an *Escherichia coli* urinary tract infection. A secondary urinary tract infection may also be seen with hyperadrenocorticism, diabetes mellitus, and pyometra.

B. **Complete blood count (CBC)**

1. An increased hematocrit in the absence of dehydration is consistent with polycythemia.

2. An inflammatory leukogram may be seen with pyelonephritis, pyometra, or an *E. coli* infection.

3. A nonregenerative anemia may be present with primary renal failure, hepatic disease, or hypoadrenocorticism.

4. The absence of a stress leukogram in an ill animal suggests possible hypoadrenocorticism.

C. **Serum biochemical profile**

1. Hyperglycemia
   a. In dogs, marked hyperglycemia is consistent with a diagnosis of diabetes mellitus.
   b. In cats, because of the transient hyperglycemia seen in response to stress, concurrent glucosuria must also be present to establish a diagnosis of diabetes mellitus.

2. Azotemia in the absence of dehydration suggests primary renal failure or pyelonephritis.

3. Hypercalcemia is diagnosed when the serum calcium level is elevated.

4. Hypokalemia is diagnosed when the serum potassium concentration is decreased.

5. Concurrent hyperkalemia and **hyponatremia** suggest hypoadrenocorticism.

6. Hypoglycemia may be seen with hypoadrenocorticism.

7. Serum alkaline phosphatase (SAP). An increase in the SAP level is common with hyperadrenocorticism.

8. Hepatic enzyme concentration
   a. Increased levels suggest hepatic disease.
   b. Mild azotemia, increased hepatic enzyme concentrations, or both can be seen with hyperthyroidism.

D. **Other tests**

1. Urine culture should be performed if bacteriuria or pyuria is present. It can also definitively rule out pyelonephritis.

2. Serum thyroxine concentration should be evaluated in a dog with a ventral cervical mass or a middle-aged or elderly cat with or without a cervical mass.

3. Abdominal radiographs or **ultrasound** can be used to rule out pyometra in the intact bitch or queen.

4. Serum bile acid concentrations, fasting and postprandial, should be assessed if the clinical signs or serum biochemical abnormalities suggest possible liver insufficiency. This test may also be considered even if polyuria and polydipsia are the only signs or laboratory abnormality.

5. Adrenocorticotropic hormone (ACTH) stimulation test
   a. This test (or another screening test) should be performed if the clinical signs or laboratory abnormalities suggest hyperadrenocorticism or hypoadrenocorticism.
   b. This test may also be considered even if polyuria and polydipsia are the only clinical signs or laboratory abnormality.

6. Creatinine clearance or another test of glomerular filtration rate (GFR) can be considered if there are any clinical findings suggestive of early primary renal failure (i.e., 2/3 renal loss with loss of concentrating ability but not the 3/4 loss associated with azotemia). If creatinine clearance is not assessed, the blood urea nitrogen (BUN) concentration should be carefully monitored if a water deprivation test is later performed.

7. A **water deprivation/vasopressin response test** (see Chapter 44 I B 2 b) should be considered if the clinical findings and results of initial laboratory tests (i.e., urinalysis, CBC, and serum biochemical profile) do not suggest a need for one of the above tests or the above tests are normal.

V. **TREATMENT** should be aimed at the primary disorder.

Chapter 15

Polyphagia

I. **DEFINITION. Polyphagia** is excessive eating. It most commonly is seen in response to a pathologic or physiologic increase in energy expenditure.

II. **CAUSES** of polyphagia are summarized in Table 15-1.

III. **CLINICAL FINDINGS** vary with the cause (see Table 15-1).

IV. **DIAGNOSTIC APPROACHES.** Concurrent weight change is often useful in narrowing the list of differential diagnoses.

A. **Concurrent weight loss** is most consistent with hyperthyroidism, diabetes mellitus, malassimilation, or feeding of a poor-quality diet.

1. **Fecal samples** should be tested for parasites, or the animal should be dewormed.

2. **Laboratory studies.** A **complete blood count (CBC), serum biochemical profile,** and **urinalysis** should be evaluated.
   a. Marked hyperglycemia and glucosuria is suggestive of diabetes mellitus.
   b. Hypoproteinemia is suggestive of malassimilation, protein-losing enteropathy or protein-losing nephropathy.
   c. Mild azotemia or increased serum hepatic enzyme concentrations may be seen with hyperthyroidism.
   d. Other abnormalities may also reveal the diagnosis.

3. **Serum thyroxine concentration** should be evaluated in middle-aged or older cats and in any dog with a palpable cervical mass.

4. **Serum trypsin-like immunoreactivity (STLI)** should also be assessed if clinical findings and other tests fail to establish a diagnosis in a dog.

5. **Gastrointestinal biopsies** should be obtained if less invasive tests fail to yield a diagnosis.

B. **Stable weight.** A stable weight is most consistent with a cold external environment, increased exercise, or hyperadrenocorticism. In the absence of increased exercise or a cold environment, a dog or cat whose weight remains stable despite polyphagia should be assessed as discussed for the animal with weight gain (see IV C).

C. **Concurrent weight gain** is most consistent with psychologic causes (e.g., competition, boredom), exogenous medication, hyperinsulinism, hypothalamic disease, or feeding of a highly palatable diet.

1. **Laboratory studies.** A CBC, serum biochemical profile, and urinalysis should be assessed for hypoglycemia (suggestive of hyperinsulinism), an increased serum alkaline phosphatase (SAP) concentration (suggestive of hyperadrenocorticism), or other abnormalities.

2. An **adrenocorticotropic hormone (ACTH) stimulation test** or other screening test for

TABLE 15-1. Causes of Polyphagia

Cause	Possible Concurrent Clinical Findings
Dietary	
Poor-quality food	None
Highly palatable food	Weight gain
Endocrinopathy	
Diabetes mellitus	Polyuria, polydipsia, weight loss, hepatomegaly, cataracts
Hyperadrenocorticism	Polyuria, polydipsia, bilaterally symmetrical truncal alopecia, "pot belly," hepatomegaly
Hyperinsulinism	Weight gain, lethargy, weakness, seizures
Hyperthyroidism	Polyuria, polydipsia, vomiting, diarrhea, weight loss, tachycardia, palpable cervical mass
Malassimilation	Diarrhea, weight loss
Medications	Variable, depending on the medication
Physiologic	
Cold environment	None
Increased exercise	None
Psychologic	
Boredom	Weight gain
Competition	Weight gain

hyperadrenocorticism [see Chapter 44 V C 3 b (4) (a)] should be performed, especially if the SAP level is increased or other signs of hyperadrenocorticism are present.

3. Serum insulin concentrations should be measured if clinical signs or laboratory evidence of hypoglycemia is present.

V. **TREATMENT.** The primary disorder should be treated. Food intake should not be restricted unless the cause of the polyphagia is psychologic.

Chapter 16

Fever and Hyperthermia

I. DEFINITIONS

A. **Hyperthermia** (i.e., an increase in body temperature) may result from excessive environmental temperature, excessive exercise, or a pathologic increase in endogenous heat production (e.g., fever, malignant hyperthermia).

B. **Fever** is an increase in body temperature that results from an increase in the hypothalamic thermoregulatory center set point. The increase in set point may be triggered by interleukins, tumor necrosis factor (TNF), or other chemical mediators.

C. **Heat exhaustion** results primarily from water and salt depletion. With heat exhaustion, the body temperature is normal or only mildly increased but clinical signs of dysfunction are seen.

D. **Heat stroke** is much more serious than heat exhaustion and is characterized by a marked increase in body temperature with concurrent dysfunction of normal physiologic temperature control. Cell damage occurs with temperatures greater than 108°F (42°C).

E. **Malignant hyperthermia** is a rapid increase in body temperature that occurs as a result of increased metabolic heat production due to abnormal cellular calcium metabolism.

II. CAUSES of hyperthermia are summarized in Table 16-1.

III. CLINICAL FINDINGS

A. **Fever.** Clinical findings vary with the underlying cause (see Table 16-1).

B. **Heat exhaustion.** Clinical findings may include weakness, tachycardia, tachypnea, nausea, vomiting, and muscle cramping.

C. **Heat stroke** or **severe hyperthermia.** Tachycardia, tachypnea, and collapse may be seen.

IV. DIAGNOSTIC APPROACHES

A. **Fever**

1. **Laboratory studies**
   a. A **complete blood count (CBC)** may show a leukocytosis (suggestive of infection or inflammation), regenerative anemia (suggestive of hemolytic anemia or blood loss), spherocytosis (suggestive of hemolytic anemia), or other abnormalities.

TABLE 16-1. Causes of Hyperthermia

Cause	Possible Concurrent Clinical Findings
Environmental	
High humidity	None
High temperature	None
Exertion	
Anxiety	Abnormal behavior
Exercise	None
Increased respiratory effort	Dyspnea, tachypnea, cough
Seizures	Neurologic abnormalities
Fever	
Immune-mediated disease	
Autoimmune hemolytic anemia (AIHA)	Anorexia, pale mucous membranes, icterus
Immune-mediated thrombocytopenia	Petechiae, other types of hemorrhage
Immune-mediated polyarthritis	Lameness, joint pain, anorexia
Polymyositis	Pain, muscle swelling or atrophy, weakness
Systemic lupus erythematosus (SLE)	Pale mucous membranes, petechiae, lameness, pain, weakness, polyuria, polydipsia
Glomerulonephritis	Weight loss, polyuria, polydipsia
Vasculitis	Anorexia, skin lesions, edema
Infection	
Bacterial	
Actinomycosis	Anorexia, dyspnea, tachypnea, lymphadenopathy, draining wound
Borreliosis (Lyme disease)	Lameness
Brucellosis	Infertility, abortion, testicular swelling or pain, discospondylitis
Discospondylitis	Anorexia, pain
Endocarditis	Anorexia, exercise intolerance, cardiac murmur
Leptospirosis	Anorexia, vomiting, polyuria or oliguria, icterus
Mycobacteriosis	Anorexia, weight loss, lymphadenopathy, cough
Nocardiosis	Anorexia, dyspnea, tachypnea, lymphadenopathy
Fungal	
Blastomycosis	Anorexia, dyspnea, cough, lymphadenopathy, lameness, weight loss
Coccidioidomycosis	Anorexia, lameness, cough, dyspnea, weight loss
Cryptococcosis	Anorexia, nasal discharge, neurologic abnormalities
Histoplasmosis	Anorexia, vomiting, diarrhea, lymphadenopathy, weight loss
Parasitic	
Babesiosis	Anorexia, vomiting, lethargy, icterus, petechiae
Cytauxzoonosis	Anorexia, dyspnea, icterus

(continued)

TABLE 16-1. *(continued)*

Cause	Possible Concurrent Clinical Findings
Dirofilariasis	Exercise intolerance, cough, weight loss, ascites
Hepatozoonosis	Anorexia, lameness, weight loss, cough
Toxoplasmosis	Icterus, anterior uveitis, anorexia, neurologic abnormalities, lymphadenopathy, pain
Rickettsial	
Hemobartonellosis	Pale mucous membranes
Ehrlichiosis	Petechiae, epistaxis, lymphadenopathy, lameness
Rocky Mountain spotted fever	Anorexia, petechiae, lymphadenopathy, lameness
Viral	
Feline leukemia virus (FeLV)	Anorexia, pale mucous membranes, diarrhea, palpable mass
Feline immunodeficiency virus (FIV)	Anorexia, oral lesions, diarrhea, other infections
Feline infectious peritonitis (FIP)	Anorexia, abdominal distention, dyspnea, icterus
Feline panleukopenia	Anorexia, vomiting, diarrhea
Feline upper respiratory disease	Anorexia, sneezing, ocular discharge, nasal discharge
Canine distemper	Ocular and nasal discharge, cough, vomiting, diarrhea, neurologic abnormalities
Canine infectious hepatitis	Anorexia, vomiting, diarrhea
Neoplasia	Variable, depending on the type and site of neoplasia
Miscellaneous causes	
Cirrhosis	Anorexia, vomiting, diarrhea, icterus, ascites
Drug reaction	Variable, depending on the medication
Inflammatory disease	Variable, depending on the type and site of inflammation
Hypothalamic disease	Depression, seizures
Malignant hyperthermia	History of anesthesia
Miscellaneous causes	
Hyperthyroidism	Polyuria, polydipsia, polyphagia, weight loss, vomiting, diarrhea, tachycardia, palpable cervical mass
Pheochromocytoma	Tachypnea, tachycardia

    b. A **serum biochemical profile** may show various abnormalities that may help localize the site of disease (e.g., azotemia, increased hepatic enzyme concentrations, panhypoproteinemia).

    c. **Urinalysis** may reveal evidence of infection (e.g., bacteriuria, pyuria) or renal disease (e.g., isosthenuria, proteinuria).

    d. A **urine culture** should be performed if there are any signs or findings of urinary tract infection and can also be useful if septicemia is suspected.

  2. **Fine needle aspiration** of any enlarged lymph nodes or any palpable masses should be performed.

   3. **Diagnostic imaging**
      a. **Radiography.** Radiographs of the thorax or abdomen may show a mass (e.g., neoplasia, granuloma, abscess), organ displacement, a decrease or increase in organ size, or the presence of fluid to help localize the disease.
      b. **Ultrasonography.** Ultrasound examination of the abdomen may identify similar abnormalities.
      c. **Echocardiography** may be helpful if a cardiac murmur is present and endocarditis is suspected.

   4. **Blood cultures** can help establish a diagnosis of bacterial septicemia.

   5. **Arthrocenteses** with cytologic analysis and possible culture of the fluid can be diagnostic for immune-mediated or septic arthritis.

   6. **Serologic tests** for infectious diseases may be useful, depending on the clinical signs and other laboratory abnormalities.

   7. **Antinuclear antibody** and **rheumatoid factor tests** may help establish a diagnosis of immune-mediated disease.

   8. **Bone marrow aspiration** can be useful if hematologic abnormalities are present.

   9. **Cerebrospinal fluid (CSF) analysis** can be helpful if neurologic abnormalities are present.

   10. **Scintigraphy** using radiolabeled leukocytes may help localize the site of inflammation.

   11. **Exploratory laparotomy** and **biopsies** should be considered if all other test results are normal.

B. **Heat exhaustion** and **hyperthermia** are both diagnosed based on the history and clinical findings.

V. TREATMENT

A. **Fever.** The underlying disease should be treated. Symptomatic fever control should not be used unless the fever is extremely high (very rare) because fever is part of the body's defense mechanism.

B. **Heat exhaustion.** Allowing the animal to rest in a cool place with provision of ample water will usually resolve heat exhaustion.

C. **Heat stroke** and **severe hyperthermia**

   1. If the body temperature is less than 104°F (40°C), no specific treatment is needed other than allowing the animal to rest in a cool place with provision of ample water.

   2. If the body temperature is greater than 104°F (40°C), intravenous fluid should be administered and supplemental oxygen supplied. The animal should be bathed in cool water and fanned for additional cooling.
      a. Careful monitoring of the temperature is required because subsequent hypothermia can occur.
      b. Cooling measures should be discontinued before the temperature returns to normal to avoid hypothermia.
      c. Any sequelae of the hyperthermia (see VI B) should be treated.

D. **Malignant hyperthermia.** The animal should be treated with **dantrolene** and external cooling measures should be instituted.

VI. PROGNOSIS

A. **Fever.** The prognosis varies with the underlying disorder.

B. **Hyperthermia.** The prognosis varies with the severity and duration of the hyperthermia. Potential sequelae include cerebral edema, disseminated intravascular coagulation (DIC), gastrointestinal hemorrhage and mucosal sloughing, hepatic failure, hyperkalemia, metabolic acidosis, renal failure, and rhabdomyolysis.

Chapter 17

Peripheral Edema

I. **DEFINITION. Peripheral edema** is an excess of interstitial fluid in body tissues. Peripheral edema may be **localized** or **generalized.** Ascites, cerebral edema, hydrothorax, and hydropericardium are specific areas of peripheral edema; the diagnostic approach to these forms of edema is discussed in more detail in other chapters.

II. **CAUSES**

A. Decreased capillary oncotic pressure, lymphatic obstruction, increased capillary hydrostatic pressure, and increased vascular permeability can all lead to abnormal fluid accumulation in body tissues.

B. Specific causes of localized and generalized peripheral edema are listed in Table 17-1.

III. **CLINICAL FINDINGS.** General signs of peripheral edema may include **pitting** of the subcutaneous tissue with light pressure, **weight gain, swelling** of the head or limbs, **abdominal distention,** and **muffled heart** or **lung sounds.** Other clinical findings are specific to the cause of the edema (see Table 17-1).

IV. **DIAGNOSTIC APPROACHES**

A. **Local peripheral edema**

1. **Laboratory study.** A **complete blood count (CBC)** may show a leukocytosis, suggestive of infection or inflammation.

2. **Imaging studies**
   a. **Radiography.** Radiographs of the affected area may show a mass or bony changes, suggestive of infection, granuloma, or neoplasia.
   b. **Angiography** may be useful to localize the site of the obstruction if venous obstruction is suspected.
   c. **Lymphography** or a **lymph scan** may be helpful if lymphatic obstruction is suspected.

3. **Biopsy** is needed if a mass is found or to identify a vasculitis if prior test results are normal.

B. **Generalized edema or fluid in a body cavity**

1. **Laboratory studies**
   a. A **CBC** may show a leukocytosis (suggestive of infection or inflammation) or hypoproteinemia (suggestive of hypoalbuminemia).
   b. A **serum biochemical profile** should be assessed for:
      (1) **Hypoalbuminemia,** which would suggest hepatic failure, protein-losing enteropathy (PLE), or protein-losing nephropathy (PLN)
      (2) **Increased hepatic enzyme concentrations,** which would suggest hepatic disease or congestion resulting from right-sided heart failure

TABLE 17-1. Causes of Peripheral Edema

Cause	Possible Concurrent Clinical Findings
Generalized peripheral edema	
Decreased capillary oncotic pressure	
Hypoalbuminemia	Ascites, dyspnea, tachypnea, other signs specific to the cause of the hypoalbuminemia
Increased capillary hydrostatic pressure	
Iatrogenic (i.e., overzealous fluid administration)	None
Pericardial disease	Anorexia, weakness, exercise intolerance, muffled heart sounds, jugular distention, dyspnea, tachypnea
Right-sided heart failure	Anorexia, weakness, exercise intolerance, dyspnea, tachypnea, ascites
Increased vascular permeability	
Infection	Variable, depending on the type and site of infection
Inflammation	Variable, depending on the type and site of inflammation
Localized peripheral edema	
Increased capillary hydrostatic pressure	
Venous obstruction or compression	
Abscess	Variable, depending on the site and cause of the abscess
Granuloma	Variable, depending on the site and cause of the granuloma
Iatrogenic (e.g., bandage, collar)	None
Neoplasia	Variable, depending on the type and site of neoplasia
Thrombus	Variable, depending on the site and cause of the thrombus
Arteriovenous fistula	Tachycardia, palpable thrill and bruit over the area
Increased vascular permeability	
Infection	Variable, depending on the type and site of infection
Inflammation	Variable, depending on the type and site of inflammation

        (3) **Hyperbilirubinemia,** which would suggest hepatic disease
        (4) **Azotemia,** which would suggest renal disease
     c. A **urinalysis** should be assessed for:
        (1) **Isosthenuria,** which would suggest renal or hepatic failure
        (2) **Proteinuria,** which would suggest PLN

  2. Imaging studies. Radiographs and **ultrasonograms** may show a mass, an increase or decrease in organ size, or the presence of fluid in a body cavity.

  3. Serology may be useful if concurrent clinical signs are suggestive of a virus- or rickettsial-induced vasculitis.

4. **Abdominocentesis, thoracocentesis,** or **pericardiocentesis** should be done if fluid is present in a body cavity, and the sample should be analyzed (see Chapters 10, 28, and 39).

5. **Angiography** may be useful to localize the site of a suspected venous obstruction.

6. **Lymphography** or a **lymph scan** may be helpful if lymphatic obstruction is suspected.

7. A **biopsy** may be needed to identify vasculitis if generalized edema is present and other test results are unremarkable.

V. TREATMENT. The primary disease should be treated. **Plasma transfusion** may be useful to prevent further edema formation while the primary disease is being treated if hypoalbuminemia is the cause of the edema and the clinical signs are severe.

Chapter 18

Weakness

I. DEFINITIONS

A. **Weakness** is a term often used synonymously with lassitude, fatigue, or lethargy; however, in this chapter, it is used to refer to **generalized muscle weakness,** which may be **persistent** or **episodic.** Weakness may be apparent after vigorous exercise, after little exertion, or at rest.

B. **Lethargy** may have a component of muscle weakness, but it also implies mental dullness.

II. CAUSES of weakness are summarized in Table 18-1.

III. CLINICAL FINDINGS associated with weakness include:

A. Reluctance to walk or run

B. Recumbency for long periods of time

C. Marked panting and trembling after mild exercise

D. Paretic gait or collapse

E. Alert or depressed mentation

F. Signs associated with other disorders

IV. DIAGNOSTIC APPROACHES

A. The initial approach should include all of the following:

   1. Thorough history and physical examination

   2. Complete blood count (CBC)

   3. Serum biochemical profile

   4. Urinalysis

B. Additional testing may include any or all of the following:

   1. Endocrine testing [e.g., adrenocorticotropic hormone (ACTH) response test, low-dose dexamethasone response test, serum thyroxine concentration]

   2. Electrocardiography

   3. Neurologic examination

   4. Radiographic examination (thoracic or abdominal)

TABLE 18-1. Causes of Weakness

Metabolic disorders
  Electrolyte disorders*
    Hypo- or hyperkalemia
    Hypo- or hypercalcemia
    Hypo- or hypernatremia
  Hypoglycemia*
    Insulin-secreting tumors
    Hypoadrenocorticism
    Glycogen storage disease
  Endocrine disorders*
    Hypoadrenocorticism
    Hyperadrenocorticism
    Hypothyroidism
    Hypo- or hyperparathyroidism
    Diabetes mellitus
  Organ dysfunction
    Renal failure and uremia
    Liver failure
Cardiovascular disorders*
  Arrhythmias
  Conduction disturbances
  Congestive heart failure (CHF)
Pulmonary disorders
  Pulmonary thromboembolism
  Pleural effusion
  Severe parenchymal disease
  Airway obstruction
Neurologic disorders
  Spinal cord or brain stem disease
  Polyneuropathies
Neuromuscular disorders*
  Myasthenia gravis
  Polymyositis
Generalized systemic disorders
  Neoplasia
  Nutritional deficiencies or excesses
  Fever
  Chronic inflammatory or infectious disorders
  Anemia
  Chronic wasting disorders (e.g., intestinal malabsorption)
  Drug therapy (e.g., anticonvulsants, vasodilators, tranquilizers)
  Overexertion

* Weakness may be episodic.

5. Ultrasound examinations (heart or abdomen)

6. Electrodiagnostic testing

7. Acetylcholine receptor antibody titer

8. Biopsy (e.g., muscle, nerve)

Chapter 19

Syncope

I. **DEFINITION.** Syncope (fainting) is a sudden and transient loss of consciousness. Syncope occurs more often in dogs than in cats.

II. **CAUSES** of syncope are summarized in Table 19-1.

A. **Cardiac arrhythmias** are a common cause of syncope in dogs.

B. **Metabolic disorders** (e.g., hypoglycemia) may also lead to syncope.

C. **Other.** In the absence of cardiac disease or hypoglycemia, there may be a historical association with one or more of the following:

1. **Excitement** is associated with vasovagal and hyperventilation-related syncope.

2. **Coughing.** In rare instances, paroxysms of coughing may increase the intrathoracic and cerebrospinal fluid (CSF) pressures to a point where cerebral blood flow is reduced.

3. **Swallowing.** Animals with esophageal disease (e.g., diverticula, neoplasia) may experience hypotension during swallowing due to stimulation of the vagal or glossopharyngeal nerve; however, this is a very rare cause of syncope.

4. **Micturition.** Rarely, syncope may occur during or shortly after micturition and is thought to be related to high vagal tone or vagal stimulation arising from the bladder.

5. **Concurrent drug administration**

III. **CLINICAL FINDINGS**

A. Syncope is usually associated with excitement or exertion. Syncope typically begins with **generalized muscle weakness,** which progresses to **ataxia, collapse,** and **loss of consciousness.** Spontaneous muscle activity or jerking is minimal, and recovery is typically rapid and complete. Vocalization, urination, and defecation may also occur with syncope but are rare.

B. **Other clinical signs may reflect the underlying cause.** For example, in a patient with syncope caused by cardiac disease, findings may include an abnormal rhythm, pulse deficits, or a murmur.

IV. **DIAGNOSTIC APPROACHES**

A. A detailed history, physical examination, complete blood count (CBC), serum biochemical profile, and urinalysis are indicated.

B. Cardiac disease may be detected and characterized with an electrocardiogram, thoracic radiographs, and a cardiac ultrasound examination. However, 24-hour continuous

TABLE 19-1. Causes of Syncope

Decreased cerebral perfusion
  Peripheral or neurogenic dysfunction (heart normal)
    Vasovagal stimulation (sudden fright or excitement)
    Postural hypotension
    Hyperventilation (excitement)
    Carotid sinus sensitivity (neoplasia, inflammation, tight collar)
    Glossopharyngeal neuralgia
    Micturition
  Cardiac dysfunction
    Obstruction to flow
      Aortic or pulmonic stenosis
      Cardiac tamponade
      Severe heartworm infection
    Rhythm disturbances
      Heart block
      Tachyarrhythmias
    Cardiopulmonary disease
      Right-to-left cardiac shunt
      Pulmonary thromboembolism
      Pulmonary hypertension
    Myocardial infarction
Metabolic disorders
  Hypoglycemia
Drug therapy
  Digoxin
  Phenothiazine tranquilizers
  Vasodilators [e.g., nitroglycerin, angiotensin-converting enzyme (ACE) inhibitors]
  Diuretics
  Quinidine
Miscellaneous
  Coughing (tussive syncope)
  Pulseless disease (e.g., obstruction of the major arteries to the head from neoplasia, thrombosis)
  Swallowing

Modified with permission from Ettinger SJ, Feldman EC (eds): *Textbook of Veterinary Internal Medicine,* 4th ed. Philadelphia, WB Saunders, 1995, p 55.

electrocardiographic monitoring (i.e., Holter monitoring) is required in some animals to detect an intermittent arrhythmia.

C. **Differential diagnoses.** It is important and sometimes difficult to differentiate syncope from seizure activity or narcolepsy–cataplexy.

  1. Narcolepsy (excessive sleep) and **cataplexy** (sudden loss of muscle tone) are rare in small animals but can be confused with syncope. Although sudden collapse and immobility occur with cataplexy, the animal is easily aroused by calling its name or touching it.

  2. Generalized seizures often occur when animals are relaxed or even sleeping and are associated with prominent tonic–clonic muscular contractions. Vocalization, urination, and defecation may occur, and postictal confusion or lethargy lasting several hours or more is common.

Chapter 20

Trembling and Shivering

I. **DEFINITIONS.** There are several terms used to describe involuntary muscle activity.

A. **Shivers (trembles, shakes, quivers, quakes).** These terms refer to an involuntary increase in skeletal muscle contraction and relaxation of moderate frequency involving the entire body, especially the trunk.

B. **Tremors** result from alternating contraction of antagonistic muscle groups.

1. **Intention tremors** appear only when an action is initiated; they are absent at rest.

2. **Postural (continuous) tremors** are persistent and most obvious at rest.

C. **Tetanus** is sustained contraction of all skeletal muscles and usually is seen as stiff and persistent limb and neck extension.

D. **Tetany** is similar to tetanus except the activity is intermittent and not continuous.

E. **Fasciculations** represent rapid contraction and relaxation of muscle fibers within a muscle group, frequently associated with nerve root irritation. When palpated, fasciculating muscle feels like a bag of writhing worms.

F. **Myoclonus** is rhythmic, involuntary contraction of one or more muscle groups and is almost pathognomonic for canine distemper virus infection.

G. **Myotonus** is sustained contraction of a muscle group.

II. **CAUSES** of trembling and shivering are summarized in Table 20-1. Shivering or trembling may be a primary disorder, or part of another disease process.

III. **DIAGNOSTIC APPROACHES**

A. A thorough history, physical, and neurologic examination are indicated.

B. Localization of the abnormality has diagnostic significance.

1. **Single limb involvement** may indicate nerve root entrapment, neoplasia, or peripheral neuritis.

2. **Rear limb involvement** may indicate senility or lumbosacral disease.

3. **Whole body tremors** may indicate toxin ingestion, electrolyte disorders, or cerebellar disease.

TABLE 20-1. Causes of Trembling and Shaking

Physiologic
   Temperature regulation (especially when the skin temperature decreases)
   Fear
   Fatigue
Pathologic
   Disorders accompanied by other signs in addition to trembling
      Intoxication
         Organophosphates
         Carbamates
         Metaldehyde
         Organochlorines
      Metabolic disorders
         Hypocalcemia
         Hyperkalemia
         Hypoglycemia
         Uremia
         Hepatopathy
         Hyperadrenocorticism
      Cerebellar disease (intention tremors)
      Nerve root disease (fasciculations)
   Disorders characterized by trembling only
      Senility
      Idiopathic tremor syndrome (white shaker dog disease)
      Cerebrospinal hypomyelinogenesis and dysmyelinogenesis

4. **Tremors in the absence of other clinical signs** would suggest:
   a. Hypo- or dysmyelinogenesis (in a young animal)
   b. Idiopathic tremor syndrome or senility (in an adult animal)

Chapter 21

Ataxia, Paresis, and Paralysis

I. ATAXIA

A. Definitions

1. **Ataxia** is incoordination without paresis, spasticity, or involuntary movement.
2. **Proprioception** is the sense of knowing where parts of the body are.

B. Causes

1. **Abnormal proprioception (sensory ataxia).** Any disease causing compression of the spinal cord or otherwise affecting proprioceptive tracts in the spinal cord or brain stem can result in proprioceptive deficits. The proprioceptive tracts are relatively superficial in the spinal cord, and proprioception is one of the first functions to be affected with compressive spinal cord lesions.
2. **Cerebellar dysfunction** (see Chapter 47) may arise from many diseases (e.g., congenital malformation, infection, abiotrophy).
3. **Vestibular disease** (see Chapter 47) is common in dogs and cats and may be idiopathic, associated with middle or inner ear disease (e.g., otitis media or interna), or associated with brain stem disease.

C. Clinical findings. Ataxia is usually associated with a **wide-based stance** and **incoordination of the limbs.**

1. **Abnormal proprioception** is indicated by the **knuckling response** (i.e., absent or delayed repositioning of the paw when it is flexed and weight is placed on its dorsal surface). Postural responses (e.g., **the hopping reaction)** may also be abnormal. **Paresis** may be associated with abnormal proprioception because of the close proximity of motor and proprioceptive tracts in the spinal cord.
2. **Cerebellar disease** is typically associated with **symmetric ataxia, dysmetria** (e.g., goose-stepping gait), and **intention tremors** (especially of the head).
3. **Vestibular disease** typically results in **asymmetric ataxia, head tilt, nystagmus,** and **falling** or **rolling to one side.**

D. Diagnostic approaches. A neurologic examination is often sufficient to localize the problem as proprioceptive, cerebellar, or vestibular. Table 21-1 outlines the signs that can be used to differentiate these disorders.

II. PARESIS AND PARALYSIS

A. Definitions

1. **Paresis** refers to partial loss of voluntary motor activity.
2. **Paralysis** refers to complete loss of voluntary motor activity.

B. Causes (Tables 21-2 through 21-5). Paresis or paralysis may result from a lesion (compressive, inflammatory, neoplastic, degenerative, traumatic, anomalous, or vascular) in the brain stem, spinal cord, peripheral nerves, or neuromuscular junction. Paresis and paralysis may be classified as resulting from either:

1. **Upper motor neuron (UMN) dysfunction** (i.e., in the spinal cord or brain stem)

TABLE 21-1. Differentiation of Ataxia Resulting from Proprioceptive Deficits, Cerebellar Deficits, and Vestibular Deficits

Clinical Sign	Abnormal Proprioception	Cerebellar Disease	Central Vestibular Disease	Peripheral Vestibular Disease
Asymmetric ataxia	Usually no	No	Yes	Yes
Head tilt	No	No	Yes	Yes
Head tremor	No	Yes	No	No
Intention tremor	No	Yes	No	No
Proprioceptive deficit	Yes	No	Yes	No
Paresis	Often	No	Often	No
Nystagmus	No	Often tremor-like	Yes	Yes
Direction of nystagmus altered with head position	...	No	Yes	No

Modified with permission from Lorenz MD, Cornelius LM (eds): *Small Animal Medical Diagnosis*, 2nd ed. Philadelphia, JB Lippincott, 1993, p 438.

    2. Lower motor neuron (LMN) dysfunction (i.e., in the peripheral spinal or cranial nerves or their cell bodies in the spinal cord or brain stem)

C. **Diagnostic approaches.** Paresis and paralysis represent two of the most common neurologic complaints in small animal practice.

    1. A neurologic examination can usually identify the cause of the paresis as UMN or LMN and localize the lesion within the spinal cord or brain stem (Tables 21-6 and 21-7).

    2. Specific diagnoses may require cerebrospinal fluid (CSF) analysis, radiography, serology, myelography, electrodiagnostic testing (e.g., electromyography, nerve conduction velocity), or computed tomography (CT) or magnetic resonance imaging (MRI).

TABLE 21-2. Causes of Monoparesis Classified According to Time Course

Type of Lesion	Acute Nonprogressive	Acute Progressive	Chronic Progressive
Degenerative	...	Disk protrusion	Lumbosacral stenosis
Neoplastic	...	...	Nerve sheath tumor, other neoplasia
Immunologic	...	Brachial plexus neuritis	...
Inflammatory	...	Rabies, abscess	...
Traumatic	Nerve injury	...	...
Vascular	Infarction	...	...

Modified with permission from Lorenz MD, Cornelius LM (eds): *Small Animal Medical Diagnosis*, 2nd ed. Philadelphia, JB Lippincott, 1993, p 431.

TABLE 21-3. Causes of Hindlimb Paresis Classified According to Time Course

Type of Lesion	Time Course		
	Acute Nonprogressive	Acute Progressive	Chronic Progressive
Degenerative	. . .	Type I disk protrusion, hemorrhagic myelomalacia	Degenerative myelopathy, type II disk protrusion, neuronopathy, demyelinating disorders, lumbosacral stenosis
Anomalous	Myelodysplasia	. . .	Spinal dysraphism
Neoplastic	. . .	Primary, metastatic, or vertebral neoplasia	Primary, metastatic, or vertebral neoplasia
Nutritional	. . .	. . .	Hypervitaminosis A
Inflammatory	. . .	Canine distemper, protozoal infection, discospondylitis	Canine distemper, feline infectious peritonitis (FIP), fungal infection, granulomatous meningoencephalitis, immune meningomyelitis
Traumatic	Spinal cord injury	. . .	. . .
Vascular	Fibrocartilaginous or septic embolism, aortic thromboembolism	. . .	. . .

Modified with permission from Lorenz MD, Cornelius LM: *Small Animal Medical Diagnosis,* 2nd ed. Philadelphia, JB Lippincott, 1993, p 431.

TABLE 21-4. Causes of Upper Motor Neuron (UMN) Tetraparesis Classified According to Time Course

Type of Lesion	Time Course		
	Acute Nonprogressive	**Acute Progressive**	**Chronic Progressive**
Degenerative	. . .	Type I disk protrusion	Cervical spondylomyelopathy, type II disk protrusion, storage diseases, neuronopathy, demyelinating diseases
Anomalous	Myelodysplasia	Atlantoaxial luxation	Vertebral malformations, spinal dysraphism
Neoplastic	. . .	. . .	Primary, metastatic, or vertebral neoplasia
Nutritional	. . .	. . .	Hypervitaminosis A
Inflammatory	. . .	Canine distemper; bacterial, fungal, or protozoal infection	Canine distemper, feline infectious peritonitis (FIP), granulomatous meningoencephalitis, fungal infection, immune meningomyelitis
Traumatic	Spinal cord injury		. . .
Vascular	Fibrocartilaginous or septic embolism, vascular malformation, hemorrhage		. . .

Modified with permission from Lorenz MD, Cornelius LM: *Small Animal Medical Diagnosis,* 2nd ed. Philadelphia, JB Lippincott, 1993, p 432.

TABLE 21-5. Causes of Lower Motor Neuron (LMN) Tetraparesis Classified According to Time Course

	Time Course		
Type of Lesion	**Episodic Nonprogressive**	**Acute Progressive**	**Chronic Progressive**
Degenerative	. . .	. . .	Neuronopathies, myopathies, axonopathies
Anomalous	. . .	Myotonia	Demyelinating diseases
Metabolic	Hypoglycemia, hyperkalemia, hypercalcemia, hypocalcemia, hyperthyroidism, hypokalemia	Hypokalemia	Diabetes mellitus, hypothyroidism, hypoadrenocorticism, hyperadrenocorticism, hypokalemia, hyperinsulinism
Nutritional	. . .	. . .	Thiamine deficiency, hypovitaminosis E
Inflammatory or immunologic	Polymyositis, myasthenia gravis	Polyneuritis, polyradiculoneuritis, polymyositis, protozoal myositis and neuritis	Polyneuritis, polymyositis
Toxic	. . .	Tick paralysis, botulism, aminoglycosides	Lead, organophosphates, miscellaneous toxins

Modified with permission from Oliver JE, Lorenz MD: *Handbook of Veterinary Neurologic Diagnosis*, 2nd ed. Philadelphia, JB Lippincott, 1993, p 174.

TABLE 21-6. Differentiation of Lower Motor Neuron (LMN) and Upper Motor Neuron (UMN) Dysfunction

	LMN	**UMN**
Motor function	Paralysis of muscle or groups of muscles	Paralysis or paresis of part of the body
Spinal reflexes	Decreased to absent	Normal to increased
Muscle tone	Decreased	Normal to increased
Muscle atrophy	Early (weeks) and severe in denervated muscles	Late (months), mild, and affects entire limb or area of body
Electromyography findings	Fibrillation potentials apparent after 5–7 days	No change

Modified with permission from Lorenz MD, Cornelius LM (eds): *Small Animal Medical Diagnosis*, 2nd ed. Philadelphia, JB Lippincott, 1993, p 424.

TABLE 21-7. Localization of Spinal Cord Lesions

Location of Lesion	Clinical Signs
C1–C5	Tetraparesis, UMN all four limbs
C6–T2 (brachial plexus)	Tetraparesis, UMN hindlimbs, LMN forelimbs
T3–L3	UMN hindlimb paresis, forelimbs normal
L4–S2 (lumbosacral plexus)	LMN hindlimb paresis, forelimbs normal
S1–S3 (pelvic plexus)	LMN bladder and urethral and anal sphincters
Cd1–Cd5	LMN paresis of tail

LMN = lower motor neuron; UMN = upper motor neuron.
Modified with permission from Lorenz MD, Cornelius LM (eds): *Small Animal Medical Diagnosis,* 2nd ed. Philadelphia, JB Lippincott, 1993, p 428.

Chapter 22

Altered Consciousness

I. DEFINITIONS

A. **Depression** is present when an animal is lethargic but still responsive to external stimuli in a near normal manner.

B. **Stupor** is present when an animal is recumbent and unaware of its surroundings but can be aroused with strong stimulation.

C. **Coma** is present when an animal is recumbent, unaware of its surroundings, and cannot be aroused.

D. A **vegetative state** is present when an animal can be aroused but is unaware of its surroundings.

II. CAUSES.
The reticular activating system in the rostral midbrain controls the level of consciousness, and any disease process that affects this area or its connections to the cerebral cortex will alter consciousness.

A. **Coma** or **stupor** results from one of **three disease processes.** Cerebral edema, brain herniation, or both may be associated with these disorders.

1. **Encephalopathy** (metabolic or toxic)

2. **Diffuse cerebral cortical disease**

3. **Disease** in the **midbrain** or **pons** (e.g., compression, destructive lesions)

B. Specific causes of stupor or coma are listed in Table 22-1.

III. CLINICAL FINDINGS

A. **Neurologic findings** can help localize the affected area or areas of the brain.

1. **Cerebral cortical disease** is indicated by **seizures, normal** or **constricted pupils** that **respond to light, roving eye movements,** and **Cheyne-Stokes respiration** (i.e., hyperpnea alternating with apnea).

2. **Midbrain disease** is indicated by **hyperventilation, loss of the oculocephalic reflex** (the normal nystagmus associated with head movement), a **negative caloric test,** and **pinpoint** or **dilated pupils** that are **unresponsive to light.**

3. **Medullary involvement** is likely if there is an **irregular respiratory pattern** or **cardiac arrhythmias** (assuming metabolic abnormalities are absent).

4. **Midbrain** and **pons.** Injury of motor tracts may cause **decerebrate rigidity** (extensor rigidity in all four limbs).

B. **Other signs.** Signs of the underlying disease may also be present.

TABLE 22-1. Causes of Stupor or Coma

Congenital
  Hydrocephalus
  Lysosomal storage diseases
  Lissencephaly
Metabolic causes
  Hepatic encephalopathy
  Hypoglycemia
  Acid–base disturbances
  Hypoxia
  Hypoadrenocorticism
  Hypothyroidism
  Diabetes mellitus
  Uremia
  Abnormal osmolality
  Heat stroke
  Hyperlipidemia
Neoplasia (primary or metastatic)
Inflammation
  Canine distemper
  Rabies
  Granulomatous meningoencephalitis
  Rocky Mountain spotted fever
  Ehrlichiosis
  Feline infectious peritonitis (FIP)
  Bacterial, protozoal and fungal infections
Toxins or Drugs
  Ethylene glycol
  Lead
  Barbiturates
  Alcohol
  Many others
Trauma
  Cranial trauma
Vascular causes
  Feline ischemic encephalopathy
  Coagulopathy
  Hypertension
Nutritional causes
  Thiamine deficiency
Miscellaneous causes
  Status epilepticus

Modified with permission from Ettinger SJ, Feldman EC (eds): *Textbook of Veterinary Internal Medicine*, 4th ed., Philadelphia, WB Saunders, 1995, p 151.

IV. DIAGNOSTIC APPROACHES

A. **History, physical examination,** and **laboratory studies.** A thorough history, physical and neurologic examinations, complete blood count (CBC), serum biochemical profile, and urinalysis (with or without blood gas analysis) are indicated.

  1. **History.** Drug administration, exposure to a toxin, preexisting disease, or a traumatic event may be the cause of the stupor or coma.

  2. **Laboratory assessment** will identify many of the metabolic causes of coma.

B. **Additional tests.** The lack of an identifiable metabolic or toxic disorder suggests primary brain disease.

1. An **electroencephalogram (EEG)** may help assess cerebral cortical function.

2. A **brain stem auditory evoked response (BAER) test** may help assess brain stem function.

3. **Invasive tests** that require general anesthesia [e.g., cerebrospinal fluid (CSF) collection, computed tomography (CT)] can be considered, but the risks versus the benefits must be considered.

V. TREATMENT

A. Coma. Immediate assessment of breathing, airway, and cardiovascular function followed by supportive care is indicated. Patients with altered consciousness require good nursing care (e.g., soft bedding, frequent turning), fluids, and nutritional support.

1. **Encephalopathy**
   a. **Toxic encephalopathies** are treated by decreasing toxin absorption (if possible), enhancing excretion, antagonizing the effects of the toxin (if possible), and providing supportive therapy.
   b. **Metabolic encephalopathies** are treated with intravenous fluids, supplemental oxygen, glucose administration, and other supportive measures.

2. **Cerebral edema** or **brain herniation** is treated with one or a combination of corticosteroids, osmotic agents, diuretics, or intubation and hyperventilation [reducing the arterial carbon dioxide tension ($Paco_2$) decreases cerebral blood flow]. If intracranial hemorrhage is likely, mannitol should be avoided because it may exacerbate bleeding.

B. Seizures. Anticonvulsant therapy may be necessary.

VI. PROGNOSIS.

Serial neurologic examinations are the best method of prognostication. Recovery is unlikely if no improvement in neurologic signs is observed within 2–3 days. Signs associated with a **poor** prognosis include:

A. Progression from stupor to coma

B. Constricted or dilated pupils that are unresponsive to light

C. Loss of the oculocephalic reflex

D. Change from normal to an abnormal respiratory pattern

E. Development of cardiac arrhythmias

F. Development of decerebrate rigidity

Chapter 23

Blindness and Anisocoria

I. ANATOMY AND PHYSIOLOGY OF VISUAL PATHWAYS

A. **Visual pathways.** The visual pathways are depicted in Figure 23-1. Table 23-1 presents the results of lesions at different levels in the visual pathway.

B. **Pupillary light responses** should be assessed in dimly lit conditions by shining a strong light into one pupil. A prompt constriction of that pupil to light (direct response) should be accompanied by pupillary constriction in the other eye (consensual response).

1. Pupillary constriction is a parasympathetic phenomenon and originates in the parasympathetic nuclei (in the midbrain) of the oculomotor nerve.

2. Pupillary dilation is a sympathetic phenomenon. Sympathetic fibers originate in the midbrain, travel down the spinal cord to the T1–T3 segments, synapse, and leave the spinal cord and course cranially in the vagosympathetic trunk. Fibers synapse in the cranial cervical ganglion and then travel to the eye.

II. BILATERAL BLINDNESS

A. Assessment

1. The **subjective assessment** of blindness can be difficult. It can be accomplished by observing the animal's navigation of an obstacle course, the animal's menace response, or the animal's ability to detect movement (e.g., of a finger or cotton ball).

2. **Electroretinograms** can be used to assess retinal function, but they do not directly assess vision.

B. **Causes.** Blindness can result from one or a combination of the following:

1. **Opacification of the ocular media,** caused by disorders of the:
   a. Cornea (e.g., keratitis)
   b. Aqueous humor (e.g., hyphema)
   c. Lens (e.g., cataracts)
   d. Vitreous humor

2. **Retinal disease** (e.g., progressive retinal atrophy, retinal detachment)

3. **Lesions in the optic nerves or tracts** (e.g., distemper encephalitis, granulomatous meningoencephalitis)

4. **Lesions in the occipital cortex** (e.g., hypoxia, trauma, granulomatous meningoencephalitis)

C. Clinical findings

1. **Opacification of the ocular media.** The fundus cannot be visualized, but the pupillary light response is usually normal.

2. **Retinal disease.** Fundoscopic examination may reveal a variety of retinal lesions. The pupillary light response is usually subnormal, and the pupils are dilated in room light.

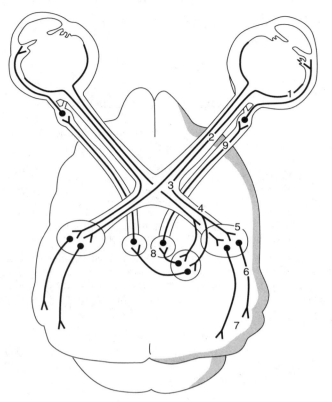

FIGURE 23-1. Pathways for vision and pupillary light reflexes: (*1*) retina; (*2*) optic nerve, (*3*) optic chiasm, (*4*) optic tract, (*5*) lateral geniculate body, (*6*) optic radiation, (*7*) occipital cortex, (*8*) parasympathetic nucleus of the oculomotor nerve [cranial nerve (CN) III] (*9*) oculomotor nerve. (Redrawn with permission from Oliver JE, Lorenz MD: *Handbook of Veterinary Medical Diagnosis.* Philadelphia, WB Saunders, 1983, p 255.)

3. **Lesions in the optic nerves or tracts**
   a. Papilledema or papillitis may be observed on fundoscopic examination.
   b. The involvement of optic nerves or tracts is inferred based on the pupillary light response, the pupil size, and the retinal examination (see Table 23-1).
   c. Bilateral optic nerve or tract involvement below the lateral geniculate body or an optic chiasm lesion will produce blindness with bilaterally dilated and unresponsive pupils.

4. **Lesions in the occipital cortex.** Cortical blindness can result from bilateral lesions in the lateral geniculate bodies, optic radiations, or occipital cortex. Typically, cortical blindness is associated with normal pupil size at rest and a normal pupillary light response.

D. **Diagnostic approaches**

1. **Ocular examination** will usually reveal any abnormalities in the ocular media or retina.

2. **Electroretinograms** may document retinal dysfunction.

3. **Routine laboratory assessment, cerebrospinal fluid (CSF) analysis, computed tomography (CT),** or **magnetic resonance imaging (MRI)** may be necessary to determine the cause of abnormalities in the optic nerves and tracts or the occipital cortex.

TABLE 23-1. Findings Associated with a Complete Lesion on the Right Side of the Visual Pathway

Structure	Vision		Resting Pupil		Pupillary Light Response	
	Right	**Left**	**Right**	**Left**	**Right**	**Left**
Retina or optic nerve	Absent	N	Slightly dilated	N	NR	BC
Optic chiasm	Absent	Absent	Dilated	Dilated	NR	NR
Optic tracts	N	Poor*	N	Slightly dilated	BC	BC
Lateral geniculate body, optic radiations, or occipital cortex	N	Poor*	N	N	BC	BC
Parasympathetic nuclei (bilateral) of cranial nerve (CN) III	N	N	Dilated	Dilated	NR	NR
CN III	N	N	Dilated	N	Left constricts	Left constricts

BC = both constrict; N = normal; NR = no response.
* Loss of sight in left visual field with partial sparing of right visual field.
Modified with permission from Oliver JE, Lorenz MD: *Handbook of Veterinary Neurologic Diagnosis*, Philadelphia, WB Saunders, 1983, p 255.

III. ANISOCORIA

A. **Definition.** Anisocoria refers to unequal pupils. The abnormal pupil may be dilated or constricted, and it may be difficult to identify which pupil is abnormal. The abnormal pupil may not respond to changes in light or may do so in a subnormal fashion when compared with the normal pupil. Blindness may be associated with anisocoria.

B. **Causes**

1. **Ocular conditions**
   a. **Iris disease** (e.g., iris atrophy, synechiae, anterior uveitis)
   b. **Intraocular pressure elevation** (i.e., glaucoma)
   c. **Drug administration** (e.g., atropine)
   d. **Corneal disease** (e.g., ulcers)
   e. **Lenticular disease** (e.g., lens subluxation, luxation, hypermature cataracts)
   f. **Unilateral retinal disease**

2. **Neurologic disease**
   a. **Unilateral optic nerve** or **tract lesions** may be associated with mild anisocoria in room light. (In a darkened room, both pupils will be equally dilated.)
      (1) **Optic nerve lesions.** The pupil ipsilateral to the site of the lesion is dilated.
      (2) **Optic tract lesions.** The pupil contralateral to the site of the lesion is dilated.
   b. **Unilateral lesions of the parasympathetic nuclei, oculomotor nerve,** or **ciliary ganglion** produce pupillary dilation ipsilateral to the lesion. The dilation is more marked than that of optic nerve or tract lesions.
      (1) **Orbital lesions** that damage both the oculomotor nerve (which has both parasympathetic and sympathetic fibers) and the ciliary body may produce a fixed and unresponsive midsized pupil.
      (2) **Feline dysautonomia** and **feline leukemia virus (FeLV)** have been associated with lesions in the parasympathetic nuclei, oculomotor nerve, or ciliary ganglia, resulting in **anisocoria** and **paradoxical anisocoria,** respectively.

(3) **Horner's syndrome** results from abnormalities in sympathetic innervation and is characterized by ipsilateral ptosis (drooped eyelid), miosis, a prolapsed third eyelid, and apparent enophthalmos. The abnormal (miotic or constricted) pupil is most obvious in dim light. Horner's syndrome can be caused by disruption at any point in the lengthy sympathetic pathway, such as disease in the midbrain, spinal cord, thorax, neck (affecting the vagosympathetic trunk), or inner or middle ear.

C. **Diagnostic approaches**

1. Ocular disease should be ruled out before proceeding to a neurologic assessment.

2. Cats with anisocoria characterized by pupillary dilation should be tested for FeLV.

3. The diagnosis of Horner's syndrome requires physical and neurologic examination and possibly pharmacologic testing to help localize the lesion.
   a. Topical hydroxyamphetamine administration in the affected eye will dilate the pupil in normal animals and in those with central lesions (i.e., in the midbrain or spinal cord) or preganglionic lesions (i.e., between the spinal cord and cranial cervical ganglion), but not in animals with postganglionic lesions.
   b. Topical phenylephrine administration will dilate the pupils only in those animals with postganglionic lesions.

4. Diagnosis of parasympathetic nuclei or optic tract lesions may require CSF analysis, CT, or MRI.

Chapter 24

Seizures

I. DEFINITIONS

A. **Seizures** represent transient paroxysmal electrical disturbances in cerebral neurons. Seizure activity indicates an abnormality in the brain rostral to the midbrain (i.e., the cerebrum and related structures). Seizures may be characterized as:

1. **Isolated** (occurring several times per year)
2. **Clustered** (many seizures occurring over several hours or a few days)
3. **Status epilepticus** (continuous seizure activity)

B. **Epilepsy** refers to recurrent seizure activity and may be idiopathic (i.e., with no identifiable intra- or extracranial cause).

II. PATHOPHYSIOLOGY

A. Seizures originate from a seizure focus, which represents an area of prolonged neuronal depolarization. Continued stimulation of neurons around the seizure focus can result in enlargement of the focus or the genesis of several foci. Once a critical level of depolarization has occurred, seizure activity is quickly propagated to other areas in the brain, resulting in a clinically recognizable seizure.

B. Seizures are classified as generalized or partial. Severe generalized seizures typically last less than 5 minutes, but partial motor or mild generalized seizures may last as long as 30 minutes.

1. **Generalized seizures** are the most common and appear as tonic–clonic muscle spasms involving the entire body (with or without sensory, autonomic, and behavioral signs).
2. **Partial seizures** are rare and occur as one of the following:
   a. **Partial motor seizure** (involving only an isolated part of the body)
   b. **Psychomotor seizure** (complex stereotypical behavior)

III. CAUSES.
There are many intracranial and extracranial causes of seizures. Many of the causative diseases are more common in animals of a certain age, which aids in the differential diagnosis (Table 24-1).

IV. CLINICAL FINDINGS

A. Seizures can be associated with **behavioral changes** (e.g., confusion, dementia, hysteria, rage, fear), **sensory changes** (exhibited by pawing at the face, tail chasing, fly-biting), **motor activity** (e.g., tonic or clonic muscle spasms, trismus, chewing, licking, running, pacing, circling), or **autonomic stimulation** (e.g., urination, defecation, salivation, vomiting). Various combinations of these signs may appear in any one animal.

TABLE 24-1. Causes and Age Distribution of Seizures in Dogs and Cats

Younger than 9 months of age
  Congenital hydrocephalus
  Lissencephaly
  Lysosomal storage diseases
  Canine distemper
  Feline infectious peritonitis (FIP)
  Other viral, bacterial, fungal, or protozoal infections
  Trauma
  Toxicity (e.g., organophosphates, lead, strychnine)
  Hypoglycemia
  Hepatic encephalopathy (e.g., portosystemic shunt)
  Other congenital metabolic disorders
  Thiamine deficiency
9 months to 5 years of age
  Canine distemper
  FIP
  Other viral, bacterial, fungal, or protozoal infections
  Steroid-responsive meningoencephalitis
  Granulomatous meningoencephalitis
  Trauma
  Toxicity
  Hypoglycemia
  Hepatic encephalopathy (e.g., portosystemic shunt, acquired liver disease)
  Other acquired metabolic disorders (e.g., hypocalcemia, renal failure)
  Inherited epilepsy (especially in the 9- to 36-month range)
  Acquired epilepsy
  Cerebral neoplasia (rare)
5 years of age and older
  Canine distemper
  FIP
  Steroid-responsive meningoencephalitis
  Granulomatous meningoencephalitis
  Trauma
  Toxicity
  Hypoglycemia (e.g, insulin-secreting tumor)
  Hepatic encephalopathy (acquired liver disease)
  Other acquired metabolic disorders
  Acquired epilepsy
  Cerebral neoplasia

Modified with permission from Ettinger SJ, Feldman EC (eds): *Textbook of Veterinary Internal Medicine,* 4th ed., Philadelphia, WB Saunders, 1995, p 153.

1. Some animals will have a behavioral change (e.g., hiding, attention seeking) a few days **(prodrome)** or a few hours **(aura)** prior to a seizure.

2. Many animals have behavioral changes (e.g., lethargy, depression, hunger, thirst, hyperactivity, pacing) that may last hours to days following a seizure.

B. Animals with idiopathic epilepsy (see Chapter 47 III H 1) do not have **clinical signs of illness between the seizure events,** whereas animals with seizures due to infectious, toxic, neoplastic, or congenital diseases often do. Animals that have seizures only a few times a year are more likely to have idiopathic epilepsy.

V. DIAGNOSTIC APPROACHES

A. **Physical** and **neurologic examination** may be normal (e.g., idiopathic epilepsy) or may reveal signs suggestive of neurologic or metabolic disease or intoxication.

B. **Laboratory** and **imaging studies**

1. Animals with multiple seizures (over a few hours, weeks, or months) should have a thorough workup [e.g., complete blood count (CBC), serum biochemical profile, urinalysis, liver function tests, possibly blood lead and serum cholinesterase levels, abdominal and thoracic radiographs]. If metabolic (e.g., hypoglycemia, liver failure) and toxic causes are ruled out, intracranial disease should be suspected and can be pursued with cerebrospinal fluid (CSF) analysis, serology, skull radiographs, and computed tomography (CT) or magnetic resonance imaging (MRI).

2. If a single seizure has occurred in an otherwise normal animal, an extensive workup may not be warranted unless further seizures occur.

VI. TREATMENT

A. **Acute treatment.** For animals presented in a state of seizure activity or status epilepticus, **intravenous diazepam** is administered in an attempt to interrupt the seizure activity. If diazepam is ineffective or if frequent administration of diazepam (due to its short duration of action) is impractical, **phenobarbital** or **sodium pentobarbital** can be given intravenously to suppress seizures for several hours.

1. Blood glucose levels should be assessed and intravenous glucose should be administered if required.

2. If an animal is under pentobarbital-induced general anesthesia, airway patency, body temperature and respiratory function should be monitored closely.

B. **Chronic treatment.** If long-term maintenance therapy is required, **phenobarbital** is the drug of choice. The treatment of idiopathic epilepsy is discussed in Chapter 47 III H 1 e.

Chapter 25
Head Tilt

I. **DEFINITIONS.** Head tilt is deviation or rotation of the head.

II. **CAUSES** of head tilt are summarized in Table 25-1.

A. **Neurologic (vestibular system) disease.** The vestibular system comprises receptors in the inner ear, the vestibular nerve [cranial nerve (CN) VIII], the vestibular nuclei in the brain stem, the flocculonodular lobes in the cerebellum, and the ascending and descending pathways.

  1. **Peripheral vestibular disease** results from dysfunction of receptors in the inner ear or the vestibular nerve.

  2. **Central vestibular disease** results from abnormalities in the vestibular nuclei, flocculo-nodular cerebellar lobes, or related neuronal pathways.

B. **Non-neurologic causes.** Head tilt (usually mild) may be associated with pain or irritation in the external ear (otitis externa) or pinna.

III. **CLINICAL FINDINGS.** Head tilt caused by vestibular disease is frequently associated with **asymmetric ataxia, falling** or **rolling to the side of the lesion,** and **spontaneous nystagmus.** Peripheral vestibular disease can usually be distinguished from central vestibular disease on the basis of clinical signs (see Table 21-1; Chapter 47 III A 5).

IV. **DIAGNOSTIC APPROACHES AND TREATMENT** are discussed in Chapter 47 III and V E.

TABLE 25–1. Causes of Head Tilt

Neurologic disease
  Peripheral vestibular disease
    Idiopathic vestibular syndrome (cats, older dogs)
    Congenital vestibular disease
    Otitis media or otitis interna
    Neoplasia of the middle or inner ear or vestibular nerve
    Drugs (e.g., aminoglycosides, metronidazole)
    Trauma to the middle or inner ear
  Central vestibular disease
    Neoplasia
    Infectious disease
    Degenerative diseases
    Toxins
Non-neurologic disease
  Pain or irritation in external ear or pinna

Chapter 26

Pain

I. **DEFINITION. Pain** is a sensation of discomfort caused by stimulation of special nerve fibers. **Pain mediators** include prostaglandins, histamine, leukotrienes, serotonin, and other substances.

II. **CAUSES** of pain are summarized in Table 26-1. General stimuli for pain include heat, ischemia, inflammation, chemicals, trauma, and mechanical forces.

III. **CLINICAL FINDINGS**

A. **General signs of pain.** In response to pain, an animal will try to remove the affected area from the cause of the painful stimulus. Other general signs may include whining, decreased activity, behavioral changes (e.g., aggression, hiding), inappetence, tachypnea, tachycardia, biting or licking at an area, limping, or hunching of the back (a sign of abdominal or back pain).

B. **Other clinical signs** are associated with the cause of the pain (see Table 26-1).

IV. **DIAGNOSTIC APPROACHES**

A. **Oral pain.** An **oral examination** should be performed, possibly followed by **radiographs** or a **biopsy.** Additional details can be found in Chapters 1, 2, and 41.

B. **Head pain**

1. **Oral, neurologic,** and **ophthalmologic examinations** should be performed. If oral pain is present, the recommendations given in IV A should be followed.

2. **Radiographs** should be considered if bony swelling or pain is present, to look for signs of trauma, neoplasia, or craniomandibular osteopathy.

3. **Electromyography** and a **muscle biopsy** should be considered if muscle pain or atrophy is present, or if the serum creatine kinase concentration is increased.

4. An **ear swab evaluation** and **culture** and **radiographs** may be needed if otitis is present, depending on the severity and chronicity of the problem.

5. **Cerebrospinal fluid (CSF) analysis** may be considered if neurologic abnormalities are found.

C. **Spinal or central nervous system (CNS) pain**

1. A thorough **neurologic examination** should be performed.

2. **CSF analysis** may be needed if diffuse pain and multiple neurologic abnormalities are present.

3. **Spinal radiographs** and a **myelogram** may be needed in addition to a CSF tap if focal pain and neurologic abnormalities are found.

4. A **biopsy** may be indicated if a bony lesion is seen.

TABLE 26-1. Causes of Pain

Cause	Possible Concurrent Clinical Signs
Generalized pain	
Meningitis	Neurologic abnormalities, fever
Polyarthritis	Anorexia, fever, lameness
Polymyositis	Anorexia, fever, lameness, weakness
Polyneuritis	Neurologic abnormalities, fever
Localized pain	
Abdominal pain	See Table 8–1
Anorectal pain	Constipation, obstipation, dyschezia, hematochezia
Head pain	
Central nervous system (CNS) disease	Neurologic abnormalities
Myositis	Muscle swelling or atrophy
Neoplasia	Variable, depending on the type and site of neoplasia
Otitis	Hyperemia, otic discharge
Trauma (e.g., fracture)	History of trauma, crepitus, swelling
Limb pain	
Hip dysplasia	Lameness
Hypertrophic osteodystrophy	Anorexia, fever, lameness
Joint disease	Lameness, joint swelling, other signs specific to the cause of the joint disease
Myositis	Anorexia, lameness, fever, muscle swelling or atrophy
Neoplasia	Variable, depending on the type and site of neoplasia
Nerve compression	Neurologic abnormalities
Osteochondritis dessicans (OCD) and other skeletal defects	Lameness
Osteomyelitis	Anorexia, fever, lameness
Panosteitis	Anorexia, fever, lameness
Thrombosis	Variable, depending on the site and cause of the thrombus
Trauma	Swelling, crepitus, history of trauma
Oral pain	Halitosis, drooling, dysphagia, dental tartar, ulceration, mass
Skin or subcutaneous pain	
Foreign body	Swelling, fever, hyperemia
Immune-mediated disease	Fever, hyperemia, ulceration
Infection	Fever, hyperemia, swelling
Panniculitis	Fever, swelling, nodules
Trauma	Swelling, erythema, history of trauma

(continued)

TABLE 26-1. (*continued*)

Cause	Possible Concurrent Clinical Signs
Spinal or CNS pain	
Atlantoaxial instability	Quadriparesis or paralysis
Cervical vertebral instability	Variable neurologic abnormalities, depending on the site and severity of the instability
Lumbosacral stenosis	Lameness, hindlimb weakness, neurologic deficits
Meningitis	Neurologic abnormalities
Neoplasia	Variable, depending on the type and site of neoplasia
Vertebral osteoarthritis	Variable neurologic deficits, depending on the site and severity of the osteoarthritis
Discospondylitis	Fever, neurologic deficits
Thoracic pain	
Musculoskeletal pain	Usually none
Pericarditis	Anorexia, exercise intolerance, tachypnea, dyspnea, ascites
Pneumothorax or hydrothorax	Dyspnea, tachypnea
Pulmonary thromboembolism	Dyspnea, tachypnea
Tracheobronchitis	Cough, fever, tachypnea

D. **Thoracic pain** is rare.

    1. Radiographs of the thorax may show an enlarged cardiac silhouette (e..g, pericardial disease), a bronchial pattern (e.g., tracheobronchitis), air or fluid in the pleural space, fractured ribs, or other abnormalities.

    2. Ultrasound examination may be helpful if pericardial disease is suspected or if fluid or a mass is seen on radiographs.

    3. Blood gas evaluation may help identify occult pulmonary disease (e.g., pulmonary thromboembolism).

    4. A **transtracheal wash** may identify infectious or inflammatory airway disease suggested by concurrent clinical signs and radiographs.

E. **Abdominal pain.** The diagnostic approach to abdominal pain is discussed in Chapter 8 IV.

F. **Anorectal pain.** The diagnostic approach to anorectal pain is discussed in Chapter 7 IV.

G. **Limb pain**

    1. Neurologic and **orthopedic examinations** should be performed.

    2. Radiographs of the affected limb may reveal a fracture, bone lysis (e.g., neoplasia, infection), periosteal reaction (e.g., inflammation, infection, neoplasia), or other bony changes.

    3. Arthrocenteses may be useful if joint pain or swelling is found.

    4. Electromyography and a **biopsy** may be considered if muscle pain is detected and there is no history of recent trauma.

    5. Angiography may be useful if poor perfusion suggests a possible thromboembolus.

H. **Cutaneous** or **subcutaneous pain.** Diagnostic tests might be unnecessary if the pain is localized and acute. However, a **biopsy** should be considered if pain is severe or persistent or if hyperemia, erythema, or swelling is present.

I. **Generalized pain**

1. **Neurologic** and **orthopedic examinations** should be performed.

2. **Multiple arthrocenteses** may be helpful to detect polyarthritis.

3. **Serum creatine kinase concentration, electromyography,** and **muscle biopsies** may reveal polymyositis.

4. **CSF analysis** should be performed to look for evidence of meningitis if spinal pain is present or neurologic abnormalities are detected.

V. **TREATMENT**

A. **Definitive therapy** entails treatment of the primary disorder.

B. **Symptomatic treatment.** Possible treatments include:

1. **Nonsteroidal anti-inflammatory drugs (NSAIDs),** such as aspirin or phenylbutazone

2. **Narcotic analgesics** (e.g., morphine, meperidine, oxymorphone)

3. **Narcotic antagonists** (e.g., butorphanol)

4. **Acupuncture**

5. **Polysulfated glycosaminoglycans** (for degenerative joint disease)

Chapter 27
Coughing

I. DESCRIPTION

A. Coughing is a protective reflex intended to remove potentially harmful material from the respiratory tract. Although coughing is beneficial, it may:

1. Exacerbate airway inflammation or irritation
2. Result in emphysema from overdistention of alveoli
3. Cause pneumothorax from the rupture of bullae or an airway
4. Produce weakness and exhaustion
5. Inadvertently aid the spread of infectious respiratory disease

B. Cough receptors are most numerous in the large airways, and they are stimulated by mechanical or chemical means. A few cough receptors are also present in the nose, paranasal sinuses, pharynx, pleura, diaphragm and pericardium. Diseases affecting these areas may be associated with coughing.

II. CAUSES of coughing are summarized in Table 27-1.

III. CLINICAL FINDINGS

A. **Patterns.** Certain diseases are associated with different patterns of coughing. For example:

1. **Cardiac disease.** Coughing often occurs initially at night.
2. **Collapsing trachea.** Coughing occurs after excitement, exertion, or drinking, or a characteristic "goose honk" cough is common.
3. **Infectious tracheobronchitis (kennel cough).** The cough is frequently loud, dry, and harsh.

B. **Systemic signs** of illness (e.g., lethargy, anorexia) and abnormal lung sounds are more common with bronchial, lower airway, pulmonary parenchymal, and cardiac disease.

IV. DIAGNOSTIC APPROACHES

A. **History.** Relevant historical information can include:

1. **Potential exposure to infectious disease** (e.g., exposure to other animals)
2. **Environmental factors**
   a. Infectious disease is less likely in indoor animals.
   b. Urban animals are more exposed to airborne pollutants.
   c. Indoor animals may be exposed to cigarette smoke.
3. **Signalment.** For example, in a toy breed, collapsing trachea may be the cause of the cough.

TABLE 27-1. Causes of Coughing in Dogs and Cats

Upper Airway	Lower Airway	Cardiovascular
Pharyngitis	Acute or chronic bronchitis	Left-sided heart failure
Tonsillitis	Bronchiectasis	Left atrial enlargement
Tracheitis	Pneumonia (e.g., aspiration)	Heartworm disease
Collapsing trachea (dogs)	Immotile cilia syndrome	Pulmonary thrombosis
Neoplasia	Pulmonary fibrosis or abscess	Pulmonary edema
Trauma	Hilar lymph node enlargement (fungal or neoplastic disease)	
	Fungal infection (e.g., histoplasmosis, blastomycosis)	
	Allergic bronchitis	
	Pulmonary infiltrate with eosinophils (PIE)	
	Lungworms	
	Trauma or physical irritation (e.g., foreign body, smoke inhalation)	
	Neoplasia	

Modified with permission from Lorenz MD, Cornelius LM (eds): *Small Animal Medical Diagnosis*, 2nd ed., Philadelphia, JB Lippincott, 1993, p 208.

    4. Geographical area or **travel history.** For example, the incidence of fungal disease or heartworm infection varies from region to region.

B. **Physical examination.** A cough can often be induced by tracheal palpation in dogs with tracheal inflammation.

C. **Laboratory tests** and **imaging studies.** The extent of the diagnostic workup depends on the severity of the coughing and other signs of respiratory disease (e.g., dyspnea) or systemic illness. Lung sounds may be abnormal and respiratory rate or effort may be increased.

    1. Thoracic radiographs are central in determining the nature of the respiratory disease.

    2. Other diagnostic tests may include a complete blood count (CBC), serum biochemical profile, urinalysis, fecal examination (routine flotation, Baermann examination), heartworm tests, electrocardiogram (ECG, with or without cardiac ultrasound), transtracheal wash, bronchoalveolar lavage, bronchoscopy, fine needle lung aspiration, or lung biopsy.

Chapter 28

Dyspnea and Tachypnea

I. DEFINITIONS

A. **Dyspnea** refers to labored breathing.

B. **Tachypnea** refers to a respiratory rate that is higher than normal. Tachypnea frequently accompanies dyspnea. If tachypnea without dyspnea is present, physiologic causes (e.g., stress, excitement, pain) should be ruled out.

II. CAUSES (Table 28-1)

A. Dyspnea and tachypnea usually develop because of the need for additional oxygen; however, compensation for metabolic acidosis, damage to the medullary respiratory centers, hyperthermia, weak or dysfunctional respiratory muscles, and pain associated with breathing (e.g., fractured ribs) may also be causes. There are four basic causes of dyspnea:

    1. Upper airway disorders (i.e., disorders affecting the nares, pharynx, larynx, or cervical trachea)

    2. Lower airway and pulmonary parenchymal disorders

    3. Restrictive disorders (e.g., pleural space disease)

    4. Miscellaneous disorders (e.g., anemia, heatstroke)

B. Tachypnea and dyspnea may be normal responses to some situations (e.g., high ambient temperature, excitement, exercise, stress).

III. CLINICAL FINDINGS. Respiratory patterns may vary, depending on the cause of the dyspnea.

A. **Inspiratory dyspnea** often results from upper respiratory disorders. It is frequently associated with a prolonged and noisy inspiratory effort.

B. **Expiratory dyspnea** often results from lower respiratory tract disorders.

C. **Inspiratory** and **expiratory dyspnea** is frequently present in animals with lower airway or pulmonary parenchymal disease.

D. **Rapid** and **shallow respiration** with muffled breath sounds on auscultation is often present with restrictive or pleural space disorders.

IV. DIAGNOSTIC APPROACHES. A thorough workup is justified in animals with dyspnea. However, if the dyspnea is severe and life threatening, diagnostic testing may need to be postponed until supplemental oxygen can be administered and the patient is stable.

TABLE 28-1. Causes of Dyspnea

Upper Airway Disorders	Lower Airway and Pulmonary Parenchymal Disorders	Restrictive Disorders	Miscellaneous Disorders
Stenotic nares	Thoracic tracheal disease (see cervical trachea)	Pleural effusion (e.g., pyothorax, right-sided heart failure)	Anemia
Nasal cavity obstruction (e.g., neoplasia)	Bronchial disease (e.g., chronic or allergic bronchitis, lungworm)	Pneumothorax	Methemoglobinemia
Elongated or edematous soft palate	Pneumonia	Congenital thoracic wall abnormalities (e.g., pectus excavatum)	Cyanosis
Nasopharyngeal polyp (cats)	Pulmonary edema	Thoracic wall trauma (e.g., fractured ribs, flail injury)	Compensation for metabolic acidosis
Laryngeal disease (e.g., neoplasia, paralysis, edema)	Pulmonary thromboembolism (e.g., heartworm disease, hyper-adrenocorticism)	Thoracic wall or mediastinal neoplasia	Heatstroke
Cervical tracheal disease (e.g., collapse, neoplasia, stenosis, foreign body, extraluminal compression)	Pulmonary contusions	Diaphragmatic hernia	Damage to central nervous system (CNS) respiratory centers (e.g., head trauma)
	Pulmonary neoplasia	Extreme obesity	Neuromuscular weakness (e.g., polyradiculo-neuritis)
	Pulmonary granulomatosis	Marked ascites	Pain (e.g., fractured ribs)
		Severe hepatomegaly	
		Large intraabdominal mass	
		Severe gastric distention	

Modified with permission from Lorenz MD, Cornelius LM (eds): *Small Animal Medical Diagnosis*, 2nd ed., Philadelphia, JB Lippincott, 1993, p 217.

A. **Radiology.** Caution is advised when performing thoracic radiographs in dyspneic animals because the stress of restraint and positioning may result in respiratory arrest and death. If pleural space disease is suspected, thoracocentesis and the removal of a significant volume of fluid or air can be lifesaving and should be performed prior to obtaining thoracic radiographs in severely dyspneic animals.

B. **Additional diagnostic workup** to identify the cause of the dyspnea is similar to that used for coughing (see Chapter 27 IV C 2).

Chapter 29

Hemoptysis and Epistaxis

I. **DEFINITION**

A. **Hemoptysis** is the coughing or spitting up of blood or blood-tinged sputum.

B. **Epistaxis** refers to hemorrhage from the nasal cavity.

II. **CAUSES**

A. **Hemoptysis.** The causes of hemoptysis are summarized in Table 29-1. Hemoptysis can be caused by any disease process that damages blood vessels in the respiratory tree. It may also occur as a result of a bleeding disorder.

B. **Epistaxis.** The causes of epistaxis are summarized in Table 29-2.

III. **DIAGNOSTIC APPROACH.** The cause of epistaxis or hemoptysis is usually revealed following evaluation of the nasal cavity, respiratory system, and cardiovascular system (see Chapters 39 and 40).

TABLE 29-1. Causes of Hemoptysis

Pulmonary thromboembolism (e.g., heartworm disease)
Severe pulmonary edema
Pneumonia (bacterial, fungal)
Bronchitis
Neoplasia (e.g., bronchogenic carcinoma)
Trauma (pulmonary contusions)
Bleeding disorder
Airway foreign body
Diagnostic procedures (e.g., transtracheal wash, fine-needle lung aspirate)
Cavitary lung lesions (e.g., abscess, parasitic cyst, tumor)

TABLE 29-2. Causes of Epistaxis

Systemic disease processes
  Bleeding disorders
    Thrombocytopenia (e.g., ehrlichiosis, immune-mediated)
    Coagulation factor deficiency (acquired or congenital)
    Platelet dysfunction (e.g., von Willebrand's disease)
  Polycythemia
  Hypertension
Local disease processes
  Neoplasia (e.g., adenocarcinoma)
  Foreign body
  Infection (e.g., aspergillosis, feline viral rhinotracheitis)
  Inflammation (e.g., lymphoplasmacytic rhinitis)
  Trauma

Chapter 30

Cyanosis

I. **DEFINITION.** Cyanosis refers to a bluish discoloration of the skin or mucous membranes. Although cyanosis implies hypoxemia, severe hypoxemia may exist without cyanosis.

II. **PATHOPHYSIOLOGY**

A. Cyanosis results from an increased concentration of **reduced** (i.e., **nonoxygenated) hemoglobin.** The development of cyanosis depends on the **absolute concentration** of reduced hemoglobin (greater than or equal to 5 g/dl or 5%) in the circulation, not on the **relative proportion** of reduced versus oxygenated hemoglobin. Therefore, the presence of cyanosis depends on hemoglobin concentration.

1. **Normal hemoglobin concentration.** Cyanosis will develop when the arterial oxygen tension (Pao_2) is less than 50 mm Hg (Pao_2 reference range = 85–100 mm Hg).

2. **Reduced hemoglobin concentration** (i.e., **anemia).** Cyanosis will not develop until the Pao_2 is much lower than 50 mm Hg. In other words, the degree of hypoxemia needs to be more severe to generate a reduced hemoglobin concentration greater than or equal to 5 g/dl.

3. **Increased hemoglobin concentration** (i.e., **polycythemia).** Cyanosis will develop when the Pao_2 is greater than 50 mm Hg.

B. Cyanosis may also result from **nonfunctioning hemoglobin** (e.g., methemoglobinemia).

III. **CAUSES** of cyanosis are summarized in Table 30-1.

A. **Central cyanosis** results from disorders that lead to hypoxemia or hemoglobin abnormalities. Central cyanosis in a young animal may indicate a congenital cardiac defect.

B. **Peripheral cyanosis** results from decreased blood flow through capillary beds (e.g., exposure to cold, poor cardiac output). It is associated with increased oxygen extraction and elevated reduced hemoglobin concentrations.

IV. **CLINICAL FINDINGS**

A. **Signs of central cyanosis**

1. Most animals will be **dyspneic** or **tachypneic,** and cyanosis will be **generalized** (i.e., skin, mucous membranes).

2. In a young animal with a reverse patent ductus arteriosus (PDA), **differential cyanosis** (i.e., pink oral membranes and cyanotic membranes elsewhere) may be noted because the shunt occurs after the exit of the carotid arteries from the aorta, leading to the admixture of unoxygenated blood.

TABLE 30-1. Causes of Cyanosis

Central cyanosis
  Hypoxemia
    Alveolar hypoventilation (e.g., airway obstruction)
    Ventilation–perfusion mismatch (e.g., pulmonary thromboembolism)
    Anatomic shunts
      Tetralogy of Fallot
      Reverse shunting (right-to-left) patent ductus arteriosus (PDA)
      Reverse shunting ventricular septal defect
      Pulmonary arteriovenous shunting (e.g., lung lobe consolidation)
    Alveolar diffusion impairment (rarely a clinical problem)
  Hemoglobin abnormalities
    Methemoglobinemia (e.g., acetaminophen ingestion or topical benzocaine application in cats)
    Sulfhemoglobinemia
Peripheral cyanosis
  Vasoconstriction
    Reduced cardiac output (e.g., myocardial failure)
    Cold exposure
    Shock
  Venous obstruction (e.g., thrombophlebitis)
  Arterial obstruction (e.g., aortic thromboembolism in cats)

B. **Signs of peripheral cyanosis.** Peripheral cyanosis is usually apparent in the extremities. Animals may have regional or generalized cyanosis (if reduced cardiac output is the cause).

C. **Other signs associated with the underlying disease** will be apparent (e.g., inspiratory stridor, abnormal lung sounds, heart murmurs, cool extremities).

V. **DIAGNOSTIC APPROACHES.** A thorough workup is justified in all cyanotic patients. Arterial blood gas analysis, thoracic radiographs, a hematocrit, and electrocardiogram (ECG) are important tests.

Chapter 31
Pallor and Shock

I. DEFINITIONS

A. **Pallor** is paleness of the skin or mucous membranes.

B. **Shock** is a clinical state that results from an inadequate supply of oxygen to the tissues or an inability of the tissues to utilize oxygen.

II. CAUSES of pallor are summarized in Table 31-1.

A. **Pallor** of mucous membranes can be caused by anemia (see Chapter 48) or decreased peripheral perfusion (i.e., shock).

B. **Shock** can be caused by hypovolemia, cardiac failure, or blood volume or flow maldistribution (see Table 31-1).

III. CLINICAL FINDINGS

A. The clinical signs of shock include **depressed mentation, weak pulses, pale mucous membranes, hypothermia, cold extremities, prolonged capillary refill time** (greater than 2 seconds), **tachycardia, tachypnea,** and **reduced urine output.**

B. **Signs of trauma** or **hypovolemia** may be apparent.

C. An **abnormal heart rhythm** or **murmur** is suggestive of cardiac disease and possibly cardiogenic shock.

IV. DIAGNOSTIC APPROACHES. Most diagnostic tests are performed during or immediately after the initial treatment of shock because of the potentially life-threatening nature of shock. Tests may include a complete blood count (CBC), serum biochemical profile, urinalysis, blood gas analysis, thoracic and abdominal radiographs, cardiac ultrasound, and an electrocardiogram (ECG).

V. TREATMENT

A. **Oxygen delivery and volume support**

1. The first goal of therapy is to ensure a patent airway and breathing. The administration of **supplemental oxygen** via face mask, an oxygen cage, or a nasal or transtracheal catheter is often necessary.

2. Measures are then instituted to restore oxygen delivery to the tissues by normalizing blood volume, blood pressure, and cardiac output.
   a. Intravenous administration of **crystalloid solutions** (e.g., 0.9% saline, lactated

TABLE 31-1. Causes of Pallor

Anemia
Decreased peripheral perfusion
Hypovolemic shock
Severe dehydration
Blood loss
Endogenous fluid loss (e.g., ascites)
Hypoadrenocorticism
Cardiogenic shock
Dilated cardiomyopathy
End-stage mitral or aortic insufficiency
Tachyarrhythmias
Cardiac tamponade
Pulmonary thromboembolism
Vasomotor shock (blood flow or volume maldistribution)
Sepsis or endotoxemia
Trauma
Systemic anaphylaxis
Neurogenic causes
Pain
Gastric dilatation–volvulus (GDV)

Ringer's) at an initial rate of 60–90 ml/kg/hour is the first measure. The administration of **hypertonic (7%) saline (with or without 6% dextran 70)** is an alternative consideration. Signs of effective treatment include restoration or strengthening of pulses, improvement in mucous membrane color and capillary refill time, or a central venous pressure of 5–12 cm H_2O.

  (1) If hypoproteinemia develops, plasma, dextran 70, or hetastarch may be used to maintain oncotic pressure within the vascular space.
  (2) Whole blood transfusions may be necessary if anemia is present or develops during therapy.
  (3) If cardiogenic shock is present, aggressive intravenous fluid therapy is contraindicated because it will exacerbate or cause pulmonary edema.
  b. If blood flow or pressure remains subnormal after volume support, **positive inotropic** or **vasoconstrictive agents** may be required (e.g., dopamine, dobutamine).

B. **Corticosteroid administration** is common for most forms of shock. Water-soluble, rapidly acting agents (e.g., prednisolone sodium succinate, dexamethasone sodium phosphate) should be administered intravenously early in the treatment effort.

C. **Other treatments**

  1. **Antibiotics.** Intravenous administration of a bactericidal, broad-spectrum antibiotic is indicated if sepsis is known or suspected.

  2. **Surgical debridement** or **drainage** may be required to remove or repair a septic focus (e.g., perforated bowel).

  3. **Intravenous glucose administration** may be required if hypoglycemia is present (more common with sepsis) and may also benefit nonhypoglycemic patients as a source of calories.

  4. **Antiarrhythmic therapy** may be necessary.

  5. **Epinephrine administration** is indicated if anaphylactic shock is suspected.

  6. **Pericardiocentesis** is indicated if pericardial effusion and cardiac tamponade are present.

  7. **Gastric decompression** is necessary if gastric dilatation–volvulus (GDV) is the cause of the shock.

Chapter 32

Dysuria

I. DEFINITIONS

A. **Dysuria** refers to painful or difficult urination.

B. **Pollakiuria** refers to frequent urination. Pollakiuria must be distinguished from **polyuria,** which may also be associated with an increased frequency of urination but in larger volumes.

C. **Stranguria** refers to slow and painful urination.

II. CAUSES of dysuria are summarized in Table 32-1.

A. Common causes include inflammatory or obstructive disease in the lower urinary tract (i.e., the bladder or urethra) or the lower genital tract (i.e., the vagina or prostate).

B. Dysuria, pollakiuria, and stranguria frequently occur together because they develop for the same reason.

III. DIAGNOSTIC APPROACHES (see also Chapter 43). Dysuria must be distinguished from urinary incontinence.

A. **Physical examination** may reveal bladder distention, suggestive of bladder atony or obstruction. Rectal palpation may reveal prostatic or pelvic urethral disease. Vaginoscopic examination may identify inflammation or mass lesions.

B. **Laboratory studies.** Urinalysis and urine culture are indicated to detect urinary tract infection.

C. **Imaging studies.** Abdominal radiography, urethrocystography, or ultrasound examination may be required to identify bladder or urethral disease (e.g., uroliths, neoplasia, or urethral strictures).

TABLE 32-1. Causes of Dysuria

Infection
Cystitis
Urethritis
Prostatitis or abscessation
Vaginitis
Inflammation
Feline lower urinary tract disease
Benign prostatic hyperplasia
Urolithiasis (bladder, urethral)
Neoplasia (bladder, urethral, prostatic, vaginal)
Trauma
Ruptured bladder
Urethral stricture
Obstruction of bladder or urethra (e.g., neoplasia, uroliths)
Reflex dyssynergia

Chapter 33

Discolored Urine

I. DEFINITIONS

A. **Normal urine** is yellow to amber in color.

B. **Abnormal urine** colors are usually either red or brown or combinations of these colors.

II. CAUSES

A. **Red discoloration** can result from:

1. **Red blood cells.** Hematuria has many causes (Table 33-1).

2. **Hemoglobin.** Hemoglobinuria is usually caused by intravascular red blood cell hemolysis and may be associated with red-tinged plasma. It may also result from the lysis of red blood cells in dilute urine or urine that has been left standing for several hours.

3. **Myoglobin.** Myoglobinuria can result from acute severe muscle trauma or necrosis. It does not discolor plasma.

4. **Food dyes**

5. **Drugs**

B. **Brown** or **red-brown discoloration** can result from:

1. **Red blood cells**

2. **Hemoglobin**

3. **Myoglobin**

4. **Methemoglobin**

5. **Drugs** (e.g., dilantin)

C. **Yellow-brown** or **orange-yellow discoloration** can be caused by bilirubin, a common urinary pigment.

III. DIAGNOSTIC APPROACHES

A. A urine dipstick test should be performed first.

1. One of the reagent pads on this stick reacts with red blood cells, hemoglobin, and myoglobin. If there is a positive reaction, the urine sediment should be examined for red blood cells.
   a. If positive for red blood cells, hematuria is present.
   b. If negative for red blood cells, hemoglobinuria or myoglobinuria is present.

2. Bilirubin can be identified by a positive reaction on one of the reagent pads.

B. If hematuria is diagnosed:

1. A thorough physical examination should be performed, paying special attention to the external genitalia, vulva, and vagina or prostate.

TABLE 33-1. Causes of Hematuria

Kidney
  Neoplasia
  Pyelonephritis
  Trauma
  Calculi
  Essential hematuria or primary renal hematuria
  Glomerulopathy
  Renal cysts
  Renal infarction
  Parasites (e.g., *Dioctophyma renale*)
Ureter, bladder, and urethra
  Neoplasia
  Calculi
  Trauma
  Feline lower urinary tract disease
  Chronic cyclophosphamide administration
  Parasites (e.g., *Capillaria plica*)
Genital tract
  Prostatic disease (e.g., infection, neoplasia)
  Uterine disease (e.g., infection, neoplasia, subinvolution)
  Estrus
  Vaginal and penile disorders (e.g., trauma, transmissible venereal tumor)
Any site
  Bleeding disorders (e.g., immune-mediated thrombocytopenia)
  Disseminated intravascular coagulation (DIC)
  Heatstroke

Modified with permission from Lorenz MD, Cornelius LM (eds): *Small Animal Medical Diagnosis,* 2nd ed. Philadelphia, JB Lippincott, 1993, p 335.

2. Localizing the source of the hematuria is aided by clinical signs.
    a. The presence of dysuria (or related signs) would suggest lower urinary tract or genital disease.
    b. The absence of dysuria would suggest disease in the ureters, kidneys, or uterus, a bleeding disorder, or a lesion on the external genitalia.
3. The timing of hematuria during urination can be helpful.
    a. Hematuria throughout urination suggests disease in the kidneys, ureters, bladder, or prostatic reflux into the bladder.
    b. Hematuria at the beginning of urination suggests disease distal to the urethral sphincter (i.e., prostate, urethra, vagina, vulva, penis).
    c. Hematuria at the end of urination can occur with bladder or prostatic disease.

C. Lower urinary tract disease can be pursued by urine culture, abdominal radiography, urethrocystography, ultrasonography, or biopsy.

D. Renal disease can be characterized with laboratory testing [i.e., complete blood count (CBC), serum biochemical profile, urinalysis], ultrasonography, intravenous pyelography (IVP), and renal biopsy.

E. Bleeding disorders can be detected by testing mucosal bleeding time, platelet count, prothrombin time (PT), and partial thromboplastin time (PTT).

Chapter 34

Urinary Retention

I. **DEFINITION.** **Urinary retention** refers to the lack of complete bladder emptying following voiding.

II. **CAUSES** of urinary retention are summarized in Table 34-1.

A. **Urinary tract obstruction** can be **mechanical** or **functional** and can occur at any level in the urinary tract (i.e., the renal pelvis, ureters, bladder, or urethra). Only those disorders that result in bladder or urethral obstruction are covered in this chapter.

B. **Bladder atony** (see Chapter 43). Bladder atony frequently results from **neurologic disease** [e.g., upper motor neuron (UMN) and lower motor neuron (LMN) disease]. It also may be caused by **disorders that directly affect the detrusor muscle.**

III. **SEQUELAE AND COMPLICATIONS**

A. **Urinary tract obstruction.** A mechanical obstruction is more likely than a functional obstruction to result in a reduction in the glomerular filtration rate (GFR) and azotemia.

1. Complete mechanical obstruction will lead to severe postrenal **azotemia, metabolic acidosis, hyperkalemia,** and if untreated, **death** within 3–5 days.

2. Partial or intermittent mechanical obstruction can result in **hydronephrosis.** If the hydronephrosis is severe, **chronic renal failure** can develop.

3. The urinary retention associated with obstruction increases the risk of **urinary tract infection.** Hydronephrosis increases the risk of **pyelonephritis.**

B. **Bladder atony.** The urine retention results in an increased risk of **urinary tract infection.**

IV. **CLINICAL FINDINGS** may include:

A. Neoplasia (in older animals)

B. Urolithiasis in breeds that are predisposed (e.g., urate urolithiasis in Dalmatians)

C. Prostatic disease (in older intact male dogs)

D. Stranguria, a thin stream, dribbling, reflex dyssynergia, dysuria, pollakiuria, or hematuria

TABLE 34-1. Causes of Urinary Retention

Bladder atony
  Neurologic disorders
    Upper motor neuron (UMN) disease
    Lower motor neuron (LMN) disease
    Reflex dyssynergia
  Detrusor muscle disorders
    Muscle damage following overdistention
    Inflammation or infiltration of neoplastic cells into the bladder wall
Urinary tract (bladder, urethra) obstruction
  Mechanical
    Neoplasia of bladder or urethra
    Uroliths
    Urethral stricture or inflammation
    Extramural intrapelvic compressive lesions (e.g., prostatic neoplasia, cysts or abscesses)
    Retroflexion of bladder (into a perineal hernia)
  Functional (increased urethral tone)
    Urethral pain or inflammation
    UMN disease
    Reflex dyssynergia

E. Signs of urinary incontinence

F. Neurologic signs (e.g., paresis or paralysis of the hindlimbs, anal sphincter, or tail with UMN or LMN causes of bladder atony)

G. An enlarged bladder, which may be turgid and painful if obstruction is present

H. Depression, lethargy, weakness, vomiting, dehydration, and cardiac arrhythmias may be present in animals with obstruction and postrenal azotemia.

V. DIAGNOSTIC APPROACHES

A. Physical and **neurologic examination**

  1. Physical examination will usually enable distinction between bladder atony and urinary tract obstruction.
     a. The bladder will be difficult to express if there is a functional or mechanical obstruction or UMN disease.
     b. The bladder is usually easy to express if LMN disease is present.

  2. The passage of a urinary catheter can also help distinguish between functional and mechanical obstructions.

  3. Rectal palpation of the prostate in males and the intrapelvic urethra in males and females may reveal masses or uroliths.

B. Laboratory studies

  1. A **urinalysis** is indicated in all animals and may help diagnose the cause or detect complicating urinary tract infections.

  2. A **complete blood count (CBC)** and **serum biochemical profile** (with or without blood gas analysis) is indicated in animals with systemic signs of illness due to urinary tract obstruction.

C. **Imaging studies**

1. Contrast radiographic (urethrocystogram) or ultrasound studies may be required to document the presence, location, and nature of an obstruction.

2. Urodynamic (e.g., cystometrography, urethral pressure profile) and radiographic (e.g., myelography, epidurography) studies may be required for identification of the specific cause of bladder atony.

VI. **TREATMENT** depends on the cause (see Chapter 43).

Chapter 35

Pruritus

I. **DEFINITION. Pruritus** is itching.

II. **CLINICAL FINDINGS**

A. **History.** Pruritus is a very common presenting complaint in small animal practice. Afflicted animals have a history of excessive scratching, chewing, rubbing, licking, and irritability.

B. **Signs.** Scratching often results in visible excoriations, erythema, alopecia, and lichenification.

III. **CAUSES** (Table 35-1). Pruritus is usually, but not always, caused by:

A. **Infection** (e.g., bacterial pyoderma, fungal infection)

B. **External parasitism** (e.g., fleas)

C. **Allergy** (e.g., atopy)

IV. **DIAGNOSTIC APPROACHES.** Identification of the type of infection or allergy or whether there is a combination of disorders can be difficult.

A. **History** and **physical examination.** Consideration of the historical and physical examination findings can help narrow the list of possible diagnoses.

  1. History
    a. Age
      (1) Flea allergy dermatitis, scabies (sarcoptic mange), demodicosis (with or without secondary pyoderma), intestinal parasite hypersensitivity, and ear mite infestations (cats) are more common in puppies and kittens.
      (2) Atopy, food allergy, pyoderma, and seborrhea are more common in adults.
    b. Breed. Certain breeds have a predisposition for specific disorders. For example:
      (1) Atopy is common in golden retrievers and many terrier breeds.
      (2) Demodicosis, pyoderma, atopy, and food allergy are common in Shar peis.
    c. Diet
      (1) Lipid-deficient diets may result in pruritus directly, or they may exacerbate other diseases associated with pruritus.
      (2) Food allergy may coexist with other skin disorders.
    d. Environment
      (1) The onset of pruritus after recent contact with other animals or animal facilities suggests a parasitism because external parasites are transmitted by contact with other animals, bedding, and grooming equipment.
      (2) Infection of human beings may help establish a parasitic cause because some external parasites (e.g., *Sarcoptes scabiei*) will transiently infect and bite humans.

TABLE 35-1. Common Causes of Pruritus

Dogs
  Flea allergy dermatitis
  Scabies (*Sarcoptes scabiei*)
  Demodicosis (*Demodex canis*)
  Pyoderma
  Seborrhea
  Atopy
  Acral lick dermatitis
Cats
  Flea allergy dermatitis
  Eosinophilic plaque
  Otodectic acariasis (ear mites)
  Food allergy

  e. **Onset**
    (1) A rapid onset of pruritus suggests flea allergy dermatitis, scabies, cheyletiellosis, chigger infestation, or drug hypersensitivity.
    (2) A slow, insidious onset is more common with atopy, food allergy, pyoderma, and seborrhea.
  f. **Intensity.** The intensity of pruritus varies. Two of the most pruritic diseases are flea allergy dermatitis and scabies.
  g. **Seasonality.** Atopy and flea allergy dermatitis are more common in the summer months.
  h. **Response to prior therapy.** Resolution of pruritus following antibiotic therapy suggests bacterial pyoderma. Food allergy is less responsive than atopy or flea allergy dermatitis to corticosteroid therapy.
2. **Physical examination findings**
  a. **External parasites.** Physical examination may reveal external parasites (e.g., fleas).
  b. **Patterns.** The distribution of skin lesions and the identification of primary (e.g., pustules) or secondary (e.g., excoriations) lesions will help determine the cause. For example:
    (1) Symmetric lesions involving the dorsal lumbosacral area and caudal thighs are very suggestive of flea allergy dermatitis (Figure 35-1).
    (2) The involvement of ear margins and elbows is common with scabies.
    (3) Head and neck lesions are typical of food allergy in cats.

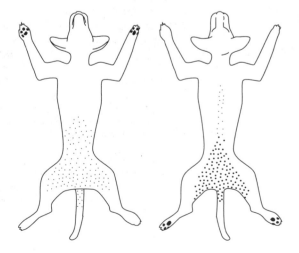

FIGURE 35-1. Typical distribution pattern for skin lesions associated with flea allergy dermatitis in dogs. (Modified and redrawn with permission from Muller GH, Kirk RW, Scott DW: *Small Animal Dermatology,* 3rd ed. Philadelphia, WB Saunders, 1983, p 127.)

B. **Diagnostic tests.** Depending on the history and physical examination findings, the following tests may be useful:

1. Skin scrapings, smears, and tape preparations to detect mites or yeast (i.e., *Malassezia pachydermatis*)

2. Fecal flotation (to detect intestinal parasites or ingested external parasites)

3. Fungal culture to detect dermatophytes (e.g., *Microsporum canis*)

4. Skin biopsy

5. Elimination diet for suspected food allergy

6. Intradermal skin testing for atopy

7. Trial therapy (e.g., with antibiotics to rule out bacterial pyoderma or parasiticides to rule out scabies or flea allergy)

Chapter 36

Alopecia

I. **DEFINITION. Alopecia** refers to the absence of hair from areas that normally have hair. Alopecia may be described as focal, multifocal, diffuse, or regional.

II. **CAUSES.** Alopecia results from primary or secondary disease of the hair follicle (Table 36-1).

III. **DIAGNOSTIC APPROACHES**

A. **History** and **physical examination.** Consideration of the signalment, history, and physical examination findings can narrow the list of possible diagnoses.

1. **Age.** External parasitism and genetic diseases are more likely to be apparent in young animals.

2. **Signalment.** There are various breed predispositions for alopecic disorders (e.g., color dilution alopecia in red-, fawn-, or blue-coated animals).

3. **Onset.** A slow onset of alopecia is suggestive of endocrine imbalance.

4. **Accompanying signs**
   a. The absence of pruritus makes intensely pruritic disorders such as scabies and flea allergy unlikely.
   b. Nonpruritic inflammatory disorders can result from pyoderma, dermatophytosis, immune-mediated disease, and neoplasia.
   c. Nonpruritic noninflammatory disorders may result from genetic disorders, endocrine imbalance, dermatophytosis, demodicosis, immune-mediated disease, and neoplasia.

5. **Distribution.** The distribution of the alopecia may be suggestive of certain disorders (Table 36-2). For example:
   a. Dorsal lumbosacral alopecia is suggestive of flea allergy dermatitis.
   b. Patchy alopecia is common in bacterial folliculitis.
   c. Diffuse, symmetrical alopecia is common with endocrine imbalances.

B. **Diagnostic tests** used to identify causes of alopecia are similar to those used in the workup for pruritus (see Chapter 35). Hematologic, serum biochemical, and hormonal testing may be needed to identify endocrine imbalances.

TABLE 36-1. Causes of Alopecia

Primary follicular disease
    Genetic disorders
        Hairless breeds of dogs and cats
        Congenital hypotrichosis
        Color dilution alopecia in red-, fawn-, and blue-coated animals
        Others
    Neoplasia
    Inflammation
        Autoimmune skin disorders (e.g., pemphigus diseases)
        Dermatophytosis
        Bacterial folliculitis
        Others
Secondary follicular disease
    Endocrine imbalances
        Hypothyroidism
        Hyperadrenocorticism
        Hyposomatotropism
        Adrenal sex hormone imbalances
    Nutritional deficiencies
        Protein/calorie malnutrition
        Vitamin A deficiency
        Fatty acid deficiency
    Stress
    Systemic disease

TABLE 36-2. Patterns of Alopecia and Associated Diseases*

Marked facial alopecia
    Demodicosis
    Dermatophytosis
    Food allergy (cats)
    Pemphigus foliaceous
    Feline and canine acne
Alopecia of the ears
    Dermatophytosis
    Sarcoptic mange
    Demodicosis
    Fly-bite dermatitis
    Pemphigus foliaceous
Alopecia of the feet
    Atopy
    Contact dermatitis
    Demodicosis
    Interdigital pyoderma
    Pemphigus diseases
Alopecia of the caudal trunk and abdomen
    Flea allergy dermatitis
    Feline endocrine alopecia
    Male feminizing syndrome
Multifocal alopecia
    Demodicosis
    Pyoderma
    Seborrhea
    Dermatophytosis
    Autoimmune skin diseases

* The listed diseases are examples only.

Chapter 37

Dermatologic Manifestations of Systemic Disease

I. **INTRODUCTION.** Dermatologic manifestations of systemic disease may include **alopecia, pruritus, erythema, petechiae, pustules** and **papules, seborrhea,** and **other abnormalities.**

II. **CAUSES.** Diseases associated with dermatologic manifestations are summarized in Table 37-1.

III. **SELECTED DISORDERS**

A. **Congenital** or **hereditary defects**

1. **Chediak-Higashi syndrome** is an autosomal recessive disorder seen in Persian cats with yellow eyes and a blue-gray haircoat.
   a. **Clinical findings.** Affected cats are more susceptible to infection and bleeding and are photophobic.
   b. **Treatment** is symptomatic only.

2. **Dermatomyositis** is an autosomal dominant disorder seen primarily in collies, Shetland sheepdogs, and crosses of these breeds.
   a. **Clinical findings.** Affected animals may develop ulceration, crusting, and alopecia of the mucocutaneous junctions, ears, tail, and front legs and local or generalized muscle atrophy by 6 months of age.
   b. **Diagnosis** is by electromyography and biopsy.

3. **Gray collie syndrome (canine cyclic neutropenia)** is a simple autosomal recessive disorder, characterized by a silver-gray haircoat and a cyclic neutropenia.
   a. **Clinical findings** commonly include decreased body size, cyclic fever, diarrhea, joint pain, conjunctivitis, and other infections. Infection is the usual cause of death in animals with this disorder.
   b. **Diagnosis** is based on the clinical findings and the presence of cyclic neutropenia.

4. A **cell-mediated immunodeficiency** occurs in which lymphocyte numbers and function are subnormal.
   a. **Clinical findings** characteristically include recurrent deep pyoderma and furunculosis.
   b. **Treatment** is with antibiotics. Use of a staphylococcal bacterin has been tried in an attempt to prevent recurrence of the infection.

B. **Endocrinopathies**

1. **Acromegaly.** In dogs, acromegaly may cause thick skin and hypertrichosis. Acromegaly is discussed in detail in Chapter 44 I E.

2. **Castration-responsive dermatopathy** may occur in younger male dogs in the absence of a Sertoli cell tumor.
   a. **Clinical findings** in affected dogs include alopecia and hyperpigmentation around the neck and over the scapulae. No other clinical signs of disease are seen.

TABLE 37-1. Systemic Diseases Organized According to Their Dermatologic Manifestations

Cause	Possible Concurrent Clinical Findings
Alopecia	
Demodicosis	Variable, depending on the underlying disease, if present
Drug eruption	Variable, depending on the medication
Estrogen-responsive dermatosis	None
Growth hormone (GH)–responsive dermatosis	None
Hyperadrenocorticism	Polyuria, polydipsia, polyphagia, "potbelly"
Hypothyroidism	Weight gain, lethargy
Ovarian imbalance type I	Pale mucous membranes, estrous cycle abnormalities, vulvar enlargement
Pituitary dwarfism	Stunted growth
Sertoli cell tumor	Feminization, pale mucous membranes
Systemic lupus erythematosus (SLE)	Pale mucous membranes, fever, petechiae, joint pain, muscle pain
Testosterone-responsive dermatosis	None
Erythema	
Demodicosis	Variable, depending on the underlying disease, if present
Drug eruption	Variable, depending on the medication
SLE	Pale mucous membranes, fever, petechiae, joint pain, muscle pain
Mucocutaneous lesions	
Cold agglutinin disease	Pale mucous membranes, lethargy
Cyclic neutropenia	Fever, anorexia, depression
Demodicosis	Variable, depending on the underlying disorder, if present
Dermatomyositis	Muscle pain, muscle atrophy, weakness
Erythema multiforme	Variable, depending on the underlying disease
Leishmaniasis	Anorexia, depression, pale mucous membranes
Staphylococcal pyoderma	Variable, depending on the severity of the infection
Superficial necrolytic dermatitis	Anorexia, icterus, vomiting
SLE	Pale mucous membranes, fever, petechiae, joint pain, muscle pain
Toxic epidermal necrolysis (TEN)	Anorexia, fever, depression
Zinc-responsive dermatosis	Anorexia, fever, depression*
Petechiae	
Babesiosis	Anorexia, icterus, vomiting, lymphadenopathy, weakness
Ehrlichiosis	Anorexia, petechiae, fever, epistaxis, lymphadenopathy
Hyperadrenocorticism	Polyuria, polydipsia, polyphagia, "potbelly"
Rocky Mountain spotted fever	Anorexia, petechiae, fever, lymphadenopathy, lameness
SLE	Pale mucous membranes, fever, petechiae, joint pain, muscle pain

(continued)

TABLE 37-1. *(continued)*

Cause	Common Concurrent Clinical Findings
Pruritus	
Atopy	Cough, conjunctivitis, vomiting, diarrhea (all uncommon)
Castration-responsive dermatosis	None
Demodicosis	Variable, depending on the underlying disease, if present
Food hypersensitivity	Diarrhea (uncommon)
Ovarian imbalance type I	Abnormal estrous cycle, vulvar enlargement, pale mucous membranes
Sertoli cell tumor	Pale mucous membranes, feminization
Staphylococcal pyoderma	Variable, depending on the severity of the infection
Recurrent pyoderma	
Atopy	Cough (uncommon)
Demodicosis	Variable, depending on the underlying disease, if present
Diabetes mellitus	Polyuria, polydipsia, polyphagia, weight loss, cataracts
Food hypersensitivity	Diarrhea (uncommon)
Hyperadrenocorticism	Polyuria, polydipsia, polyphagia, "potbelly"
Hypothyroidism	Lethargy, weight gain
Zinc-responsive dermatosis	Anorexia, fever, depression*
Scrotal dermatitis	
Brucellosis	Fever, testicular pain and swelling, anorexia
Cold agglutinin disease	Pale mucous membranes, lethargy
Rocky Mountain spotted fever	Anorexia, fever, petechiae, lymphadenopathy, lameness
Seborrhea	
Castration-responsive dermatosis	None
Demodicosis	Variable, depending on the underlying disease, if present
Estrogen-responsive dermatosis	None
Food hypersensitivity	Diarrhea (uncommon)
Hyperadrenocorticism	Polyuria, polydipsia, polyphagia, "potbelly"
Hypothyroidism	Weight gain, lethargy
Ovarian imbalance type I	Estrous cycle abnormalities, vulvar enlargement, pale mucous membranes
Staphylococcal pyoderma	Variable, depending on the severity of the infection
Systemic lupus erythematosus	Pale mucous membranes, fever, petechiae, joint pain, muscle pain
Testosterone-responsive dermatosis	None
Zinc-responsive dermatosis	Anorexia, fever, depression*

* One of two syndromes.

    b. Diagnosis is based on ruling out other dermatopathies and on response to therapy.

3. Diabetes mellitus rarely causes dermatologic abnormalities but may predispose the animal to pyoderma, seborrhea, demodicosis, or xanthoma formation.

4. Estrogen-responsive alopecia and **testosterone-responsive alopecia**
    a. Clinical findings. Alopecia is seen in the perineal region in spayed or neutered dogs. No other clinical signs of disease are present.
    b. Diagnosis is based on ruling out other endocrinopathies and on response to therapy.

5. Growth hormone (GH)–responsive dermatosis occurs in adult dogs.
    a. Clinical findings characteristically include truncal alopecia and hyperpigmentation.
    b. Diagnosis and **treatment** are discussed in Chapter 44 I A 2 d and e.

6. Hyperadrenocorticism may cause bilaterally symmetrical truncal alopecia, thin skin, seborrhea, hyperpigmentation, comedones, calcinosis cutis, frequent bruising, poor wound healing, and increased susceptibility to secondary pyoderma, dermatophytosis, or demodicosis. In cats, alopecia and skin fragility are most common. Hyperadrenocorticism is discussed in more detail in Chapter 44 V C and D.

7. Hyperestrogenism in the female dog (ovarian imbalance type I) is rare and can occur with an ovarian cyst, an ovarian tumor, or exogenous estrogen administration. Bilaterally symmetrical alopecia beginning in the perineal region is usually seen.

8. Hypothyroidism. Clinical findings may include bilaterally symmetrical truncal alopecia; seborrhea; hyperpigmentation; thickened skin; dry, brittle hair; increased susceptibility to secondary pyoderma; dermatophytosis; otitis externa; and numerous other dermatologic abnormalities. Other clinical signs, diagnosis, and treatment are discussed in Chapter 44 III A.

9. Pituitary dwarfism. Clinical findings often include truncal alopecia, a soft "puppy coat," hyperpigmentation, and seborrhea. Other clinical findings, diagnosis, and treatment are discussed in Chapter 44 I A 1.

10. Sertoli cell tumors may cause bilaterally symmetrical truncal alopecia and feminization in male dogs. Other clinical findings, diagnosis, and treatment are discussed in Chapter 45 II B 3 f.

C. **Hypersensitivity disorders**

1. Atopy is a common skin disorder in the dog.
    a. Clinical findings. Most affected dogs first show pruritus at 1–3 years of age. Secondary pyoderma, seborrhea, and self-induced skin lesions may be seen on the face, feet, and ventrum. Other clinical signs may include otitis externa, conjunctivitis, rhinitis, asthma, and vomiting or diarrhea.
    b. Diagnosis is based on ruling out other disorders and on results of intradermal skin testing.
    c. Treatment. A management plan may include avoidance of the inciting allergens, bathing, antihistamines, glucocorticoids, and hyposensitization.

2. Drug eruption can occur in response to any medication.
    a. Clinical findings. It may appear as seborrhea, papules, bullae, alopecia, petechiae, erythema, erosions, or any other form of dermatopathy.
    b. Diagnosis is based on resolution of the lesions following discontinuation of the medication; however, it may take several weeks (or months) for the lesions to resolve.

3. Food hypersensitivity may occur in response to a dietary protein, carbohydrate, preservative, or food additive.
    a. Clinical findings. Affected animals are usually younger than 3 years of age at the time of onset. Pruritus, dermatitis, diarrhea, or all three may be seen.

    b. Diagnosis is made by ruling out other causes of the diarrhea and by observation of response to an elimination diet.

  4. Internal parasite hypersensitivity
    a. Clinical findings. This condition may be seen as pruritic dermatitis or pruritus in the absence of gross skin lesions. Other clinical signs will vary with the parasite.
    b. Diagnosis is based on fecal examinations and response to antiparasitic treatment.
    c. Treatment. Symptoms can be treated with glucocorticoids; bathing may also be needed if the pruritus is severe.

  5. Urticaria and **angioedema (hives)** can occur with infection, immune-mediated disease, neoplasia, medication, and many other causes.
    a. Clinical findings. Erythematous wheals, swelling (localized or generalized), or both many be seen with possible concurrent pruritus.
    b. Treatment. Symptomatic emergency treatment requires administration of epinephrine, glucocorticoids, or both. The underlying disorder should be treated and the inciting cause removed or avoided.

D. **Immune-mediated disorders**

  1. Cold agglutinin disease. Clinical findings may include cyanosis, erythema, ulceration, and necrosis of the extremities.

  2. Erythema multiforme is an acute dermatopathy that can occur in association with infection, neoplasia, medications, or other disorders.
    a. Clinical findings. Erythematous annular "target" lesions are often seen.
    b. Diagnosis is by biopsy; the underlying disease should be identified, if possible.
    c. Treatment is aimed at the primary disease.

  3. Systemic lupus erythematosus (SLE). Clinical findings may include cutaneous ulcers, erythema, crusting, and depigmentation of the mucocutaneous junctions and footpads. SLE is discussed in more detail in Chapter 48 V B 4.

  4. Toxic epidermal necrolysis (TEN) is a rare disorder that can occur in association with bacterial infection, drug eruption (see III C 2), neoplasia, or other disease. Clinical findings include severe bullae formation and, later, ulceration. The superficial layer of the adjacent skin can be easily rubbed away (Nikolsky sign). Anorexia, fever, and depression are also seen.

  5. Vasculitis can occur with SLE, Rocky Mountain spotted fever, and other disorders, or it may be idiopathic. Clinical findings may include cutaneous bullae, ulcers, purpura, anorexia, fever, depression, and signs of the primary disorder.

E. **Infections**

  1. Bacterial infections
    a. *Brucella canis* infection (brucellosis) can result in a secondary scrotal dermatitis caused by the dog's licking in response to the pain of orchitis and epididymitis (see also Chapter 49 I E).
    b. *Yersinia pestis* infection (plague). Clinical findings include fever and subcutaneous abscesses in cats (see also Chapter 49 I K).
    c. Staphylococcal infection may be primary or can occur secondary to allergic disorders, an endocrinopathy, external parasites, or immunosuppression (e.g., neoplasia, immunosuppressive medications). Treatment requires antibiotics and control or resolution of the underlying problem.
    d. Cutaneous actinomycosis, tuberculosis, and **nocardiosis** (see also Chapter 49 I B, I 1, and J). Pyogranulomatous skin lesions are seen.

  2. Fungal infections
    a. Systemic mycoses (e.g., **blastomycosis, cryptococcosis, coccidioidomycosis).** Cutaneous granulomas or draining tracts may be seen in addition to systemic signs of illness (see also Chapter 49).

    b. Candidiasis can occur secondary to immunosuppression.
      (1) Diagnosis is by cytology and culture.
      (2) Treatment requires resolution of the underlying disorder in conjunction with topical nystatin, miconazole, or clotrimazole.
    c. Prototothecosis (see also Chapter 41 IV C 5 c). Clinical findings may include only cutaneous nodules, or cutaneous nodules in addition to systemic signs of disease.
    d. Sporotrichosis (see also Chapter 49 II I). Clinical findings include cutaneous ulcerated nodules, ulcerated lymph nodes, or deeper infection.

3. Parasitic infections
    a. Demodicosis is most common in immunocompromised patients. Young animals may have a defect in cell-mediated immunity. Adult animals may be predisposed to clinical *Demodex* infection by diabetes mellitus, hyperadrenocorticism, hypothyroidism, immunosuppressive drug therapy, or neoplasia.
      (1) Diagnosis is by skin scrapings.
      (2) Treatment is with amitraz. Concurrent antibacterial therapy may also be indicated. The underlying disorder should be treated.
    b. Dirofilariasis (see also Chapter 39 VI). Occasionally, a cutaneous nodule or a pruritic dermatitis is seen.
    c. Hookworm larval migrans may cause erythema, swelling, and crusting of the feet and ventrum.
    d. Leishmaniasis (see also Chapter 49 III I). Clinical findings may include pruritic ulcerated hyperemic nodules (alone or in addition to systemic signs of illness). Erythema, alopecia, and ulceration of the ears and mucocutaneous junctions can also occur.

4. Rickettsial disease. Rocky Mountain spotted fever can cause petechiae and erythema, and possibly ulceration of the mucous membranes, in addition to systemic signs of illness (see also Chapter 49 IV E).

5. Viral disease
    a. Canine distemper virus (see also Chapter 49 V B). Dermatologic manifestations include hyperkeratosis of the footpads.
    b. Feline leukemia virus (FeLV) and **feline immunodeficiency virus (FIV) infection** may predispose the cat to secondary bacterial pyoderma or other infections.
    c. Feline upper respiratory virus infection (see also Chapter 40 I C 1). Dermatologic manifestations may include oral and cutaneous ulceration and swelling.

F. **Neoplastic disease**

    1. Internal or systemic neoplasia may cause a dull dry haircoat or mild seborrhea.

    2. Tumors of the skin are discussed in Chapter 50 II Q.

G. **Nutritional disorders**

    1. Pansteatitis, which results from vitamin E deficiency, may be seen in cats fed a diet containing a high level of red fish or cod liver oil.
      a. Clinical findings. Painful nodules are present in the subcutaneous and abdominal fat. Fever, anorexia, and depression may also be seen.
      b. Treatment requires correction of the diet, vitamin E supplementation, and prednisone.

    2. Zinc-responsive dermatosis can appear as two syndromes.
      a. One syndrome is seen in puppies fed a diet oversupplemented with vitamins and minerals.
        (1) Clinical findings include crusting of the head, trunk, and limbs with possible concurrent anorexia, fever, and depression.
        (2) Treatment requires correction of the diet.
      b. The other syndrome is seen primarily in Alaskan malamutes and Siberian huskies and is thought to result from inadequate zinc absorption.

(1) **Clinical findings** include crusting and alopecia on the face, mucocutaneous junctions, footpads, and abdomen.

(2) **Treatment** requires zinc supplementation.

3. **Other nutrient-responsive dermatoses** and **dermatologic problems secondary to nutritional deficiencies** can occur, but systemic signs of illness are not usually seen.

H. Miscellaneous disorders

1. **Cutaneous depigmentation and uveitis in dogs (Vogt-Koyanagi-Harada–like syndrome)** is a rare syndrome of unknown etiology.

a. **Clinical signs** characteristically include uveitis and depigmentation of the nose, lips, eyelids, and sometimes the anus and footpads. Blindness is a common sequela.

b. **Treatment.** There is no definitive treatment, but glucocorticoid treatment of the uveitis may prevent blindness.

2. **Dalmatian bronzing syndrome** is a disease of unknown etiology.

a. **Clinical findings** characteristically include pruritus, a reddish-brown coloration of the hair, folliculitis, and secondary pyoderma. Affected dogs also often have hyperuricosuria, urate crystals, and a urinary tract infection.

b. **Treatment.** The skin lesions require symptomatic treatment. The abnormal uric acid metabolism is managed as discussed for urate calculi (see Chapter 43 Part I:VIII E 3).

3. **Panniculitis** is a rare disorder that can occur with infection or immune-mediated disease, or it may be idiopathic.

a. **Clinical findings** characteristically include inflammation of the subcutaneous fat. Deep cutaneous nodules may form, which later ulcerate and drain.

b. **Diagnosis** is by excisional biopsy and subsequent appropriate tests to rule out an underlying infectious or immune-mediated cause.

c. **Treatment** with glucocorticoids, vitamin E, or both may cause remission of idiopathic disease.

4. **Superficial necrolytic dermatitis (hepatocutaneous syndrome)** is a rare dermatologic disorder seen in conjunction with hepatic disease. Erythema, alopecia, and crusting of the face and extremities and ulceration of the footpads may occur.

Chapter 38

Ocular Manifestations of Systemic Disease

I. **INTRODUCTION.** Systemic diseases can affect any of the ocular structures. Examples of systemic diseases that can involve structures from the eyelids to retina are presented in Tables 38-1 through 38-6.

II. **SELECTED DISORDERS**

A. **Infections**

1. **Toxoplasmosis** is caused by the protozoal organism *Toxoplasma gondii*. The cat is the definitive host and normally, the infection remains within the intestine. Systemic infection can occur in both cats and dogs and may affect the gastrointestinal (GI) and respiratory tracts, muscle, eye, and central nervous system (CNS).
   a. Ocular lesions are more common in cats than in dogs.
   b. The most common ocular lesion is a multifocal posterior chorioretinitis, which may or may not be accompanied by retinal detachment. An exudative or granulomatous anterior uveitis is also common.

2. **Ehrlichiosis** is a rickettsial infection of dogs caused by *Ehrlichia canis*. In the acute stage, typical signs include fever, lethargy, and thrombocytopenia. If untreated, the chronic stage can develop and is characterized by bone marrow injury and pancytopenia. Ocular signs are common and include anterior uveitis, hyphema, and corneal opacities (cellular precipitates). Focal subretinal hemorrhages are also common. A nongranulomatous chorioretinitis may also occur, which can later manifest as focal or diffuse retinal atrophy. Retinal detachment may occur.

3. **Blastomycosis** is a common systemic fungal infection in dogs caused by *Blastomyces dermatitidis*. It is uncommon in cats. Infection of the lungs, skin, eyes, and bones or joints is common. Ocular lesions occur in up to 40% of infected animals. Anterior uveitis, exudative retinal detachment, severe granulomatous chorioretinitis, optic neuritis, and secondary glaucoma can be observed.

4. **Canine distemper.** Ocular abnormalities associated with distemper are, in order of decreasing frequency, conjunctivitis, chorioretinitis, keratoconjunctivitis sicca, and optic neuritis.
   a. A serous, progressing to mucopurulent, conjunctivitis is usually present in the acute stage of the disease. Inclusion bodies may be evident in conjunctival epithelial cells when a scraping is obtained.
   b. Retinal lesions may occur in the acute, generalized form of distemper or may occur as an isolated finding in older dogs.
      (1) Retinitis is estimated to be present in 60% of dogs with distemper.
      (2) Acute retinal lesions are associated with hyporeflective, hazy areas of retinitis and perivascular infiltration. These areas become atrophic and hyperreflective ("medallion lesions") after several weeks.

5. **Feline infectious peritonitis (FIP),** caused by a coronavirus, is characterized by a widespread vasculitis and pyogranulomatous inflammation in many organs, including the eye. Ocular lesions are more common with the noneffusive (dry) form of the disease and may develop before signs of systemic illness.
   a. The predominant ocular lesion is a severe pyogranulomatous anterior uveitis.
   b. Keratitic precipitates are common.
   c. Other lesions may include focal retinal hemorrhages, perivascular edema, chorioretinitis, and, occasionally, retinal detachment.

TABLE 38-1. Examples of Systemic Disorders that Affect the Eyelids

> Sarcoptic mange
> Demodicosis
> Pyoderma
> Juvenile cellulitis
> *Microsporum canis* blepharitis
> Zinc deficiency
> Immune-mediated dermatoses (e.g., pemphigus diseases)
> Uveodermatologic syndrome
> Atopy
> Lymphoma

TABLE 38-2. Examples of Systemic Disorders that Affect the Conjunctiva and Third Eyelid

> **Inflammatory diseases**
>   Ehrlichiosis
>   Rocky Mountain spotted fever
>   Herpesvirus infection (cats)
>   Mycoplasmosis (cats)
>   Chlamydiosis (cats)
>   Calicivirus infection (cats)
>   Canine distemper
>   Keratoconjunctivitis sicca (immune-mediated)
>   Drug allergy
> **Neurologic disease**
>   Horner's syndrome
>   Tetanus
> **Hematologic or oncologic disease**
>   Anemia
>   Polycythemia
>   Icterus
>   Cyanosis
>   Bleeding disorders (hemorrhage)
>   Lymphoma

TABLE 38-3. Examples of Systemic Disorders that Affect the Cornea

> Rocky Mountain spotted fever
> Infectious canine hepatitis
> Canine distemper
> Herpesvirus infection (cats)
> Hyperlipidemia
> Hypercalcemia
> Infectious canine hepatitis

TABLE 38-4. Examples of Systemic Disorders that Affect the Lens

Metabolic cataract
  Diabetes mellitus
Postinflammatory cataract (e.g., following uveitis)
Toxic cataract
  Selenium
  Antimitotic drugs
Nutritional cataract (e.g., following use of a milk replacer)

TABLE 38-5. Examples of Systemic Disorders that Affect the Uvea

Infectious disease
  Toxoplasmosis
  Ehrlichiosis
  Rocky Mountain spotted fever
  Leptospirosis
  Brucellosis
  Blastomycosis
  Cryptococcosis
  Histoplasmosis
  Coccidioidomycosis
  Feline infectious peritonitis (FIP)
  Feline leukemia virus (FeLV) infection
  Feline immunodeficiency virus (FIV) infection
  Infectious canine hepatitis
  Tuberculosis
Uveodermatologic syndrome
Autoimmune uveitis (e.g., associated with SLE, uveodermatologic syndrome)
Lymphoma
Metastatic tumors

SLE = systemic lupus erythematosus.
Modified with permission from Ettinger SJ, Feldman EC (eds): *Textbook of Veterinary Internal Medicine,*
4th ed. Philadelphia, WB Saunders, 1995, p 525.

6. **Feline immunodeficiency virus (FIV) infection.** Approximately 40% of cats with FIV infection have ocular lesions. Focal retinal degeneration, retinal hemorrhages, and anterior uveitis are the most common abnormalities. Transient conjunctivitis may also occur.

B. **Metabolic and nutritional disorders**

1. **Diabetes mellitus** is commonly associated with bilateral cataract formation in dogs. (Cataract formation is very uncommon in cats with diabetes.)
    a. Cataracts are thought to develop from the diffusion of large amounts of glucose into the lens. Normal intralenticular metabolic pathways are overwhelmed and the excess glucose is metabolized to sorbitol, a hydrophilic alcohol that cannot diffuse out of the lens. Water is drawn osmotically into the lens, which swells, rupturing the lens fibers and resulting in cataract formation.
    b. Mild retinal and vascular lesions can also occur in dogs with diabetes.

2. **Hyperlipidemia** due to inherited lipid metabolism disorders or secondary to metabolic disease (e.g., hypothyroidism) can result in corneal lipid deposits (lipid keratopathy), lipid-laden (diffusely opaque) aqueous humor, or lipemia retinalis.
    a. Corneal lipid deposits must be differentiated from corneal calcium deposits. In addition to being a sequela to hyperlipidemia, lipid deposits may result from corneal

TABLE 38-6. Examples of Systemic Disorders that Affect the Retina

Blood vessel abnormalities (± hemorrhages, secondary retinal detachment)
  Systemic hypertension
  Bleeding disorders
  Lipemia retinalis
  Anemia
  Polycythemia
  Hyperviscosity syndrome
Inflammatory retinal lesions
  Toxoplasmosis
  Ehrlichiosis
  Cryptococcosis
  Blastomycosis
  Histoplasmosis
  Feline infectious peritonitis (FIP)
  Feline leukemia virus (FeLV) infection
  Feline immunodeficiency virus (FIV) infection
  Canine distemper
  Systemic hypertension
  Multiple myeloma
  Lymphoma
  Metastatic neoplasia
Retinal degeneration
  Taurine deficiency
  Vitamin E deficiency

Modified with permission from Ettinger SJ, Feldman EC (eds): *Textbook of Veterinary Internal Medicine,*
4th ed. Philadelphia, WB Saunders, 1995, p 526.

inflammation and degeneration or occur as an inherited disorder in some breeds
(e.g., Siberian husky).
  b. Lipemia retinalis is uncommon but can occur secondary to hypercholesterolemia.
  The retinal vessels appear pink or cream colored and may be distended.
3. Taurine deficiency in cats can result in bilateral central or panretinal degeneration
  and dilated cardiomyopathy. Most commercial diets contain adequate taurine; therefore, taurine deficiency is most often seen in cats who eat homemade diets or dog
  food.

C. **Bleeding disorders** commonly result in ocular hemorrhages that can appear as small retinal petechial hemorrhages or subretinal hemorrhage and detachment, hyphema, and scleral hemorrhage.

D. **Hypertension.** Ocular disease (e.g., acute blindness) is one of the most common clinical
presentations of hypertension, which characteristically results in retinal hemorrhage and
detachment. Other ocular signs may include a nongranulomatous chorioretinitis, exudative retinal detachment, "cotton wool spots" (areas of microinfarct that cause edema of
the nerve fiber layer), sclerosis of the retinal vasculature, vitreous hemorrhage, secondary
uveitis, and glaucoma.

E. **Neoplasia.** Anterior uveitis commonly accompanies lymphosarcoma in dogs. Many neoplasms metastasize to the eye.

PART II

DISEASES OF ORGAN SYSTEMS

Chapter 39

Cardiovascular Diseases

I. **CLINICAL EVALUATION**

A. Signalment, clinical signs, and physical examination

1. **Signalment**

   a. **Age.** Some cardiac diseases have a wide age range associated with them (e.g., cardiomyopathy), whereas others are more likely in animals of a certain age.

      (1) **Young animals** with cardiovascular disease are likely to have **congenital defects** [e.g., patent ductus arteriosus (PDA)].

      (2) **Older animals** are usually afflicted with **degenerative conditions** (e.g., mitral valve insufficiency).

   b. **Sex and breed.** Many congenital defects and acquired cardiac diseases have sex and breed associations (Table 39-1).

2. **Clinical signs**

   a. **Coughing** is the most common sign associated with heart disease or failure. **Cardiac causes** include **left ventricular failure** (leading to pulmonary venous congestion, edema, or both), **enlargement of the left atrium** (causing impingement of the left mainstem bronchus), and **heartworm infection** (leading to pulmonary vascular disease and pneumonitis). Pulmonary edema rarely causes coughing in cats; however, coughing can be a sign of heartworm infection in this species.

   b. **Exercise intolerance** may be one of the first indications of heart disease. It is more often noted in dogs than in cats because of the latter's aversion to athletic activity.

   c. **Ascites** can be caused by **right ventricular failure.**

   d. **Dyspnea** associated with heart disease is usually caused by either **pulmonary edema** or **pleural effusion.**

      (1) In cats, dyspnea and tachypnea (rather than coughing) is the usual manifestation of pulmonary edema or pleural effusion.

      (2) Severe pulmonary edema usually results in a mixed respiratory or dyspneic pattern (i.e., difficulty on both inspiration and expiration).

   e. **Syncope** resulting from heart disease may be caused by **brady-** or **tachyarrhythmias, outflow obstructions,** conditions characterized by **cyanosis** or **impaired forward flow, cardiac tamponade,** and therapy with **diuretics** or **vasodilators.**

   f. **Other signs**

      (1) **Polyuria** and **polydipsia** may be caused by diuretic therapy or concurrent renal disease.

      (2) **Brownish** or **reddish urine** could indicate hemoglobinuria and may be associated with postcaval syndrome as a result of heartworm infection.

      (3) **Regurgitation** can result from esophageal constriction caused by a congenital vascular ring anomaly.

      (4) **Hindend paresis** may result from aortic thromboembolism in cats with cardiomyopathy.

      (5) **Hemoptysis** can be associated with pulmonary embolism secondary to heartworm infection or severe pulmonary edema.

3. **Physical examination**

   a. **General appearance.** The animal's **demeanor, strength, respiratory pattern,** and **conformation** should be noted.

      (1) Dyspneic animals are often **anxious** and either **stand, sit,** or **lie in sternal recumbency** with their elbows abducted to allow for maximal excursion of the chest wall.

TABLE 39-1. Sex and Breed Associations of Common Cardiac Disorders

Disorder	Sex and Breed Associations	
	Sex	Breed
Patent ductus arteriosus (PDA)	Female	Poodles, collies, Pomeranians, Shetland sheepdogs, Maltese, cocker spaniels, English springer spaniels, German shepherds, keeshonds, bichon frises, Irish setters
Subaortic stenosis (SAS)	. . .	Newfoundlands, golden retrievers, German shepherds, boxers, rottweilers, Samoyeds, bulldogs, Great Danes
Pulmonic stenosis	. . .	English bulldogs, Samoyeds, mastiffs, beagles, miniature schnauzers, cocker spaniels, West Highland white terriers
Dilated cardiomyopathy	Male	Large and giant dog breeds
Acquired mitral valve insufficiency	Male	Small dog breeds
Hypertrophic cardiomyopathy	Male	Cats

     (2) Open mouth breathing, especially in cats, is a sign of severe dyspnea.
  b. Evaluation of the mucous membranes. The mucous membranes should be evaluated for **color** and **capillary refill time.** Oral as well as vulvar or preputial mucous membranes should be evaluated to rule out differential cyanosis as a result of reverse PDA.
  c. Evaluation of the jugular veins. The jugular veins are evaluated with the animal standing and the head in a normal position. Normal jugular veins are not distended and may have a pulse wave that does not extend more than one third up the neck.
    (1) Jugular venous distention results from increased central venous pressure, which is most often caused by right ventricular failure or cranial vena caval obstruction.
    (2) Abnormal jugular pulsation may be caused by tricuspid insufficiency, right ventricular hypertrophy, cardiac arrhythmias, or heartworm disease.
  d. Evaluation of arterial pulses
    (1) Pulse deficits (i.e., a heart beat with no corresponding pulse) indicate the presence of a cardiac arrhythmia. Auscultation or palpation of the heart beat while assessing the pulse allows detection of pulse deficits.
    (2) Weak pulses are caused by reduced cardiac output and can be associated with dilated cardiomyopathy, subaortic or pulmonic stenosis, pericardial effusion, or hypovolemia. Poor femoral pulses may be associated with aortic thromboembolism.
    (3) Strong pulses can result from excitement, fever, hyperthyroidism, or hypertrophic cardiomyopathy. Very strong **("bounding") pulses** are associated with PDA and fever.
  e. Precordial palpation. The precordium is palpated by placing one hand on either side of the chest wall in the region of the fifth intercostal space. Normally, the **precordial impulse** (i.e., the heart beat) is felt most intensely on the left side at the level of the costochondral junction just after the first heart sound [S_1; see I A 3 g (1)].
    (1) The **intensity** may be decreased by obesity, poor cardiac contractions, pericardial or pleural effusion, intrathoracic masses, or pneumothorax.
    (2) The **location** of the precordial impulse may be shifted to the right side by right ventricular enlargement, displacement by a mass in the left thorax, lung atelectasis, or a chest wall deformity.

f. Detection of fluid accumulation
  (1) Pleural fluid. Significant amounts of pleural fluid decrease breath sounds and result in varying degrees of dyspnea.
  (2) Peritoneal fluid. Accumulation of fluid in the peritoneum distends the abdomen. Ballottement causes a fluid wave.
g. Thoracic auscultation. The heart and lungs should be auscultated separately in a systematic manner.
  (1) Heart sounds
    (a) Normal heart sounds heard in dogs and cats consist of S_1 **(closure of the tricuspid and mitral valves)** and S_2 **(closure of the aortic and pulmonic valves).**
      (i) Decreased intensity. Obesity, pericardial effusion, diaphragmatic hernia, pleural effusion, and hypovolemia can decrease the intensity of the heart sounds.
      (ii) Increased intensity
        —A thin body wall, arterial hypertension, high sympathetic tone, tachycardia, or a shortened PR interval can increase the intensity of S_1.
        —Pulmonary arterial hypertension, such as that caused by heartworm disease or cor pulmonale, can increase the intensity of S_2.
      (iii) Splitting of S_1 or S_2 may occur if there is asynchronous closure of either the atrioventricular (AV) valves or semilunar valves. Arrhythmias, conduction disturbances (e.g., bundle branch block), and pulmonary arterial hypertension can lead to splitting of heart sounds.
    (b) Abnormal heart sounds (S_3 and S_4). The third and fourth heart sounds, which represent the end of rapid ventricular filling and atrial contraction, respectively, occur during diastole (i.e., the interval between S_2 and S_1) and are not normally heard. When either is audible, a **gallop rhythm** is detected.
      (i) Dilated cardiomyopathy can produce an audible S_3.
      (ii) Increased ventricular stiffness (e.g., hypertrophic cardiomyopathy) or ventricular hypertrophy can be associated with an audible S_4.
  (2) Murmurs are generated by turbulent blood flow.
    (a) Classification of murmurs. A variety of characteristics are used to describe murmurs. The timing, intensity, and location of the murmur are the most important assessments.
      (i) Timing. Murmurs are described according to when they occur within the cardiac cycle (e.g., systolic, diastolic, continuous) as well as by when they occur during specific phases of the cardiac cycle (e.g., early, late, holosystolic, mid-diastolic).
      (ii) Intensity. The grades of intensity range from 1/6 to 6/6 (Table 39-2).

TABLE 39-2. Grading of Heart Murmur Intensity

Grade	Characteristics
1	Very soft; heard only after minutes of careful listening
2	Soft but easily detected
3	Moderate
4	Loud but not accompanied by a palpable precordial thrill
5	Loud; accompanied by a palpable precordial thrill
6	Very loud; accompanied by a palpable precordial thrill that can be heard with the stethoscope held several millimeters away from the chest wall

Modified with permission from Nelson RW, Couto CG: *Essentials of Small Animal Internal Medicine,* St. Louis, Mosby-Yearbook, 1992, p 10.

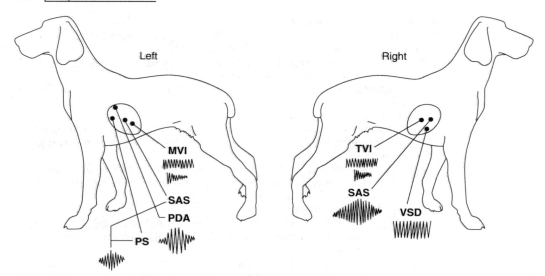

FIGURE 39-1. The usual location of the point of maximal intensity (PMI) and phonocardiographic shape of various congenital and acquired murmurs. *MVI* = mitral valve insufficiency; *PDA* = patent ductus arteriosus; *PS* = pulmonic stenosis; *SAS* = subaortic stenosis; *TVI* = tricuspid valve insufficiency; *VSD* = ventricular septal defect. (Redrawn with permission from Fenner W: *Quick Reference to Veterinary Medicine.* Philadelphia, JB Lippincott, 1991, p 136.)

      (iii) Location. The **point of maximal intensity (PMI)** may be described as being in the right or left hemithorax, or associated with a valve region (Figure 39-1).

      (iv) Pattern of radiation. Murmurs can be described according to where and how far the sound spreads.

      (v) Sound. Murmurs may be described by their quality and pitch (e.g., harsh, musical).

      (vi) Shape (Figure 39-2). Murmurs produce distinctive shapes on the phonocardiogram (e.g., plateau, crescendo–decrescendo).

    (b) Types of murmurs

      (i) Systolic murmurs, the most common type of murmur, can be caused by outflow tract narrowing, AV valve insufficiency, and congenital cardiac shunts. **Functional murmurs** occur in the absence of cardiac pathology and include **innocent murmurs** (i.e., transient murmurs heard most often in puppies) and **physiologic murmurs,** which can be associated with anemia, fever, hypoproteinemia, peripheral arteriovenous fistulae, hyperthyroidism, and athletic hearts.

      (ii) Diastolic murmurs are uncommon and result from mitral or tricuspid valve stenosis and pulmonic or aortic valve insufficiency.

      (iii) Continuous murmurs occur during both systole and diastole and are caused by extracardiac arteriovenous shunts (e.g., PDA). Continuous murmurs are sometimes referred to as **machinery murmurs** because of the variability in the intensity of the sound during systole and diastole.

B. Electrocardiography

    1. Indications. Electrocardiography is used to:

      a. Detect and identify cardiac arrhythmias

      b. Assess changes in the size of cardiac chambers (although it is much less sensitive than thoracic radiographs or echocardiography)

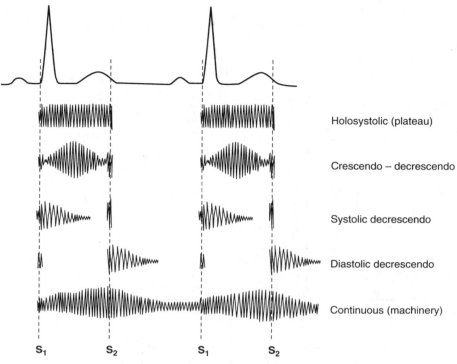

Holosystolic (plateau)

Crescendo – decrescendo

Systolic decrescendo

Diastolic decrescendo

Continuous (machinery)

S_1 S_2 S_1 S_2

FIGURE 39-2. Timing, description, and phonocardiographic shape of murmurs within the cardiac cycle. S_1 and S_2 refer to the first and second heart sounds, which represent closure of the atrioventricular (i.e., mitral and tricuspid) and semilunar (i.e., aortic, pulmonic) valves, respectively. (Redrawn with permission from Nelson RW, Couto CG: *Essentials of Small Animal Internal Medicine.* St. Louis, Mosby-Yearbook, 1992, p 11.)

    c. Monitor the effectiveness or toxicity of antiarrhythmic therapy and screen for electrolyte abnormalities (especially hyperkalemia)

2. Evaluation of the electrocardiogram (ECG)
    a. The **normal ECG pattern** (Figure 39-3) consists of **three waveforms** (P, QRS, T), **two intervals** (PR, QT), and **one segment** (ST). Normal values are listed in Table 39-3.
        (1) Waveforms. The P, QRS, and T waves represent atrial depolarization, ventricular depolarization, and ventricular repolarization, respectively.
        (2) Intervals
            (a) The **PR interval** is the time it takes for the impulse generated in the sinoatrial (SA) node to travel through the atrium and conduction system (i.e., the AV node, bundle of His, bundle branches, and Purkinje system) before the onset of ventricular depolarization.
            (b) The **QT interval** is the time it takes for ventricular systole (depolarization and repolarization) to occur.
    b. Evaluation of the ECG should be performed in a systematic fashion.
        (1) Identify waveforms.
        (2) Estimate the heart rate by counting the number of RR intervals in 3 seconds and multiplying by 20 (paper speed = 50 mm/sec).
        (3) Determine the mean electrical axis (MEA). The MEA describes the **orientation of the ventricular depolarization wave** and is useful in the **assessment of ventricular enlargement.** It can be estimated by identifying the isoelectric lead (i.e., I, II, III, aVR, aVL, or aVF) and then determining the lead perpendicular to the isoelectric lead in the frontal plane (using a hexaxial lead diagram). If the QRS complex in the perpendicular lead is positive, then the

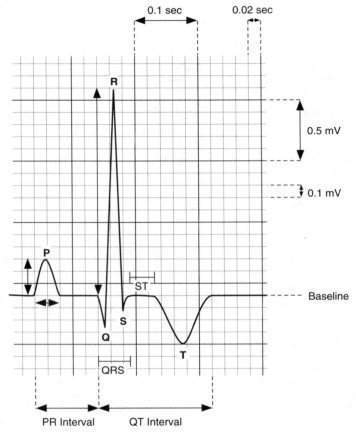

FIGURE 39-3. A normal canine P–QRS–T complex with waveforms and intervals identified. The duration and amplitude values indicated for the grid boxes are based on a paper speed of 50 mm/sec and a sensitivity setting of 1 cm = 1 mV. (Redrawn with permission from Tilley LP: *Essentials of Canine and Feline Electrocardiography— Interpretation and Treatment*, 3rd ed. Baltimore, Williams & Wilkins, 1992, p 48.)

MEA is oriented to the positive pole of this lead (and vice versa if the QRS complex is negative). The MEA (measured from 0° to ± 180°) corresponds to the value noted at the positive or negative pole of the perpendicular lead. The normal MEA is +40° to +100° in dogs and 0° to +160° in cats.

(4) Assess rhythm.
   (a) Is there a P wave for every QRS complex (i.e., is the PR interval normal and constant from complex to complex)?
   (b) Is the atrial rate the same as the ventricular rate?
   (c) Are the RR and PP intervals regular or irregular?
(5) Assess the P–QRS complex, ST segment, and T wave.
   (a) The P waves and QRS complexes should have normal morphology.
   (b) The duration and amplitude of the P wave and QRS complex and the duration of the PR and QT intervals should be measured.
   (c) The ST segment and T wave should be subjectively assessed, looking for depression or elevation from baseline, coving, or slurring.
c. Abnormal ECG patterns
   (1) Arrhythmias are discussed in X.
   (2) Chamber enlargement
      (a) Left atrial enlargement. The width of the P wave exceeds normal values **(P mitrale).**

TABLE 39-3. Normal Canine and Feline ECG Values*

	Canine	Feline
Heart rate	Puppy: 70–220 bpm	120–240 bpm
	Toy breeds: 70–180 bpm	
	Standard: 70–160 bpm	
	Giant breeds: 60–140 bpm	
Rhythm	Sinus rhythm	Sinus rhythm
	Sinus arrhythmia	
	Wandering pacemaker	
P wave		
Height	Maximum: 0.4 mV	Maximum: 0.2 mV
Width	Maximum: 0.04 sec (0.05 sec in giant breeds)	Maximum: 0.04 sec
PR interval	0.06–0.13 sec	0.05–0.09 sec
QRS complex		
Height	Large breeds: 3.0 mV maximum†	0.9 mV maximum
	Small breeds: 2.5 mV maximum	
Width	Large breeds: 0.06 sec maximum	0.04 sec maximum
	Small breeds: 0.05 sec maximum	
ST segment		
Depression	No more than 0.2 mV	None
Elevation	No more than 0.15 mV	None
QT interval	0.15–0.25 sec at a normal heart rate	0.12–0.18 sec at a normal heart rate
T waves	Positive, negative, biphasic	Usually positive
	Amplitude range: ±0.05–1.0 mV in any lead or not more than ¼ height of R wave	Amplitude range: <0.3 mV
Mean electrical axis (MEA)	+40° to +100°	0° to +160°
Chest leads		
CV$_5$RL (rV$_2$)	T positive; R < 3.0 mV	. . .
CV$_6$LL (V$_2$)	S < 0.8 mV; R < 3.0 mV	R < 1.0 mV
CV$_6$LU (V$_4$)	S < 0.7 mV; R < 3.0 mV	R < 1.0 mV
V$_{10}$	QRS negative; T wave negative except in Chihuahuas	T negative; R wave: Q wave <1

Modified with permission from Miller MS, Tilley LP: *Manual of Canine and Feline Cardiology,* 2nd ed. Philadelphia, WB Saunders, 1995, p 54.
ECG = electrocardiogram; sec = second.
* Measurements made in lead II unless specified otherwise.
† Not valid for thin, deep-chested dogs younger than 2 years of age.

    (b) Right atrial enlargement. The height of the P wave exceeds normal values **(P pulmonale).**
    (c) Left ventricular enlargement
        (i) The **MEA** is less than +40° in dogs and 0° in cats (left axis deviation).
        (ii) In dogs, the **R wave** is greater than 3.0 mV (2.5 mV in small breeds) in leads II and aVF and greater than 1.5 mV in lead I. In cats, the R wave is greater than 0.9 mV in lead II.

TABLE 39-4. ECG Changes Associated with Selected Drug Toxicities and Electrolyte Imbalances

Disturbance	ECG Changes
Hyperkalemia	Large, spiked (±tented) T waves; QT interval abbreviation; flat or absent P waves; widened QRS complex; ST segment depression
Hypokalemia	ST segment depression; small, biphasic T waves; QT interval prolongation; tachyarrhythmias
Hypercalcemia	Abbreviated QT interval; prolonged conduction; tachyarrhythmias
Quinidine or procainamide	QT interval prolongation; AV block; ventricular tachyarrhythmias; widened QRS complex; sinus arrest
Lidocaine	AV block; ventricular tachycardia; sinus arrest
Barbiturates or thiobarbiturates	Ventricular bigeminy
Halothane or methoxyflurane	Sinus bradycardia, ventricular arrhythmia
Digoxin	PR interval prolongation; second- or third-degree AV block; sinus bradycardia or arrest; ventricular premature complexes (VPCs) or bigeminy; ventricular tachycardia; paroxysmal atrial tachycardia with block; atrial fibrillation with a slow ventricular rate
Xylazine	Sinus bradycardia; sinus arrest; SA block; AV block; ventricular tachyarrhythmias

Adapted with permission from Nelson RW, Couto CG: *Essentials of Small Animal Internal Medicine*, St. Louis, Mosby-Yearbook, 1992, p 25.
AV = atrioventricular; ECG = electrocardiogram; SA = sinoatrial.

      (iii) The **QRS complex** is widened and **ST segment coving** or **slurring** is evident.
    (d) **Right ventricular enlargement** is associated with an MEA that is greater than +100° in dogs and +160° in cats (right axis deviation). S waves are prominent in leads I (dogs > 0.05 mV), II (dogs > 0.35 mV), III, and aVF.
  (3) **Drug toxicities and electrolyte imbalances.** ECG changes associated with selected drug toxicities and electrolyte imbalances are summarized in Table 39-4.
  (4) **Other conditions**
    (a) **Elevation of the ST segment** can be associated with myocardial hypoxia, pericardial effusion, pericarditis, digitalis toxicity (in cats), and transmural myocardial infarction.
    (b) **Depression of the ST segment** may be caused by myocardial hypoxia, hyper- or hypokalemia, subendothelial myocardial infarction, and digitalis toxicity.
    (c) **Large T waves** are associated with myocardial hypoxia, interventricular conduction disturbances, ventricular enlargement, metabolic abnormalities or drug toxicities, and respiratory disease.

C. **Radiology**

  1. General considerations
    a. At least two views [e.g, the lateral view and either the dorsoventral (DV) or ventrodorsal (VD) view] should be obtained. Ideally, radiographs should be taken during inspiration.
    b. Chest conformation should be considered when evaluating the heart shadow.
      (1) In barrel-chested dogs, the heart has more sternal contact on the lateral view and is oval-shaped on the DV or VD view.
      (2) In breeds with deep and narrow chests, the heart is more upright and elon-

TABLE 39-5. Common Differential Diagnoses for Radiographic Signs of Cardiomegaly and Vessel Abnormalities

Radiographic Sign	Differential Diagnoses
Generalized enlargement of the cardiac shadow	Dilated cardiomyopathy, mitral and tricuspid insufficiency, pericardial effusion, pericardioperitoneal diaphragmatic hernia, tricuspid dysplasia, ventricular septal defect, patent ductus arteriosus (PDA)
Left atrial enlargement	Early mitral valve insufficiency, hypertrophic cardiomyopathy, early dilated cardiomyopathy (especially in Doberman pinschers), subaortic stenosis (SAS)
Left atrial and ventricular enlargement	Dilated cardiomyopathy, hypertrophic cardiomyopathy, mitral valve insufficiency, aortic valve insufficiency, ventricular septal defect, PDA, SAS
Right atrial and ventricular enlargement	Advanced heartworm disease, chronic, severe pulmonary disease, tricuspid valve insufficiency, pulmonic stenosis, tetralogy of Fallot, atrial septal defect, reverse shunts
Enlarged aorta	Subaortic stenosis, PDA
Enlarged pulmonary arteries	Heartworm disease, pulmonary thromboembolism, cor pulmonale, pulmonic stenosis, PDA
Enlarged pulmonary veins	Left-sided heart failure

Adapted with permission from Nelson RW, Couto CG: *Essentials of Small Animal Internal Medicine,* St. Louis, Mosby-Yearbook, 1992, p 28.

gated on the lateral view and has a small, more circular shape on the DV or VD view.

    c. Heart size can be reduced by disease states that decrease venous return (e.g., hypovolemia).

2. Evaluation of radiographs

    a. Cardiac chamber enlargement. Table 39-5 summarizes common differential diagnoses for radiographic evidence of cardiomegaly.

        (1) Left atrial enlargement

            (a) Lateral view. There is dorsal elevation of the caudal trachea, separation of the mainstem bronchi, straightening and enlargement of the dorsocaudal cardiac silhouette, and loss of the caudal waist.

            (b) DV view. There is enlargement of the auricular appendage (manifested as a bulge at the 2 to 3 o'clock position). In cats, the cardiac margin is enlarged at the 2 to 3 o'clock position. A double opacity may be observed over the caudal aspect of the cardiac silhouette.

        (2) Left ventricular enlargement

            (a) Lateral view. There is loss of the caudal waist and the caudal cardiac margin may become straighter and more upright or more convex. The caudal trachea (carina) is elevated.

            (b) DV view. There is rounding and enlargement in the 2 to 5 o'clock position and the cardiac apex is shifted to the right.

        (3) Right atrial enlargement

            (a) Lateral view. Bulging of the cranial heart border and a widening of the cardiac silhouette are evident. The trachea may be elevated over the cranial aspect of the heart.

            (b) DV view. Bulging may be observed in the 9 to 11 o'clock position.

        (4) Right ventricular enlargement

            (a) Lateral view. The convexity of the cranioventral cardiac silhouette and sternal contact may be increased. Elevation of the trachea over the cranial heart is also evident.

            (b) DV view. There is enlargement at the 6 to 11 o'clock position, a shift of the cardiac apex to the left, and, if left-sided enlargement is mild or absent, a "reverse D" shape may be observed.

b. Vessel abnormalities. Differential diagnoses for radiographic evidence of vessel abnormalites are given in Table 39-5.

(1) Enlargement of the aorta is observed as a widening of the craniodorsal aspect of the cardiac silhouette on the lateral view and an extension of the cardiac margin at the 11 to 1 o'clock position on the DV view.

(2) Enlargement of the main pulmonary trunk manifests as a protrusion of the craniodorsal heart border on the lateral view and as a bulge in the 1 to 2 o'clock position on the DV view.

(3) Abnormalities of the pulmonary veins and artery. The pulmonary veins are located ventral and caudal to the pulmonary artery and bronchus. Normally, they are the same size as the artery and do not exceed the width of the fourth rib at its narrowest point (i.e., near the rib head).

(a) Pulmonary vein enlargement is a result of chronic venous hypertension.

(b) Enlargement of both pulmonary arteries and veins produces an **overcirculation pattern.** The increased perfusion results in a generalized haziness in the lung fields.

(c) Constriction of both pulmonary arteries and veins produces an **undercirculation pattern,** characterized by radiolucent lung fields and narrowed pulmonary artery and veins.

c. Pulmonary edema is characterized radiographically by a generalized haziness of the lung fields.

(1) Increased density in the lung fields and air bronchograms are observed.

(2) Pulmonary structures (e.g., vessels) begin to lose their definition.

(3) Saturation of the interstitial space causes fluid to flow into the alveolar spaces, producing fluffy or mottled fluid densities that coalesce as more fluid accumulates. Fluid infiltrates from cardiogenic edema in dogs tend to localize in a symmetric fashion in the dorsal and perihilar areas; however, in cats, the interstitial and alveolar infiltrates tend to have a patchy, uneven distribution throughout the lung fields.

d. Pericardial effusion results in a globoid (rounded) cardiac silhouette. The normal cardiac margins and bulges are obscured, helping to differentiate generalized cardiomegaly from pericardial effusion. There is usually elevation of the trachea and caudal vena cava.

D. **Echocardiography (cardiac ultrasound)** is a noninvasive method of assessing chamber size, wall thickness, wall motion, valve conformation, valve function, and structures adjacent to the heart (e.g., great vessels, pericardial space).

1. Indications for cardiac ultrasound examination include congenital heart disease, murmurs in large breed dogs, left- or right-sided heart failure, murmurs or gallop rhythms in cats, arrhythmias not related to trauma or metabolic disturbances, and suspected pericardial effusion, cardiac neoplasia, or bacterial endocarditis.

2. Types

a. M-mode echocardiography gives a **one-dimensional** view of the heart. As the heart beats, a linear tracing is generated that reflects tissue interfaces. Typically, the M-mode tracing is used to measure parameters such as left ventricular and interventricular wall thickness during systole and diastole. From these parameters, indicators of myocardial function (e.g., fractional shortening) can be calculated.

b. Two-dimensional echocardiography generates a recognizable cardiac image with length and width. It allows assessment of chamber size, shape, width, and valvular action and can detect the presence of masses in or around the heart or on the valves. In addition, it allows subjective assessment of contractile function and is a sensitive means of detecting pericardial fluid.

c. Doppler echocardiography is used to assess blood flow patterns and velocity. It is useful for assessing valvular insufficiency, stenotic lesions, and cardiac shunts.

E. **Special techniques**

1. **Nonselective angiocardiography** is performed by rapidly administering a bolus of radiocontrast agent into a large central vein. Nonselective angiocardiography aids in the evaluation of cardiac chamber size and thickness, congenital shunts or other malformations, and pulmonary vascular disease. Echocardiography can provide much of this information in a less invasive manner, but nonselective angiocardiography provides superior evaluation of the pulmonary vasculature.

2. **Selective angiocardiography (cardiac catheterization).** Catheters are advanced into the left and right heart chambers. Dye injections, blood pressure measurements, and blood gas analyses can be performed in each of the cardiac chambers, the pulmonary artery, or the aorta. This procedure is used most often to identify and quantify the severity of congenital cardiac defects if echocardiographic examination fails to provide enough information.

3. **Endomyocardial biopsy** is performed using a special biopsy instrument that is passed into the right ventricle via the jugular vein. Samples can be examined histologically or used to investigate myocardial metabolic abnormalities.

II. **HEART FAILURE**

A. **Introduction.** Heart failure occurs when circulation to the peripheral tissues is inadequate because of cardiac disease.

1. **Pathophysiology.** Cardiovascular priorities are, in order of importance, the maintenance of arterial blood pressure, cardiac output, and normal venous and capillary pressure. When the arterial pressure drops as a result of heart failure, vasoconstriction increases, increasing the peripheral resistance (i.e., afterload) to maintain perfusion pressure. However, maintenance of perfusion pressure occurs at the expense of cardiac output. To enhance cardiac output, salt and water retention occurs to increase the venous (filling) pressure (i.e., preload). Eventually, the venous pressure reaches a point where congestion, edema, and effusions develop.

2. **Compensatory mechanisms.** Various compensatory mechanisms are activated in response to heart failure to maintain perfusion and cardiac output. Regardless of the cause of heart failure, the compensatory response is the same. However, aspects of the response vary in importance depending on the cause of heart failure.

   a. **Neurohormonal response**

   (1) **Increased sympathetic tone.** When blood pressure decreases, activation of the sympathetic nervous system results in an increase in heart rate and contractility. However, the beneficial effect of β_1 -**receptor stimulation** on contractility is short-lived because the receptors down-regulate within a few days. Despite this, norepinephrine concentrations progressively increase as heart failure worsens.

   (2) **Renin-angiotensin-aldosterone system activation.** The renin-angiotensin-aldosterone system is primarily activated by a decrease in arterial pressure, but the sympathetic nervous system also participates in its activation.

   (a) **Angiotensin II,** a potent vasoconstrictor, plays a significant role in the increased peripheral resistance and afterload associated with heart failure.

   (b) **Aldosterone** is secreted by the adrenal cortex and enhances sodium and water reabsorption in the kidney, leading to increased vascular volume, venous pressure, and preload.

   (3) **Vasopressin (antidiuretic hormone, ADH) release** is stimulated by an increase in plasma osmolality. Significant declines in arterial pressure, sympa-

thetic nervous system stimulation, and angiotensin II levels can also contribute to vasopressin secretion. Vasopressin, which acts on the collecting tubules of the kidney to maximize water reabsorption, causes increases in vascular volume, venous pressure, and preload.

b. Cardiac hypertrophy develops in response to chronic increases in myocardial wall stress.

(1) Eccentric hypertrophy is characterized by enlargement of the heart and the ventricular chamber. Increased venous and filling pressures (i.e., preload) increase the end-diastolic volume, leading to eccentric hypertrophy. Chronic AV valve insufficiency is a major cause of eccentric hypertrophy.

(2) Concentric hypertrophy occurs when the ventricular wall becomes thicker and the chamber becomes smaller. Concentric hypertrophy occurs when there is outflow resistance (e.g., aortic or pulmonic stenosis).

B. **Etiology.** Causes of heart failure can be grouped into one of four pathophysiologic groups. Treatment principles are the same within each group.

1. Myocardial failure occurs when myocardial contractility is significantly reduced, either by primary myocardial disease (e.g., idiopathic dilated cardiomyopathy) or as a complication of other types of heart failure (e.g., volume–flow or pressure overload).

2. Volume–flow overload occurs when there is a leak across an incompetent valve (e.g., mitral valve insufficiency) or a congenital shunt. The ventricle has to pump an abnormally large volume of blood to achieve normal cardiac output because a portion of the stroke volume is redirected. The ventricle undergoes eccentric hypertrophy to increase chamber size and stroke volume. As venous pressures rise to maintain cardiac output, edema and effusions result. Myocardial contractility is usually normal until late in the course of the disease.

3. Pressure overload occurs as a result of outflow resistance (e.g., aortic stenosis). The ventricle undergoes concentric hypertrophy to maintain cardiac output. Myocardial contractility and stroke volume are normal but may decrease late in the course of the disease. Ventricular tachyarrhythmias cause sudden death in many dogs.

4. Restricted ventricular filling results from either myocardial disease (e.g., hypertrophic cardiomyopathy) or pericardial disease. The noncompliant ventricle requires increased venous or filling pressure to maintain cardiac output. As the venous pressure increases, edema and effusions result.

C. **Descriptive terminology**

1. Systolic versus diastolic

a. Systolic failure. Systolic function (i.e., the ability to eject blood) is impaired in heart failure that is associated with myocardial failure, volume–flow overload, or pressure overload.

b. Diastolic failure. Diastolic function is impaired in those diseases that interfere with ventricular filling (e.g., hypertrophic cardiomyopathy, pericardial effusion).

2. Left versus right. These terms are usually used to describe abnormal function of the ventricles. Right and left ventricular failure may coexist.

a. Left ventricular failure causes an increase in left atrial size and pressure, which is followed by the development of pulmonary venous congestion, edema, and, occasionally, pleural effusion.

b. Right ventricular failure elevates the central venous pressure, causing pleural effusion, ascites, hepatomegaly, jugular venous distention, and, rarely, subcutaneous edema.

3. Backward versus forward

a. Backward (congestive) heart failure occurs when tissue congestion and edema develop as a result of elevated atrial and ventricular filling pressures. Systolic or diastolic dysfunction can cause backward heart failure.

    b. Forward (low-output) heart failure. Arterial pressure, tissue perfusion, and tissue oxygenation are reduced, leading to exercise intolerance, weakness, pale mucous membranes, and lactic acidosis. Low-output heart failure is usually associated with systolic dysfunction.

D. **Diagnosis**

  1. Clinical signs
    a. Coughing. Dogs commonly develop a cough as the result of pulmonary edema or left atrial enlargement.
    b. Tachypnea, dyspnea, or **orthopnea** may be caused by pulmonary edema or pleural effusion. Pulmonary edema usually causes dyspnea, rather than a cough, in cats.
    c. Exercise intolerance may be noted early in the course of heart failure but is frequently overlooked by owners with cats or inactive dogs.

  2. Physical examination
    a. Weakness, pale mucous membranes, a prolonged capillary refill time, ascites, pitting subcutaneous edema, and jugular venous distention may be observed.
    b. The pulse rate and character are variable and pulse deficits may be detected if arrhythmias are present.
    c. When pulmonary edema is severe, audible crackles may develop. Because auscultation is an insensitive means of detecting mild to moderate pulmonary edema, thoracic radiographs should be taken if pulmonary edema is suspected. Lung sounds are muffled by moderate amounts of pleural fluid.
    d. Gallop rhythms may be heard. Murmurs accompany valvular insufficiencies, congenital shunts, and stenotic lesions.

  3. Radiographic findings. Cardiomegaly (left, right, or generalized) is usually present; however, heart failure may develop without any visible change in cardiac size or shape (e.g., constrictive pericarditis).
    a. Left-sided failure. Early left-sided failure results in pulmonary venous distention. As heart failure worsens and pulmonary venous pressures increase, interstitial and then alveolar edema patterns emerge. Occasionally, left-sided failure is associated with pleural effusion.
    b. Right-sided failure usually causes pleural effusion, ascites, and hepatomegaly.

  4. Echocardiography will not help diagnose heart failure but is extremely useful in identifying the cause of the failure.

  5. Electrocardiography is not required to diagnose heart failure but is helpful in identifying arrhythmias or conduction disturbances that may require specific therapy.
    a. Severe left atrial enlargement can result in the development of atrial fibrillation.
    b. Myocardial diseases are frequently associated with ventricular arrhythmias (especially in Dobermans and boxers).

E. **Therapy**

  1. Symptomatic therapy
    a. Preload reduction (i.e., **relieving congestion** and **edema**)
      (1) Reduced-salt diets. Reduction of sodium intake reduces vascular volume, venous congestion, and edema. Because of poor palatability, some animals will not eat reduced-salt diets.
      (2) Diuretic therapy is usually the most effective way to reduce congestion and edema.
        (a) Agents
          (i) Loop diuretics (e.g., **furosemide**) are the most commonly used agents. The dose and route of administration are dictated by the severity of the congestion and edema.
          (ii) Thiazide diuretics (e.g., **hydrochlorothiazide, chlorothiazide**) are less potent and are used less frequently.
        (b) Side effects of diuretic therapy include dehydration, hypokalemia, and

dilutional hyponatremia. Although hypokalemia is the most common electrolyte disturbance associated with diuretic therapy, it rarely occurs in animals that are eating well.

    (3) Venodilators (e.g., **nitroglycerin**) decrease venous pressures and preload by increasing the capacitance (storage capacity) of the venous system. Venodilators are used most often in conjunction with other agents to rapidly reverse severe pulmonary edema. Occasionally, they are used on a chronic basis when diet and diuretic therapy are no longer effective.

  b. Afterload reduction (i.e., **increasing forward flow**). Arterial **vasodilators** reduce the cardiac workload and improve forward flow, prolonging survival. Mixed (balanced) vasodilators dilate both arteries and veins. Abrupt cessation of vasodilator therapy can result in an acute rebound of arterial or venous pressures and worsen clinical signs.

    (1) Angiotensin-converting enzyme (ACE) inhibitors (e.g., **captopril, enalapril**) are the most commonly used vasodilators in dogs and cats; most veterinary cardiologists feel their use is associated with prolonged survival.

      (a) Mechanism of action. ACE inhibitors dilate both arteries and veins by blocking the conversion of angiotensin I to angiotensin II in the pulmonary vasculature. Consequently, angiotensin II concentrations decline, resulting in arterial and venous dilation and reduced salt and water retention. As a result, ACE inhibitors reduce both afterload and preload.

      (b) Indications. ACE inhibitors are best used for long-term, rather than acute or emergency, therapy.

      (c) Side effects include anorexia, vomiting, diarrhea, hypotension, and azotemia.

    (2) Other vasodilators

      (a) Hydralazine is a potent arteriodilator that has been shown to have beneficial effects in dogs with heart failure caused by mitral regurgitation. It is also used when the use of ACE inhibitors is cost-prohibitive or for cases that are refractory to ACE inhibitors.

      (b) Sodium nitroprusside is a potent arterial and venous dilator that is used intravenously in critical care situations when an acute reduction of afterload and preload is required. Sodium nitroprusside is titrated to effect while monitoring arterial blood pressure.

  c. Enhancement of myocardial contractility

    (1) Indications

      (a) Dilated cardiomyopathy. Increasing myocardial contractility is almost always indicated in dogs and cats with dilated cardiomyopathy.

      (b) Mitral valve disease. Reduced myocardial function does not occur until late in the course of the disease in small dogs with congestive heart failure caused by mitral valve regurgitation. However, large dogs that develop heart failure secondary to mitral valve disease may develop myocardial failure sooner.

    (2) Contraindications. Augmenting myocardial contractility in dogs and cats with **hypertrophic cardiomyopathy** is contraindicated.

    (3) Agents

      (a) Digitalis compounds (e.g., **digoxin, digitoxin**) are the only positive inotropic agents currently available for long-term oral use.

        (i) Mechanism of action. Digitalis compounds exert their positive inotropic effects by binding to myocardial cell membrane Na^+-K^+-ATPase. Binding to Na^+-K^+-ATPase results in increased intracellular calcium concentrations, which directly increases contractile function.

        (ii) Toxicity. Digoxin has a narrow margin of safety; therefore, adverse effects (e.g., myocardial toxicity, gastrointestinal toxicity) are common.

      (b) Bipyridine compounds (e.g., **amrinone, milrinone**) are potent positive inotropic agents. They are more effective than digoxin for increasing contractile function and are also arterial vasodilators.

        (i) Amrinone is administered intravenously for short-term support in dogs and cats with severe heart failure that is refractory to other therapies.

        (ii) Milrinone is administered orally. It is not marketed for use in dogs; long-term studies of its use in human beings with chronic heart failure have documented decreased survival.

    (c) Catecholamines (e.g., **dopamine, dobutamine**) can be used for short-term positive inotropic support in animals with severe heart failure. Because dopamine and dobutamine are rapidly metabolized, they are administered by continuous intravenous infusion.

        (i) Dopamine, which increases blood pressure and heart rate and is arrhythmogenic in a dose-dependent fashion, is used most often in animals with cardiogenic shock associated with anesthesia or following cardiopulmonary resuscitation (CPR).

        (ii) Dobutamine, a synthetic analog of dopamine, is used in animals with severe heart failure caused or complicated by myocardial failure. At appropriate doses, it increases myocardial contractility and improves coronary and skeletal muscle blood flow but does not elevate heart rate and blood pressure. However, cats can be particularly sensitive to dobutamine and may develop vomiting and seizures.

d. Promoting myocardial relaxation and filling. β-adrenergic blockers (e.g., **propranolol, atenolol**) and **calcium channel blockers** (e.g., **diltiazem**) are used when congestive heart failure develops because of restricted ventricular filling associated with hypertrophic cardiomyopathy.

2. Treatment protocols

  a. Heart disease but no signs of failure [New York Heart Association (NYHA) functional class I]. Many small breed dogs have a detectable murmur caused by mitral valve insufficiency but no signs of failure. In general, **no treatment is indicated** at this stage.

  b. Mild heart failure (NYHA class II)

    (1) Signs of heart failure occur only after heavy exertion. No other signs are present.

    (2) Treatment. Strenuous exercise should be avoided. If this is not possible or signs become associated with light exercise, low-dose furosemide or ACE inhibitor therapy (or both) should be considered.

  c. Moderate heart failure (NYHA class III)

    (1) Signs of heart failure appear after light exercise or at night.

    (2) Treatment. Furosemide and ACE inhibitor therapy is indicated. Digoxin may be indicated if myocardial dysfunction is present. A reduced-salt diet should be considered.

  d. Severe heart failure (NYHA class IV)

    (1) Signs. Coughing, dyspnea, and weakness occur at rest. Obvious pulmonary congestion and edema are detectable radiographically.

    (2) Treatment. Moderate to high doses of furosemide should be administered until pulmonary edema has been resolved; lower doses may be sufficient for long-term maintenance. ACE inhibitor therapy should be initiated, and digoxin should be considered if myocardial dysfunction is present. A reduced-salt diet is recommended.

  e. Fulminant heart failure is usually an emergency situation.

    (1) Signs. Dogs have severe dyspnea due to pulmonary edema and may cough up blood-tinged foam.

    (2) Treatment

      (a) Ensure adequate ventilation. The patency of the airway should be checked, and supplemental oxygen administered. If frothing is evident, nebulization with 20% ethanol should be considered. Intubation and mechanical ventilation may be necessary.

      (b) Reduce pulmonary edema or pleural effusion.

(i) High doses of furosemide (administered either intramuscularly or intravenously) should be initiated.

(ii) Venodilation with nitroglycerin may further reduce preload.

(iii) Morphine. In dogs, morphine may help redistribute blood out of the venous compartment and reduce anxiety associated with dyspnea.

(iv) Thoracocentesis may rapidly improve respiratory function in animals with large amounts of pleural fluid.

(c) **Reverse bronchoconstriction. Aminophylline** may be administered to reverse bronchoconstriction.

(d) **Reduce anxiety.** Morphine (dogs only), acepromazine, or diazepam are useful for reducing anxiety.

(e) **Reduce afterload.** Vasodilators (e.g., ACE inhibitors, hydralazine) will reduce afterload.

(f) **Increase myocardial contractility.** Digoxin or, if more immediate cardiac support is required, dobutamine, dopamine, or amrinone can be used to increase myocardial contractility if necessary.

(g) **Monitor the patient.** If dehydration necessitates intravenous fluid therapy, reduced-sodium or sodium-free fluids should be cautiously administered. Reduced-sodium fluids should not be used if significant hyponatremia (i.e., serum sodium ≤ 130 mEq/L) is present.

III. ACQUIRED VALVULAR DISEASE

A. **Mitral valve endocardiosis (insufficiency)** is the most common valvular (and cardiovascular) disease in dogs. (Valvular disease of any kind is rare in cats.) Although mitral valve incompetence is usually caused by endocardiosis and occurs as a distinct clinical entity, it may accompany other cardiac diseases (e.g., dilated or hypertrophic cardiomyopathy, endocarditis).

1. **Signalment**
   a. **Age.** Prevalence increases with age, ranging from 5% in dogs younger than 1 year of age to 75% in dogs older than 16 years of age.
   b. **Sex.** Males are affected one and one half times more often than females.
   c. **Breed.** Miniature and small breed dogs are affected much more commonly than large breed dogs. In cavalier King Charles spaniels, mitral valve insufficiency is detected in approximately 33% of dogs aged 2–3 years and in 60% of dogs over 4 years of age.

2. **Pathophysiology**
   a. Proliferation of fibroblastic tissue and the deposition of glycosaminoglycans in the middle layers of the mitral valve result in the formation of nodules along the free margins of the valve leaflets. The nodules enlarge and coalesce, causing **thickening, irregularity,** and **shortening of the leaflets.** There is no inflammation associated with this process.
      (1) Thickening, shortening, or rupture of the chordae tendineae, dilation of the mitral valve annulus, fibrosis or necrosis of the papillary muscles, dilation and rupture of the left atrium, or dilation of the left ventricle may accompany valvular endocardiosis.
      (2) The mitral valve is the only valve affected in approximately 62% of dogs with endocardiosis. Mitral and tricuspid endocardiosis occur in 33% of cases and the tricuspid valve is solely affected in only 1% of cases.
   b. Endocardiosis compromises mitral valve function so that during systole, blood regurgitates across the valve into the left atrium, generating a midsystolic murmur.
      (1) Increases in left atrial pressure are blunted by **left atrial dilation.** Valvular endocardiosis usually produces a slow increase in regurgitant flow, which

allows left atrial enlargement to attenuate pressure increases. A rapid increase in regurgitant volume will produce a higher atrial pressure because there is inadequate time for the atrium to dilate.

    (2) Once **maximal left atrial dilation** has occurred, left atrial pressure increases and **pulmonary venous congestion** and **edema** result. That is, **congestive heart failure** develops as a result of volume–flow overload (see II B 2). It has been estimated that mitral valve insufficiency accounts for 75% of cases of congestive heart failure in dogs of all breeds and 95% of cases in small breed dogs.

        (a) Several years may elapse between the detection of a mitral valve murmur and the development of congestive heart failure.

        (b) The main **factors that affect the development of congestive heart failure** are the **volume of regurgitant flow** and the **left atrial pressure.** The volume of regurgitant flow is determined by the afterload (i.e., the peripheral resistance) and the severity of the valvular incompetence.

    (3) **Pulmonary arterial hypertension** can develop late in the course of mitral valve insufficiency, causing right ventricular hypertrophy and, possibly, concomitant right ventricular failure.

3. **Diagnosis** of mitral valve incompetence is usually straightforward and is based on signalment, clinical signs, and physical examination.

  a. **Clinical signs**

    (1) **Coughing** is the most common presenting complaint. The cough is usually deep and resonant and is worse at night or after exercise. Causes include left atrial enlargement and pulmonary congestion and edema. Care must be taken to establish a cardiac cause for the cough because chronic airway disease is also common in middle-aged to older small breed dogs.

    (2) **Signs related to congestive heart failure** (e.g., dyspnea, orthopnea, exercise intolerance, weakness, lethargy, inappetence) may be present.

    (3) **Syncope** may occur as a result of poor forward flow and may be related to episodes of coughing **(post-tussive syncope).**

  b. **Physical examination**

    (1) A **midsystolic murmur** over the left apex of the heart is present.

        (a) Although systolic murmurs are often first detected in middle-aged dogs, clinical signs of heart failure are uncommon before 10 years of age in small breeds.

        (b) The intensity and duration of the murmur increase as the valvular disease progresses. A palpable thrill may be detected when the murmur is severe.

    (2) **Crackles, snaps,** and **pops** may be heard, especially at end-inspiration in dogs with pulmonary edema. **Heart sounds may be muffled** if significant amounts of pleural or pericardial fluid are present.

    (3) **Pulse deficits** (related to cardiac arrhythmias), **weak pulses** (related to advanced heart failure), or **gray** or **cyanotic mucous membranes** may be detected.

    (4) **Ascites** and **jugular venous distention** may occur if right ventricular failure is present.

  c. **Radiographic findings.** As the valvular insufficiency worsens, progressive enlargement of the left atrium occurs. Left ventricular enlargement develops concomitantly. Pulmonary venous dilation followed by interstitial, then alveolar, edema develops as the left atrial pressure increases.

    (1) On the lateral projection, there is loss of the caudal waist, elevation of the thoracic trachea, and dorsal displacement of the left bronchus relative to the right.

    (2) On the DV view, left atrial enlargement is seen as a bulge at the 2 to 3 o'clock position. This is the first and most consistent radiographic feature observed with mitral insufficiency.

  d. **Echocardiographic findings**

    (1) **Left atrial** and **ventricular dilation** are evident.

    (2) Mitral valve incompetence can be assessed by spectral or color flow Doppler.

    (3) Valve thickening or **prolapse** may be observed, as well as torn chordae tendinea.

    (4) Myocardial contractile function is usually normal until late in the course of the disease. Because regurgitation across the mitral valve leads to less overall outflow resistance, the ventricles can contract more easily. Therefore, measures of contractile function (e.g., fractional shortening, ejection fraction) are often increased, making the objective assessment of contractile function in dogs with mitral regurgitation difficult. It has been suggested that a fractional shortening of less than 35% or an increased left ventricular end-systolic minor axis dimension indicates reduced contractility in dogs with mitral regurgitation.

  e. Electrocardiographic findings

    (1) An **increased QRS duration, tall R waves,** and **left axis deviation** are indicative of left atrial and ventricular enlargement, but the ECG may be normal.

    (2) There may be **evidence of supraventricular arrhythmias** (e.g., atrial premature contractions, tachycardia, or fibrillation), **ventricular ectopy,** or **sinus tachycardia.**

4. Therapy

  a. In animals with **left mainstem bronchial compression but no pulmonary venous congestion** or **edema,** the main goal is to **reduce the size of the left atrium.** The following therapies are employed in a stepwise manner, starting with arterial vasodilators (with or without digoxin), followed by another vasodilator, and then diuretics. At least 1–2 weeks should be allowed between therapies to evaluate clinical effect. Caution is advised with the concomitant use of more than one vasodilator or a vasodilator and a diuretic because hypotension and reduced renal function may result.

    (1) Reducing peripheral resistance by using an **arterial vasodilator** (e.g., an ACE inhibitor or hydralazine) is the most effective way to increase forward flow through the aorta and decrease regurgitant flow into the left atrium.

    (2) The use of **digoxin** in this setting is controversial but it may reduce regurgitant flow by tightening the mitral valve annulus and improving left ventricular emptying.

    (3) Diuretics and **reduced-salt diets** may help to decrease total blood volume, thereby decreasing the size of the left atrium and ventricle.

  b. In animals with **pulmonary congestion** and **edema,** the blood volume and preload must be reduced.

    (1) Mid-range to **high doses of furosemide** are used during the first 2–3 days to alleviate the clinical signs associated with pulmonary edema. Over the next 2 weeks, the dose is lowered to a level that will control clinical signs.

    (2) Venodilators may be considered for short-term support in cases of severe or refractory pulmonary edema.

    (3) Administration of arterial vasodilators (e.g., enalapril) and a reduced-salt diet should be employed to reduce left atrial pressure.

    (4) Digoxin may reduce regurgitant flow, decrease reflex tachycardia, normalize baroreceptor reflexes, and antagonize central sympathetic nervous system activation. However, its use in patients with mitral valve insufficiency that is not accompanied by reduced myocardial contractility is controversial.

5. Complications associated with mitral insufficiency

  a. Right ventricular failure can be caused by long-standing pulmonary hypertension.

    (1) Pathogenesis. Chronically elevated left atrial pressures and pulmonary congestion-induced hypoxemia are thought to induce constriction of the pulmonary arterioles, resulting in hypertension.

    (2) Signs include exertional weakness and syncope and ascites.

    (3) Treatment is difficult but includes the use of **supplemental oxygen** to reduce the hypoxia-induced arteriolar constriction, taking **measures to reduce left atrial pressure** and **edema,** administration of **bronchodilators,** and **severe exercise restriction.** Although most arterial vasodilators do not work well on pulmonary vasculature, hydralazine may have some effect.

b. **Ruptured chordae tendineae**

(1) **Pathogenesis.** The main hemodynamic consequence of chordal rupture is an acute increase in regurgitant flow and left atrial pressure, which results in the sudden development or exacerbation of pulmonary edema (depending on which chordae and valve leaflet are affected).

   (a) Rupture of a first-order chordae attached to the septal mitral valve leaflet results in severe incompetence and fulminant pulmonary edema. In contrast, rupture of a second-, third-, or even a first-order chordae on the free wall leaflet may induce only mild or no signs.

   (b) Ruptured chordae may occur in asymptomatic dogs or in those with advanced disease and congestive heart failure.

(2) **Signs** include the acute onset of severe dyspnea, reduced intensity of the systolic murmur, lack of a significant change in left atrial size from previous evaluations, and echocardiographic evidence of a prolapsed valve leaflet and ruptured chordae.

(3) **Treatment**

   (a) In severely affected animals, treatment requires intensive care, supplemental oxygen, and the use of high doses of diuretics to reduce the pulmonary edema.

   (b) The use of venodilators (with blood pressure monitoring) can also be considered.

   (c) Dobutamine or dopamine may aid ventricular emptying and reduce left ventricular dilation and the size of the mitral valve annulus.

(4) **Prognosis.** Dogs with rupture of a first-order chordae on the septal leaflet usually do not survive. Less serious chordal ruptures may be stabilized and then managed long-term.

c. **Tachyarrhythmia.** Dogs with left atrial enlargement are prone to supraventricular arrhythmias. Supraventricular (atrial or junctional) tachycardia and atrial flutter or fibrillation are the most common rhythm disturbances.

(1) **Pathogenesis.** Cardiac output is compromised if the ventricular rate exceeds 180 bpm. When this occurs, left atrial pressure rises and **pulmonary edema develops** or **worsens.**

(2) **Treatment**

   (a) **Arrhythmia. Digoxin** is indicated to reduce the heart rate to less than 150–160 bpm. If digoxin does not lower the heart rate, then **diltiazem** or a **β-adrenergic blocker** can be added. The drugs should be started at a low dose and gradually increased to effect. Some patients depend on a relatively high heart rate to ensure adequate cardiac output and may not tolerate rates below 150 bpm.

   (b) The **pulmonary edema** is treated as described in III A 4 b.

d. **Left atrial rupture** results in acute hemopericardium, cardiac tamponade, and, usually, sudden death.

(1) **Pathogenesis**

   (a) Left atrial rupture occurs rarely and is thought to be preceded by **endocardial splitting,** often at the site of a previous jet lesion on the caudal atrial endocardium. Endocardial splitting and atrial rupture are more likely in dogs with severe left atrial dilation.

   (b) **Rupture of a first-order chordae** has been observed in many of these dogs on postmortem examination.

(2) **Signs**

   (a) Acute onset of weakness, ascites, jugular venous distention, muffled heart sounds, and weak femoral pulses are characteristic clinical signs, provided the dog lives long enough to be examined.

   (b) A globoid-shaped heart shadow may be observed radiographically.

   (c) Pericardial effusion is detected echocardiographically.

       (d) Reduced amplitude of the QRS complex and electrical alternans may be detected on an electrocardiogram.

    (3) Treatment consists of pericardiocentesis to remove a small amount of fluid (25–50 ml) with the goal of relieving enough intrapericardial pressure to allow improved right ventricular function without encouraging further hemorrhage. Fresh whole blood transfusions may help reduce bleeding. Emergency thoracotomy to repair the atrial tear could be considered, but the prognosis is poor.

B. **Bacterial endocarditis** is a rare disorder.

  1. Predisposing factors

    a. Signalment. Large breed, male dogs and German shepherds are overrepresented.

    b. Dogs with **congenital heart defects** (e.g., subaortic stenosis, ventricular septal defects) may be predisposed. Other risk factors include **indwelling catheters, reduced immune function,** and **sepsis.** Mitral valve endocardiosis does not appear to be a strong risk factor.

  2. Etiology. *Staphylococcus aureus, Escherichia coli,* and *β*-hemolytic streptococci account for approximately 70% of the infections in dogs, although other bacteria and fungi have been documented. Gram-positive organisms cause approximately 60% of infections.

  3. Pathogenesis

    a. Bacteremia is a prerequisite for endocarditis. Common sources of bacteria include heavily colonized mucosal surfaces [e.g., the oral cavity, gastrointestinal (GI) tract, and urogenital tract] and localized infections that allow bacterial entry into local veins and lymphatics.

    b. Colonization

      (1) Bacterial colonization and damage occur most often on the **mitral valve** and to a lesser extent, on the **aortic valve;** however, other valves, supporting structures, and the myocardium may also be affected.

      (2) Most bacteria colonize **previously damaged endothelium,** but some bacteria (e.g., *S. aureus)* secrete **proteases** that allow them to colonize endothelial surfaces directly. Tissue destruction by infecting organisms can cause **severe valve pathology, destruction of surrounding structures, damage and rupture of chordae tendineae,** left atrial or ventricular **septal perforation,** and **damage to the interventricular conduction system.**

      (3) The accumulation of platelets and fibrin at the site of colonization produces the characteristic **vegetative lesions** observed on valve leaflets. Fragments of vegetative valve lesions can break off and embolize to various areas of the body. The spleen and kidney are most commonly affected, but **embolization** to the joints, central nervous system (CNS), and other organs can occur.

    c. Gram-positive infections have a **subacute to chronic course,** which increases the likelihood that an antibody response will develop. The antibody response may lead to the **development of immune complex disease** that can affect the kidneys (glomerulonephritis) and joints (polyarthritis). Gram-negative infections tend to produce a more fulminant clinical course.

  4. Diagnosis is based on positive blood cultures, evidence of cardiac disease, and consistent physical, echocardiographic, and laboratory findings. In the absence of positive blood cultures, a tentative diagnosis can be based on echocardiographic findings and evidence of systemic embolization.

    a. Clinical signs

      (1) Fever, lethargy, shock, and **joint** and **muscle pain** can result from sepsis.

      (2) Lameness, arrhythmias, seizures, or **sudden death** can result from septic embolism.

      (3) Heart failure, arrhythmias, weakness, syncope, and **exercise intolerance** are signs of cardiac abnormalities.

b. **Physical examination.** Fever, a recently acquired murmur, and lameness are commonly reported signs of endocarditis but there is marked variability in the clinical presentation of this disorder. A murmur or fever is not detected in all dogs.

(1) **Murmurs**

    (a) **Mitral valve involvement** produces a **systolic murmur.**

    (b) **Aortic valve insufficiency** produces a **diastolic murmur.**

        (i) A systolic component may also be heard, producing a "to and fro" sound.

        (ii) The detection of a diastolic murmur in the setting of congestive heart failure is quite suggestive of bacterial endocarditis with aortic valve involvement.

(2) **Pulse deficits** may be detected if arrhythmias are present. Water-hammer (bounding) pulses may be audible in the presence of aortic valve incompetence.

(3) **Pulmonary crackles** may be heard if pulmonary edema has developed.

c. **Laboratory findings**

(1) **Blood cultures** are positive in only 72% of the cases.

    (a) Negative cultures may result from prior antimicrobial therapy, chronic endocarditis, isolated right-sided infection, failure to culture for anaerobic agents, or a nonbacterial or noninfective cause for the endocarditis.

    (b) The recommended protocol for blood culture collection is three samples from three different sites taken within a 24-hour period and at least 1 hour apart. The blood bacteria concentration is usually very low, so prolonged periods of culture (up to 3 weeks) may be required before a negative culture can be assured.

(2) **Other findings**

    (a) **Leukocytosis** and **monocytosis** are present in approximately 80% of cases.

    (b) A **normocytic, normochromic, nonregenerative anemia, hematuria, pyuria,** and **proteinuria** are present in just over 50% of cases.

    (c) **Azotemia** and **hypoglycemia** are present in 31% and 22% of dogs, respectively.

    (d) **Disseminated intravascular coagulation (DIC)** can occur in rare cases.

d. **Radiographic findings**

(1) **Mitral valve incompetence** is associated with **left atrial** and **ventricular enlargement.**

(2) **Aortic valve incompetence** is primarily associated with **left ventricular enlargement.**

(3) **Pulmonary venous dilation** and **edema** may be evident.

e. **Echocardiographic findings.** Echocardiography allows **detection of vegetative lesions** on valve leaflets or on mural surfaces and **assessment of the site** and **degree of valvular incompetence.**

(1) Valve lesions may not be observed if they are small or if it is early in the course of infection (less than 2 weeks).

(2) Small lesions on the mitral valve may be difficult to distinguish from nodules and fibrosis associated with endocardiosis.

(3) Vegetative lesions often remain unchanged for months following successful antimicrobial therapy.

f. **Electrocardiographic findings.** Conduction disturbances or arrhythmias [commonly ventricular premature complexes (VPCs)] are observed in up to 75% of dogs with endocarditis.

5. **Therapy**

a. **Goals** are to sterilize the vegetative lesions, remove the source of infection (if possible), manage the effects of sepsis (particularly with Gram-negative infection), control signs of congestive heart failure, and support organ function compromised by embolic damage. Early and aggressive therapy is required.

b. **Antimicrobial therapy** should be carefully chosen, initiated early, and administered for an extended period of time.

(1) **Selection** of an antibiotic should be based on blood culture results, but therapy may have to be initiated before the results are known. Empiric therapy with an aminoglycoside (e.g., gentamicin) and a penicillin is effective against most Gram-positive and Gram-negative organisms, as well as anaerobic organisms.

(2) **Duration.** Initially, antimicrobial therapy should be administered intravenously for 5–10 days and continued for a minimum of 6–8 weeks. The antimicrobial agent selected for prolonged use should be bactericidal and have as few side effects as possible. Aminoglycoside antibiotics should not be administered for longer than 7–10 days.

(3) **Follow-up.** Patients should be monitored closely for response, relapse, or drug-induced complications (e.g., renal failure). If a relapse occurs after cessation of antimicrobial therapy, it usually occurs within 1–2 months.

6. **Prognosis.** The long-term prognosis is poor to grave. Animals die from congestive heart failure, septic embolization, or renal failure.

   a. Aortic valve infection is particularly onerous because it leads to the rapid development of intractable congestive heart failure. Mitral valve infection carries a better prognosis, with approximately 50% of dogs surviving in one study.

   b. Infections caused by Gram-negative organisms have a poorer prognosis than those caused by Gram-positive organisms.

IV. CARDIOMYOPATHY.
Cardiomyopathies may be classified as either primary or secondary (Table 39-6). Primary cardiomyopathies have no identifiable cause; these are the focus of this section.

A. Canine cardiomyopathy

1. **Dilated cardiomyopathy** is a slowly progressive disorder that results in the diminution of systolic myocardial function (i.e., reduced contractility) and the develop-

TABLE 39-6. Classification of Cardiomyopathies

Primary	Secondary
Dilated	Metabolic
Hypertrophic	Endocrine disturbances
Restrictive	Hyperthyroidism
Intermediate	Acromegaly
	Pheochromocytoma
	Nutritional
	Taurine deficiency
	L-Carnitine deficiency
	Toxic
	Doxorubicin
	Lead
	Cobalt
	Inflammatory or infectious
	Viral
	Bacterial
	Protozoal (trypanosomiasis, toxoplasmosis)
	Infiltrative
	Neoplasia
	Glycogen storage diseases
	Other
	Muscular dystrophy

Adapted with permission from: Miller MS, Tilley LP: *Manual of Canine and Feline Cardiology,* 2nd ed. Philadelphia, WB Saunders, 1995, p 146.

ment of congestive heart failure. Arrhythmias commonly accompany this syndrome (with or without heart failure) and sudden death is not infrequent.

a. Signalment

(1) Breed. Dilated cardiomyopathy is predominantly a disease of large and giant breed dogs; however, a form of this disease has been described in American cocker spaniels. The prevalence among the large and giant breeds ranges from 0.9% in Old English sheepdogs to 6.0% in Scottish deerhounds.

(2) Sex. Males seem to be at higher risk than females.

(3) Age. The prevalence increases with age and ranges from approximately 1% at 1–2 years of age to 8%–10% at 7–10 years of age.

b. Etiology. The etiology is unknown. However, the lack of significant inflammation and myocardial damage suggests a cellular or subcellular defect, and the breed predispositions point to possible genetic factors. L-Carnitine and taurine deficiency have been investigated as a cause of dilated cardiomyopathy in dogs, but evidence suggests that nutritional deficiencies are not factors in the development of dilated cardiomyopathy in the majority of cases.

c. Pathophysiology. Myocardial lesions consist of scattered areas of myofiber atrophy, degeneration, or necrosis and fibrosis and are mild compared with the degree of functional impairment. Mitral or tricuspid valve incompetence may contribute to the functional impairment, but usually is not of major significance.

(1) The progressive deterioration of systolic function (following marked dilation of all of the heart's chambers) leads to elevation of the end-diastolic left ventricular and left atrial pressures and the pulmonary venous pressure, causing pulmonary venous congestion and edema.

(2) Cardiac output is low as a result of impaired myocardial function. Atrial fibrillation or paroxysmal episodes of ventricular tachycardia may also significantly reduce cardiac output.

d. Diagnosis

(1) Clinical signs

(a) Occult (asymptomatic) dilated cardiomyopathy is common in breeds with a predisposition for the disease (especially Doberman pinschers).

(b) Signs of right- or left-sided congestive heart failure may be present.

(i) Giant breed dogs tend to develop right-sided signs (e.g., abdominal distention, anorexia, weight loss, and fatigue).

(ii) Doberman pinschers and boxers tend to develop left-sided signs (e.g., exercise intolerance, coughing, dyspnea, and lethargy).

(c) Syncope may occur, especially if ventricular arrhythmias are a factor.

(2) Physical examination

(a) Gallop rhythms, soft systolic murmurs (1/6 to 3/6) over the mitral or tricuspid valves, irregular heart beats, and pulmonary crackles may be heard. Ventricular dilation can result in an audible S_3.

(b) Weak pulses and pulse deficits caused by arrhythmias are common.

(c) Mucous membrane pallor and a prolonged capillary refill time may be present.

(d) Weight loss and muscle wasting may be evident.

(3) Laboratory abnormalities. Azotemia may result from reduced renal perfusion. Mild elevations in liver enzymes can be related to hepatic congestion. Mild hyponatremia, hyperkalemia, and hypoproteinemia may accompany congestive heart failure.

(4) Radiographic findings

(a) Pulmonary venous congestion and **edema** will be present if congestive heart failure has developed.

(b) Left atrial and **ventricular enlargement** is seen in Dobermans and boxers. The magnitude of these changes may not be marked, although severe pulmonary edema may be present.

(c) Marked, generalized cardiomegaly is more common in giant breeds and is often accompanied by signs of biventricular or right ventricular failure (e.g., pleural effusion, hepatomegaly).

(5) Echocardiographic findings
  (a) A key finding is the detection of **left ventricular hypokinesis** (i.e., reduced contractility).
  (b) Left ventricular systolic performance indices (e.g., **ejection fraction, left ventricular shortening fraction)** are **reduced.**
(6) Electrocardiographic findings
  (a) Arrhythmias
    (i) Atrial fibrillation is present in 75%–80% of giant breed dogs with dilated cardiomyopathy.
    (ii) VPCs and **ventricular tachycardia** are more common in Doberman pinschers and boxers, putting these breeds at a high risk of sudden death. Approximately 80% of Dobermans in congestive heart failure have ventricular arrhythmias.
  (b) Alterations in chamber size will also be reflected on the ECG.
  e. Therapy consists primarily of controlling signs of congestive heart failure in symptomatic dogs (see II E). Therapy is individualized because all dogs do not respond or tolerate the drugs in a consistent manner.
  (1) Preload reduction. Although difficult in some animals, sufficient preload reduction (to alleviate pulmonary edema) must be induced without a major reduction in cardiac output and organ perfusion. Judicious use of low-sodium intravenous fluids may be required to prevent marked dehydration.
    (a) Diuresis. The amount and rapidity of preload reduction required will dictate the amount and route of administration of **furosemide.** Dogs with dilated cardiomyopathy may be asymptomatic or near death with fulminant pulmonary edema. In dogs with the latter, parenteral administration of high doses of furosemide is required.
    (b) Venodilation. Additional preload reduction with the use of a venodilator (e.g., nitroglycerin) may be required.
    (c) Reduced-salt diets and **ACE inhibitors** aid in preload reduction over the long term.
  (2) Afterload reduction. Although the goal of afterload reduction is to decrease peripheral resistance and increase cardiac output, a failing myocardium may not be able to increase cardiac output to maintain blood pressure. Afterload reduction may have to be delayed until cardiac output can be supported by positive inotropic agents.
    (a) ACE inhibitors are the primary means of reducing afterload.
    (b) A **combination of hydralazine** and **nitroglycerin** can be considered for patients that do not tolerate or are refractory to ACE inhibitors.
    (c) Nitroprusside will provide rapid and profound vasodilation when life-threatening left ventricular failure is present, but its use requires continuous blood pressure monitoring in an intensive care setting.
  (3) Enhancement of myocardial contractility. Positive inotropic agents (e.g., digoxin) are indicated in all dogs with dilated cardiomyopathy to improve the strength of myocardial contraction.
  (4) Antiarrhythmic therapy
    (a) VPCs and **ventricular tachycardia.** Antiarrhythmic therapy is indicated in dogs with frequent VPCs or ventricular tachycardia, but may not significantly reduce the risk of sudden death caused by ventricular arrhythmias in dogs with heart failure.
      (i) Procainamide (or in acute situations, **lidocaine)** is commonly used initially. If these drugs are ineffective, the addition of **propranolol** to the regimen may control the arrhythmia.
      (ii) Alternatively, **quinidine, mexiletine,** or **tocainide** can be considered.
    (b) Atrial fibrillation. Digoxin is indicated for atrial fibrillation. If the heart rate cannot be reduced with digoxin alone, then a β-**adrenergic blocker** (e.g., propranolol, atenolol) or **calcium channel blocker** (e.g., diltiazem) can be added.
  f. Prognosis. Dilated cardiomyopathy is a **uniformly fatal disease.**

(1) Most dogs with signs of heart failure die within 6 months to 2 years. Dogs with severe signs of heart failure may not survive the initial hospitalization period.

(2) Doberman pinschers have an even worse prognosis; once congestive heart failure has developed, survival time usually ranges from 1–3 months. Sudden death is common in Dobermans and boxers.

2. Hypertrophic cardiomyopathy is a rare disease in dogs. It is characterized by marked hypertrophy of the left ventricular myocardium and impaired diastolic (i.e., filling) function. In addition, in some dogs, abnormal motion of the mitral valve toward the interventricular septum during systole leads to the development of dynamic obstruction of the left ventricular outflow tract.

a. Diagnosis

(1) Clinical signs. Many dogs are asymptomatic, but when signs are present, they are indicative of left-sided heart failure (e.g., exercise intolerance, cough, pulmonary edema). Ventricular arrhythmias may cause syncope or sudden death.

(2) Echocardiographic examination reveals concentric left ventricular hypertrophy without identifiable fixed aortic outflow obstruction (i.e., subaortic stenosis).

b. Therapy is similar to that for cats with hypertrophic cardiomyopathy (see IV B 2 e).

B. Feline cardiomyopathy

1. Dilated cardiomyopathy was common in cats before 1987, when it was discovered that the majority of cats suffering from this disorder were deficient in the amino acid taurine. Since that time, most commercial cat foods have been supplemented with taurine, making dilated cardiomyopathy a rare diagnosis in cats. The pathophysiology is similar to that described in dogs with dilated cardiomyopathy (see IV A 1 c).

a. Signalment. Dilated cardiomyopathy typically affects middle-aged and older cats. There is no sex or breed predisposition.

b. Diagnosis

(1) Clinical signs

(a) Dyspnea (usually caused by pleural effusion), **lethargy, weakness,** and **inappetence** are common. The **onset of signs appears to be acute** to owners because cats will restrict their physical activity until their respiratory function is very compromised. As such, most of these cats are in a very fragile state and can easily die when stressed from excessive diagnostic or therapeutic manipulation.

(b) Signs of posterior paresis may be present if aortic thromboembolism, a common complication of cardiomyopathy, has occurred (see XII A 2).

(2) Physical examination findings usually reflect biventricular failure and include pale or ashen mucous membranes with a prolonged capillary refill time, weak femoral pulses, a gallop rhythm, a systolic murmur, rhythm irregularities with pulse deficits, and hypothermia. Jugular vein distention with abnormal pulses may also be present.

(3) Laboratory findings

(a) Azotemia. Many cats are azotemic as the result of decreased renal perfusion.

(b) Plasma taurine concentration is decreased in most cats with dilated cardiomyopathy.

(c) Pseudochylous and **chylous effusions** may occur, although pleural fluid is usually a modified transudate.

(d) Elevations in serum alanine aminotransferase (SALT), serum aspartate aminotransferase (SAST), creatine phosphokinase, and **glucose** often accompany thromboembolism (see XII A 2).

(4) Radiographic findings. Generalized cardiomegaly and pleural effusion are the most common abnormalities. Pulmonary venous congestion and patchy pulmonary edema are less common.

   (5) **Echocardiographic findings** are similar to those found in dogs with dilated cardiomyopathy and are characterized by left atrial and ventricular dilation with reduced myocardial contractility. Thrombi are occasionally visualized in the left atrium.

   (6) **Electrocardiographic findings.** Ventricular arrhythmias are common. Cardiac chamber size alterations (especially left atrial and ventricular enlargement) may also be evident.

  c. Therapy

   (1) **Basic therapy** is similar to that for dogs with dilated cardiomyopathy (see IV A 1 e). Diuretics must be used judiciously because cats are more prone to volume depletion than dogs. Similar caution should be observed when administering intravenous fluids to cats with pulmonary edema because the edema can be easily exacerbated.

   (2) **Thoracentesis** is indicated to remove pleural effusion when large volumes are present and can be lifesaving. Therapeutic thoracentesis may need to precede stressful procedures (e.g., radiography).

   (3) **Taurine supplementation** is indicated in all cats regardless of plasma taurine status. Cats that have idiopathic dilated cardiomyopathy not related to taurine deficiency will either not respond to therapy or relapse after a transient improvement.

   (a) Improvement in clinical signs usually takes 2–3 weeks, and echocardiographic abnormalities usually improve within 3–6 weeks. One third to one half of affected cats die within the first 2 weeks as a result of heart failure.

   (b) In those cats that respond to taurine, therapy for heart failure can usually be discontinued after 2–3 months. These cats are effectively cured of dilated cardiomyopathy and experience few long-term negative effects. Taurine supplementation is discontinued after 2–3 months as long as the cat is placed on an adequately supplemented diet.

  d. Prognosis. The prognosis is good if taurine deficiency is the cause and if the cat survives the first few weeks of therapy. If taurine deficiency is not the cause, the prognosis is poor.

2. **Hypertrophic cardiomyopathy** is one of the most common cardiac diseases of cats and is characterized by left ventricular hypertrophy and impaired diastolic function.

  a. Signalment

   (1) **Age** at the time of diagnosis ranges from 1–16 years, with a mean age of 6–7 years.

   (2) **Sex.** Males (intact and neutered) are predisposed.

   (3) **Breed.** There are no marked breed predilections, but a familial association has been documented in Maine coon cats.

  b. Etiology

   (1) **Primary hypertrophic cardiomyopathy** has no known cause although genetic factors, abnormal catecholamine metabolism, abnormal calcium transport, and circulating trophic factors have been considered as possible causes.

   (2) **Secondary hypertrophic cardiomyopathy** may be caused by hyperthyroidism, acromegaly, and hypertension.

  c. Pathophysiology. Concentric ventricular hypertrophy and ischemic myocardial fibrosis reduce the size of the left ventricular lumen and hinder myocardial relaxation, leading to reduced ventricular filling. Consequently, left atrial pressure and size increase, which leads to pulmonary congestion and edema.

  d. Diagnosis

   (1) **Clinical signs.** Cats with hypertrophic cardiomyopathy usually present in one of three ways:

  (a) **Asymptomatic;** diagnosed after discovery of a systolic murmur or gallop rhythm during a routine physical examination

  (b) **Acute onset of dyspnea** and **lethargy** following the development of heart failure and pulmonary edema

  (c) **Acute onset of hindend paresis** as a result of aortic thromboembolism (see XII A 2)

 (2) **Physical examination**

  (a) A **soft 2/6 to 3/6 systolic murmur** that is loudest over the aortic or mitral valve region is present in approximately 66% of affected cats.

  (b) **Gallop rhythms** and **arrhythmias** are detected in approximately 40% and 25% of affected cats, respectively.

  (c) **Mild to marked dyspnea** will be present if pulmonary edema has developed.

 (3) **Radiographic findings** may vary from minimal in asymptomatic cats to obvious left atrial enlargement, cardiomegaly, pulmonary venous distention, and interstitial and alveolar edema in cats with congestive heart failure.

 (4) **Echocardiographic findings**

  (a) **Concentric left ventricular hypertrophy is the main diagnostic criterion** for hypertrophic cardiomyopathy. Left ventricular hypertrophy is usually symmetric (i.e., both the septum and the free wall are equally affected) but asymmetric hypertrophy is also seen occasionally. The most common variant is disproportionate hypertrophy of the interventricular septum.

  (b) **Left atrial enlargement** is a consistent feature. Thrombi are occasionally visualized in the left atrial lumen.

  (c) **Dynamic left ventricular outflow obstruction** may be caused by systolic anterior motion of the mitral valve.

  (d) **Mitral valve regurgitation** may be detected using Doppler techniques.

 (5) **Electrocardiographic findings**

  (a) **Cardiac size-induced alterations** include P mitrale, increased R-wave amplitude, increased QRS width, and left axis deviation.

  (b) **Sinus tachycardia, ventricular arrhythmias,** and **conduction abnormalities** (i.e., left anterior fascicular block) are common.

 e. **Therapy**

 (1) **Symptomatic cats**

  (a) **Relief of pulmonary edema.** The treatment of cats with pulmonary edema includes the use of **supplemental oxygen, diuretics** (with or without **venodilators),** and **cage rest. Bronchodilators** (e.g., aminophylline, theophylline) may be of benefit in acute cases.

  (b) **In an effort to slow heart rate, improve myocardial relaxation,** and **increase ventricular filling,** a nonselective β-adrenergic blocker (e.g., **propranolol**) or a calcium channel blocker (e.g., **diltiazem**) should be administered.

   (i) Controversy exists as to which drug is superior for the treatment of hypertrophic cardiomyopathy in cats. A small study showed diltiazem to be superior to propranolol; however, propranolol may be better at reducing dynamic left ventricular outflow obstruction.

   (ii) Propranolol should not be used in the presence of pulmonary edema or thromboembolism. **Atenolol,** a β_1-specific receptor blocker, has less effect on airways and vessels and may provide an alternative to propranolol.

  (c) **Prophylaxis for thromboembolism** is indicated in all cats with hypertrophic cardiomyopathy. **Aspirin** is used most commonly and is administered at a low dose, once every 3 days.

  (d) **Treatment of ventricular arrhythmias. Propranolol** is often used initially. **Lidocaine** given at low doses is an alternative, but it has a narrow therapeutic index in cats.

 (2) **Asymptomatic cats.** Appropriate therapy for asymptomatic cats is unknown. However, if significant myocardial alterations are present, then

treatment with either **propranolol or diltiazem** in conjunction with **prophylaxis for thromboembolism** is probably justified.

    (3) Contraindications

        (a) Arterial vasodilators (e.g., ACE inhibitors, hydralazine) are not used commonly to treat hypertrophic cardiomyopathy because they may aggravate dynamic outflow obstruction.

        (b) Positive inotropic drugs (e.g., digoxin) are contraindicated.

  f. Prognosis

    (1) Asymptomatic cats without marked myocardial changes may live for years following diagnosis.

    (2) Symptomatic cats. Approximately 70% of cats presented in heart failure die within 1 year of diagnosis. If thromboembolism is present, few cats survive longer than 6 months as a result of the high rate of recurrence. Sudden death may also occur.

3. Restrictive cardiomyopathy is a rare disorder.

  a. Signalment. There is a wide age range with no sex or breed predilection.

  b. Pathogenesis. Restrictive cardiomyopathy is characterized by endocardial, subendocardial, and myocardial fibrosis that predominantly affects the left ventricle, impairing diastolic function. Abnormal left ventricular geometry, papillary muscle fibrosis, and distortion of the mitral valve apparatus (leading to mitral regurgitation) contribute to the development of congestive heart failure.

  c. Diagnosis

    (1) Clinical signs. The clinical features of this disorder are not well defined. Cats present with signs similar to those of hypertrophic cardiomyopathy.

    (2) Radiographic findings include pleural effusion, pulmonary venous congestion and edema, marked left atrial and, occasionally, biatrial enlargement, and normal or moderately enlarged ventricles.

    (3) Echocardiographic findings are variable and can include marked left atrial dilation, a normal or moderately dilated left ventricle, various patterns of regional myocardial hypertrophy, and variable enlargement of the right side of the heart. There is little to distinguish restrictive cardiomyopathy from hypertrophic cardiomyopathy unless extensive areas of hyperechoic endocardium (indicative of fibrosis) or a marked alteration in left ventricular geometry is observed. However, these are uncommon findings.

  d. Therapy. Treatment is similar to that for hypertrophic cardiomyopathy. Extensive fibrosis renders β-adrenergic and calcium channel blockers ineffective for improving diastolic function, but these drugs may still be beneficial because they reduce heart rate and suppress arrhythmias.

  e. Prognosis is difficult to predict because of the paucity of information on this disorder. A high incidence of thromboembolism, refractory congestive heart failure, and arrhythmias has been reported by some authors. Response to therapy is the most useful predictor at present.

4. Intermediate (unclassified) cardiomyopathy refers to disorders that do not fit the diagnostic criteria for either dilated or hypertrophic cardiomyopathy.

  a. Etiology. Many of these cats present in congestive heart failure but it is not known if these cases represent a single disease entity, a transition from one disease to another, congenital or acquired disease, or primary or secondary myocardial disease. Information suggests these cats have abnormal diastolic function similar to that seen in hypertrophic and restrictive cardiomyopathy.

  b. Diagnosis

    (1) Clinical signs are similar to those seen in cats with hypertrophic or restrictive cardiomyopathy.

    (2) Radiographic findings are similar to those of restrictive cardiomyopathy and can include left or biatrial enlargement, pulmonary venous congestion and edema, and less often, pleural effusion.

    (3) Echocardiographic findings are quite variable.

        (a) Marked left atrial dilation is a consistent feature.

        (b) The left ventricle may be normal or slightly dilated and in some cases, areas of mild regional myocardial hypertrophy are detected in the interventricular septum and left ventricular free wall.

    (c) Variable degrees of mitral or tricuspid insufficiency may be present.

    (d) Right heart enlargement may vary from minimal to marked.

  c. Treatment for congestive heart failure is similar to that for other cardiomyopathies. However, guidelines on more specific therapy are lacking at this time.

  d. Prognosis. Asymptomatic cats without marked left atrial enlargement may have a good long-term prognosis. In general, cats presented in congestive heart failure or with aortic thromboembolism have a poor prognosis.

V. CONGENITAL HEART DISEASE

A. Introduction

1. Causes

  a. Insults during gestation (e.g., exposure to drugs, toxins, or infectious agents) can lead to cardiac malformation.

  b. Genetic mechanisms may be responsible. Congenital cardiac defects known to have an inherited basis include PDA in poodles, subaortic stenosis (SAS) in Newfoundlands, tetralogy of Fallot in keeshonds, and pulmonic stenosis in beagles.

2. Prevalence

  a. Dogs. Most congenital cardiac defects occur in **purebred dogs.**

    (1) Breed predispositions for congenital cardiac defects in dogs are listed in Table 39-7.

    (2) The most common cardiac defects in dogs, in approximate order of frequency, are PDA, SAS, and pulmonic stenosis. There is some degree of variation from one geographic region to another.

  b. Cats. Cardiac malformation is less common in cats and breed predispositions are not a prominent feature.

    (1) The most common congenital cardiac defect in cats is ventricular septal defect, which may occur as part of an anomaly referred to as an endocardial cushion defect. Atrial septal defect or malformation of one or both AV valves may also be involved in an endocardial cushion defect.

    (2) Other defects in cats include PDA, SAS, isolated AV dysplasia, and endocardial fibroelastosis (primarily in certain lines of Burmese and Siamese cats).

3. Clinical signs

  a. Most congenital heart disease is diagnosed in dogs and cats younger than 6 months of age after a **murmur** is detected during a routine physical examination.

    (1) Unlike murmurs associated with cardiac defects, innocent murmurs are usually systolic, soft (i.e., 1/6 to 3/6) and may vary in intensity with exercise, body position, phase of respiration or from day to day. Innocent murmurs usually disappear by 6 months of age.

    (2) Murmurs that are loud (i.e., greater than 4/6) or have a diastolic component are likely pathologic.

  b. Other clinical signs that may suggest a cardiac defect include **poor growth, exercise intolerance, cyanosis,** and **syncope.**

B. PDA

1. Signalment. Miniature poodles, German shepherds, collies, Pomeranians, Shetland sheepdogs, and toy breeds are predisposed. PDA is more common in females than in males.

TABLE 39-7. Breed Predilections for Congenital Heart Disease

Breed	Defect
Basset hound	Pulmonic stenosis
Beagle	Pulmonic stenosis
Bichon frise	Patent ductus arteriosus (PDA)
Boxer	Subaortic stenosis, pulmonic stenosis, atrial septal defect
Boykin spaniel	Pulmonic stenosis
Bull terrier	Mitral dysplasia, aortic stenosis
Chihuahua	PDA, pulmonic stenosis
Chow chow	Cor triatriatum dexter, pulmonic stenosis
Cocker spaniel	PDA, pulmonic stenosis
Collie	PDA
Doberman pinscher	Atrial septal defect
English bulldog	Tetralogy of Fallot, ventricular septal defect, pulmonic stenosis
English springer spaniel	PDA, ventricular septal defect
German shepherd	Subaortic stenosis, mitral and tricuspid valve dysplasia, PDA
German shorthair pointer	Subaortic stenosis
Golden retriever	Subaortic stenosis, tricuspid and mitral valve dysplasia
Great Dane	Mitral and tricuspid valve dysplasia, subaortic stenosis
Keeshond	Tetralogy of Fallot, PDA
Labrador retriever	Tricuspid valve dysplasia, PDA, pulmonic stenosis
Maltese	PDA
Mastiff	Pulmonic stenosis, mitral valve dysplasia
Newfoundland	Subaortic stenosis, mitral valve dysplasia, pulmonic stenosis
Pomeranian	PDA
Poodle	PDA
Rottweiler	Subaortic stenosis
Samoyed	Pulmonic stenosis, atrial septal defect, subaortic stenosis
Schnauzer	Pulmonic stenosis
Shetland sheepdog	PDA
Terrier breeds	Pulmonic stenosis
Weimaraner	Tricuspid valve dysplasia, peritoneopericardial hernia
West Highland white terrier	Pulmonic stenosis, ventricular septal defect
Yorkshire terrier	PDA

Modified with permission from Bonagura JD, Darke PGG: Congenital heart disease. In *Textbook of Veterinary Internal Medicine,* 4th ed. Edited by Ettinger SJ, Feldman EC. Philadelphia, WB Saunders, 1995, p 893.

2. **Etiology.** Because PDA is thought to be inherited, affected animals should not be used for breeding.

3. **Pathophysiology.** PDA occurs when the fetal ductus arteriosus fails to close within 2–3 days of birth. Because the pressure in the aorta is higher than that in the pulmonary artery, **left-to-right shunting** of blood occurs. Volume overload of the pulmonary circulation, left atrium, and ventricle follows.

   a. If the shunt is large and the aortic-to-pulmonary artery pressure differential is high, then marked volume overload occurs, which may lead to **left-sided congestive heart failure.**

b. Infrequently, the excessive blood flow into the pulmonary circulation results in vascular changes and the development of **pulmonary hypertension.** Pulmonary arterial pressure may become high enough to cause **right-to-left shunting (reverse PDA).**

- **(1)** Normally, the pulmonary circulation can accept large quantities of blood without an increase in pulmonary artery pressure. However, in some instances, the increased blood flow induces **irreversible intimal changes** (i.e., thickening, medial hypertrophy) in pulmonary arterioles, increasing resistance and elevating the pulmonary artery pressure. In response, the **right ventricle hypertrophies.**
- **(2)** Ultimately, the right ventricular and pulmonary arterial pressures exceed the left ventricular and aortic pressures, causing the blood flow to reverse direction. Unoxygenated blood starts to enter the systemic arterial circulation in varying amounts.

4. Diagnosis

a. Clinical signs and physical examination

- **(1) PDA**
  - **(a)** Dogs may be asymptomatic or present with signs of congestive heart failure.
  - **(b)** Because the shunt is extracardiac, blood flow continues throughout the cardiac cycle, generating a murmur during both systole and diastole (i.e., a continuous or **"machinery" murmur**). This murmur is very suggestive of a PDA.
    - **(i)** It is **loudest on the left side.** Because it is occasionally restricted to the left heart base, it may be overlooked if only the apex is ausculted.
    - **(ii)** A **precordial thrill** often accompanies the murmur.
  - **(c)** Rapid diastolic pressure runoff in the arterial system leads to a large pulse pressure differential and results in a hyperkinetic or **"water-hammer"** pulse.
- **(2) Reverse PDA**
  - **(a)** Because a PDA is distal to the carotid arteries, admixture of unoxygenated blood occurs after the exit of the carotid arteries from the aorta, giving rise to **differential cyanosis** (i.e., normal or pink oral mucous membranes and cyanotic membranes elsewhere). Reversed intracardiac shunts (e.g., those seen in tetralogy of Fallot) are associated with cyanosis in all mucous membranes.
  - **(b)** **Hyperviscosity** (due to hypoxia-mediated polycythemia) may reduce the intensity of, or entirely abolish, the murmur.
  - **(c)** A **loud** or **split** S_2 can be associated with pulmonary hypertension.

b. Radiographic findings

- **(1) PDA**
  - **(a)** Pulmonary overcirculation and mild to moderate left atrial and ventricular enlargement are characteristic.
  - **(b)** On the DV view, a triad of bulges at the 1, 2, and 3 o'clock positions representing the pulmonary trunk, aorta, and left auricle, respectively, may be observed in some animals.
  - **(c)** Pulmonary congestion and edema may be detected if congestive heart failure has developed.
- **(2) Reverse PDA.** The development of pulmonary hypertension is usually associated with right ventricular enlargement, dilation of the main pulmonary trunk, and widened and tortuous pulmonary arteries. Left ventricular enlargement may be observed as well.

c. Echocardiographic findings

- **(1) PDA.** Left atrial and ventricular dilation are characteristic. The presence of a shunt can usually be documented using Doppler studies.
- **(2) Reverse PDA.** Right ventricular hypertrophy is usually visible.

d. Electrocardiographic findings
  (1) **PDA.** Findings are consistent with left-sided heart enlargement (i.e., increased R wave amplitude, increased QRS duration, P mitrale, and left axis deviation). Deep Q waves may be present in leads II, III, and aVF. Atrial and ventricular arrhythmias may accompany congestive heart failure.
  (2) **Reverse PDA.** The ECG usually shows signs of right ventricular, and possibly, right atrial enlargement.
e. Cardiac catheterization is rarely necessary to demonstrate the defect but may be indicated if more than one defect is suspected.

5. **Therapy**
  a. **PDA. Surgical ligation** of the shunt as soon as possible (usually when the animal is between 2–4 months of age) is the preferred treatment.
    (1) Dogs that have developed congestive heart failure should be stabilized (e.g., furosemide, cage rest, reduced-salt diet, possibly digoxin) before surgery.
    (2) If advanced failure or atrial fibrillation is present, the anesthetic risk is high.
  b. **Reverse PDA.** Treatment is limited to **exercise restriction** and **phlebotomy** as needed to maintain the packed cell volume (PCV) at 55%–65%.
    (1) **Surgery is contraindicated.** Closure of the ductus in this situation will result in acute right ventricular failure and death.
    (2) Most arterial dilators work on systemic, but not pulmonary, vessels. Therefore, the use of arterial vasodilators to ameliorate pulmonary hypertension is not very successful, and systemic hypotension is a potential side effect.

6. **Prognosis**
  a. **Treated PDA.** The prognosis is very good in uncomplicated cases (i.e., those that have not progressed to heart failure) treated with surgical ligation.
    (1) The surgical mortality rate in uncomplicated cases is usually less than 8%.
    (2) Dogs that have undergone successful surgery for PDA will have a lifespan close to that of normal dogs.
    (3) Recanulation of the ductus occurs in approximately 2% of cases.
  b. **Untreated PDA.** If the PDA is left untreated, approximately 60% of dogs will die within the first year of life. Occasionally, untreated dogs will survive longer than 10 years.
  c. **Reverse PDA.** The prognosis for animals with reverse PDA is poor.

C. SAS

1. **Signalment.** The condition is inherited in Newfoundland dogs. Breeds that are predisposed include golden retrievers, German shepherds, boxers, bull terriers, and in some areas, rottweillers, Samoyeds, and Great Danes.

2. **Pathogenesis**
  a. In **dogs,** SAS usually results from a **subvalvular fibrous ring** in the left ventricular outflow tract. In **cats,** the stenosis is **supravalvular.**
  b. The impediment to blood ejection results in **pressure overload-induced left ventricular (concentric) hypertrophy.**
    (1) The increased ventricular wall thickness, decreased capillary density, and increased wall tension contribute to the development of **myocardial hypoxia,** which predisposes the animal to **ventricular arrhythmias.** The reasonably high incidence of sudden death in SAS is related to fatal arrhythmias.
    (2) Left ventricular hypertrophy **may interfere with diastolic filling** or result in **AV valve insufficiency.** These factors plus arrhythmias may all contribute to the development of congestive heart failure. Animals with SAS are at **increased risk for bacterial endocarditis** of the aortic valve.

3. **Diagnosis**
  a. **Clinical signs.** Dogs may be asymptomatic, or they may exhibit exercise intolerance, syncope, or other signs of congestive heart failure. Sudden death may be the first sign.

    b. Physical examination. All dogs have a **systolic, ejection-type murmur heard loudest over the aortic valve.** Femoral pulses are often weak.

    c. Radiographic findings. Left ventricular enlargement and poststenotic dilation of the ascending aorta are observed; the degree corresponds to the severity of the stenosis. Left atrial enlargement may be present if mitral valve incompetence complicates the condition.

    d. Echocardiographic findings

        (1) Varying degrees of left ventricular hypertrophy and dilation of the ascending aorta are observed.

        (2) A fibrous subvalvular ring may be detected.

        (3) Mitral or aortic valve insufficiency and left atrial dilation may be documented.

        (4) Doppler examination can estimate the pressure gradient across the stenosis based on blood flow velocity through the defect.

    e. Electrocardiographic findings. The ECG may be unremarkable. Signs of left ventricular enlargement (i.e., increased R wave amplitude, left axis deviation) may be present. Ventricular or supraventricular arrhythmias may be detected.

4. Therapy

    a. Mild SAS (i.e., that characterized by a pressure gradient less than 30 mm Hg) does not require treatment; however, these dogs should not be bred.

    b. Severe SAS is characterized by gradients that exceed 100 mm Hg.

        (1) Surgery or **balloon catheter dilation** is required. Surgery carries a high mortality rate and therefore is not frequently performed.

        (2) Administration of *β*-adrenergic blockers may reduce the incidence of arrhythmias.

        (3) Congestive heart failure should be treated as discussed in II E.

        (4) Prophylactic antibiotics should be administered when warranted (e.g., prior to dental procedures) because of the risk of bacterial endocarditis.

5. Prognosis. Dogs with minimal left ventricular hypertrophy, a mild degree of stenosis, and a pressure gradient less than 75 mm Hg will likely live a normal lifespan. Dogs with gradients greater than 125 mm Hg will usually develop congestive heart failure (especially if mitral incompetence is present) or die suddenly.

D. Pulmonic stenosis

1. Signalment. Pulmonic stenosis is more common in small breed dogs (especially fox terriers, miniature schnauzers, and Chihuahuas), but English bulldogs, beagles, Samoyeds, Labrador retrievers, mastiffs, Newfoundlands, and basset hounds may be affected as well.

2. Pathophysiology. Pulmonic stenosis usually results from **dysplastic changes in the pulmonic valve** (i.e., thickening and partial fusion of valve cusps and hypoplasia of valve annulus). Sequelae depend on the severity of the stenosis and are similar to those seen with SAS, except that the right side is affected.

    a. Right ventricular hypertrophy develops, frequently accompanied by **tricuspid valve insufficiency** and **right atrial dilation.**

    b. These changes predispose to the development of **right-sided congestive heart failure.**

3. Diagnosis

    a. Clinical signs. Animals may be asymptomatic, or they may be presented for exercise intolerance or syncope.

    b. Physical examination

        (1) Heart sounds. A **systolic ejection murmur** is heard high on the left heart base and may be accompanied by a **palpable precordial thrill.** A **split S$_2$,** which represents delayed closure of the pulmonic valve, may be heard. A **systolic murmur associated with tricuspid insufficiency** may also be present.

        (2) Femoral pulses are usually near normal.
        (3) If right-sided heart failure is present, **jugular venous distention** with **abnormal pulsation** may be evident.
    c. Radiographic findings can include right atrial and ventricular enlargement, enlargement of the main pulmonary artery segment (i.e., poststenotic dilation), and decreased pulmonary vascularity.
    d. Echocardiographic findings
        (1) Right ventricular hypertrophy and **dilation and flattening of the interventricular septum** (as a result of the increased right ventricular pressure) are evident.
        (2) If the stenosis is valvular, **thickened** and **immobile valve cusps** may be observed in addition to a poststenotic dilation of the main pulmonary artery.
        (3) Doppler examination can determine the pressure gradient across the stenotic area.
    e. Electrocardiographic findings are consistent with right ventricular enlargement (i.e., deep S waves in leads I, II, and III; right axis deviation; possibly P pulmonale). Arrhythmias are uncommon.

4. Therapy
    a. Mild cases. Animals with mild pressure gradients (i.e., less than 30 mm Hg) do not require treatment.
    b. Severe cases. Animals with gradients that exceed 70–100 mm Hg and that exhibit significant cardiac changes are candidates for either surgery (i.e., **patch graft, valvulotomy, conduit**) or **balloon valvuloplasty.** The degree of subvalvular muscular hypertrophy that may accompany valvular stenosis and contribute to the ventricular outflow obstruction affects the choice of procedure. If congestive heart failure is present, appropriate therapy is indicated (see II E).

5. Prognosis
    a. Animals with mild stenosis may have a normal lifespan without therapy.
    b. Those with severe stenosis that is not treated usually die within a few years of diagnosis from congestive heart failure or sudden death.
    c. There is little information on the long-term survival of animals treated surgically or with balloon valvuloplasty.

E. **Ventricular septal defects** usually occur high in the interventricular septum (i.e., in the membranous area) and vary in size. They may occur alone, in conjunction with other cardiac defects (e.g., PDA) or as part of a complex anomaly (e.g., tetralogy of Fallot).

1. Signalment
    a. Ventricular septal defect is one of the most common congenital cardiac defects in cats and may be part of an endocardial cushion defect.
    b. Ventricular septal defect is inherited in keeshonds. English bulldogs, English springer spaniels, and West Highland white terriers are predisposed.

2. Pathophysiology. The pathophysiology is similar to that of PDA. Left-to-right shunting of blood results in volume overload of the pulmonary circulation, left atrium, and left ventricle.
    a. If **left-sided congestive heart failure** develops, it frequently does so before the animal reaches 4 months of age. Biventricular congestive heart failure is not uncommon in cats with moderate to severe defects.
    b. If **pulmonary hypertension** develops or another anomaly such as pulmonic stenosis increases ventricular outflow resistance, right ventricular hypertrophy may increase right ventricular pressure enough to result in **right-to-left shunting.**

3. Diagnosis
    a. Clinical signs may not be evident with small defects, whereas larger defects may produce signs of left-sided congestive heart failure (e.g., exercise intolerance, coughing). Signs associated with right-to-left shunting [see V B 4 a (2)] may be present.
    b. Physical examination

    (1) A **harsh, holosystolic murmur** is typically heard **over the right sternal border** (second to fourth intercostal space).

    (2) Additional murmurs may be heard over the pulmonic or aortic valves.

        (a) **Murmurs over the pulmonic valve** are systolic and indicative of functional pulmonic stenosis as a result of volume overload.

        (b) **Murmurs over the aortic valve** are diastolic and indicative of aortic insufficiency as a result of aortic valve cuff instability.

  c. **Radiographic findings** may be normal. If the shunt is large enough, enlargement of the left atrium and ventricle and main pulmonary artery (as a result of functional pulmonic stenosis) as well as pulmonary overcirculation may be apparent. Right ventricular enlargement may be visible if pulmonary hypertension develops.

  d. **Echocardiographic findings** typically include left atrial and ventricular dilation and absence of the interventricular septum, usually in the membranous portion. Doppler examination helps to confirm shunting of blood though this area.

  e. **Electrocardiographic findings** may be normal or reveal left atrial enlargement or left, right, or biventricular enlargement. There may be evidence of a right bundle branch block.

4. Therapy

  a. **Small defects.** Animals with small ventricular septal defects usually require no therapy. Small defects may spontaneously close within the first 2 years of life.

  b. **Moderate to severe defects.** Therapy for dogs with moderate to severe defects includes **pulmonary artery banding** (to increase right ventricular pressure and decrease the degree of left-to-right shunting) and **surgical closure of the defect.**

    (1) Surgical closure requires **open heart surgery,** which is not widely available.

    (2) **Both banding and surgical correction are contraindicated if right-to-left shunting has developed.**

5. Prognosis

  a. A normal lifespan can be expected for animals with small ventricular septal defects. The outlook is also good for animals that have undergone surgery to repair the defect.

  b. The development of congestive heart failure or right-to-left shunting is associated with a poor prognosis.

F. **Atrial septal defects** occur in the interatrial septum and are often associated with other cardiac defects (e.g., mitral valve insufficiency).

1. Pathophysiology. The defect usually occurs high in the septum in dogs and lower in cats. Blood shunts from left to right and results in volume overload of the right atrium, ventricle, and pulmonary arteries. The development of pulmonary hypertension or the coexistence of pulmonic stenosis may result in right-to-left shunting and cyanosis.

2. Diagnosis

  a. **Clinical signs.** Historical signs may be few and nonspecific. Signs of heart failure may be evident.

  b. **Physical examination**

    (1) A **soft systolic murmur** is usually present **over the pulmonic and tricuspid valves** and the S_2 **is often split.**

    (2) A **systolic murmur** caused by functional pulmonic stenosis (related to volume overload) may be heard over the **left heart base.**

    (3) Occasionally, a **soft diastolic murmur over the right hemithorax** is caused by functional tricuspid stenosis related to volume overload.

  c. **Radiographic findings.** With severe shunts, **right-sided enlargement** (with or without pulmonary artery dilation) and **pulmonary overcirculation** are seen. The left side of the heart is usually normal unless another defect (e.g., mitral insufficiency) is present.

  d. **Echocardiographic findings.** Right atrial and ventricular dilation and the septal defect are usually observed. Doppler examination will help verify the presence of a shunt.

e. Electrocardiographic findings. The ECG may be normal. P pulmonale is indicative of right atrial enlargement. Deep S waves in leads I, II, and III and right axis deviation are indicative of right ventricular enlargement.

3. Therapy. Surgical correction of the defect can be considered in animals with large shunts, but open heart surgery is required.

4. Prognosis is variable and depends on the size of defect and the presence of other cardiac defects, congestive heart failure, or pulmonary hypertension (right-to-left shunting).

G. Mitral valve dysplasia

1. Signalment. Large breed dogs (e.g., Great Danes, German shepherds, and bull terriers) are predisposed. Mitral valve dysplasia is a reasonably common congenital defect in cats.

2. Etiology. Mitral valve dysplasia may result from elongated or shortened chordae tendineae, attachment of a valve cusp to a papillary muscle, upwardly displaced papillary muscles, cleft or shortened valve cusps, or dilation of the mitral valve annulus.

3. Pathophysiology. The pathophysiologic sequelae are identical to those of severe acquired mitral valve insufficiency (see III A 2).

4. Diagnosis. The clinical, electrocardiographic, radiographic, and echocardiographic findings are identical to those of acquired mitral insufficiency (see III A 3).

5. Therapy is identical to that for acquired mitral insufficiency (see III A 4).

6. Prognosis. The prognosis is poor for animals with clinical signs of heart failure. Animals with mild mitral insufficiency without clinical signs of failure may survive for several years.

H. Tricuspid valve dysplasia

1. Signalment. Male Old English sheepdogs, German shepherds, weimaraners, and Labrador retrievers are more commonly affected than other breeds.

2. Pathophysiology. The structural abnormalities associated with tricuspid valve dysplasia are similar to those observed with mitral valve dysplasia. In addition, fusion of the papillary muscles, patent foramen ovale, atrial septal defect, and fibrinous epicarditis over the dilated right atrium have been documented. Tricuspid valve incompetence leads to progressive increases in the end-diastolic right atrial and ventricular pressures, leading to the eventual development of right-sided congestive heart failure.

3. Diagnosis
   a. Clinical signs include exercise intolerance, dyspnea, and weight loss.
   b. Physical examination. A **holosystolic murmur** is heard **over the tricuspid area.** Ascites and jugular venous distention may be evident.
   c. Radiographic findings. Right atrial and ventricular enlargement are usually seen and if heart failure is present, pleural effusion, ascites, hepatomegaly, and distention of the caudal vena cava may also be present.
   d. Echocardiography reveals right atrial and ventricular dilation. A malformed tricuspid valve may be visualized. The severity of insufficiency can be assessed by Doppler examination.
   e. Electrocardiographic findings. Atrial arrhythmias (especially atrial fibrillation) are common. Signs of right atrial and ventricular enlargement and ventricular conduction disturbances (i.e., bundle branch blocks) may be observed.

4. Therapy is focused on managing the congestive heart failure and any arrhythmias that should develop. Periodic thoracentesis may also benefit some patients if pleural fluid accumulation is unresponsive to diuretic and dietary therapy.

5. Prognosis. In general, the prognosis is poor but some patients may remain asymptomatic or have reasonably well controlled heart failure for years.

I. **Tetralogy of Fallot** consists of ventricular septal defect, pulmonic stenosis, right ventricular hypertrophy, and dextropositioning (i.e., overriding) of the aorta.

1. **Signalment.** Tetralogy of Fallot is inherited in keeshonds and occurs more commonly in English bulldogs, miniature poodles, miniature schnauzers, and wire-haired fox terriers.

2. **Pathophysiology.** The pulmonic stenosis and resultant right ventricular hypertrophy lead to increased right ventricular pressure and right-to-left shunting through the ventricular septal defect. Admixture of unoxygenated blood with the systemic arterial circulation results in varying degrees of hypoxemia and cyanosis. Polycythemia can result from hypoxemia-stimulated erythropoietin release from the kidney. When the PCV is greater than 65%, blood viscosity increases and may result in microvascular sludging, poor tissue oxygen delivery, intravascular thrombosis, stroke, seizures, hemorrhage, or, rarely, arrhythmias.

3. **Diagnosis**
   a. **Clinical signs** include poor growth, exercise intolerance, cyanosis, syncope, and seizures. **Cyanosis,** which is visible on all mucous membranes, may not be present at rest but can usually be induced with mild exercise.
   b. **Physical examination.** A systolic murmur associated with pulmonic stenosis may be heard over the left heart base. A systolic murmur associated with the ventricular septal defect will be heard over the right sternal border. A precordial thrill may be palpated over either area. Hyperviscosity may reduce the intensity of the murmur to an inaudible level.
   c. **Radiographic findings.** Variable right heart enlargement with pulmonary under-circulation is often observed.
   d. **Echocardiographic findings.** Anomalies associated with tetralogy of Fallot (e.g., right ventricular hypertrophy, malpositioning of the aorta, ventricular septal defect, pulmonary stenosis) are usually detectable. Doppler examination can help confirm the presence of a shunt and its directional flow.
   e. **Electrocardiographic findings.** Signs of right ventricular enlargement are usually present. Arrhythmias are uncommon.

4. **Treatment**
   a. **Definitive correction** of all the defects **requires open heart surgery** and is rarely performed in dogs and cats.
   b. **Palliative surgical techniques.** Anastomosis of the subclavian artery or ascending aorta to the pulmonary artery increases pulmonary blood flow, thereby increasing the amount of oxygenated blood entering the systemic circulation by creating a left-to-right shunt.
   c. **Phlebotomy.** If polycythemia is present, periodic phlebotomy may be required to maintain the PCV at 55%–65%. Care should be taken not to reduce the PCV any further because tissue oxygen delivery may be compromised in these animals.
   d. **β-adrenergic blockade** (e.g., with propranolol) may benefit some animals by decreasing dynamic right ventricular outflow obstruction and increasing peripheral vascular resistance (which may decrease the magnitude of right-to-left shunting).

5. **Prognosis.** Outcome depends primarily on the severity of the pulmonic stenosis and polycythemia.
   a. Mildly affected animals or those with a successful palliative surgery may live 4–7 years.
   b. Many animals succumb to the effects of hypoxemia and polycythemia or experience sudden death. Occasionally, congestive heart failure develops.

J. **Vascular ring anomalies** are malformations of the large vessels over the heart base. They become clinically significant if they entrap the esophagus as it passes over the heart base. In dogs, the most common anomaly of this type is **persistent right aortic arch (PRAA).** Other vascular ring anomalies include **double aortic arch, left aortic arch with right-sided ligamentum arteriosum,** and **anomalies associated with retroesophageal subclavian arteries.** Vascular ring anomalies are very rare in cats.

1. **Signalment.** PRAA may be more common in German shepherds, Great Danes, and Irish setters, but any breed can be affected.

2. **Pathophysiology.** In PRAA, the esophagus is encircled by the PRAA dorsally and to the right, by the ligamentum arteriosum to the left, and by the heart base ventrally. Constriction of the esophagus leads to frequent regurgitation, poor growth, and, possibly, the development of aspiration pneumonia.

3. **Diagnosis**
   a. **Clinical signs. Regurgitation** is the **hallmark sign** and usually begins shortly after weaning. Aspiration pneumonia is evidenced by fever, tachypnea, dyspnea, and coughing.
   b. **Radiographic findings**
      (1) A **dilated esophagus** is visualized **cranial to the heart base.** Occasionally, esophageal dilation extends caudal to the heart.
      (2) Barium studies document an area of **esophageal constriction over the heart base.**
      (3) A **bronchoalveolar pattern** in dependent lobes, with or without consolidation, may be visible if pneumonia has developed.

4. **Therapy.** In PRAA, **surgical division of the ligamentum arteriosum** relieves the esophageal constriction. (Division of a vessel is usually required in most other anomalies.)
   a. If surgery is performed soon after recognition of clinical signs, esophageal motility has a greater chance of returning to normal.
   b. Medical management of the esophageal disease before or after surgery entails frequent feedings of small portions of semisolid or liquid food from an elevated position.

5. **Prognosis.** The prognosis for animals with PRAA is generally good, but long-term success depends on esophageal function. Some dogs experience persistent regurgitation after surgical treatment.

VI. HEARTWORM DISEASE

A. **Canine heartworm disease**

1. **Introduction**
   a. **Incidence and transmission**
      (1) **Incidence** varies with geographic region.
         (a) In the United States, infection rates of up to 45% have been reported along the Atlantic and Gulf coasts and along the Mississippi river and its tributaries. Infection rates of approximately 5% are reported for most of the remainder of the continental United States and parts of southern Canada.
         (b) Endemic areas also exist in Australia and Japan.
      (2) **Transmission.** Female mosquitoes of several different species act as the intermediate host for *Dirofilaria immitis* and are infected after a blood meal is taken from a dog with circulating microfilaria (larval stage L_1). Transmission of heartworm in an area is governed by the length and timing of the mosquito season; however, transmission still declines between December and February in areas of the continental United States with a year-round mosquito season.
   b. **Life cycle of *D. immitis***

    (1) L$_1$ larvae ingested by a mosquito reach the L$_3$ stage within 2–2.5 weeks and are transmitted to dogs via mosquito bites.

    (2) The L$_3$ larvae enter the bite wound, migrate through body tissues, and develop into L$_5$ larvae in approximately 100 days. The L$_5$ larvae then enter the vascular system and migrate to the pulmonary artery.

    (3) After gaining access to the pulmonary artery, the L$_5$ larvae mature, releasing microfilaria (L$_1$ larvae) into the bloodstream.

        (a) The **prepatent period** (i.e., the time from infection to the appearance of circulating microfilaria) is approximately 6 months

        (b) The number of circulating microfilaria increases during the next 6 months and then declines.

  c. Occult heartworm disease refers to the presence of adult heartworms without circulating microfilaria. It is estimated that 57%–85% of occult infections result from prepatent or unisex infections; other causes include drug-induced sterilization of adult worms and immune-mediated removal of microfilaria.

    (1) The overall incidence of occult infection varies by region and ranges from 5%–67%.

    (2) Occult disease has been associated with some of the most severe manifestations of heartworm infection. Complications are related to long-standing undetected infection (which can lead to severe pulmonary artery disease and right-sided heart failure) and pulmonary inflammation associated with immune-mediated microfilaria removal [see VI A 5 b].

2. Pathophysiology. Heartworm infection is primarily a disease of the pulmonary arterial vasculature and is the most common cause of pulmonary hypertension in dogs. The severity of disease is related to the number of worms present, the duration of the infection, and the host response.

  a. The presence of adult heartworms in the pulmonary arteries causes **endothelial sloughing.** Aggregation of platelets and leukocytes and the release of growth factors results in proliferation of arterial smooth muscle cells and the development of **villous hypertrophy** on endothelial surfaces.

  b. The combination of villous hypertrophy and the obstruction by worms can severely impede blood flow in the smaller arterioles. If worm burdens are high or if the inflammatory reaction (in the lungs) is severe, **pulmonary hypertension** develops.

    (1) As a result of increased pressure, the **pulmonary arteries become dilated and tortuous,** especially in the caudal and accessory lobes.

    (2) The increased afterload induces **right ventricular hypertrophy,** which may progress to **myocardial failure** and **right-sided congestive heart failure.**

3. Diagnosis

  a. Signalment. Large breed, male, outdoor dogs that have not been receiving prophylactic treatment are most commonly affected. The average age at diagnosis is 4–8 years.

  b. Clinical signs. Dogs may be asymptomatic or exhibit signs of severe pulmonary disease (e.g., mild paroxysmal to severe coughing, exercise intolerance, dyspnea, hemoptysis), right-sided congestive heart failure (e.g., exercise intolerance, syncope, weight loss), or both.

    (1) Asymptomatic infection is more common with infections of short duration.

    (2) Severe disease is a consequence of long-standing infection and is more likely in dogs with occult infection or those who have not been tested for several years, if ever.

  c. Physical examination

    (1) Moist crackles can be heard in dogs with severe pulmonary arterial pathology.

    (2) If right-sided congestive heart failure has developed, ascites, hepatomegaly, jugular venous distention, and a gallop rhythm may be detected.

    (3) Splitting of the S$_2$ may accompany pulmonary hypertension. Occasionally, a systolic murmur associated with tricuspid insufficiency (related to pulmonary hypertension or right-sided heart failure) may be heard.

    d. Laboratory findings. Diagnosis is made based on compatible clinical features and a positive result on any of the following laboratory tests.

      (1) Detection of circulating microfilaria. A negative result on either of the following tests does not rule out infection.

        (a) A **direct blood smear** may detect microfilaria in heavily infected dogs.

        (b) Concentration tests (e.g., the **modified Knott's** or **filter** tests) are capable of detecting microfilaria at much lower concentrations and are more sensitive than a direct blood smear.

          (i) If this test is negative, a heartworm antigen test [see VI A 3 d (2)] should be performed to rule out occult infection.

          (ii) All dogs should be tested using a concentration test prior to initiating prophylactic therapy, especially if diethylcarbamazine (DEC) is to be used.

          (iii) An animal will not test positive unless the adult heartworms have started to produce microfilaria (i.e., 6–6.5 months postinfection).

      (2) Heartworm antigen tests detect adult heartworm antigen in serum. Antigen is primarily derived from female worms (especially gravid ones).

        (a) Animals will not test positive until approximately 7 months postinfection.

        (b) Heartworm antigen tests are very specific and false-positive tests are rare. False-negative results are infrequent (less than 5%) but may occur if:

          (i) Only immature worms (i.e., those younger than 7 months old) are present

          (ii) The number of worms is small

          (iii) No gravid female worms are present

    e. Radiographic findings

      (1) The caudal lobar pulmonary arteries (visualized best on a DV projection) are most affected. In severe infection, the arteries are dilated, tortuous, and peripherally blunted.

      (2) Right-sided heart enlargement and **dilation of the main pulmonary artery** may also be observed. The combination of these findings with **dilated, tortuous caudal lobar pulmonary arteries** is very characteristic (some say pathognomonic) of heartworm infection.

    f. Echocardiographic findings may include variable right ventricular dilation and reduced contractility (with or without interventricular septal thickening and flattening), right atrial enlargement, pulmonic valve insufficiency, and enlargement of the main pulmonary artery. If the infection is severe, worms may be observed in the main pulmonary artery and right ventricle.

    g. Electrocardiographic findings. In most dogs, the ECG is normal. Features of right ventricular enlargement may be present in dogs with severe pulmonary hypertension. Atrial arrhythmias are uncommon but may occur in dogs with marked right atrial enlargement.

  4. Therapy

    a. Adulticide therapy (asymptomatic dogs)

      (1) Thiacetarsamide, an arsenical, is administered via a peripheral vein every 8–12 hours for four treatments, using either a butterfly or an indwelling catheter. Before each thiacetarsamide injection, a physical examination should be performed, the animal should be fed (30–60 minutes prior) to observe appetite, and the urine should be checked for bilirubinuria.

        (a) Side effects of thiacetarsamide include **tissue necrosis** and **sloughing** (if extravasation of the drug occurs) and **hepatotoxicity.** If hepatotoxicity (e.g., bilirubinuria, icterus) develops, treatment should be stopped and the animal should be given supportive care for 1 month. If the animal is healthy when reevaluated 4 weeks later, adulticide treatment is repeated. Few dogs develop toxicity on the second treatment.

(b) Indications to stop thiacetarsamide therapy include persistent vomiting, lethargy, and anorexia or the development of icterus, marked bilirubinuria, or azotemia.

(c) Drug interactions. Concurrent use of glucocorticoids will decrease the worm kill.

(2) Melarsamine dihydrochloride has shown superior efficacy and fewer side effects and is easier to administer than thiacetarsamide.

b. Microfilaricide therapy is initiated 4–6 weeks after adulticide therapy. Although not approved for this use, **ivermectin** and **milbemycin** are used as microfilaricides.

(1) Potentially fatal side effects may be observed in collies following the use of either drug.

(2) Side effects in other dogs are uncommon (less than 5%) and seem to be more likely when high concentrations of microfilaria are present.

(a) Signs usually appear within 2 hours of treatment and consist of vomiting and lethargy. In rare instances, shock (evidenced by pale mucous membranes, tachycardia, and tachypnea) may occur. With appropriate treatment (i.e. intravenous fluids, glucocorticoids), death is an infrequent occurrence.

(b) Occasionally, anorexia and lethargy may occur 2 days after microfilaricide treatment.

c. Confirmation of treatment success

(1) Microfilaria concentration testing should be performed 3 weeks after microfilaricide therapy. If positive, ivermectin treatment is repeated. If negative, prophylactic therapy is initiated.

(2) A **heartworm antigen test** should be performed 3 months after adulticide therapy to confirm removal of adult parasites.

d. Complications of adulticide therapy. Post-adulticide thromboembolic lung disease is potentially life threatening and occurs most often in dogs with moderate to severe pulmonary arterial disease.

(1) Pathogenesis. Fragments of dead worms shower the pulmonary vasculature and block the small arteries, reducing perfusion to affected lobes (especially the caudal lobes) and inducing granulomatous inflammation, villous hypertrophy, and lung lobe consolidation.

(a) Ventilation–perfusion mismatching can be severe.

(b) Pulmonary arterial resistance can increase dramatically and induce **right-sided heart failure.**

(2) Diagnosis

(a) Clinical signs usually occur 1–3 weeks after adulticide administration and include fever, severe coughing, tachypnea, dyspnea, hemoptysis, tachycardia, and pale mucous membranes.

(b) Radiographic findings include patchy areas of alveolar infiltrate and air bronchograms, mostly in the caudal lobes.

(c) Laboratory findings. Thrombocytopenia, prolonged clotting times, and increased amounts of fibrin degradation products are indicative of low-grade DIC.

(3) Therapy consists of strict cage rest, corticosteroids, supplemental oxygen, and possibly bronchodilators. Heparin should be administered if low-grade DIC is present. Aspirin is beneficial (although heparin may be superior) and can be administered for 2–4 weeks if significant thrombocytopenia is not present.

5. Complicated heartworm infection

a. Severe pulmonary arterial disease is associated with enlarged and tortuous pulmonary arteries. Seventy percent of affected dogs have occult disease.

(1) Pathogenesis. Secondary parenchymal lung disease, right-sided congestive heart failure, hemolysis, hemoglobinuria, pulmonary hypertension, and pulmonary arteriolar obstruction (associated with platelet aggregation and consumption, fibrin deposition, and thromboembolism) can occur.

(2) Diagnosis. Clinical signs include coughing, exercise intolerance, weight loss, syncope, dyspnea, hemoptysis, audible pulmonary crackles, fever, and signs of right-sided congestive heart failure. Thrombocytopenia, low-grade DIC and an inflammatory leukogram may be present if significant thromboembolism has occurred.

(3) Therapy. If there is secondary parenchymal disease, a short course of corticosteroids should be administered to alleviate some of the clinical and radiographic signs. Because conventional treatment regimens (as outlined in VI A 4) are associated with a high mortality rate in animals with severe pulmonary artery disease (mostly as a result of marked thromboembolism caused by the death of a large number of adult worms), three alternative treatment regimens have been proposed:

(a) Surgical removal of the worms. Special alligator forceps are inserted into the pulmonary artery via the jugular vein using fluoroscopic guidance.

(b) Melarsamine dihydrochloride (RM 340). A reduced dose is administered to kill only a portion of the worm population.

(c) Prolonged cage confinement and aspirin. Aspirin is administered for 2–3 weeks before, during, and 3 weeks after thiacetarsamide administration. The use of heparin instead of aspirin has been associated with improved survival.

b. Allergic pneumonitis occurs in approximately 10%–15% of dogs with occult disease and is caused by immune-mediated removal of microfilaria.

(1) Pathogenesis. Antibody-mediated leukocyte adhesion to microfilaria results in their deposition in pulmonary capillaries. The ensuing inflammatory reaction is intensely eosinophilic.

(2) Diagnosis

(a) Clinical signs usually progress over weeks to months and are characterized by coughing and dyspnea.

(b) Physical examination. Crackles may be heard over the caudal lung lobes.

(c) Radiographic findings typically consist of diffuse, bilateral linear interstitial and alveolar infiltrates in the caudal lung lobes.

(d) Laboratory findings

(i) Eosinophilia and basophilia may be present.

(ii) Cytologic evaluation of transtracheal aspiration fluid reveals eosinophilic inflammation.

(iii) A heartworm antigen test is positive.

(3) Therapy consists of a short course (i.e., 3–5 days) of **corticosteroids,** which usually results in complete resolution of the radiographic and clinical abnormalities. Adulticide therapy should follow.

c. Caval syndrome results from very heavy worm burdens (i.e., greater than 75 to 100 worms) and is rare except in highly endemic heartworm areas.

(1) Pathogenesis. Ordinarily, most heartworms live in the pulmonary artery and right ventricle. When the number of worms is high, they move into the right atrium and vena cava, causing acute cardiovascular collapse, shock, icterus, intravascular hemolysis, and hemoglobinuria.

(2) Diagnosis. Dogs often present with acute collapse with no prior signs of heartworm infection. Findings relate to acute right-sided heart failure (weakness, tachypnea, dyspnea, pale mucous membranes, tricuspid murmur, jugular venous distention), intravascular hemolysis (regenerative anemia, hemoglobinuria), abnormal liver function (icterus), and DIC. The detection of worms by cardiac ultrasound provides a definitive diagnosis.

(3) Therapy consists of **surgical removal of the worms** via the jugular vein. The objective is to remove at least 50% of the worms, continuing until no more can be retrieved on repeated attempts.

(a) Supportive care and **treatment for DIC** (if present) are indicated.

> **(b)** **Adulticide therapy** can be initiated 2 weeks after recovery from the acute episode. Aspirin and cage rest are recommended before, and for 3–4 weeks following, adulticide therapy.
>
> **(4)** **Prognosis.** The survival rate is approximately 50% when animals are treated surgically by an experienced veterinarian.

> **d.** **Renal disease** associated with heartworm infection is usually caused by mild immune-complex glomerulonephritis. However, in some instances, glomerulonephritis is severe or amyloidosis may develop, both of which are associated with marked proteinuria. The nephrotic syndrome (with or without renal failure) may develop. Renal failure precludes adulticide therapy with thiacetarsamide.

6. Prognosis

  a. Asymptomatic dogs or those with only mild signs usually have an excellent prognosis.

  b. The prognosis is good for moderately affected dogs (i.e., those with mild to moderate exercise intolerance, frequent coughing, and radiographically detectable but not marked arterial changes).

  c. In those dogs with severe pulmonary artery disease or congestive heart failure, the mortality rate with standard therapy is 40%–60%. With modifications to treatment protocols [see VI A 5 a (3)], the mortality rate can be reduced to less than 20%.

7. Prevention

  a. **Routine screening** (using either a concentration or antigen test) is recommended in areas where heartworm infection is prevalent and prior to the administration of prophylactic treatment.

  (1) In areas with a year-round mosquito season, screening should be done in March and April and again in late summer.

  (2) In areas with a cold winter season, annual testing should occur in the spring before the onset of mosquito season.

  b. **Prophylaxis** is indicated for all dogs in an endemic area. All dogs should be free of microfilaria before starting prophylactic therapy.

  (1) **Agents.** Three agents are available for heartworm prevention.

  (a) **DEC** is administered daily. Potentially life-threatening reactions can occur if microfilaria are present.

  (b) **Ivermectin** is administered monthly and can usually be administered to dogs with circulating microfilaria without adverse effects. However, both ivermectin and milbemycin can cause iatrogenic occult heartworm disease because they will clear microfilaria within approximately 6 months at prophylactic doses.

  (c) **Milbemycin** is administered monthly. Adverse reactions may occur if milbemycin is administered to dogs with high numbers of microfilaria.

  (2) **Timing**

  (a) In areas with a cold winter climate, administration is initiated in the spring, 1 month before the onset of the mosquito season, and continued for 2 months after the first frost (usually about 6 months total).

  (b) In areas with a warm climate year-round, administration may continue all year. Prophylaxis may not be necessary in December and January in North America because transmission is minimal during these months.

B. **Feline heartworm disease**

1. Incidence. The regional occurrence of heartworm disease in cats parallels that of dogs but at a much lower infection rate. Cats appear to be more resistant to infection because they are infected with fewer, smaller, and shorter-lived adult worms as compared with dogs.

2. Pathophysiology. The pulmonary arterial changes that occur in response to heartworms in dogs are similar but exaggerated in cats. The incidence of acute pulmonary or neurologic disease is higher in cats.

3. **Diagnosis**
   a. **Signalment.** Male, outdoor cats 3–6 years of age are most frequently diagnosed.
   b. **Clinical signs.** Cats may be asymptomatic, experience sudden death, or present with acute or chronic signs.
      (1) **Acute signs.** Acute pulmonary disease and thromboembolism can cause coughing, dyspnea, and shock. Aberrant larval migration can produce CNS signs (e.g., seizures, dementia, blindness, ataxia).
      (2) **Chronic signs** relate to right-sided congestive heart failure caused by pulmonary hypertension or recurrent pulmonary disease characterized by eosinophilic infiltrates. Intermittent vomiting may be the only sign in some cats.
      (3) **Laboratory findings**
         (a) Eosinophilia is present in less than 33% of cats, and basophilia is even less common.
         (b) A nonregenerative anemia attributed to chronic disease develops in approximately 33% of cats.
         (c) A polyclonal gammopathy is detected in 33%–50% of cats.
         (d) Variable biochemical abnormalities associated with right-sided congestive heart failure may be evident (e.g., prerenal azotemia, mild to moderate liver enzyme elevation, electrolyte abnormalities).
         (e) **Detection of infection.** Most cats do not have circulating microfilaria at the time of diagnosis. The prepatent period is approximately 7 months, but the microfilaria produced disappear after 6–8 weeks.
            (i) **Adult antigen tests** used for dogs may be used for cats and are specific and reasonably sensitive. The test is usually not positive until 7–8 months postinfection. False-negative results may arise from low worm numbers or the absence of female or gravid female worms. False-positive results are extremely unlikely if the test is properly performed.
            (ii) **Antibody to heartworm antigen.** The detection of circulating antibody to heartworm antigen in cats is very sensitive and may be considered if other diagnostic tests are inconclusive. False-positive results can occur.
      (4) **Radiographic findings** are similar to those in dogs but are more difficult to detect and interpret in cats.
         (a) Caudal lobar arteries are prominent and may be blunted and tortuous.
         (b) Right ventricular enlargement and diffuse or focal pulmonary infiltrates may be observed.
         (c) Pleural effusion (transudate or pseudochylous) is seen more commonly in cats and is associated with right-sided heart failure.
      (5) **Echocardiographic findings.** A cardiac ultrasound examination may reveal worms in the pulmonary artery, right ventricle, right atrium, or vena cava. Right ventricular enlargement may be present if pulmonary hypertension is developing.
      (6) **Electrocardiographic findings.** The ECG is often normal. Signs of right ventricular enlargement may be seen in cats that develop pulmonary hypertension and right-sided heart failure.
      (7) **Nonselective angiography findings.** Nonselective angiography may be indicated for cats with mild or inconclusive radiographic findings, a negative antigen test, and no visible worms on cardiac ultrasound. The finding of dark, linear filling defects associated with the presence of worms confirms the diagnosis.

4. **Therapy**
   a. **Surgical removal of worms.** In cats with high worm numbers, surgical removal via the jugular vein could be considered.
   b. **Adulticide therapy.** The **use of thiacetarsamide in cats is controversial** because of the risk of peracute, potentially life-threatening adverse drug effects (i.e., acute, fulminant pulmonary edema) and the high incidence of severe post-

adulticide thromboembolic disease. The manifestations of post-adulticide thromboembolic disease are similar to those in dogs and are treated similarly.

(1) Infection may be self-limiting (because of the shorter life spans of worms in cats) and adulticide therapy may not be required in asymptomatic cats or those with mild clinical signs.

(2) Thiacetarsamide should probably be reserved for cats with persistent or severe clinical signs (e.g., pulmonary hypertension, congestive heart failure) when surgical removal cannot be performed.

(3) Cats occasionally develop an allergic pneumonitis similar to that seen in dogs and are treated with a short course of corticosteroids before adulticide therapy is considered.

   c. Microfilaricide therapy is unnecessary in cats because few have circulating microfilaria. Heartworm prophylaxis using either ivermectin or milbemycin should be considered for cats in endemic areas.

VII. **PERICARDIAL DISEASE** accounts for only 1% of cardiovascular disease in dogs and cats.

  Pericardial effusion is the most common pericardial disorder in dogs and cats.

1. **Etiology**
   a. **Transudative effusions** are associated with congestive heart failure, hypoalbuminemia, and peritoneopericardial hernias (see VII C).
   b. **Exudative effusions** can be caused by infectious agents or uremia, or they may be idiopathic. Feline infectious peritonitis (FIP) is the most common cause of pericardial effusion in cats.
   c. **Hemorrhagic effusions** are associated with neoplasia [e.g., **hemangiosarcoma,** chemodectoma (heart base tumor), lymphosarcoma], thoracic trauma, and left atrial rupture. They may also be **idiopathic.** Hemorrhagic effusion (either idiopathic or as a result of neoplasia) accounts for approximately 90% of the pericardial effusions diagnosed in dogs.

2. **Pathogenesis.** As fluid accumulates, the right side of the heart, which has a lower pressure and thinner walls, is easily compressed (i.e., cardiac tamponade occurs). Filling of the right atrium and ventricle is greatly reduced, producing central venous congestion, reduced cardiac output, and signs of right-sided heart failure.
   a. If fluid accumulation is slow, the pericardial sac can dilate to considerable size. Very large pericardial sacs may compress the lungs, main airways, or esophagus.
   b. High intrapericardial pressures may develop acutely (e.g., as the result of left atrial rupture). In this instance, only small volumes of fluid are required to elevate the intrapericardial pressure because the pericardial sac cannot dilate to accommodate the fluid and reduce pressure. Rapid accumulation of fluid leads to compression of the heart and reduced filling to the point where shock and death occur.

3. **Diagnosis**
   a. **Signalment.** Pericardial effusion is diagnosed most often in large breed dogs older than 5 years of age. **German shepherds** and **golden retrievers** are overrepresented because they are predisposed to hemangiosarcoma and idiopathic hemorrhagic pericardial effusion. **Brachycephalic breeds** are more prone to develop pericardial effusion from heart base tumors.
   b. **Clinical signs** of pericardial effusion will not become evident until the intrapericardial pressure equals or exceeds the cardiac filling pressure. Most dogs are presented because of exercise intolerance, weakness, abdominal distention from ascites, coughing, lethargy, or dyspnea.

    c. Physical examination. The combination of muffled heart sounds, weak femoral pulses, and signs of right-sided congestive heart failure is very suggestive of pericardial effusion.

        (1) Muffled heart sounds. Moderate to marked amounts of pericardial fluid will muffle heart sounds.

        (2) Decreased respiratory sounds. Pleural effusion may decrease respiratory sounds.

        (3) Weak pulses are common. **Pulsus paradoxus** (i.e., a decrease in pulse pressure during inspiration) is occasionally detected.

        (4) Tachypnea, tachycardia, pale mucous membranes, and **prolonged capillary refill times** are common.

    d. Laboratory findings. Abnormalities may reflect dehydration and poor renal perfusion or hepatic congestion. Dogs with hemangiosarcoma may have a regenerative anemia, schistocytosis, or thrombocytopenia. Hemorrhagic pericardial fluid from dogs with idiopathic or neoplastic disease usually is "port wine" in color and contains many erythrocytes and reactive mesothelial cells. It is very uncommon to identify exfoliated neoplastic cells in pericardial fluid.

    e. Radiographic findings. With the accumulation of moderate to marked amounts of pericardial fluid, the heart shadow takes on a globoid or rounded shape. The trachea may be elevated dorsally. Distention of the caudal vena cava, hepatomegaly, pleural effusion, and ascites may also be observed.

    f. Echocardiographic findings. Ultrasound examination is very sensitive; it can detect small volumes and confirm the presence of pericardial effusion.

        (1) An **echo-free (anechoic) area** is observed between the epicardium and pericardial sac.

        (2) Overall cardiac chamber size may be decreased as a result of reduced filling.

        (3) Collapse of the right atrium or **ventricle** indicates marked intrapericardial pressure elevation.

        (4) Cardiac or intrapericardial masses can be detected.

    g. Electrocardiographic findings that are suggestive of pericardial effusion include **decreased amplitude of the R wave (< 1 mV), ST segment elevation,** and **electrical alternans.**

4. Therapy

    a. Pericardiocentesis is the treatment of choice when significant amounts of pericardial fluid are present.

        (1) Fluid removal often brings about rapid resolution of the signs of right-sided heart failure.

        (2) Drainage of the pericardial sac is curative in 50% of dogs with idiopathic hemorrhagic effusion. Many clinicians advocate a 2- to 4-week course of glucocorticoids to help prevent recurrence of the effusion.

        (3) Pericardiocentesis is palliative when neoplasia is the cause of the effusion.

    b. Subtotal pericardectomy. If repeated removal of pericardial fluid fails to resolve the effusion in dogs with idiopathic disease, a subtotal pericardectomy often provides long-term relief. Subtotal pericardectomy may also be considered a palliative procedure in dogs with neoplastic effusions.

5. Prognosis

    a. Dogs with idiopathic hemorrhagic effusion generally have a good prognosis following pericardiocentesis or subtotal pericardectomy. Occasionally, dogs with long-standing idiopathic effusion may develop exuberant fibrosis within the pericardial sac, leading to constrictive pericardial disease.

    b. The prognosis is poor if the effusion is related to hemangiosarcoma because tumor metastasis has probably already occurred. If the effusion is related to a chemodectoma or another slow-growing neoplasm, a subtotal pericardectomy may provide palliative relief for many months to a few years.

B. **Constrictive pericardial disease** is a rare disease in both dogs and cats.

1. **Pathophysiology.** Thickening and fusion of the visceral and parietal pericardium can lead to obliteration of the pericardial space. Histologically, fibrous tissue proliferation with variable amounts of inflammatory cell infiltration is present. Right and left atrial and ventricular filling is restricted.

2. **Diagnosis**
   a. **Signalment.** Middle to large breed, male dogs are more likely to be affected. German shepherds may be predisposed.
   b. **Clinical signs** are related to right-sided congestive heart failure and are similar to those described with pericardial effusion.
   c. **Physical examination.** A diastolic pericardial knock (from the abrupt deceleration of the ventricle during filling) may be heard in some dogs.
   d. **Radiographic findings.** The heart shadow is moderately enlarged. Pleural effusion, distention of the caudal vena cava, hepatomegaly, and ascites may also be observed.
   e. **Echocardiographic findings.** An echodense, thickened pericardial sac, diminished cardiac chamber size, abnormal septal motion, and flattening of the left ventricular endocardium during diastole may be observed. It may be difficult to differentiate constrictive pericardial disease from restrictive cardiomyopathy.
   f. **Electrocardiographic findings** include diminished amplitude of the R waves and P mitrale.

3. **Therapy**
   a. **Surgical removal of the pericardial sac** is the treatment of choice. If the pericardial sac is the primary constricting structure, then the response to therapy should be good.
   b. **Epicardial stripping.** If there is extensive epicardial fibrosis, sac removal may not be beneficial and epicardial stripping may have to be considered. This procedure is associated with high morbidity and mortality rates.

C. **Peritoneopericardial diaphragmatic hernia (PDH)** is the **most common congenital malformation affecting the pericardium** in dogs and cats. Other congenital defects such as sternal malformations, umbilical hernias, and cardiac defects (e.g., ventricular septal defect) may accompany PDH.

1. **Pathogenesis.** An error in embryonic development results in a connection along the ventral floor of the thorax between the pericardial sac and peritoneal cavity, which allows the abdominal contents to herniate into the pericardial sac. Strangulation of the herniated contents can lead to shock and collapse. Cardiac tamponade occurs rarely.

2. **Diagnosis**
   a. **Clinical signs** are dictated by the amount of abdominal contents herniated into the pericardial sac. Signs may include vomiting, diarrhea, anorexia, weight loss, abdominal discomfort, cough, dyspnea, and wheezing.
   b. **Physical examination** may reveal muffled heart sounds (on one or both sides), displacement or absence of a precordial impulse, and an abdomen that feels "empty" (if some abdominal organs are herniated).
   c. **Radiographic findings** are usually characteristic and can include an enlarged cardiac silhouette, dorsal displacement of the trachea, overlap of the caudal cardiac silhouette and the diaphragmatic shadow, and bowel loops or abnormal fat or gas densities within the pericardial sac. The abdomen may appear relatively empty. Oral barium administration can help outline abnormally located bowel loops.
   d. **Echocardiographic findings.** Ultrasound can definitively identify abnormal pericardial contents.

3. **Therapy** entails **surgical closure of the hernia.**

4. **Prognosis** is good in uncomplicated cases.

VIII. **COR PULMONALE** is the development of right-sided heart disease (i.e. hypertrophy, dilation, or failure) as a consequence of pulmonary arterial hypertension induced by airway, pulmonary parenchymal, pulmonary vascular, or thoracic cage disease.

A. **Etiology**

1. **Acute cor pulmonale.** The most common cause of acute cor pulmonale is **pulmonary thromboembolism,** which can occur secondary to hypercoagulable states (e.g., hyperadrenocorticism, nephrotic syndrome) [see also Chapter 40 IV H].

2. **Chronic cor pulmonale** is usually caused by **heartworm disease** or **chronic obstructive pulmonary disease (COPD).**

B. **Pathophysiology.** There are two main routes to cor pulmonale.

1. **Reduced blood flow.** Pulmonary embolization can reduce blood flow to pulmonary vascular beds. The reduced blood flow, in addition to local hypoxia-induced vasoconstriction, leads to the development of pulmonary hypertension.
   a. If hypertension is of sufficient magnitude and duration, **right-sided heart failure** may develop (acutely or chronically).
   b. If a large cross-sectional area of pulmonary vasculature is blocked (e.g., by a main pulmonary artery thrombus or an embolic showering of a large number of smaller arteries), severe ventilation–perfusion mismatching leads to **marked systemic hypoxia.**

2. **Reduced airflow.** COPD can reduce airflow to regions of the lung, thereby inducing local hypoxic vasoconstriction. Hypercapnia and the development of local acidosis intensifies this vasoconstriction, leading to chronic pulmonary hypertension and the development of right-sided heart disease.

C. **Diagnosis**

1. **Clinical signs** include exercise intolerance, dyspnea, syncope, cyanosis, and other signs of right-sided heart failure. Clinical signs specific to the underlying disorder may also be apparent. Significant pulmonary thromboembolism can result in acute dyspnea and should be suspected in patients that are in a hypercoagulable state.

2. **Physical examination.** Auscultation of animals with pulmonary hypertension may reveal splitting of the S_2, a gallop rhythm, or a murmur of tricuspid insufficiency.

3. **Laboratory findings.** Systemic hypoxemia may be detected on blood gas analysis, especially if thromboembolism is the cause.

4. **Radiographic findings**
   a. **Acute cor pulmonale as a result of pulmonary thromboembolism.** The combination of dyspnea, hypoxia, and a **dearth of thoracic radiographic abnormalities** is indicative of main pulmonary artery thrombosis. **Selective or nonselective pulmonary angiography** can help confirm the presence of thromboembolism (i.e., filling defects in arteries, blunted arteries, reduced or absent opacification of pulmonary tissue).
   b. **Chronic cor pulmonale** will be accompanied by signs of **right ventricular enlargement.** The **thoracic radiographs** of animals with COPD may reveal **hyperinflation,** a **bronchointerstitial pattern,** or **bronchiectasis.**

5. **Echocardiographic findings** consistent with cor pulmonale include right atrial dilation, right ventricular hypertrophy, and paradoxical motion of the interventricular septum.

6. **Electrocardiographic findings.** Signs of right ventricular enlargement may be detected. Elevation or depression of the ST segment may occur if myocardial hypoxia is present.

D. **Therapy**

1. The major goal is to identify and **treat the underlying disorder.**
   a. **Right-sided heart failure** should be treated as outlined in II E.
   b. **Pulmonary thromboembolism.** The treatment of pulmonary thromboembolism (unrelated to heartworm) is difficult.
      (1) The use of **heparin** followed by **warfarin** to prevent additional thrombus growth is indicated, as is therapy for the underlying cause.
      (2) Definitive removal of the thrombus, either surgically or with thrombolytic agents, is rarely attempted in dogs and cats.
   c. **COPD.** Animals with COPD are treated with bronchodilators (e.g., terbutaline, aminophylline) to improve gas exchange and attenuate hypoxia-induced pulmonary vasoconstriction. Other measures include weight control, coupage, humidification, antitussives, antibiotics, and anti-inflammatory drugs (e.g., prednisone).

2. **Adjunctive therapy**
   a. **Hydralazine** may have some dilatory effect on pulmonary vasculature, but systemic hypotension may be a problem.
   b. **Supportive care** (e.g., cage rest, supplemental oxygen) may be necessary for severely affected animals.

E. **Prognosis**

1. The outlook for animals with cor pulmonale caused by thromboembolism depends on how much vascular obstruction is present and the nature and reversibility of the underlying disorder. The prognosis may range from poor to fair.

2. The long-term prognosis for animals with cor pulmonale caused by COPD is usually poor because the pulmonary disease is not readily reversed.

IX. MISCELLANEOUS DISORDERS AFFECTING THE HEART

A. **Neoplasia**

1. **Incidence**
   a. **Primary** tumors of the myocardium are rare. The only primary tumor that occurs with any frequency is **hemangiosarcoma,** which usually arises from the right atrium. German shepherd and German shepherd–crossbred dogs are affected more frequently than other breeds.
   b. **Secondary.** Many types of tumors may metastasize to the heart, but **hemangiosarcoma in dogs** and **lymphosarcoma in cats** are the most common.

2. **Pathogenesis.** Tumors may disrupt cardiac function by infiltrating the ventricular wall or obstructing ventricular in- or outflow. Cardiac tamponade or arrhythmias can result.

3. **Diagnosis**
   a. **Clinical signs** vary considerably, depending on the nature of the cardiac dysfunction. Signs may include those consistent with pericardial effusion (i.e., exercise intolerance, ascites, muffled heart sounds, weak pulses), right- or left-sided congestive heart failure, or arrhythmias (i.e., syncope, pulse deficits).
   b. **Radiographic findings.** A globoid heart shadow may be visualized if pericardial effusion is present. Mass lesions (e.g., right atrial hemangiosarcoma) may protrude from the cardiac silhouette.
   c. **Echocardiographic findings.** Ultrasound is very useful for identifying thickened areas, mass lesions, and pericardial effusion.
   d. **Electrocardiographic findings.** The ECG may reveal reduced complex size, atrial or ventricular arrhythmias, or conduction disturbances (e.g., bundle branch blocks, AV blocks).

4. Therapy. Tumors of the heart are rarely resectable.
   a. Pericardiocentesis may provide palliative relief from signs of right-sided heart failure.
   b. Chemotherapy. Chemoresponsive tumors (e.g., lymphosarcoma) may respond to treatment.
   c. Adjunctive therapy entails treating arrhythmias (although they tend to be resistant to therapy) and addressing the signs of congestive heart failure.

5. Prognosis. The prognosis is generally poor.

B. Infectious diseases

1. Borreliosis (Lyme's disease) is caused by the spirochete *Borrelia burgdorferi,* which is transmitted to dogs and humans by ticks of the *Ixodes* species.
   a. In dogs, borreliosis is primarily a disease of the joints, but occasionally, cardiac involvement occurs and most frequently results in AV block.
   b. Therapy requires **antibiotics** and is successful in most animals. A short course of **corticosteroids** may help resolve the heart block if antibiotics alone do not.

2. Trypanosomiasis (Chagas' disease) is caused by *Trypanosoma cruzi* and is a rare cause of heart disease in the southeastern United States.
   a. Pathogenesis. The organism directly infects the myocardium and causes acute right- or left-sided heart failure when the trypomastigotes rupture from the myocardial cells. If the animal survives, a chronic stage ensues where myocardial degeneration results in the development of dilated cardiomyopathy.
   b. Diagnosis. Clinical signs may include sudden death, anorexia, diarrhea, lymphadenopathy, and signs of right-sided or left-sided congestive heart failure. Diagnosis can be made by the identification of trypomastigotes on a blood film during the acute stage or by identification of antibodies during the chronic stage.
   c. Therapy with antiprotozoal agents is often unrewarding by the time clinical signs become established.

3. Parvovirus is an extremely rare cause of heart disease in dogs. Infection of puppies younger than 2 weeks of age that have no maternal antibodies can lead to viral myocarditis. Sudden death is common. If puppies survive the acute infection, most will die of either arrhythmias or dilated cardiomyopathy before they reach 1 year of age.

C. Toxins

1. Toad poisoning. Dogs and cats can be poisoned by ingesting or playing with either Colorado river toads (*Bufo alvaritus*) or marine toads (*Bufo marinus*). These toads secrete a digitalis-like toxin from their parotid glands that is quickly absorbed across the mucous membranes of animals. Coma and death can occur within 30 minutes.
   a. Diagnosis. Clinical signs appear within minutes and may include hypersalivation, vomiting, weakness, pulmonary edema, and seizures. The ECG will reveal atrial or ventricular arrhythmias, which may progress to ventricular fibrillation.
   b. Therapy. The animal's mouth should be rinsed thoroughly (atropine may help decrease hypersalivation). Propranolol is quite effective for tachyarrhythmias, and it may be necessary to administer anticonvulsants. Supportive care should be provided.

2. Chocolate poisoning. Tachycardia and ventricular arrhythmias result from catecholamine release induced by theobromine, an ingredient in chocolate. The LD_{50} is approximately 0.6 to 1.3 oz of dark (baking) chocolate/kg body weight.
   a. Diagnosis. Clinical signs include hyperactivity, diarrhea, muscle tremors, ataxia, hyperthermia, coma, and death.
   b. Therapy entails decreasing absorption and increasing excretion of the toxicant, treating arrhythmias, controlling seizures, and providing supportive care.

3. Doxorubicin toxicity. Doxorubicin is a chemotherapeutic drug used for the treatment of many different malignancies in dogs and cats. Chronic toxicity results in the development of dilated cardiomyopathy or arrhythmias, but usually occurs only if the cumulative dose has exceeded 240 mg/m². Arrhythmias may also occur during the intravenous administration of doxorubicin. Animals being treated with doxorubicin should be monitored electrocardiographically and echocardiographically.

X. CARDIAC ARRHYTHMIAS

A. **Introduction**

1. **Approach to arrhythmias**
   a. **What is the identity of the arrhythmia?** The ECG should be evaluated in a systematic fashion, as described in I B 2 b.
   b. **What is the cause of the arrhythmia?**
      (1) **Cardiac causes.** Any acquired cardiac disease may be associated with arrhythmias, but left atrial enlargement, cardiomyopathy, and trauma are particularly common causes. Breed-associated cardiac abnormalities that result in arrhythmias are summarized in Table 39-8.
      (2) **Noncardiac causes** include acidosis; alkalosis; electrolyte disturbances; hypoxia; excessive parasympathetic or sympathetic nervous system activity; respiratory, GI, or brain disease; drug toxicity; endocrinopathies; shock; hypothermia; sepsis; neoplasia; and mechanical stimulation.
   c. **Is the arrhythmia clinically significant?**
      (1) Is the arrhythmia associated with **clinical signs of reduced cardiac output?** Clinical signs usually observed include syncope, weakness, seizures, personality changes, or in rare instances, signs of congestive heart failure.
      (2) Is the arrhythmia **electrically unstable?** In other words, does the potential for the arrhythmia to progress to a more severe or lethal arrhythmia (e.g., ventricular fibrillation) exist? This is most often a concern with ventricular arrhythmias with characteristics such as very frequent VPCs, runs of VPCs, multifocal or multiform VPCs, or the presence of R on T events (i.e., a VPC occurring within the QT interval of a previous beat).

2. **General treatment principles**
   a. **Underlying causes** (e.g., electrolyte and acid–base abnormalities) **should be treated before therapy with antiarrhythmic agents is initiated,** unless the arrhythmia is associated with clinical signs or is electrically unstable.
   b. **Drugs with the potential to cause arrhythmias should be discontinued.** Examples include digoxin, xylazine, procainamide, quinidine, and acepromazine.

TABLE 39-8. Breed Predispositions to Arrhythmias

Abnormality	Predisposed Breeds
His bundle degeneration (second- and third-degree atrioventricular (AV) block	Doberman pinschers
Persistent atrial standstill	English springer spaniels
Sick sinus syndrome	Miniature schnauzers, dachshunds, cocker spaniels
Sinus node disease	Pugs, dalmatians
His bundle stenosis and degeneration (second- and third-degree AV block)	Pugs
Ventricular tachyarrhythmias and sudden death	German shepherds

    c. **Attention should be paid to antiarrhythmic drug indications, contraindications, dosages, side effects,** and **interactions with other drugs.** For example, the concomitant use of digoxin and quinidine can increase the risk of digoxin toxicity.

B. **Sinus rhythms.** Sinus rhythm is a **normal cardiac rhythm.** All waveforms are present with normal amplitudes and interval durations. There is less than 10% variability in the RR interval.

1. **Sinus arrhythmia** is a normal arrhythmia resulting from variation in vagal tone associated with respiration (i.e., heart rate increases with inspiration and slows with expiration). Cyclic changes in the height of the P wave (i.e., taller during inspiration, shorter during expiration) may be observed and are referred to as a **wandering pacemaker.**

2. **Sinus tachycardia** is a normal sinus rhythm with a heart rate exceeding the acceptable limits for the size or species of animal. Sinus tachycardia is common and can be associated with physiologic states (e.g., excitement or pain), drug therapy, or pathologic states (e.g., fever, hyperthyroidism, anemia, hypoxia, heart failure, shock).

3. **Sinus bradycardia** is a normal sinus rhythm with a heart rate below acceptable limits for the size and species of animal.
    a. **Causes** include hypothermia, hypothyroidism, pre- or postcardiac arrest status, drug therapy, brainstem lesions, increased intracranial pressure, ocular or carotid sinus pressure, severe metabolic disease (e.g., uremia), and SA node disease. Sinus bradycardia may be normal in very athletic dogs.
    b. **Therapy.** The underlying disorder should be treated.
        (1) **Atropine** or **glycopyrrolate** can be used initially if the bradycardia is related to clinical signs (e.g., weakness, syncope).
        (2) **Potent sympathomimetic agents** (e.g., dopamine, dobutamine, isoproterenol) may be required if bradycardia is related to cardiac arrest.
        (3) **Artificial pacing** is considered when medical therapy is unsuccessful.

4. **Sinus arrest** occurs when sinus node impulse formation fails. Sinus arrest may be associated with sick sinus syndrome or result from vagal stimulation or drug therapy.
    a. **Appearance on the ECG.** Long intervals with no P–QRS complexes occur on the ECG. An RR interval greater than twice the normal interval is present and junctional or ventricular escape beats may occur.
    b. **Therapy** is unnecessary if clinical signs are absent. If the animal is symptomatic and responds to atropine, chronic therapy with oral anticholinergics or theophylline may be useful. Failure of medical therapy may necessitate pacemaker implantation.

C. **Abnormal impulse formation** may be supraventricular or ventricular.

1. **Supraventricular**
    a. **Supraventricular premature complexes**
        (1) **Types**
           (a) **Atrial premature complexes** arise from an impulse formed in the atrium outside the SA node but above the AV node.
           (b) **Junctional premature complexes** arise in the AV junctional area.
        (2) **Causes.** Supraventricular premature complexes may be incidental or they may result from atrial pathology (e.g., left atrial dilation) or acid–base and electrolyte abnormalities.
        (3) **Appearance on the ECG**
           (a) An ectopic P' wave occurs prematurely and has an abnormal conformation. It may be negative if it arises in the junctional area.
           (b) The QRS complex occurs prematurely but it has a normal configuration.

(c) A noncompensatory pause occurs where the interval between the QRS complexes bracketing the atrial premature complex is less than the interval between three consecutive normal impulses.

(4) Therapy. If the number of premature complexes exceeds 20–30 per minute and the premature complexes are associated with clinical signs or underlying cardiac disease, antiarrhythmic drug therapy should be considered (e.g., digoxin, propranolol, diltiazem).

b. Supraventricular tachycardia is a sustained period (paroxysm) of supraventricular premature complexes (atrial or junctional). The onset of supraventricular tachycardia is often sudden and may be preceded by an atrial premature complex. The clinical significance of the arrhythmia varies. It may cause weakness, syncope or exercise intolerance.

(1) Causes. Supraventricular tachycardia may be caused by repetitive firing of an ectopic focus or by reentry phenomenon (i.e., the abnormal conduction of a normal atrial impulse in a continuous circuit). Likely etiologies are similar to those associated with atrial premature complexes and include stress, hypoxia, atrial disease, Wolff-Parkinson-White syndrome, hyperthyroidism, systemic hypertension, cor pulmonale, and digitalis toxicity.

(2) Appearance on the ECG (Figure 39-4A)

(a) The heart rate is rapid (greater than 160 bpm in large breed dogs, 180 bpm in toy breed dogs, and 240 bpm in cats) and regular unless there are multiple ectopic atrial foci.

(b) The morphology of the QRS complexes is normal unless a concomitant bundle branch block is present.

(c) The morphology of the P' wave is different from the normal sinus P wave. The P' wave may be obscured by the preceding QRS complex when the heart rate is rapid.

(3) Treatment

(a) A **vagal maneuver** (e.g., applying ocular or carotid sinus pressure) can terminate paroxysmal atrial or junctional tachycardia. This procedure increases parasympathetic tone, which can slow sinus rate and prolong AV node conduction.

(b) **Medical treatment**

(i) If the animal is in congestive heart failure, digoxin should be used initially. If the heart rate cannot be decreased with digoxin alone, propranolol, atenolol, or diltiazem can be added. However, the addition of diltiazem or a β blocker to the regimen will have negative inotropic effects and may exacerbate congestive heart failure. In cats with hypertrophic cardiomyopathy and heart failure, β blockers or diltiazem should be used first.

(ii) If the animal is not in congestive heart failure, propranolol, diltiazem, or adenosine can be used.

(iii) Digoxin should be avoided if a reentry mechanism is the suspected cause of the supraventricular tachycardia. Reentry mechanisms are evidenced by signs of ventricular preexcitation on the ECG and rapid termination of the tachycardia following the performance of a vagal maneuver.

(c) **Electrophysiologic pacing methods** or **direct current (DC) cardioversion** may be necessary to resolve refractory atrial tachycardia, but these techniques should only be employed by experienced specialists.

c. Atrial flutter. Rapid atrial discharge (i.e., an atrial rate greater than 300–350 discharges per minute) results in a variable ventricular rate, depending on how many atrial discharges transverse the AV node. Atrial flutter is not a stable arrhythmia; it often changes to atrial fibrillation or back to sinus rhythm.

(1) Causes are similar to those of supraventricular tachycardia.

(2) Appearance on the ECG. Atrial flutter produces a sawtooth pattern in the ECG baseline between normal QRS complexes.

(3) Therapy is similar to that for atrial fibrillation [see X C 1 d (3)].

A.

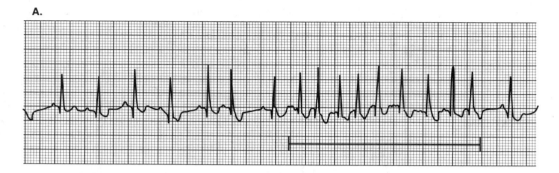

B.

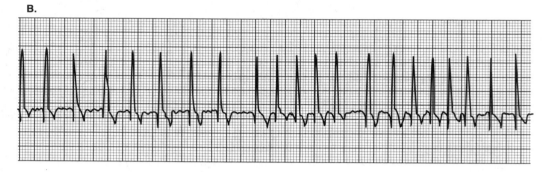

C.

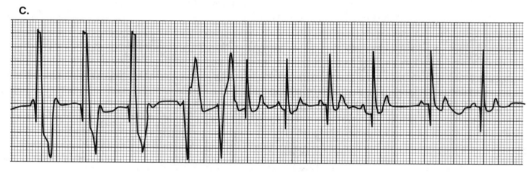

D.

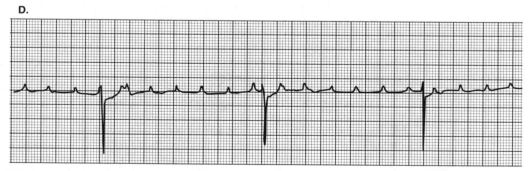

FIGURE 39-4. Electrocardiographic appearance of common arrhythmias in the dog. (*A*) Paroxysm of atrial tachycardia preceded and followed by a normal sinus rhythm. P′ waves are buried in preceding complexes. Note the normal conformation of the QRS complex. (*B*) Atrial fibrillation. Note the characteristic undulating baseline, variable RR interval, and rapid ventricular rate. (*C*) Paroxysm of multiform ventricular tachycardia followed by a normal sinus rhythm. The two different conformations of the ventricular premature complexes (VPCs) indicate that the impulses are arising from at least two different foci. (*D*) Third-degree (complete) atrio-ventricular (AV) block. Note the P waves are unrelated to the QRS complexes as indicated by the variable PR interval. A ventricular escape rhythm is present. Paper speed = 25 mm/sec. Sensitivity = 1 cm/mV.

d. **Atrial fibrillation** is a common arrhythmia. Organized atrial impulses and significant atrial contraction are lacking. The AV node conducts as many of these disorganized impulses as possible, resulting in an irregular and rapid ventricular rate.

   (1) **Causes.** The causes of atrial fibrillation are similar to those of supraventricular tachycardia. Atrial fibrillation is usually associated with marked atrial disease and enlargement.

   (2) **Appearance on the ECG** (Figure 39-4B). Atrial fibrillation is characterized by an absence of P waves and small undulations (i.e., fibrillation waves) in the ECG baseline between normal QRS complexes.

   (3) **Therapy**

     (a) **Decrease ventricular rate.** The main objective is to decrease the ventricular rate to below 140–160 bpm.

       (i) **Digoxin** is the drug of choice. **Diltiazem** can be used simultaneously if a more rapid reduction in ventricular rate is required (digoxin may take several days to decrease the rate).

       (ii) **Diltiazem** or **propranolol** can be added if digoxin alone does not reduce the ventricular rate. Propranolol should be started at a low dose and increased slowly because its negative inotropic effects may adversely affect animals in congestive heart failure.

     (b) **Convert to sinus rhythm.** The use of digoxin, diltiazem, and propranolol in animals with congestive heart failure rarely results in the conversion of atrial fibrillation to sinus rhythm. In animals with no cardiomegaly or signs of congestive heart failure, conversion to a sinus rhythm can be attempted with **quinidine** or **diltiazem.**

2. Ventricular

  a. **VPCs** result from an impulse generated by an ectopic focus below the AV node and are followed by a compensatory pause. The compensatory pause occurs because the ectopic ventricular impulse is not transmitted retrograde through the AV node and does not affect the normal SA node discharge and rate. The heart rate is usually normal but irregular.

   (1) **Causes** of VPCs include myocardial disease (e.g., cardiomyopathy, trauma, neoplasia, congestive heart failure), hypoxia, anemia, uremia, sepsis or endotoxemia, gastric dilatation–volvulus (GDV), pancreatitis, and various drugs (e.g., digoxin, anesthetic agents, atropine). An inherited syndrome of ventricular tachyarrhythmias and sudden death occurs in German shepherds.

   (2) **Appearance on the ECG.** The QRS complex is wide and abnormal. The RR interval between the P–QRS complex before and after the VPC is exactly twice the normal length because of the compensatory pause. Multiple ectopic foci (i.e., multifocal or multiform VPCs) are indicated by variations in the configuration of the VPCs. There is no P wave associated with a VPC.

   (3) **Therapy.** If clinical signs are present or there are more than 20–30 VPCs per minute, frequent runs of VPCs, a multifocal VPC pattern, or the presence of R on T events, therapy should be considered. Treatment is similar to that for ventricular tachycardia [see X C 2 b (3)].

  b. **Ventricular tachycardia** refers to a continuous series or paroxysm of VPCs. The rhythm within the string of VPCs is regular and often has a rate that exceeds 100 bpm. **Fusion beats** occur when both the SA node and an ectopic focus initiate ventricular discharge simultaneously.

   (1) **Causes.** The causes of ventricular tachycardia are similar to those of VPCs. Ventricular tachycardia is usually an indicator of significant cardiac or systemic disease. Ventricular tachycardia may result in weakness or syncope if cardiac output drops significantly during the arrhythmia.

   (2) **Appearance on the ECG.** There are no P waves related to the VPCs. Fusion beats, which appear as the melding of a normal P–QRS complex with a

VPC, can help distinguish supraventricular tachycardia with abnormal conduction (resulting in abnormal QRS configuration) from ventricular tachycardia (Figure 39-4C).

(3) **Therapy.** Frequent ECG monitoring is indicated to see how the arrhythmia is responding to the drug therapy.

(a) **Acute therapy**

(i) **Dogs.** In dogs, intravenous **lidocaine** (without epinephrine) is used initially. **Procainamide** or **quinidine** can be considered if lidocaine is ineffective. β **blockers** followed by **mexiletine** or **tocainide** can be tried next.

(ii) **Cats.** In cats, **propranolol** is used initially, followed by a low dose of **lidocaine** if the propranolol is ineffective.

(b) **Chronic therapy.** If ventricular arrhythmias have been abolished or are extremely well controlled, antiarrhythmic therapy can be tapered off over a 2- to 3-week period (with regular monitoring). Gradual withdrawal from therapy will determine if ongoing drug administration is necessary. If chronic therapy is indicated, **oral procainamide** is the first choice for dogs, propranalol for cats.

c. **Ventricular fibrillation** is a **lethal** arrhythmia characterized by a lack of organized electrical or mechanical activity. Ventricular fibrillation results in a loss of consciousness, collapse, pupillary dilation, and no respiration, audible heart sounds, or palpable pulses.

(1) **Causes** include severe systemic or cardiac disease, electric shock, hypoxia, anoxia, shock, hypothermia, electrolyte disturbances, and untreated ventricular tachycardia.

(2) **Appearance on the ECG.** Ventricular fibrillation produces an irregularly undulating baseline on the ECG.

(3) **Therapy. Cardiopulmonary resuscitation (CPR)** must be initiated immediately. **Electrical defibrillation** is the treatment of choice. Occasionally, an **external blow to the chest, open-chest cardiac massage,** or **intratracheal lidocaine or propranolol** can convert fibrillation to sinus rhythm.

d. **Ventricular asystole** is associated with no electrical or mechanical cardiac activity.

(1) **Causes** are similar to those of ventricular fibrillation.

(2) **Appearance on the ECG.** The ECG has a flat baseline. Some P waves may be observed.

(3) **Therapy. CPR** must be initiated immediately. **Epinephrine** is administered either intravenously or intratracheally. If ventricular fibrillation can be induced and then followed by electrical defibrillation, sinus rhythm may be reestablished.

e. **Escape rhythms** are a protective mechanism to ensure continued pump activity when higher pacemakers are not functioning. Escape rhythms can arise from the atria, AV node area, or ventricles and are regular with a slower rate than those initiated by the SA node (junctional escape rhythms = 40–60 bpm, ventricular escape rhythms = < 40–50 bpm in dogs; < 100 bpm in cats).

(1) **Appearance on the ECG.** The configuration of the escape complex corresponds to where the impulse arose. It is important to distinguish escape complexes and rhythms from supraventricular and ventricular complexes or tachycardia.

(2) **Antiarrhythmic therapy is contraindicated for escape complexes because they are maintaining cardiac function in the absence of higher pacemaker activity. Abolishing them will result in cardiac arrest.**

D. **Conduction disturbances**

1. **SA block** is an interruption of impulse conduction out of the SA node. It cannot be distinguished from sinus arrest on the ECG. Causes include vagal stimulation, drugs, or sick sinus syndrome (see X E).

2. **Atrial standstill** occurs because of an absence of atrial depolarization. Atrial standstill may be temporary or persistent.
   a. **Causes.** Hyperkalemia may cause atrial standstill. Persistent atrial standstill has been observed in dogs with various types of muscular dystrophy (especially English springer spaniels) and in cats with cardiomyopathy.
   b. **Appearance on the ECG.** There are no P waves and a junctional or ventricular escape rhythm is present.
   c. **Therapy** entails treating the underlying cause.

3. **Ventricular preexcitation syndrome (Wolff-Parkinson-White syndrome)** occurs when conduction through the AV node is bypassed; the impulse is transferred directly to the ventricles or bundle of His. The heart rate and rhythm may be normal or marked tachycardia (> 300 bpm) may be present.
   a. **Causes** include congenital malformation and, in cats, hypertrophic cardiomyopathy.
   b. **Appearance on the ECG.** Ventricular preexcitation syndrome is characterized on the ECG by a shortened PR interval and a notched or slurred upswing of the R wave (i.e., a delta wave).
   c. **Therapy** may be unnecessary unless tachycardia is present. Tachycardia is treated with vagal maneuvers, digoxin, lidocaine, propranolol, quinidine, verapamil, or DC cardioversion. Digoxin is useful in narrow-QRS complex Wolff-Parkinson-White syndrome but may exacerbate tachycardia if used in wide-QRS complex Wolff-Parkinson-White syndrome.

4. **AV block**
   a. **First-degree AV block** occurs when conduction through the AV node is prolonged.
      (1) Causes include drug therapy, electrolyte imbalances, vagal stimulation, and chronic degenerative changes in the conduction system.
      (2) Appearance on the ECG. The PR interval is lengthened.
      (3) Therapy entails discontinuing potentially causative drug therapy and correcting any electrolyte imbalances.
   b. **Second-degree AV block** is characterized by an intermittent failure of conduction through the AV node.
      (1) Causes include drug therapy and electrolyte imbalances.
      (2) Appearance on the ECG. Occasional P waves without corresponding QRS complexes are seen.
         (a) Mobitz type I (Wenckebach phenomenon) second-degree AV block occurs when there is progressive prolongation of the PR interval until a P wave is not conducted. Mobitz type I blocks are thought to be caused by disorders of the AV node or high vagal tone.
         (b) Mobitz type II second-degree AV block is characterized by constant PR intervals until a P wave is blocked unexpectedly. A fixed ratio of P waves to QRS complexes (e.g., 2:1) may be present. Type II blocks are thought to be caused by abnormalities in the lower part of the conduction system (i.e., the bundle of His or bundle branches).
      (3) Therapy
         (a) Mobitz type I AV blocks usually do not require specific therapy. Potentially causative drug therapy should be stopped or the dosage reduced.
         (b) Mobitz type II AV blocks may require therapy if they are associated with clinical signs (e.g., weakness, syncope). **Atropine, theophylline, isoproterenol,** or **pacemaker implantation** (temporary or permanent) may be indicated.
   c. **Third-degree AV block (complete heart block)** arises when there is no conduction through the AV node. The atria and ventricles beat independently of one another: the atria at the rate of SA node firing and the ventricles at the rate established by a ventricular escape rhythm. The atrial rate exceeds the ventricular rate.
      (1) Causes include digoxin toxicity, AV nodal disease (neoplasia, amyloid deposition), fibrosis, borreliosis, and hyperkalemia.

      (2) Appearance on the ECG (Figure 39-4D). The P waves are regular but have no relation to the QRS complexes. The configuration of the QRS complex varies depending on where the ventricular pacemaker is located— it will appear to be near normal if the ventricular pacemaker is close to the junction or wide and bizarre if the pacemaker is in the conduction system or ventricle.

      (3) Therapy. Assuming there is no reversible underlying disease, implantation of a **permanent cardiac pacemaker** is usually the only effective treatment in animals with clinical signs. Medical therapy can include atropine, theophylline, isoproterenol, and corticosteroids (if an inflammatory lesion is suspected).

   5. Bundle branch block. Blockage of the left or right common bundles or the left anterior or posterior fascicle results in an abnormal sequence of ventricular excitation. Therapy for all bundle branch blocks entails treating the underlying condition.

    a. Left bundle branch block results in depolarization of the right ventricle before the left.

      (1) Causes. Left bundle blocks may arise from myocardial disease, neoplasia, fibrosis, or congenital defects. They do not cause significant alterations in cardiac output or function.

      (2) Appearance on the ECG. The QRS complex is wide and positive in leads I, II, III, and aVF. This pattern may be confused with that produced by VPCs; however, the P wave consistently precedes each QRS complex in left bundle branch block but does not in VPCs.

    b. Left anterior fascicular block results in an alteration of the sequence of left ventricular depolarization.

      (1) Causes. Left anterior fascicular block has been associated with hypertrophic cardiomyopathy (in cats), left ventricular hypertrophy, ischemic cardiomyopathy, cardiac surgery, and hyperkalemia.

      (2) Appearance on the ECG. Left anterior fascicular block is characterized by a normal QRS width, left-axis deviation, small Q and tall R waves in leads I and aVL, and deep S waves in leads I, II, III, and aVF.

    c. Right bundle branch block results in delayed depolarization of the right ventricle.

      (1) Causes. Right bundle branch block may be normal in some animals or associated with congenital, valvular, or neoplastic heart disease, trypanosomiasis, heartworm disease, hypokalemia, or pulmonary embolism.

      (2) Appearance on the ECG. Right bundle branch block produces a wide QRS complex with a wide and large S wave in leads I, II, III, and aVF. As with left bundle branch blocks, right bundle blocks may be confused with VPCs.

E. **Sick sinus syndrome** represents an abnormality in both impulse formation and conduction. It encompasses several abnormalities, including sinus bradycardia, sinus arrest, SA block, alternating sinus bradycardia–tachycardia, and various conduction disturbances (e.g., AV blocks, bundle branch blocks).

   1. Signalment. Sick sinus syndrome is most common in older females and in the following breeds: miniature schnauzers, cocker spaniels, dachshunds, pugs, and West Highland white terriers.

   2. Causes. Sick sinus syndrome may be idiopathic, hereditary, or associated with myocardial disease (e.g., ischemia, fibrosis, neoplasia, inflammation).

   3. Therapy. Animals with mild or no clinical signs may not require therapy. If significant clinical signs are apparent, **atropine** or **oral anticholinergics** (e.g., propantheline) may help. **Cardiac pacemaker implantation** is usually required for the long-term control of bradyarrhythmias. **Digoxin** and **diltiazem** may control tachyarrhythmias.

XI. CARDIOPULMONARY ARREST

A. Etiology. Anticipating and preventing cardiopulmonary arrest is of prime importance because few animals are successfully resuscitated following cardiac arrest. Clinical situations where cardiopulmonary arrest should be anticipated include severe cardiac disease, severe respiratory disease (associated with hypoxemia), severe trauma (especially thoracic trauma or that involving significant blood loss), marked acid–base disturbances, hyperkalemia, hypocalcemia, sepsis or endotoxemia, ventricular tachycardia with R on T events or a multiform pattern, ventricular flutter, prolonged seizures, electric shock, and cardiovascular surgery or techniques (e.g., angiocardiography, pericardiocentesis). Marked increases in parasympathetic tone may also precipitate cardiac arrest and can be associated with vomiting, endotracheal intubation, and laryngeal, pharyngeal, ocular, and abdominal surgery.

B. Clinical signs

1. **Signs of impending cardiac arrest** include slowing of the respiratory or heart rate, irregular or gasping respirations, weakness, deteriorating consciousness, progressive T wave enlargement, depression or elevation of the ST segment (indicative of myocardial hypoxia), or the development of cardiac (especially ventricular) arrhythmias.

2. **Signs of cardiac arrest** include the absence of palpable pulses; an audible heart beat and respirations; loss of consciousness; and dilated, fixed pupils.

C. Therapy. An algorithm for the management of cardiopulmonary arrest is presented in Figure 39-5.

1. **CPR.** The goals of CPR are to restore ventilation, establish effective circulation to the heart and brain, and normalize cardiac rhythm and output.
   a. **A— Airway.** An unobstructed airway should be secured immediately.
      (1) **Remove foreign objects.** The mouth and oropharynx should be inspected for the presence of foreign objects.
      (2) **Endotracheal intubation** is the most efficient way of securing an airway. If laryngeal damage or obstruction is present, an emergency tracheostomy may be required. The percutaneous insertion of a large-bore needle into the trachea distal to the obstruction allows oxygen to be administered while preparing for a tracheostomy.
      (3) **Mouth-to-nose** (or **face mask) ventilation** may be used if endotracheal intubation is not immediately available.
   b. **B— Breathing.** After securing the airway, the veterinarian should check for spontaneous respiration.
      (1) If respiration is not immediately apparent, the animal should be ventilated with **100% oxygen** using either an Ambu bag (connected to oxygen) or an anesthetic machine (after ensuring that the breathing circuit has been well flushed of anesthetic gases). If 100% oxygen is unavailable, room air can be administered through an Ambu bag or via a mouth-to-tube technique.
      (2) **Two initial, deep breaths** should be given, and then a rate of **25–35 breaths/minute** should be established.
   c. **C— Circulation**
      (1) If no pulses are palpable, **external cardiac massage** should be initiated.
         (a) **Cats** and **small dogs.** External cardiac massage is best done in **lateral recumbency** for cats and small dogs.
         (b) **Large dogs.** In larger dogs, compression of the thoracic cavity propels the blood. Therefore, **dorsal recumbency** may provide superior thoracic cavity compression in dogs that weigh more than 10–15 kg. A V-trough or other support aids patient stability in this position. The chest cavity is compressed by 25%–30% by placing the hands over the caudal third of the sternum.
         (c) Chest compressions in cats and dogs should be delivered at a rate of at

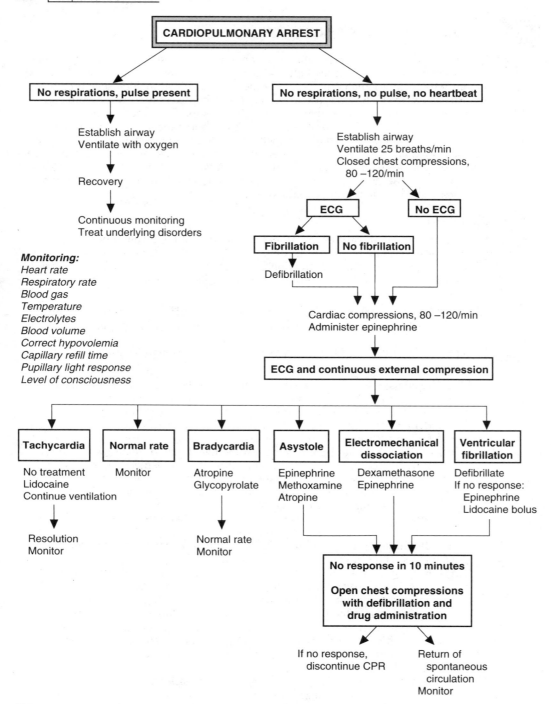

FIGURE 39-5. An algorithm for the management of cardiopulmonary arrest. CPR = cardiopulmonary resuscitation; *ECG* = electrocardiogram. (Redrawn with permission from Labato MA: Cardiopulmonary arrest and resuscitation. In *Textbook of Small Animal Internal Medicine,* 4th ed. Edited by Ettinger SJ and Feldman EC. Philadelphia, WB Saunders, 1995, p 74.)

least **60–80 compressions/minute,** although a rate of 80–120 compressions/minute may be superior.

    (2) If external cardiac massage has not generated a palpable peripheral pulse or improved mucous membrane color within 2–3 minutes, **internal (open chest) cardiac massage** should be considered. Additional indications for internal massage include flail chest, severe obesity, pleural space disease (e.g., effusion, pneumothorax, diaphragmatic hernia), pericardial effusion, large or barrel-chested dog breeds, and severe hypovolemia.

        (a) A strip of hair is clipped over the fifth or sixth intercostal space on the left side, the skin is briefly swabbed with antiseptic solution, and the thoracic cavity is opened with a skin incision.

        (b) The pleural space is entered with the tips of Mayo scissors and the incision is extended to a length sufficient to allow entry of the fingers or hands (depending on the size of the animal). The internal thoracic artery just lateral to the sternum and the intercostal artery just caudal to the rib should be avoided.

        (c) The pericardial sac is incised with scissors along its apex. The heart is lifted out of the pericardial sac and massaged at a rate of **60–100 compressions/minute.**

            (i) Massage is accomplished with the fingers of one hand or both hands, depending on the size of the animal.

            (ii) Care should be taken not to rotate or displace the heart from its normal position, which can lead to occlusion or tearing of blood vessels.

    (3) Supporting effective volume

        (a) After cardiac compression has been initiated, an intravenous line should be established and lactated Ringer's or a comparable solution should be administered. The rate is determined by the volume status of the patient (usually shock dosages).

        (b) The placement of a caudal abdominal wrap can help prevent peripheral pooling of blood. Occlusion of the distal aorta during internal massage can improve blood flow to the brain.

2. Electrocardiography. An ECG should be performed as soon as a patent airway, breathing, and circulation have been reestablished to help determine the nature of the cardiac arrhythmia (usually either ventricular fibrillation, asystole, or electromechanical dissociation) and to gauge response to drugs or defibrillator therapy.

3. Defibrillation

    a. Electrical (DC) defibrillation is the best treatment for ventricular fibrillation. The sooner a fibrillating myocardium can be defibrillated, the better the chance of success. In external defibrillation, the paddles are placed on each side of the chest over the heart. Internal defibrillation involves placing special paddles directly on the heart.

    b. Chemical defibrillation using **potassium chloride** (with or without acetylcholine) can be attempted but is rarely successful.

4. Drug therapy

    a. Agents

        (1) Epinephrine is indicated for ventricular asystole, electromechanical dissociation, and to change ventricular fibrillation from fine to coarse prior to defibrillation. Epinephrine has both α- and β-adrenergic effects.

            (a) The α-adrenergic effects result in peripheral vasoconstriction and help maintain arterial blood pressure and venous return.

            (b) The β-adrenergic effects increase heart rate and myocardial contractility.

        (2) Atropine is used to treat bradycardia. Excessive parasympathetic tone may inhibit SA node automaticity.

        (3) Lidocaine is used pre- or postcardiac arrest if high-risk ventricular arrhythmias are present.

        (4) Sodium bicarbonate should be administered according to the measured acid–base status of the patient. Adequate CPR should control acidosis in patients that were normal prior to cardiac arrest. Sodium bicarbonate is more likely to be required after CPR has been performed for longer than 10–15 minutes.

    (5) Calcium administration during CPR is not recommended unless hypocalcemia was present prior to cardiac arrest, or if hyperkalemia or calcium channel blocker overdosage is present.

  b. Routes of drug administration

    (1) Intravenous. A central vein is preferred, but a peripheral vein is acceptable.

    (2) Intratracheal administration is a fast and effective method of administration for most drugs. Sodium bicarbonate should not be given intratracheally.

    (3) Interosseous administration can be established by placing a bone marrow or spinal needle into the medullary cavity of the proximal femur, humerus, tibia, or wing of the ilium. All drugs can be administered by this route (including fluid therapy) and distribution to the heart is rapid.

    (4) Intracardiac. The intracardiac route is the least preferred route because of the risk of myocardial injury and lung laceration.

5. Aftercare

  a. Monitoring. Rearrest is common in resuscitated patients; therefore, close patient monitoring is necessary. Regular assessment of vital signs, mentation, ECG activity, blood gases, electrolytes, urine output, and blood pressure should be performed.

  b. Controlling sequelae. Hypoxic damage to the CNS leading to seizures, coma, and blindness is a common sequela of cardiac arrest. Cerebral edema induced by hypoxia should be suspected if unconsciousness persists longer than 15–30 minutes after resuscitation. Dexamethasone, mannitol, and furosemide are commonly used to reverse cerebral edema, although success is variable.

D. **Prognosis.** Good post-resuscitation prognostic indicators include improved mentation, spontaneous respiration, and responsive pupils. The prognosis for recovery is poor if unconsciousness and nonreactive pupils persist longer than 6–24 hours.

XII. VASCULAR DISORDERS

A. **Thrombotic disorders**

1. Thrombosis

  a. Etiology (Table 39-9). Thrombosis is caused by disorders that result in endothe-

TABLE 39-9. Diseases Associated with Thrombosis

Bacterial endocarditis
Hypercoagulable states
Nephrotic syndrome
Hyperadrenocorticism
Disseminated intravascular coagulation (DIC)
Polycythemia (hyperviscosity)
Immune-mediated hemolytic anemia
Severe thrombocytosis
Heartworm infection
Vasculitis or arteritis
Physical or chemical injury to a vessel
Venous stasis or obstruction

lial damage, blood stasis, increased blood viscosity, or alterations in the concentration of blood constituents (e.g., decreased antithrombin III concentration).

  b. Diagnosis

    (1) Clinical findings. Typically, thrombosis results in an acute onset of nonprogressive clinical signs that reflect the organs involved. The heart, limbs, CNS, kidneys, adrenal glands, liver, spleen, or skin may be involved.

      (a) Cardiac involvement is reflected by ECG changes and arrhythmias.

      (b) Involvement of the extremities may be manifested as weakness, pain, and coolness to the touch.

      (c) Involvement of the spinal cord may be reflected as paresis, and involvement of the brain may be reflected as seizures or changes in mentation.

      (d) Involvement of the kidneys may be reflected by renal failure.

      (e) Adrenal gland involvement may be manifested as hypoadrenocorticism.

    (2) Other findings. Radiography, angiography, ultrasonography, or radionuclide studies may be necessary to confirm the diagnosis.

  c. Therapy

    (1) Specific treatment for the underlying disorder should be instituted. ˙

    (2) Supportive care (i.e., intravenous fluids, care of damaged tissue) and the use of **anticoagulants** are indicated. Heparin is commonly used when pulmonary arterial or aortic thrombosis has occurred. Aspirin or, less frequently, warfarin, is used for long-term prophylaxis.

    (3) Surgical embolectomy or the use of **thrombolytic agents** (e.g., streptokinase) is uncommon due to the inaccessibility of many vessels, serious drug-related side effects, and the poor long-term success of these modalities.

2. Aortic thromboembolism occurs most commonly with feline hypertrophic cardiomyopathy and restrictive cardiomyopathy (10%–20% of cases).

  a. Etiology. The formation of clots in the left atrium or apex of the left ventricular lumen may be caused by sluggish blood flow (especially in an enlarged left atrium), altered or damaged endocardial surfaces, and enhanced platelet aggregability.

  b. Pathophysiology

    (1) Ninety percent of clots lodge at the aortic trifurcation. Less common sites include the renal, mesenteric, pulmonary, cerebral, and brachial arteries.

    (2) Mere obstruction of the distal aorta will not significantly impair blood flow to the hind limbs because of the presence of collateral vessels. However, if a clot is responsible for the obstruction, the elaboration of various vasoactive substances from platelets (e.g., serotonin, thromboxane) results in vasoconstriction of collateral vessels and severe diminution of blood flow to the hindlimbs.

  c. Diagnosis

    (1) Clinical findings

      (a) Obstruction of the distal aorta results in **posterior paresis.**

        (i) The muscles of the hindlimbs may be painful and contracted (especially the gastrocnemius and cranial tibial muscles).

        (ii) The legs are cool to the touch, femoral arterial pulses are absent or much diminished, and foot pads and nail beds are pale or cyanotic. Hindlimb signs may be lateralized to a degree.

        (iii) Signs of congestive heart failure (e.g., dyspnea) may be present.

      (b) Embolization to areas other than the distal aorta will generate the expected clinical signs (i.e., brachial artery— forelimb paresis, cerebral arteries— acute neurologic signs, pulmonary artery— acute dyspnea, renal arteries— acute renal failure).

    (2) Laboratory findings

      (a) Extensive muscle injury leads to marked elevation of serum creatine phosphokinase and, to a lesser extent, SAST and SALT levels.

      (b) Prerenal azotemia may be present if congestive heart failure or dehydration are present. Renal azotemia or acute renal failure may occur if both renal arteries become obstructed.

       (c) Metabolic acidosis, DIC, or hyperkalemia (from muscle reperfusion or acute renal failure) may also occur.

    (3) Radiographic and **echocardiographic findings.** Occasionally, clots may be visualized within the left atrium, ventricle, or distal aorta. The location of the clot may be documented by selective or nonselective angiography but this is seldom necessary unless surgical intervention is being contemplated.

d. Therapy. The main goals are to treat the congestive heart failure (if present), provide supportive care (i.e. fluid therapy, maintenance of body temperature, physiotherapy), and prevent further thrombus formation or growth.

    (1) Heparin. Following a thromboembolic event, heparin is commonly used for the initial inhibition of coagulation. Heparin does not dissolve an established thrombus but should prevent additional growth or the formation of new thrombi.

       (a) The effective dose of heparin is the amount that prolongs the activated partial thromboplastin time (APTT) by 1.5 times.

       (b) The major side effect of heparin administration is hemorrhage.

    (2) Aspirin given at low doses every 3 days inhibits platelet aggregation and is frequently used for chronic maintenance therapy.

    (3) Warfarin. The use of warfarin instead of aspirin for maintenance therapy is advocated by some. However, the risk of significant hemorrhage is greater and requires closer patient monitoring.

    (4) Streptokinase and **recombinant tissue plasminogen activator (TPA).** Pharmacologic dissolution of the clot can be attempted with streptokinase or recombinant TPA; however, results have not been encouraging. This therapy should probably be reserved for those animals with thrombi in critical areas (renal, cerebral, mesenteric, or pulmonary arteries) because:

       (a) A 50% mortality rate, mostly attributable to reperfusion abnormalities (i.e., hyperkalemia, metabolic acidosis), was reported in one study with the use of TPA.

       (b) The induction of a bleeding tendency and hemorrhage are likely.

       (c) Expense can be considerable, especially with TPA.

    (5) Surgical removal of clots can be considered but is associated with a high mortality rate because of anesthetic complications related to heart failure and the effects of reperfusion.

    (6) Vasodilators. The use of vasodilators (e.g., acepromazine, hydralazine) may improve collateral circulation. However, beneficial effects have not been clearly documented and hypotension is a potential side effect.

e. Prognosis

    (1) If the signs of congestive heart failure can be managed, many cats treated conservatively (i.e., supportive care, heparin, aspirin, possibly vasodilators) will regain some degree of motor function in their hind limbs. Improvement should be noted within 1–2 weeks and some cats become clinically normal in 1–2 months. Nevertheless, residual deficits are common and the prognosis is still poor because of the high rate of recurrent thromboembolism.

    (2) Embolization of the renal, pulmonary, cerebral or mesenteric arteries carries a grave prognosis.

B. **Hypertensive disorders**

1. Etiology

    a. Primary or **essential (systemic) hypertension** is not associated with an underlying cause and is rare in dogs and cats.

    b. Secondary (systemic) hypertension is the most common form of hypertension in dogs and cats and has been associated with renal disease (especially glomerular), hyperadrenocorticism, hyperthyroidism, pheochromocytoma, drugs (e.g., α-adrenergic agonists) and CNS disease.

    c. Pulmonary hypertension. The causes of pulmonary hypertension are discussed in VIII B.

2. **Signalment.** Most hypertensive dogs and cats are middle aged to older. Greyhounds normally have higher resting blood pressure than other breeds. Male dogs and obese animals may be at increased risk.

3. **Diagnosis** is based on compatible clinical signs and an abnormally elevated blood pressure.
   a. **Clinical findings** are related to the **underlying disorders** (e.g., polyuria, polydipsia, weight loss, ascites, edema) and to **pressure-induced injury to end-organs** (e.g., the eye, kidney, cardiovascular system, cerebrovascular system).
      (1) **Blindness** may result from retinal hemorrhage or detachment. Animals with acute blindness of short duration (1–2 days) due to hypertension may regain vision with the successful control of blood pressure.
      (2) **Seizures, syncope, paresis,** or **collapse** can result from damage to cerebral vasculature or vascular accidents (stroke).
      (3) **Epistaxis** can result from rupture of vessels in the nasal mucosa .
      (4) A low-grade **systolic murmur** (associated with mitral insufficiency) or a **gallop rhythm** (associated with left ventricular hypertrophy) can occur.
   b. **Physical examination findings.** Although the upper limit of a normal blood pressure is somewhat controversial, most would agree that a systolic pressure greater than 180 mm Hg and a diastolic pressure greater than 100 mm Hg (in a resting dog or cat with a normal heart rate) is indicative of hypertension.
      (1) Blood pressure can be measured using direct (arterial puncture) or indirect (oscillometric or Doppler flow) techniques.
      (2) Multiple abnormal measurements should be obtained before conclusively diagnosing hypertension.

4. **Treatment**
   a. The underlying disorder should be treated.
   b. A stepwise approach using a diuretic (e.g., furosemide) and dietary salt restriction followed by a vasodilator (e.g., enalapril, prazosin) or a β-adrenergic blocker (e.g., propranolol, atenolol) is commonly recommended. Moderate to severe hypertension will require the use of both a diuretic and a vasodilator to normalize pressures.
   c. Regular monitoring of blood pressure is central to successful management. The patient should be monitored for signs of drug-induced hypotension (e.g., weakness, depression, syncope).

DIRECTIONS: Each of the numbered items or incomplete statements in this section is followed by answers or by completions of the statement. Select the ONE numbered answer or completion that is BEST in each case.

1. Which one of the following clinical signs is most commonly observed in cats that develop pulmonary edema as a result of congestive heart failure?

(1) Syncope
(2) Frequent coughing
(3) Dyspnea
(4) Exercise intolerance
(5) Muffled lung sounds

2. A 7-year-old, male, neutered golden retriever is brought to the veterinarian because of exercise intolerance and abdominal enlargement. Physical examination findings include ascites (i.e., a fluid wave was ballotted), jugular venous distention, and abnormal jugular pulsation. These findings are consistent with:

(1) right-sided heart failure.
(2) liver disease.
(3) left-sided heart failure.
(4) mitral valve insufficiency.
(5) systemic hypertension.

Questions 3–4

A 9-year-old, female, spayed poodle is presented because of a 2-month history of frequent coughing, especially at night. A 3/6 systolic murmur is present over the left cardiac apex. Thoracic radiographs reveal moderate left atrial and mild left ventricular enlargement. The pulmonary vasculature and lung fields are normal.

3. What is the most likely cause of the clinical and radiographic signs?

(1) Dilated cardiomyopathy
(2) Tricuspid valve endocardiosis and insufficiency
(3) Left-sided congestive heart failure
(4) Bacterial endocarditis of the mitral valve
(5) Mitral valve endocardiosis and insufficiency

4. Which one of the following treatments would be the best initial choice to decrease left atrial size and reduce the frequency of coughing in this dog?

(1) Furosemide administration
(2) Reduced-salt diet
(3) Hydrochlorothiazide administration
(4) Enalapril administration
(5) Digoxin administration

5. Which would be the most efficacious treatment for pulmonary congestion and edema associated with left-sided heart failure?

(1) Administration of furosemide
(2) Administration of digoxin
(3) Feeding a reduced-salt diet
(4) Administration of an angiotensin-converting enzyme (ACE) inhibitor
(5) Administration of a nonselective β-adrenergic blocker

6. An 8-year-old male Doberman pinscher is presented with dyspnea and an irregular heart beat with pulse deficits. Extensive crackles are heard over the lung fields. The most likely diagnosis is:

(1) end-stage mitral valve insufficiency with left-sided heart failure.
(2) pericardial effusion.
(3) dilated cardiomyopathy with left-sided heart failure.
(4) hypertrophic cardiomyopathy with left-sided heart failure.
(5) heartworm infection.

7. A 10-year-old, female, spayed, domestic short-hair cat is brought to the veterinarian because of lethargy and dyspnea. Physical and radiographic findings include weakness, poor pulses, generalized cardiomegaly, and pleural effusion. Cardiac ultrasound reveals left atrial and ventricular dilation with poor myocardial contractility. In addition to a diuretic, vasodilator, and a positive-inotropic drug, therapy should include:

(1) aggressive intravenous fluid administration.
(2) taurine administration.
(3) L-carnitine administration.
(4) vitamin B administration.
(5) arginine administration

8. A gallop rhythm is detected in a 6-year-old, male, neutered, domestic long-haired cat during a routine physical examination. Mild left atrial enlargement is visible on thoracic radiographs. Echocardiographic findings consist of moderate concentric left ventricular hypertrophy with no visible outflow obstructions. The best treatment would be:

(1) digoxin and furosemide.
(2) furosemide, enalapril, and low-dose aspirin.
(3) diltiazem and low-dose aspirin.
(4) reduced-salt diet and low-dose aspirin.
(5) diltiazem and enalapril.

9. A 4/6 continuous murmur, loudest over the heart base, is heard in a 4-month-old, male German shepherd. The likely diagnosis is:

(1) ventricular septal defect.
(2) aortic valve insufficiency.
(3) pulmonic stenosis.
(4) tetralogy of Fallot.
(5) patent ductus arteriosus (PDA).

10. A 6-month-old female Border collie is brought to the veterinarian because of exercise intolerance. Physical examination reveals oral mucous membrane cyanosis that worsens with exercise. A 3/6 systolic murmur is heard over the left heart base. The clinical findings would be most consistent with:

(1) right-to-left shunting patent ductus arteriosus (PDA).
(2) left-to-right shunting ventricular septal defect.
(3) heart failure.
(4) tetralogy of Fallot.
(5) left-to-right shunting atrial septal defect.

11. If a dog is infected with heartworm in May, a concentration test (e.g., a modified Knott's test) should become positive in:

(1) June.
(2) November.
(3) February.
(4) August.
(5) September.

12. Which one of the following findings would be most suggestive of heartworm infection?

(1) Tortuous and blunted caudal lobar pulmonary arteries
(2) Right-sided heart enlargement and ascites
(3) Peripheral eosinophilia and basophilia
(4) Exercise intolerance and a split second heart sound (S_2)
(5) Jugular venous distention, pleural effusion, and hepatomegaly

13. A 5-year-old male Labrador retriever is brought to the veterinarian because of abdominal enlargement and lethargy. The veterinarian determines that the abdominal enlargement is due to ascites. The heart sounds are muffled and the femoral pulses are weak. A large, rounded heart shadow is present on thoracic radiographs. These findings suggest a diagnosis of:

(1) right-sided heart failure as a result of heartworm infection.
(2) right-sided heart failure as a result of dilated cardiomyopathy.
(3) left-sided heart failure as a result of dilated cardiomyopathy.
(4) right-sided heart failure as a result of pericardial effusion.
(5) left-sided heart failure as a result of mitral valve insufficiency.

14. The two most common causes of hemorrhagic pericardial effusion in dogs are:

(1) septic pericarditis and idiopathic causes.
(2) disseminated intravascular coagulation (DIC) and atrial hemangiosarcoma.
(3) atrial hemangiosarcoma and idiopathic causes.
(4) trauma and idiopathic causes.
(5) atrial hemangiosarcoma and von Willebrand's disease.

15. Atrial fibrillation is diagnosed in a 7-year-old male Great Dane with dilated cardiomyopathy. The ventricular rate is 180 bpm. The best initial treatment to reduce the ventricular rate would be:

(1) propranolol.
(2) vagal maneuver.
(3) diltiazem.
(4) digoxin.
(5) atropine.

16. What is the initial treatment for ventricular tachycardia?

(1) Lidocaine
(2) Procainamide
(3) Quinidine
(4) Digoxin
(5) Epinephrine

DIRECTIONS: Each of the numbered items or incomplete statements in this section is negatively phrased, as indicated by a capitalized word such as NOT, LEAST, or EXCEPT. Select the ONE numbered answer or completion that is BEST in each case.

17. Which one of the following routes of drug administration is the LEAST preferred during cardiopulmonary resuscitation (CPR)?

(1) Intratracheal
(2) Intracardiac
(3) Intravenous via a peripheral vein
(4) Intravenous via a central vein
(5) Interosseous

1. The answer is 3 [I A 2 d (1)]. Dyspnea is the most common sign of congestive heart failure in cats. Frequent coughing is common in dogs, but not cats, with pulmonary edema. Exercise intolerance is usually not detected in cats because of their sedentary lifestyle. Muffled lung sounds more often accompany pleural effusion, and syncope is not usually a manifestation of pulmonary edema in dogs or cats.

2. The answer is 1 [I A 2 c, 3 c, f; II D 2]. Right-sided heart failure causes increased central venous pressure, which results in jugular venous distention and abnormal pulsation as well as fluid accumulation in the abdomen, thoracic cavity, and subcutis. Liver disease could be associated with ascites but not jugular venous distention. Left-sided heart failure is associated with pulmonary venous congestion and edema, but not with ascites or jugular venous distention. Mitral valve insufficiency is associated with signs of left-sided failure. Systemic hypertension does not appreciably affect venous pressures and would not result in the clinical signs present in this dog.

3–4. The answers are: 3-5 [III A 3 a, b, c], **4-4** [III A 4 a]. Mitral valve endocardiosis and insufficiency is a very common disorder of middle-aged to older small breed dogs. Compromise of the mitral valve leads to regurgitation of blood into the left atrium during systole, generating a midsystolic murmur and leading to enlargement of the left atrium. Left-sided congestive heart failure is not present (yet) because there is no pulmonary venous dilation and congestion. Dilated cardiomyopathy is rare in small breed dogs. The location of the murmur and the radiographic signs are not consistent with tricuspid valve disease. Bacterial endocarditis is a rare condition and systemic signs of illness would probably be present.

Enalapril, an angiotensin-converting enzyme (ACE) inhibitor, is the most effective way to decrease left atrial size (in patients with mitral valve insufficiency) because it reduces the regurgitant flow across the incompetent mitral valve by lowering the aortic outflow resistance (i.e., by dilating the systemic arteries). Furosemide, hydrochlorothiazide,

and a reduced-salt diet may decrease left atrial size in this setting but to a lesser extent. Digoxin may also reduce regurgitant flow but again, to a lesser extent than enalapril will.

5. The answer is 1 [II E 1 a (2)]. Administration of furosemide or another potent diuretic is the most effective way to promptly reduce vascular volume, preload, and pulmonary edema. Reduced-salt diets and angiotensin-converting enzyme (ACE) inhibitors (e.g., enalapril) will also reduce preload, but to a more modest extent and with a longer onset of action. Digoxin has little if any direct effect on preload or pulmonary edema. Nonselective β-adrenergic blockers (e.g., propranolol) may actually exacerbate dyspnea associated with pulmonary edema because they cause bronchoconstriction.

6. The answer is 3 [IV A 1 d (1) (b) (ii), (2)]. Dilated cardiomyopathy is a common disorder and predominantly affects large and giant breed male dogs. Doberman pinschers are commonly affected with dilated cardiomyopathy and tend to develop left-sided heart failure (as indicated by the crackles heard over the lung fields, suggestive of pulmonary edema) and ventricular arrhythmias (as indicated by the irregular heart beat and pulse deficits). Mitral valve insufficiency is uncommon in large breed dogs. Hypertrophic cardiomyopathy is rare in dogs. Pericardial effusion and heartworm infection would produce signs of right-sided heart failure.

7. The answer is 2 [IV B 1 c]. The clinical description is consistent with dilated cardiomyopathy, which can be caused by taurine deficiency in cats. Therefore, taurine supplementation should be included in the treatment plan for all cats with this disorder. Aggressive intravenous fluid support would aggravate signs of congestive heart failure. L-Carnitine deficiency has been linked to some cases of dilated cardiomyopathy in dogs, but not in cats. Vitamin B would not hurt but would not necessarily help a cat with dilated cardiomyopathy. Arginine is an essential amino acid in cats, but arginine deficiency is not linked to dilated cardiomyopathy and most diets are formulated with adequate amounts.

8. The answer is 3 [IV B 2 e (2)]. The clinical description is consistent with a diagnosis of hypertrophic cardiomyopathy. Although the most beneficial therapy for asymptomatic cats is not known, if myocardial changes are significant, most clinicians would prescribe either diltiazem, propranolol, or atenolol and prophylaxis for thromboembolism (i.e., low-dose aspirin). Positive-inotropic drugs such as digoxin are contraindicated in patients with hypertrophic cardiomyopathy. Furosemide and a reduced-salt diet are not necessary because heart failure is not present. Enalapril (or any vasodilator) is generally avoided when treating cats with hypertrophic cardiomyopathy because it may aggravate any dynamic left ventricular obstruction.

9. The answer is 5 [V B 4 a (1) (b)]. A continuous ("machinery") murmur is very suggestive of patent ductus arteriosus (PDA), especially in German shepherds. None of the other cardiac disorders listed (ventricular septal defect, aortic valve insufficiency, pulmonic stenosis, and tetralogy of Fallot) is associated with a continuous murmur.

10. The answer is 4 [V I 3]. Tetralogy of Fallot is the most common congenital defect that causes cyanosis. A reverse (i.e., right-to-left shunting) patent ductus arteriosus (PDA) would produce differential cyanosis (i.e., the oral mucous membranes appear normal). Left-to-right shunting ventricular septal defects or atrial septal defects will not result in cyanosis because there is no admixture of unoxygenated blood in the systemic circulation. Advanced heart failure may be accompanied by cyanosis, but the Border collie does not have other clinical signs consistent with heart failure.

11. The answer is 2 [VI A 3 d (1) (b)]. The prepatent period (i.e., the time from infection to the appearance of circulating microfilaria) is approximately 6 months. Concentration tests do not produce positive results until the adult heartworms start to produce microfilaria; therefore, a dog infected in May will not test positive until November.

12. The answer is 1 [VI A 3 e]. Tortuous and blunted caudal lobar pulmonary arteries are very suggestive of heartworm infection. Signs of right-sided heart failure (i.e., ascites, exercise intolerance, jugular venous distention, pleural effusion, hepatomegaly) may accom-

pany severe heartworm infection, but right-sided heart failure may also be caused by other diseases. A split second heart sound (S_2) can be indicative of pulmonary hypertension, which can be associated with heartworm infection, but again, there are many other causes of pulmonary hypertension.

13. The answer is 4 [VII A 3 c]. The combination of muffled heart sounds (caused by pericardial fluid accumulation), weak pulses, a rounded heart shadow, and signs of right-sided heart failure are suggestive of pericardial effusion. Muffled heart sounds usually do not accompany dilated cardiomyopathy or heartworm infection. Signs of left-sided heart failure are not present.

14. The answer is 3 [VII A 1 c]. Approximately 90% of the cases of pericardial effusion in dogs are due to idiopathic causes or hemangiosarcoma. Septic pericarditis is very rare in dogs. Coagulopathies such as disseminated intravascular coagulation (DIC) and von Willebrand's disease are rare causes of pericardial effusion. Trauma is an uncommon cause of pericardial effusion.

15. The answer is 4 [X C 1 d (3) (a)]. Digoxin is the preferred drug for animals with cardiac disease and atrial fibrillation. It slows atrioventricular (AV) conduction and is usually successful at slowing the ventricular rate in response to rapid atrial discharges. Diltiazem and propranolol are usually added if the ventricular rate cannot be lowered with digoxin alone. Vagal maneuvers have little effect on atrial fibrillation. Atropine may actually increase the ventricular rate by reducing any parasympathetic suppression of AV conduction.

16. The answer is 1 [X C 2 b (3) (a)]. The administration of lidocaine intravenously is the initial treatment of choice for ventricular tachycardia. Procainamide and quinidine are considered if lidocaine is ineffective. Digoxin and epinephrine may aggravate ventricular arrhythmias.

17. The answer is 2 [XI C 4 b (4)]. The intracardiac route is the least preferred route of drug administration during cardiopulmonary resuscitation (CPR) due to the risk of myocardial damage and lung laceration.

Chapter 40

Respiratory Diseases

I. NASAL DISORDERS

A. Clinical manifestations

1. **Sneezing** is an acute response associated with inflammation or irritation of the nasal mucosa. It often subsides with time, but its disappearance does not necessarily indicate resolution of the causative disorder.

2. **Reverse sneezing** is bouts of noisy, stertorous inspiration, a few seconds to a few minutes in duration, which occur most frequently in healthy, small-breed dogs. It may result from entrapment of the epiglottis under the soft palate and is usually a lifelong disorder that does not progress. Massaging the neck may help stop the episode.

3. **Nasal discharge** is a nonspecific response to irritation or inflammation of the nasal mucosa. Occasionally, pulmonary disorders or coagulopathies can result in nasal discharge.
   a. **Location**
      (1) **Bilateral** discharge results from infectious or allergic disorders, or coagulopathies.
      (2) **Unilateral** discharge typically results from foreign bodies, neoplasia, polyps, or the extension of an oral disease process (e.g., tooth root abscess).
      (3) **Initial unilateral** discharge with **secondary bilateral** involvement may occur with neoplasia or fungal infections.
   b. **Physical characteristics**
      (1) **Serous nasal discharge** can be normal, associated with upper respiratory viral infection in cats, or precede a mucopurulent discharge.
      (2) **Mucopurulent nasal discharge** is associated with inflammation and can accompany any nasal disease (i.e., viral, bacterial, fungal, or parasitic infection; foreign body; neoplasia; nasopharyngeal polyp; allergic rhinitis; or an extension of an oral disease process).
      (3) **Hemorrhagic nasal discharge** can be associated with trauma, fungal infection, neoplasia, foreign body, or systemic diseases (e.g., coagulopathies, systemic hypertension, hyperviscosity syndrome, vasculitis, polycythemia).

4. **Stertorous respiration**

5. **Facial deformity**

6. **Systemic signs** (e.g., anorexia, lethargy)

7. **Central nervous system (CNS) signs** (from extension of a disease process through the cribriform plate)

B. Diagnostic approaches and techniques

1. **Physical examination**
   a. **Decreased air flow** in one or both sides of the nasal cavity indicates obstructive disease.
   b. **Facial deformity** or **exophthalmus** may indicate neoplasia.
   c. **Oral abnormalities** (e.g., dental tartar, gingivitis, pus in the gingival sulcus, sensitivity to pressure, oronasal fistula) may indicate tooth root abscess.
   d. **Ophthalmologic abnormalities** such as retinal detachment may indicate hypertension, and active chorioretinitis may indicate cryptococcosis or lymphoma.
   e. **Petechiation** on skin or mucous membranes may indicate a coagulopathy.

2. **Laboratory tests**
   a. **Nasal cytology.** Parasites, fungal elements, or bacteria may be seen. Rarely, neoplastic cells are apparent.
   b. **Culture.** The normal flora of the nasal cavity makes interpretation difficult.

    c. Serology
      (1) Titers may indicate exposure to *Aspergillus* and *Penicillium* species, Rocky Mountain spotted fever, or ehrlichiosis.
      (2) Latex agglutination capsular antigen test (LCAT). This test can detect *Cryptococcus neoformans* infection.
    d. Other tests may include a complete blood count (CBC), platelet count, coagulation profile, and serum biochemical profile.

  3. Radiography. Radiographic studies should be performed before any invasive procedures, which might induce hemorrhage.
    a. Plain films. Lateral, ventrodorsal (VD), intraoral, and frontal sinus views should be obtained. Plain films may reveal increased fluid density, loss or lysis of turbinates, lysis of facial bones, radiodense foreign bodies, lucency near tooth roots, or fracture of the nasal bones.
      (1) Loss of turbinate detail and the presence of a fluid density is common with fungal infections.
      (2) The presence of a soft-tissue density, especially in the caudal aspect of the nasal cavity, associated with turbinate (and possibly facial bone) lysis suggests neoplasia.
    b. Computed tomography (CT) provides excellent detail of the nasal cavity and turbinates. It is the most accurate method of determining the extent of tumor involvement.

  4. Rhinoscopy is indicated for dogs and cats with a chronic nasal discharge or a suspected foreign body. It reveals the presence and extent of inflammation, mass lesions, turbinate destruction, fungal plaques, and parasites. It also aids in the retrieval of foreign bodies, nasal biopsies, and specimens for culture.

  5. Nasal flush. A nasal flush is performed to retrieve samples for cytology and, occasionally, histopathology. Nasal flush may also help remove accumulated mucus and debris and improve airflow through the nasal cavity.

  6. Biopsy procedures are valuable in providing a definitive diagnosis in animals with a chronic nasal discharge.
    a. Traumatic nasal flush. A stiff polypropylene catheter attached to a syringe is raked against the nasal mucosa to obtain tissue samples for histopathology. Samples are collected in the syringe or are flushed and filtered out.
    b. Pinch biopsy usually provides a larger and deeper tissue sample and allows for more directed biopsies (i.e., tissue from a certain area).
    c. Core biopsy is best suited for visible and accessible mass lesions and allows a large tissue sample to be collected directly from the mass.
    d. Surgical turbinectomy is both diagnostic and therapeutic. In addition to retrieving high-quality samples for histopathology, surgical entry into the nose allows the placement of drains (for the administration of antifungal agents), debridement of necrotic or diseased turbinates, and the excision or debulking of mass lesions.

C. | **Diseases**

  1. Feline upper respiratory tract infection
    a. Agents. In 80%–90% of cases, **feline rhinotracheitis virus (FRV, feline herpesvirus-1)** or **feline calicivirus (FCV)** is the cause of the infection. *Chlamydia psittaci,* *Mycoplasma* species, and *Bordetella bronchiseptica* are implicated less often.
    b. Transmission occurs mostly by **direct contact** with infected animals or fomites (e.g., contaminated cages). **Aerosol transmission** can occur, but only over a relatively short distance (i.e., less than 4 feet). Susceptibility is highest in young kittens, unvaccinated cats, and cats in catteries or multicat households.
      (1) The **average survival time of the virus outside of the animal** is 18–24 hours for FRV and 8–10 days for FCV.
      (2) Most cats become **subclinical carriers** after recovery and serve as **reservoirs for the virus.**
        (a) FRV. Cats shed FRV intermittently for the rest of their lives, often coincid-

TABLE 40-1. Clinical Signs Associated with Upper Respiratory Virus Infection in Cats

	Feline Rhinotracheitis Virus (FRV)	**Feline Calcivirus (FCV)**
Incubation period	3–5 days	1–3 days
Duration	5–10 days	5–7 days
Anorexia and depression	Severe and frequent	Mild and inconsistent
Fever	Frequent	Inconsistent
Nasal signs	Sneezing (severe), marked nasal discharge, ulcerated nares, turbinate necrosis	Sneezing (mild), mild or absent nasal discharge, ulcerated nares
Ocular signs	Severe conjunctivitis, ulcerative keratitis (punctate, oval, or dendritic ulcers), panophthalmitis (neonates)	Mild conjunctivitis
Oral signs	Hypersalivation ulcers (rare)	Oral ulcers (tongue, palate)
Pulmonary signs	Bacterial pneumonia (rare)	Viral pneumonia (infrequent)
Other signs	Abortion, peracute neonatal death	Polyarthritis, interdigital ulcers, enteritis

Modified with permission from Birchard SJ, Sherding RG (eds): *Saunders Manual of Small Animal Practice,* Philadelphia, WB Saunders, 1994, p 101.

ing with stress. Viral shedding lasts for a couple of weeks and may be associated with mild clinical signs.

    (b) FCV. Cats shed FCV persistently for months to years following recovery from the acute infection.

  c. Clinical findings are most severe in kittens and include anorexia, lethargy, oculonasal discharge, and sneezing. Table 40-1 compares the clinical signs associated with FRV and those associated with FCV.

    (1) FRV usually produces severe oculonasal signs and corneal ulceration.

    (2) FCV often produces oral ulceration.

    (3) *C. psittaci* infection is often characterized by chronic uni- or bilateral mucopurulent ocular discharge and mild rhinitis.

  d. Diagnosis is usually based on consistent clinical signs. Identification of the infectious agent is usually not necessary.

    (1) Conjunctival biopsies or **scrapings** may reveal inclusion bodies, which can be associated with FRV or *C. psittaci* infection.

    (2) Serology

      (a) Fluorescent antibody staining of conjunctival or nasal mucosal scrapings may detect FRV.

      (b) Acute and convalescent neutralizing antibody titers can also be performed, but this is rarely done.

    (3) Virus isolation or polymerase chain reaction (PCR) can also detect FRV.

    (4) Tests for **feline leukemia** and **feline immunodeficiency virus (FIV) infection** should be done when infection is persistent, recurrent, or unusually severe.

  e. Treatment is mostly supportive because the disease is usually self-limiting, with signs lasting 5–7 days. Cats should be treated as outpatients if possible to reduce contamination of the hospital environment.

    (1) Symptomatic therapy. Relief of nasal congestion or obstruction is accomplished by **removing dried exudate** from the external nares and providing **adequate hydration** and **airway humidification.** Nasal **decongestants** (e.g., phenylephrine, oxymetazoline) may also be helpful.

    (2) Antibiotic therapy

      (a) Secondary bacterial infection. If the nasal discharge is purulent, antibiotic therapy with ampicillin or amoxicillin may be indicated to treat secondary bacterial infection.

(b) *Chlamydia* or *Mycoplasma* infections are treated with chloramphenicol, tetracycline, or doxycycline.

(3) Treatment of oral lesions. Irrigation with **topical chlorhexidine solution** can be used on necrotic oral lesions.

(4) Treatment of ocular lesions

  (a) FRV infection. Corneal ulceration associated with FRV infection is treated with a **topical broad-spectrum antibiotic ophthalmic ointment** and **atropine.** Antiviral agents (e.g., **idoxuridine, trifluridine**) may also be considered to treat FRV-induced corneal ulceration.

  (b) *C. psittaci* infection. Ocular lesions associated with *C. psittaci* infection are treated with **topical tetracycline ointment.**

(5) Supportive therapy (e.g., intravenous fluid therapy, enteral hyperalimentation, supplemental oxygen) may be required for severely ill cats.

(6) Treatment of complications. Chronic rhinitis or sinusitis may develop from persistent local FRV infection, turbinate ulceration, osteolysis and necrosis, or secondary bacterial infection.

  (a) Chronic intermittent or **prolonged antibiotic therapy.** "Chronic snufflers" are usually treated with chronic intermittent or prolonged antibiotic therapy.

  (b) Surgical turbinectomy (with or without frontal sinus ablation) may be considered in select cases.

 f. Prognosis is good. Most cats will not develop chronic symptomatic infection, but those that do still have a reasonably good quality of life.

 g. Prevention

(1) Vaccination usually prevents clinical illness but does not eradicate the carrier state or stop virus shedding.

  (a) Vaccine products do not protect against all strains of FCV.

  (b) Vaccination should begin at 8–9 weeks of age with a booster at 12 weeks of age. Yearly revaccination is recommended.

(2) Isolation of all cats for 3 weeks before entering a multicat environment is recommended. It is also important to ensure that the new cat has been vaccinated before entering the household.

(3) Minimize stress. Clean, warm, well-ventilated facilities with adequate space will reduce susceptibility in catteries.

(4) Disinfection of potential fomites (e.g., food dishes, blankets, cages) will decrease disease transmission.

 2. Nasal mycoses

  a. Aspergillosis

(1) Etiology

  (a) Organisms. *Aspergillus fumigatus,* a normal inhabitant of the nasal cavity, is the most common cause of aspergillosis. Other *Aspergillus* species, such as *A. nidulans, A. niger,* and *A. flavus,* may also cause aspergillosis. Infection with *Penicillium* species can also produce identical clinical signs.

  (b) Predisposing factors. Depressed immune function, underlying nasal disease (e.g., neoplasia), or excessive exposure to the organism may be predisposing factors. In dogs, nasal aspergillosis has no age or breed specificity. It is rare in cats.

(2) Pathogenesis. Infection results in invasion, destruction, and necrosis of the nasal mucosa and turbinates.

(3) Clinical findings. The most common signs are facial pain, profuse uni- or bilateral sanguinopurulent nasal discharge, and ulceration of the external nares.

(4) Diagnosis

  (a) Radiography

   (i) Turbinate destruction is revealed as increased radiolucency in most dogs. Some have a mixed pattern of lucent and fluid dense areas.

   (ii) Frontal sinus involvement occurs in most dogs.

(b) **Laboratory findings**

(i) **Cytologic examination** and **bacterial** or **fungal culture** are usually not rewarding. Fungal elements are rarely visualized and *Aspergillus* or *Penicillium* species can be successfully cultured in approximately 40% of healthy animals.

(ii) **Serologic detection** of infection can be useful, but false-positive results occur in 6%–15% of cases, and negative results can occur.

(iii) **Biopsies** may reveal fungal invasion accompanied by chronic inflammation. Multiple biopsies and special stains may be necessary.

(c) **Rhinoscopic findings.** Erosion, loss of nasal turbinates, and **fungal plaques** (i.e., fluffy patches of fungal growth) may be observed. The absence of characteristic rhinoscopic findings does not rule out fungal infection.

(5) **Treatment**

(a) **Enilconazole,** administered twice daily into each nasal cavity for 7–10 days, is associated with an 80%–90% cure rate. The drug is diluted in water and instilled into each nasal cavity through fenestrated tubing placed into each frontal sinus and extending into the nasal cavity. Repeat treatments may be necessary.

(b) **Ketoconazole, thiabendazole,** and **fluconazole** may be administered orally but are less effective. Studies on the oral administration of **itraconazole** are ongoing.

(c) **Clotrimazole.** A regimen involving a single installation of clotrimazole into the frontal sinuses and nasal cavity may be effective.

b. **Cryptococcosis**

(1) **Etiology.** Cryptococcosis is caused by **Cryptococcus neoformans,** which is found in the soil, especially in areas contaminated with pigeon droppings.

(2) **Clinical findings.** In cats, infection of the nasal cavity, CNS, eyes, skin, or subcutaneous tissue can occur. In dogs, infection occurs less frequently and usually involves the CNS. Subclinical pulmonary infections are common in both dogs and cats.

(a) **Sneezing** and **uni- or bilateral mucopurulent nasal discharge** is the most common sign.

(b) A **polyp-like mass** within the nares or **swelling over the bridge of the nose** is present in many cats.

(c) **Submandibular lymphadenopathy** is common.

(d) **Cutaneous** or **subcutaneous lesions** (e.g., papules, nodules, ulceration) are present in approximately 40% of cats.

(e) **Neurologic signs** may include **seizures, depression, ataxia,** and **paresis.**

(f) **Ophthalmologic signs** can include **anterior uveitis** and **blindness,** which may result from exudative retinal detachment, granulomatous chorioretinitis, panophthalmitis, or optic neuritis.

(g) **Systemic signs** may include **anorexia, lethargy,** and **weight loss.**

(3) **Diagnosis**

(a) **Cytologic samples** may be taken from nasal discharge, draining tracts, lymph node aspirates, or cerebrospinal fluid (CSF). The diagnosis is usually made by identifying the organism in cytologic samples.

(b) **Radiography.** Findings include increased soft tissue density within the nasal cavity and some turbinate destruction.

(c) **Rhinoscopy** reveals inflamed mucosa.

(d) **Serologic testing** using the LCAT is sensitive and specific for cryptococcal infection and can also be used to monitor response to therapy.

(e) **Histologic examination** of tissue biopsies or culture of CSF (when CNS involvement is suspected) can be performed if cytology or serology fail to detect the organism.

(4) **Treatment**

(a) **Ketoconazole** is the preferred antifungal agent and is administered for 1–2 months following the resolution of clinical signs (i.e., for a total of

3–6 months). Cryptococcal antigen titers monitored on a monthly basis can help assess response to therapy. Side effects include anorexia, vomiting, liver enzyme elevations, and hyperbilirubinemia.

    (b) Amphotericin B alone or in combination with **flucytosine** or **ketoconazole** is another treatment option.

    (c) Fluconazole and **itraconazole** are newer antifungal agents under investigation.

  (5) Prognosis. With an adequate duration of treatment, recovery in cats is fair to good. CNS involvement is associated with a poorer prognosis.

3. Bacterial rhinitis

  a. Etiology. Bacterial rhinitis is **usually secondary to an underlying nasal disorder** (e.g., neoplasia in dogs, viral rhinitis in cats).

  b. Clinical findings. Bacterial rhinitis produces a **mucopurulent nasal discharge.**

  c. Diagnosis

    (1) Cytology forms the basis for diagnosis and usually reveals neutrophilic inflammation with intra- and extracellular bacteria.

    (2) Bacterial culture from deep within the nasal cavity is indicated but can be difficult to interpret. Heavy growth of one or two bacterial species may be significant.

  d. Treatment. Antibiotic selection should be based on sensitivity testing.

    (1) If the response is good within 1 week, therapy should be continued for a total of 4–6 weeks.

    (2) If the response is poor, another antibiotic or additional diagnostic evaluation should be considered.

  e. Prognosis. Long-term resolution depends on the presence and nature of any underlying disorders.

4. Nasopharyngeal polyps are pink polypoid growths that arise from a stalk attached near the auditory (eustachian) tube in the nasopharynx. They may extend into the middle ear and external ear canal as well as into the nasopharynx. Kittens and young adult cats are most often affected.

  a. Clinical findings

    (1) Stertorous respiration, upper airway obstruction, and a **serous** to **mucopurulent nasal discharge** may be observed.

    (2) Signs of otitis externa, media, or **interna** may also be present.

  b. Diagnosis is based on finding a soft tissue mass above the soft palate, in the nasopharynx, or in the external ear canal.

    (1) Deep otoscopic examination and **radiographs** of the tympanic bulla help to determine the extent of involvement.

    (2) Histologic examination of polyps reveals a mixture of inflammatory and fibrous connective tissue covered by epithelium.

  c. Treatment

    (1) Surgical excision must remove all of the mass, or regrowth will occur (usually within 1 year).

    (2) Bulla osteotomy may have to be performed if there is middle ear involvement.

  d. Prognosis is excellent.

5. Nasal neoplasia usually occurs in older animals, especially mid- to large-breed dogs (especially Airedale terriers, collies, Old English sheepdogs, basset hounds, German shepherds, keeshonds, German short-haired pointers, Scottish terriers.)

  a. Types

    (1) Most nasal tumors in dogs and cats are malignant. In dogs, **adenocarcinoma** and **undifferentiated carcinoma** are very common. **Squamous cell carcinoma, lymphosarcoma** (more common in cats), and **fibrosarcoma** also occur.

    (2) Benign tumors may include **adenomas, papilloma, transmissible venereal tumors,** and **fibromas.**

  b. Clinical findings include obstruction to airflow in one or both nasal cavities and a uni- or bilateral chronic serous to mucopurulent (possibly bloody) nasal discharge.

(1) Ulcerated, draining tracts or facial deformity may result from erosion of the overlying facial bones.

(2) Changes in mentation or behavior and seizures may result if the cribriform plate is breached and the tumor or associated inflammation extends into the cranial vault.

(3) Exophthalmus may be observed if the orbit has been invaded.

(4) Secondary bacterial rhinitis is common.

c. **Diagnosis** is usually based on histopathologic examination of tissue biopsies obtained during rhinoscopy.

(1) **Rhinoscopic examination** may reveal mass lesions. Adenocarcinomas tend to involve the caudal aspect of the nasal cavity and may be difficult to visualize.

(2) **Radiography.** Findings can include an increased soft tissue density in one or both nasal cavities; turbinate, septal, or facial bone destruction; frontal sinus opacification; and periosteal bone formation. Pulmonary metastasis is uncommon. Adenocarcinomas tend to be locally aggressive and do not metastasize until late in the course of the disease.

(3) **CT** can be used to more accurately assess the extent of tumor infiltration.

d. **Treatment**

(1) **Surgical debulking** of the tumor followed by **radiation therapy** is associated with the longest survival times in patients with malignant tumors (54% survival rates at 1 year and 35% at 3 years). Survival time is not increased if surgical excision alone is used.

(2) **Combination chemotherapy** or **radiation therapy** may achieve a reasonable response in patients with lymphosarcoma. **Chemotherapy** alone (e.g., with cisplatin) may elicit a partial response from other tumor types.

e. **Prognosis.** In general, the prognosis is poor if malignant neoplasia is present.

6. **Lymphocytic/plasmacytic rhinitis** is a rare inflammatory condition of the nose.

a. **Clinical findings** include sneezing and serous, mucopurulent, or hemorrhagic nasal discharge.

b. **Diagnosis** is based on finding lymphocytic/plasmacytic inflammation on nasal mucosal biopsies after an extensive search has failed to identify other disorders (e.g., neoplasia, fungal infection). Radiographically, increased soft-tissue density and turbinate destruction may be observed in the nasal cavity.

c. **Treatment** with **prednisone** at immunosuppressive doses usually produces improvement within 2 weeks. The dose should then be tapered to the lowest effective dose.

d. **Prognosis.** The long-term prognosis is unknown.

7. **Allergic rhinitis** is an uncommon and not well-described syndrome in dogs and cats.

a. **Etiology.** The development of allergic rhinitis is usually associated with allergen exposure (e.g., new kitty litter, furniture, or carpet; recent use of cleaning agents in the house; cigarette smoking; seasonal changes).

b. **Clinical findings** include sneezing and a serous or mucopurulent nasal discharge.

c. **Diagnosis** is based on a history of allergen exposure and clinical signs. Nasal biopsy reveals eosinophilic inflammation. Thorough evaluation does not reveal an underlying nasal disease.

d. **Treatment** consists of removal of the allergen (if possible) and treatment with antihistamines (e.g., chlorpheniramine) or antiinflammatory doses of corticosteroids (i.e., prednisone).

e. **Prognosis** is good if the animal responds promptly to treatment.

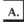 **LARYNGEAL DISORDERS**

A. **Clinical manifestations.** With most disorders, signs develop slowly over a few weeks to months.

1. **Inspiratory dyspnea** is common and results from upper airway obstruction. Inspira-

tory dyspnea may also be caused by diseases of the pharynx (e.g., masses), trachea (e.g., strictures), or pleural space (e.g., effusion). The dyspnea may not be evident until the respiratory rate is increased.

2. **Stridor** (a harsh, high-pitched sound heard during inspiration) is a common sign but may not be evident until the respiratory rate is increased.

3. A **change in the dog's bark** may be noted.

4. **Syncope** and **life-threatening respiratory distress** can result from severe laryngeal disease and upper airway obstruction.

B. **Diagnostic approaches and techniques**

1. **Radiography** may reveal radiodense foreign bodies (e.g., needles) and masses in the laryngeal area.

2. **Laryngoscopy**
   a. Direct visualization of the larynx and related structures and assessment of the function of the arytenoid cartilages and vocal folds can be performed with the animal under light anesthesia. A detailed examination (with the animal under a deeper plane of anesthesia) of the soft palate, pharynx, nasopharynx, and larynx should follow.
   b. Scrapings or swabs for cytologic examination and tissue biopsies can be collected; however, bacterial cultures are difficult to interpret due to the presence of normal bacterial flora.

C. **Diseases**

1. **Laryngeal paralysis** is characterized by poor or absent abduction of the arytenoid cartilages during inspiration and is primarily a disease of large-breed dogs. Both cartilages are usually involved if clinical signs are present.
   a. **Etiology**
      (1) **Idiopathic.** Most cases of laryngeal paralysis in dogs are idiopathic.
      (2) **Congenital** laryngeal paralysis occurs in Bouvier des Flanders, Siberian huskies, Dalmatians, and bull terriers.
      (3) **Other causes** include trauma, inflammation, or neoplasia involving the ventral cervical region or cranial thorax (i.e., disruption of the recurrent laryngeal nerves) and polymyopathy or polyneuropathy resulting from immune-mediated or hormonal disorders (e.g., hypothyroidism).
   b. **Clinical findings** relate to upper airway obstruction and include **inspiratory dyspnea** and **stridor**. Dyspnea may be exacerbated by the development of edema and inflammation in the larynx, pharynx, or, occasionally, the lungs. **Syncopal episodes** or **severe respiratory distress** and **cyanosis** may develop in severely affected dogs.
   c. **Diagnosis** is established by visualization of inadequate arytenoid cartilage abduction while the dog is under light anesthesia. Further evaluation to identify any underlying disease is indicated (e.g., cervical and thoracic radiographs, thyroid and adrenal testing, electrodiagnostic testing).
   d. **Treatment**
      (1) **Treatment of the underlying disease** is appropriate; however, it rarely results in significant reversal of the laryngeal paralysis.
      (2) **Surgical intervention** (e.g., arytenoid lateralization, partial arytenoidectomy) produces the best long-term improvement. These procedures attempt to enlarge the laryngeal opening without significantly increasing the risk of aspiration.
      (3) **Supportive treatment**
         (a) **Corticosteroids** are indicated if laryngeal inflammation and edema are present.
         (b) **Supplemental oxygen, endotracheal intubation,** or **tracheostomy tube** placement may be required for animals with severe respiratory distress.
   e. **Prognosis.** For uncomplicated cases, the prognosis with surgical treatment is fair. Concurrent alteration of pharyngeal or esophageal motility (e.g., megaesophagus) will increase the risk of aspiration pneumonia.

2. **Brachycephalic syndrome** is a collection of upper airway abnormalities commonly observed in brachycephalic dogs and, to a lesser extent, cats (e.g., Persians, Himalayans). Abnormalities may occur in various combinations and include **stenotic nares, elongated soft palate, everted laryngeal saccules,** and **laryngeal collapse. Tracheal hypoplasia** may also occur in English bulldogs.
   a. **Clinical findings** relate to upper airway obstruction and include **inspiratory dyspnea, stridor,** and, in severe cases, **syncope** and **cyanosis.** Long-standing inspiratory difficulties can result in edema and inflammation of the larynx and eversion of the laryngeal saccules, both of which exacerbate the upper airway obstruction.
   b. **Diagnosis** is based on the animal breed and the presence of stenotic nares, an elongated soft palate, or laryngeal abnormalities.
   c. **Treatment**
      (1) **Surgical intervention** to improve airflow (e.g., widening of the external nares, resecting an elongated soft palate or removing everted laryngeal saccules) is necessary to achieve long-term relief.
      (2) **Supportive treatment**
         (a) **Corticosteroid therapy** may improve signs temporarily.
         (b) **Supplemental oxygen, endotracheal intubation,** or **tracheostomy tube placement** may be required in animals with severe respiratory distress.
   d. **Prognosis**
      (1) The prognosis is good if abnormalities are surgically corrected early. The upper airway obstruction tends to progress, and related problems (e.g., laryngeal edema and inflammation, everted saccules) develop unless corrective measures are employed.
      (2) The prognosis is poor for animals with laryngeal collapse or severe tracheal hypoplasia.

3. **Laryngeal neoplasia** is uncommon.
   a. **Types**
      (1) Squamous cell carcinoma in dogs and lymphosarcoma in cats are the most common tumor types. Infiltration of adjacent tumors (e.g., thyroid carcinoma) may also occur.
      (2) Other tumor types include mast cell tumors, carcinomas, melanomas, sarcomas, and benign tumors.
   b. **Clinical findings** are similar to those seen with other laryngeal disorders.
   c. **Diagnosis.** Radiography and laryngoscopy help establish the diagnosis; definitive diagnosis is based on histopathology or cytology. **Differential diagnoses** include nasopharyngeal polyps, granuloma (e.g., from a foreign body), abscess, and granulomatous laryngitis (a corticosteroid-responsive inflammatory condition of unknown etiology).
   d. **Treatment**
      (1) **Surgery**
         (a) **Surgical excision** is usually effective for benign tumors. Generally, malignant tumors are not resectable, although debulking the tumor may temporarily improve airflow.
         (b) **Total laryngectomy** with a **permanent tracheostomy** can also be considered in select cases.
      (2) **Radiation therapy** or **chemotherapy** can be considered, depending on the type of tumor.
   e. **Prognosis** is poor with malignant tumors.

III. TRACHEAL AND BRONCHIAL DISORDERS

A. **Clinical manifestations**
   1. **Cough** (see Chapter 27) and **dyspnea** (see Chapter 28) are common.
   2. **Nonspecific signs** include **anorexia, fever, lethargy,** and **weight loss.**

B. Diagnostic approaches and techniques

1. **Physical examination**
   a. **Auscultation**
      (1) Auscultation of the **larynx** and **trachea** may reveal areas of stertor or stridor indicative of obstructive lesions.
      (2) Auscultation of the **right** and **left lung fields** may reveal **crackles** and **wheezes.**
         (a) **Crackles** are nonmusical, discontinuous sounds (similar to paper being crumpled) that are associated with pulmonary edema or exudate in airways.
         (b) **Wheezes** are musical, continuous sounds associated with airway narrowing (e.g., bronchoconstriction, extraluminal compression, exudate, masses within airways).
   b. **Lung sounds.** Decreased lung sounds may indicate the presence of pleural effusion, pneumothorax, diaphragmatic hernia, or large masses.

2. **Imaging techniques**
   a. **Radiography**
      (1) **Lungs.** The lungs should be examined for the presence of vascular, bronchial, alveolar, or interstitial patterns as well as mass lesions, cysts, or lung lobe torsions. Causes of different lung patterns are summarized in Figure 40-1.
      (2) **Extrathoracic structures** (e.g., the ribs, sternum, ventral column) should be assessed.
   b. **Ultrasonography** is useful for evaluation of mass lesions close to the thoracic wall and can determine if the mass is solid, cystic, or fluid filled. It can also be used to guide aspiration or tissue biopsy procedures.
   c. **Nonselective angiography** can be used to diagnose heartworm infection in cats and pulmonary artery thromboembolism.

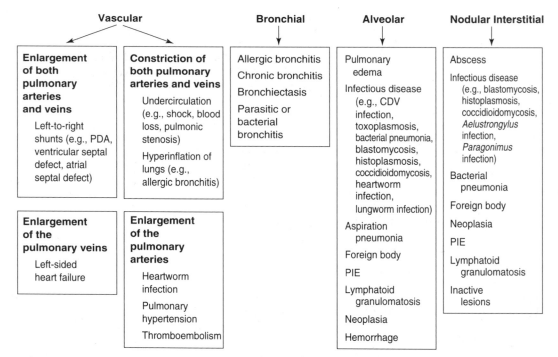

FIGURE 40-1. Differential diagnoses for radiographic lung patterns. *CDV* = canine distemper virus; *PDA* = patent ductus arteriosus; *PIE* = pulmonary infiltrates with eosinophils.

   d. Nuclear imaging can be used to assess ventilation and perfusion of different regions of the lung.

3. **Transtracheal wash** is indicated for animals with a chronic cough or pulmonary parenchymal disease.
   a. The diagnostic yield is best for animals with airway disease, but the procedure may help characterize some parenchymal disorders.
   b. Cytologic examination of samples can characterize inflammatory processes and may yield infectious agents (e.g., *Histoplasma, Blastomyces, Cryptococcus*), parasitic eggs or larvae, or, rarely, neoplastic cells. The sample can also be cultured for bacteria.

4. **Bronchoalveolar lavage** is useful if transtracheal wash has failed to provide a diagnosis. The fluid and cells collected reflect disease processes in the interstitium and alveoli.
   a. General anesthesia is required to perform this procedure.
   b. Transient hypoxemia (especially in cats) is a complication of the procedure, but patients usually respond well to supplemental oxygen.
   c. Bronchoalveolar lavage is contraindicated for animals in severe respiratory distress.

5. **Arterial blood gas analysis** can be used to assess pulmonary function. Venous blood gas measurements do not adequately reflect pulmonary gas exchange.
   a. **Arterial oxygen tension (Pao$_2$)** and **arterial carbon dioxide tension (Paco$_2$) assessments**
      (1) A **decreased Pao$_2$ and an increased Paco$_2$ can be caused by:**
         (a) **Hypoventilation** resulting from upper airway obstruction, pleural space disease (e.g., effusion, pneumothorax, chest wall disorder), reduced respiratory muscle function (e.g., anesthesia, CNS disease, polyneuropathy, polymyopathy), and severe emphysema
         (b) **Severe thromboembolic disease**
         (c) **Inadvertent venous sampling**
      (2) A **decreased Pao$_2$** and a **normal** or **decreased Paco$_2$** can be caused by:
         (a) **Ventilation–perfusion mismatching** (i.e., areas of the lung are ventilated but not perfused, or vice versa)
         (b) **Pulmonary parenchymal disease**
         (c) **Lung lobe consolidation** or **collapse**
         (d) **Pulmonary thromboembolism**
   b. **Alveolar–arterial (A-a) oxygen gradient.** The A-a oxygen gradient is used to differentiate hypoventilation from ventilation–perfusion mismatch.
   c. **Acid–base status** can also be assessed with blood gas measurements (see Chapter 43 Part II:V).

6. **Bronchoscopy** allows visualization of structural abnormalities (e.g., collapsing trachea), mass lesions, and foreign bodies and can be used to obtain samples (e.g., biopsies, brushings) from the lower airways. It is contraindicated in animals with severe respiratory distress unless a retrievable foreign body is present.

7. **Biopsy**
   a. **Needle aspiration** or **biopsy of the lung** should be performed only if less invasive procedures are not diagnostic.
      (1) These procedures are indicated for diffuse pulmonary parenchymal disorders or discrete mass lesions adjacent to the chest wall.
      (2) They are contraindicated in animals with pulmonary hypertension or a coagulopathy. Complications include pneumothorax, hemothorax, and pulmonary hemorrhage. Suspected cysts or abscesses should not be aspirated.
   b. **Bronchial biopsies** consist primarily of mucosa unless taken at the bifurcation of two small airways, in which case small samples of bronchial wall and some pulmonary parenchyma may be obtained. Complications are few, but small sample size limits the usefulness of this procedure.
   c. **Open-chest lung biopsy.** A thoracotomy can be performed to collect biopsy samples and to excise localized lesions. The biopsy sample is of very high quality,

and other structures such as regional lymph nodes may also be biopsied. It is considered for pulmonary parenchymal disorders when other less invasive tests are not diagnostic or if a surgically reversible disorder is present or suspected.

C. Diseases

1. **Infectious tracheobronchitis (kennel cough)** is the most common respiratory infection in dogs. Frequently, there is a history of recent contact with other dogs (e.g., boarding at a kennel or attending a dog show 2–10 days prior to the onset of clinical signs).
   a. **Etiology.** Agents include *Bordetella bronchiseptica, parainfluenza virus, Mycoplasma,* **canine adenovirus types 1** and **2, canine herpesvirus, reovirus,** and **canine distemper virus (CDV),** alone or in combination.
   b. **Clinical findings**
      (1) Infectious tracheobronchitis is characterized by the acute onset of a **honking cough** (i.e., a frequent, severe cough that may or may not be productive) that is exacerbated by exercise or excitement. The cough is inducible on tracheal palpation.
      (2) Complications such as secondary bacterial infection are rare, but dogs with collapsing trachea, chronic bronchitis, or immotile cilia syndrome may be at increased risk.
   c. **Diagnosis**
      (1) In uncomplicated cases, diagnosis is based on the history and physical examination. Systemic illness is absent and physical examination findings are minimal.
      (2) In cases that are persistent or complicated by systemic disease, additional diagnostic tests (e.g., CBC, serum biochemical profile, thoracic radiographs, transtracheal wash) are indicated.
   d. **Treatment.** Uncomplicated infectious tracheobronchitis is self-limiting, and signs usually resolve within 1–2 weeks.
      (1) **Antibiotic treatment. Tetracycline, amoxicillin** with **clavulanic acid,** and **chloramphenicol** are usually effective against *B. bronchiseptica.*
      (2) **Supportive treatment**
         (a) **Rest** and restricted activity will help reduce coughing.
         (b) **Prednisone** at anti-inflammatory doses for 5–7 days can rapidly diminish the severity and frequency of the cough.
         (c) **Narcotic antitussive drugs** (e.g., butorphanol, hydrocodone bitartrate) can be effective but should be avoided if the cough is productive or if significant airway secretions are present. Nonnarcotic antitussive drugs (e.g., dextromethorphan) are of variable effectiveness.
         (d) **Nebulization** with saline to help mobilize secretions can also be considered in dogs with complicated infections.
   e. **Prevention**
      (1) **Avoidance of exposure, good husbandry, routine disinfection,** and **well-ventilated housing** will help decrease the risk of infection or at least reduce the severity of the disease. If dogs with infectious tracheobronchitis are hospitalized, they should be quarantined and personnel should take appropriate precautions to avoid transmission to other patients.
      (2) **Vaccination** will also decrease risk of infection and severity of disease.
         (a) Dogs that are not exposed to other dogs on a routine basis should receive annual vaccination with modified-live virus vaccines for parainfluenza virus and canine adenovirus type 2.
         (b) Dogs that are exposed to other dogs should receive a vaccine against *B. bronchiseptica,* using either an injectable or intranasal product. Intranasal products rapidly induce local immunity and can overcome maternal immunity in pups older than 3 weeks; however, intranasal vaccination can result in mild clinical signs.

2. **Collapsing trachea** is characterized by flattened cartilaginous tracheal rings and the development of a loose redundant dorsal tracheal membrane. Tracheal narrowing

and airway obstruction results. The intra- or extrathoracic trachea or mainstem bronchi may be affected.

    a. Clinical findings. Collapsing trachea is primarily a disorder of middle-aged miniature and toy breed dogs. Signs begin in adulthood and slowly progress over months to years.

        (1) A **honking, nonproductive cough** associated with excitement, exercise, or pressure on the trachea (i.e., a leash) is a characteristic finding. The cough may be elicited on tracheal palpation, and an end-expiratory click or snap may be heard if intrathoracic tracheal collapse is occurring.

        (2) Respiratory distress may develop in animals with severe disease.

        (3) Systemic signs of illness are **absent.** Concurrent diseases such as chronic bronchitis, left atrial enlargement, or heart failure may exacerbate clinical signs.

    b. Diagnosis is based on clinical findings and cervical and thoracic radiographs.

        (1) Radiography. Cervical radiographs taken on inspiration will demonstrate collapse of the extrathoracic trachea. **Thoracic radiographs** taken on expiration will show collapse of the intrathoracic trachea.

        (2) Fluoroscopy may also be used to demonstrate collapse.

        (3) Bronchoscopy. Bronchoscopic visualization of a flattened tracheal lumen with a dorsal redundant membrane provides a definitive diagnosis but is not necessary in most cases.

        (4) Other tests (e.g., inspiratory thoracic radiographs, transtracheal wash, cardiac ultrasound) may be warranted if concurrent disease is suspected.

    c. Treatment

        (1) Nonmedical therapy, such as weight reduction (if the animal is obese), use of a harness instead of a collar, and the avoidance of excitement, overheating, or strenuous exercise, is sufficient for most dogs.

        (2) Medical therapy

            (a) Cough suppressants (e.g., dextromethorphan, butorphanol) can be considered if the cough is unrelenting and nonproductive.

            (b) Bronchodilators (e.g., aminophylline, theophylline, terbutaline) may be beneficial in some patients.

            (c) Antimicrobials are indicated if bacterial infection is present.

            (d) Corticosteroids are indicated for the acute management of animals in respiratory distress or for dogs with a severe, unrelenting cough that has not responded to other therapy.

        (3) Surgical procedures (e.g., plication of the dorsal tracheal membrane or the use of plastic supportive prostheses placed around and sutured to the trachea) to reverse severe tracheal collapse can be considered. Extrathoracic tracheal collapse is easier than intrathoracic collapse to treat surgically.

3. Allergic bronchitis is characterized by airway obstruction that can result from the accumulation of mucus or exudate in airways, bronchospasm, inflammatory cell infiltration into bronchial walls, and epithelial hyperplasia and hypertrophy of bronchial smooth muscle. Cats appear to be affected with allergic bronchitis (feline asthma) more frequently than dogs. Animals are usually affected as young to middle aged adults.

    a. Etiology. Allergic bronchitis results from a hypersensitivity reaction to inhaled allergens, infectious agents, neoplasia, or unknown antigens. Primary allergic bronchitis is diagnosed when no infectious agent or neoplastic disease is found and the allergen is unknown or suspected to be inhaled.

    b. Clinical findings are usually slowly progressive.

        (1) Cough is the most common clinical sign in both dogs and cats. However, cats may experience bouts of respiratory distress (from bronchospasm), which may be life-threatening.

        (2) Wheezing may be reported by owners. Expiratory wheezing and crackles may be heard by the clinician.

        (3) Systemic signs of illness are **usually not present** in primary allergic bronchitis.

    c. **Diagnosis** is based on clinical findings, thoracic radiographs, and transtracheal wash results. **Differential diagnoses** include **heartworm** or **lungworm infection.**
       (1) **Thoracic radiographs** may reveal a bronchial pattern and occasionally a reticular interstitial pattern, hyperinflation of the lungs, or right middle lung lobe collapse. Negative radiographic findings do not rule out the disease.
       (2) **Transtracheal wash fluid** usually reveals eosinophilic inflammation; however, nonseptic neutrophilic inflammation may occur in some cats.
    d. **Treatment**
       (1) **Acute respiratory distress** in cats should be treated with a rapid-acting injectable **glucocorticoid** (i.e., prednisolone sodium succinate), **supplemental oxygen,** and possibly a **bronchodilator** (e.g., aminophylline). Subcutaneous **epinephrine** injection may be necessary to help reverse bronchospasm.
       (2) **Long-term therapeutic measures** include removal of the offending allergen (if possible), corticosteroids (i.e., prednisone) and bronchodilators (e.g., aminophylline, terbutaline).
    e. **Prognosis.** The prognosis is good for the control of clinical signs, but a cure is unlikely unless an underlying cause is found and eliminated.

  4. **Chronic bronchitis** is an irreversible disease characterized by fibrosis, glandular hypertrophy, epithelial hyperplasia, mucus accumulation, and chronic inflammation in the airways. **Bronchiectasis** (i.e., permanent dilation of the airways) may be a complication of chronic bronchitis. Bronchiectasis usually affects all major airways, but is occasionally localized. Chronic bronchitis tends to be a disease of middle-aged and older small-breed dogs.
    a. **Etiology.** The initiating cause is seldom found, but chronic inflammation from infectious agents or hypersensitivities could be responsible.
    b. **Clinical findings**
       (1) **Chronic cough.** The development of a slowly progressive, productive or nonproductive chronic cough (i.e., present on most days for over 2 consecutive months) is the **hallmark feature** of this disease.
       (2) **Increased bronchovesicular sounds, crackles,** and **wheezes** may be heard.
       (3) **Systemic signs of illness are usually absent,** but exercise intolerance may be associated with severe disease.
    c. **Diagnosis** is based on a history of chronic cough and compatible radiographic and airway cytologic findings. Common **differential diagnoses** for a chronic cough in a small-breed dog include **collapsing trachea** and **mitral valve insufficiency.**
       (1) **Radiography. Thoracic radiographs** usually reveal a **bronchial pattern** with a variable **increase in interstitial markings.** Bronchiectasis and right middle lung lobe collapse are detected in some patients.
       (2) **Transtracheal wash** or **bronchial brushings** typically reveals chronic inflammation dominated by **nondegenerate neutrophils.** Chronic bronchitis may be complicated by bacterial infection, which would result in degenerate neutrophils and visible intra- and extracellular bacteria.
       (3) **Bronchoscopy** is not required to diagnose chronic bronchitis in most cases but if performed, usually reveals **roughened, granular, erythematous and edematous mucosa** in most airways. **Abundant mucus** is often present and may plug small airways. **Airway collapse** may be observed if cartilaginous support has been weakened by chronic inflammation. **Airway dilation** may be detected if bronchiectasis is present.
    d. **Treatment** is mainly symptomatic and focuses on decreasing the frequency of the cough, minimizing airway inflammation, and treating complications (e.g., bacterial infection).
       (1) **Nonmedical therapy**
         (a) **Limiting exercise** or **weight reduction** (in obese animals) may help some patients.
         (b) **Mobilization of airway secretions.** Good hydration and airway humidification (e.g., by placing the animal in a steamy bathroom), vaporization, or nebulization can help mobilize airway secretions.

(2) Medical therapy

(a) Corticosteroids (e.g., prednisone) may reduce airway inflammation. They should be tapered to the lowest effective dose over a 2-month period and avoided if bacterial infection is suspected or detected.

(b) Bronchodilators (e.g., albuterol, terbutaline, aminophylline, theophylline) are beneficial in some dogs with chronic bronchitis.

(c) Cough suppressants (e.g., dextromethorphan, butorphanol, dihydrocodeine) should be used only in those patients with a dry, nonproductive, unrelenting cough. Suppression of a productive cough will interfere with the clearance of airway secretions and exacerbate the disease process.

(d) Antibiotics should be administered if bacterial infection is suspected or confirmed. (Bacterial infection is more common in animals with bronchiectasis.) Drug selection should be based on bacterial culture and sensitivity testing.

e. **Prognosis.** The prognosis for chronic bronchitis is fair to good if signs and complications can be adequately managed. Recurrent bacterial infection is common in dogs with bronchiectasis.

5. **Tracheal neoplasia** is uncommon.

a. **Types.** Tumor types include squamous cell carcinoma, lymphosarcoma, adenocarcinoma, osteoma, osteosarcoma, chondroma, chondrosarcoma, and leiomyoma.

b. **Clinical findings.** Tracheal masses result in **dyspnea, stridor,** or **raspy respiration.**

c. **Diagnosis**

(1) Radiography. Lateral radiographs of the trachea will frequently detect soft-tissue masses within the tracheal lumen. Extraluminal compression from a mass outside the trachea may also be observed.

(2) Bronchoscopy can be used to visualize or take biopsy samples from masses within the tracheal lumen.

d. **Treatment** may involve **surgical resection, bronchoscopic removal** (if tumors are small and benign), or **chemotherapy.**

e. **Prognosis** depends on the type of tumor and the extent of involvement.

6. **Tracheal trauma**

a. **Etiology.** Bite wounds, gunshot injuries, or diagnostic procedures (e.g., transtracheal wash, misguided jugular venipuncture) can lead to penetration of the trachea.

b. **Clinical findings.** Injuries can result in air leakage and the development of subcutaneous emphysema, which may spread to involve the entire body.

c. **Treatment.** If the emphysema is stable or regressing and there is no respiratory distress from tracheal obstruction, treatment consists of cage rest. However, if the emphysema persists, surgical closure of the tracheal injuries may be necessary.

7. **Primary ciliary dyskinesia (immotile cilia syndrome)** is a rare disorder characterized by defective clearance of respiratory secretions due to dysfunctional cilia on respiratory epithelial cells, resulting in chronic bacterial rhinitis and bronchitis. **Situs inversus** (transposition of thoracic and abdominal viscera from left to right) and **bronchiectasis** may be present. Primary ciliary dyskinesia is most often seen in young dogs.

a. **Clinical findings**

(1) Respiratory signs include **chronic mucopurulent nasal discharge** and a **productive cough.**

(2) Other signs. Abnormal ciliary function is present in all ciliated cells and can result in otitis media, deafness, male infertility (as a result of defective sperm motility), hydrocephalus, and dilated renal tubules.

b. **Diagnosis.** The disorder should be suspected if bacterial rhinitis or pneumonia occurs in a dog with situs inversus, bronchiectasis, or infertility. Definitive diagnosis requires electron microscopic evaluation of respiratory mucosal biopsies.

c. **Treatment.** Antibiotics are indicated to control bacterial airway infections. Cough suppressants or glucocorticoids are contraindicated.

d. **Prognosis** is guarded.

8. **Bronchial foreign bodies** are uncommon.
   a. **Etiology.** The aspiration of grass awns by hunting dogs is the most common cause.
   b. **Clinical findings**
      (1) **Large objects.** Respiratory distress will result if the foreign object is large enough to obstruct a large airway.
      (2) **Small objects.** An **acute, nonproductive cough** results from smaller objects. If dogs with grass awn foreign bodies are not treated, the cough often subsides after 2 weeks and is followed by the development of **bronchopulmonary abscesses, fever, lethargy,** and **anorexia.**
   c. **Diagnosis** is made by **bronchoscopic visualization** of the foreign body. Radiographs may reveal a radiodense object within an airway. Radiolucent foreign bodies such as grass awns will not be detected, but the associated inflammation will often produce localized bronchial, interstitial, or alveolar lung patterns.
   d. **Treatment** consists of **foreign body removal** via bronchoscope or surgery and appropriate **antibiotic therapy.**
   e. **Prognosis.** If the foreign body can be identified and removed, the prognosis is good. The prognosis is guarded to grave if grass awn foreign bodies migrate through tissues, resulting in pyothorax, pneumothorax, discospondylitis, or diffuse pleuropneumonia.

9. **Parasitic infections** are discussed in IV D.

IV. PULMONARY PARENCHYMAL DISORDERS

A. Viral pneumonia

1. **Dogs.** CDV is the most common cause of viral pneumonia in dogs (see also Chapter 49 V B). CDV infection can occur in dogs of any age, but unvaccinated puppies (usually between the ages of 3 and 6 months) or those with poor colostral antibody protection are particularly susceptible.
   a. **Pathogenesis.** CDV infects epithelial tissues throughout the gastrointestinal (GI) tract, respiratory tract, CNS, and eyes. Involvement of the respiratory tract is usually associated with severe disease.
   b. **Clinical findings**
      (1) It has been estimated that 25%–75% of dogs infected with CDV develop subclinical infection and clear the virus.
      (2) In dogs with clinical signs, lethargy, anorexia, bilateral serous to mucopurulent nasal discharge, conjunctivitis, and cough may be followed by vomiting and diarrhea. Neurologic signs can occur a few weeks later. Chorioretinitis may be detected on fundoscopic examination. Crackles may be heard over the lung fields.
   c. **Diagnosis.** The combination of respiratory and GI signs in a young, unvaccinated puppy is suggestive of CDV infection. The coexistence of chorioretinitis with or without neurologic signs would be highly suggestive of CDV infection.
      (1) **Thoracic radiographs** usually reveal a generalized interstitial pattern, which commonly progresses to an alveolar pattern as bacterial infection occurs.
      (2) **Transtracheal wash cytology** reveals acute nonseptic inflammation if bacterial infection has not occurred. Respiratory epithelial cells present in transtracheal wash samples may have inclusion bodies. The cells may also be used to detect CDV antigen with fluorescent antibody staining.
   d. **Treatment** is primarily supportive with the addition of antibiotics if bacterial infection is present.
   e. **Prognosis.** Some dogs will survive severe clinical disease, but approximately 50% of these dogs will develop neurologic signs later. The prognosis is guarded in dogs that develop significant clinical signs associated with CDV infection.
   f. **Prevention.** Vaccination programs are highly effective (see Chapter 49 V B 5).

2. Cats. FCV and the **feline infectious peritonitis (FIP) virus** occasionally cause viral pneumonia in cats.

B. | **Bacterial pneumonia** occurs with low to moderate frequency in dogs, and is rare in cats.
   1. Etiology
      a. Secondary infection with opportunistic bacteria (e.g., *Escherichia coli, Streptococcus, Staphylococcus, Pseudomonas,* and *Klebsiella* species) is the **most common cause** of bacterial pneumonia. Predisposing conditions include viral infection, bronchial foreign body, pulmonary neoplasia, mycotic pneumonia, immunodeficiency (e.g., as a result of chemotherapy, feline leukemia or immunodeficiency virus infection), lung or airway parasite infection, megaesophagus, primary ciliary dyskinesia, chronic bronchitis, bronchiectasis, and bronchoesophageal fistula.
      b. Primary bacterial pneumonia can be caused by *B. bronchiseptica* and possibly *Streptococcus zooepidemicus,* but is uncommon. Mycobacterial infections are a rare cause of pneumonia in dogs and cats.
   2. Clinical findings may include mucopurulent nasal discharge, productive cough, dyspnea, exercise intolerance, fever, anorexia, lethargy, and weight loss. Cyanosis may be observed in severely affected animals. Auscultation usually reveals crackles over most lung fields, especially the cranioventral areas.
   3. Diagnosis is based on thoracic radiographs and cytologic examination of transtracheal wash samples.
      a. Radiographs characteristically reveal an alveolar pattern and possibly lung lobe consolidation in the cranioventral lung fields. Increased bronchial and interstitial markings are common. Predisposing abnormalities (e.g., megaesophagus, bronchiectasis) may be observed.
      b. Airway cytology typically reveals septic inflammation with abundant degenerate neutrophils and visible intra- and extracellular bacteria; however, neutrophils may be nondegenerate and bacteria may not be visible in some cases.
      c. Laboratory studies. A **CBC** may reveal a neutrophilic leukocytosis.
      d. Bronchoscopy or **bronchoalveolar lavage** may be indicated for localized disease.
   4. Treatment
      a. Medical therapy
         (1) Antibiotics. Drug selection should be based on culture and sensitivity testing or gram stains.
            (a) Gram-positive cocci are usually sensitive to trimethoprim/sulfonamide, chloramphenicol, and cephalosporins.
            (b) Gram-negative rods are often sensitive to trimethoprim/sulfonamide, chloramphenicol, enrofloxacin, and gentamicin.
            (c) *B. bronchiseptica* infections usually respond to treatment with tetracycline, chloramphenicol, or enrofloxacin.
         (2) Bronchodilators (i.e., theophylline) are most effective in patients with suspected bronchoconstriction (more common in cats) and in animals with aspiration pneumonia. Bronchodilators should be used with caution because they may interfere with the inflammatory response and contribute to ventilation–perfusion mismatching.
         (3) Drugs to avoid include diuretics, corticosteroids, and cough suppressants.
      b. Supportive therapy
         (1) Airway hydration reduces the viscosity of airway secretions and improves removal by coughing and mucociliary clearance. Maintenance of systemic hydration, placing animals in humidified rooms (e.g., a steamy bathroom), and saline nebulization are methods to consider.
         (2) Physiotherapy should include coupage, mild exercise (if possible), and frequent turning of recumbent animals.
         (3) Supplemental oxygen is indicated in patients with cyanosis, a Pao_2 that is less than 60 mm Hg, a $Paco_2$ that is greater than 60–75 mm Hg, or increased respiratory effort in conjunction with a deterioration in mental status or cardiac arrhythmias.

5. **Prognosis** will vary from poor to good, depending on the bacterial species, appropriate antibiotic selection, quality of supportive care, and presence of underlying diseases.

C. Mycotic pneumonia

1. **Histoplasmosis** (see also Chapter 49 II F)
   a. **Pathogenesis.** *Histoplasma capsulatum* enters the body through the respiratory tract and results in either an asymptomatic, self-limiting infection of the lungs or severe pulmonary disease with dissemination to other organs.
   b. **Clinical findings.** Dogs are most often presented with gastrointestinal signs, whereas cats are most often presented with nonspecific signs (e.g., weight loss, fever, anorexia).
      (1) **Respiratory signs** can include dyspnea, coughing, and abnormal lung sounds.
      (2) **Gastrointestinal signs.** Large bowel diarrhea and chronic weight loss are the most common presenting signs in dogs. Hepatomegaly, splenomegaly, icterus, visceral lymphadenopathy, and ascites may also be present.
      (3) **Neurologic** and **ocular involvement** (i.e., granulomatous chorioretinitis, retinal detachment) may also occur.
   c. **Diagnosis** is confirmed by detection of the organism in cytology or biopsy samples collected from the respiratory tract or other affected organ systems.
      (1) **Radiography.** Thoracic radiographs usually reveal a miliary interstitial pattern and, in severe infection, an alveolar pattern, areas of consolidation, and hilar lymphadenopathy.
      (2) **Transtracheal wash cytology** may be normal, may have various patterns of inflammation (e.g., neutrophilic, eosinophilic), or may be hemorrhagic. Macrophages should be scrutinized for intracellular *Histoplasma* organisms.
      (3) **Fungal culture** or **serology** may be useful.
   d. **Treatment.** Aggressive therapy is required for animals with disseminated disease and usually involves the combined use of **amphotericin B** and **ketoconazole** or **itraconazole.** Corticosteroids should be avoided unless acute, severe respiratory distress and cyanosis are present.
   e. **Prognosis.** The prognosis for animals with disseminated disease is guarded, but for those animals with mild, localized respiratory disease, the prognosis is good.

2. **Blastomycosis** (see also Chapter 49 II B) is rare in cats but reasonably common in dogs.
   a. **Pathogenesis.** *Blastomyces dermatitidis* primarily infects the lung and may disseminate to the skin, eyes, bone, lymph nodes, and CNS.
   b. **Clinical findings**
      (1) **Respiratory signs** are present in approximately 50% of affected dogs. Lung sounds are harsh.
      (2) **Other signs** can include anorexia, weight loss, lameness, blindness, uveitis, retinal detachment, peripheral lymphadenopathy, and skin lesions.
   c. **Diagnosis**
      (1) **Radiography.** Radiographically detectable pulmonary disease, which may include a miliary to nodular interstitial pattern, an alveolar or bronchial pattern, and hilar lymphadenopathy is found in approximately 85% of dogs.
      (2) **Transtracheal wash, fine needle lung aspirate,** or **bronchoalveolar lavage** may be used to detect the organism and confirms the diagnosis.
      (3) **Fungal culture** or **serology** may be required in some cases.
   d. **Treatment** involves the use of **amphotericin B, ketoconazole,** or **itraconazole.**
   e. **Prognosis.** Animals with severe pulmonary involvement or CNS signs have the worst prognosis.
      (1) Most dogs that die do so during the first week of therapy. Cure rates range from 65%–88% in animals that survive initial treatment.
      (2) Female dogs have a higher survival rate than males but suffer from more recurrent infections. Most recurrent infections occur within the first 6 months of treatment.

3. Coccidioidomycosis (see also Chapter 49 II C) is rare in cats.
   a. Etiology. Coccidioidomycosis is caused by *Coccidioides immitis* and occurs primarily in the southwestern United States (including the San Joaquin valley in California), Mexico, and Central and South America.
   b. Pathogenesis. Infection occurs first in the lungs and may disseminate to (in order of decreasing frequency) the bone, joints, visceral organs, pericardium, testicles, eyes, brain, and spinal cord.
   c. Clinical findings
      (1) Asymptomatic or mild self-limiting respiratory infection is common.
      (2) Clinical illness is usually a result of progressive pulmonary or disseminated disease, exhibited by a **cough** (productive or nonproductive), **dyspnea** (possibly due to bronchial compression from enlarged tracheobronchial lymph nodes), fluctuating or persistent fever, anorexia, weight loss, lethargy, weakness, localized peripheral lymphadenopathy, lameness, draining skin lesions, keratitis, uveitis, acute blindness, and diarrhea.
   d. Diagnosis
      (1) Radiography. Radiographic changes in the lungs are similar to those of histoplasmosis and blastomycosis but may also reveal pleural thickening or effusion.
      (2) Transtracheal wash, fine needle lung aspirate, bronchoalveolar lavage, or **pleural fluid** samples may be used to detect the organism and confirm the diagnosis.
   e. Treatment
      (1) Ketoconazole or **itraconazole** are recommended.
      (2) Amphotericin B may be used to hasten response to therapy in severely affected dogs or when other drugs are not tolerated, but *C. immitis* is more resistant to amphotericin B than are other fungal organisms.
   f. Prognosis. The prognosis is good for dogs with only pulmonary involvement and more guarded for those with disseminated disease. Relapses are common.

D. | **Parasitic infections**

   1. *Oslerus (Filaroides) osleri* is a metastrongyle parasite that infects wild canids and occasionally, domestic dogs. Most affected dogs are younger than 2 years of age.
   a. Transmission. The organism produces fibrous nodules in the trachea at the bifurcation of the bronchi. Infective L_1 larvae are coughed up and passed in the feces.
      (1) Pups can be infected by the dam from grooming or regurgitative feeding.
      (2) Transmission in kennels can also occur following contamination of the environment with L_1 larvae. The prepatent period is 10–18 weeks.
   b. Clinical findings. Affected dogs may be asymptomatic or demonstrate a chronic cough, dyspnea, exercise intolerance, or debilitation. Inspiratory wheezes may be heard.
   c. Diagnosis. A definitive diagnosis is usually made by **bronchoscopic visualization** of cream-colored nodules, 1–5 mm in diameter, at the tracheal bifurcation, and the identification of L_1 larvae in brushings or biopsies of the nodules.
      (1) Radiographs may reveal tracheal nodules, if they are large.
      (2) Transtracheal wash may allow the detection of L_1 larvae or eggs.
      (3) Fecal floatation (i.e., Baermann technique) may occasionally detect L_1 larvae.
   d. Treatment. There is no consistently successful treatment.
      (1) Levamisole, diethylcarbamazine, thiacetarsamide, thiabendazole, fenbendazole, albendazole, and **ivermectin** may be effective.
      (2) Surgical or **bronchoscopic removal** of a very large obstructive nodule may be indicated in rare instances.

   2. Aelurostrongylus abstrusus is the most common lungworm infection in cats.
   a. Transmission. Infection occurs through ingestion of an intermediate host (snail, slug) or by predation of a paratenic host (i.e., rodents, birds). The prepatent period is about 4–6 weeks. Adult worms live in the pulmonary parenchyma and bronchioles. L_1 larvae are coughed up, swallowed, and passed in the feces.

b. Clinical findings. The majority of infections are asymptomatic. When clinical signs occur, they range from mild coughing to severe wheezing and dyspnea. Lethargy, anorexia, and weight loss can also occur.

c. Diagnosis can be made in 90% of cases by demonstration of L_1 larvae in the feces using the **Baermann technique.**

(1) Radiography. Thoracic radiographs usually reveal small, nodular, ill-defined densities throughout the lung field that are worst in the caudal areas. Bronchial, interstitial, and alveolar patterns may also be present. Radiographic changes can mimic pulmonary neoplasia, mycotic pneumonia, and feline asthma.

(2) Transtracheal wash cytology most commonly demonstrates eosinophilic inflammation; acute, chronic, or mixed inflammatory responses and L_1 larvae may also be seen.

(3) Laboratory studies. A **CBC** may reveal peripheral eosinophilia.

d. Treatment. Infection is usually self-limiting and treatment may not be necessary if clinical signs are absent or minimal.

(1) Fenbendazole or **ivermectin** may be used to treat moderate to severe infections.

(2) Corticosteroids, with or without **bronchodilators,** may be indicated for short-term use in cats with severe respiratory signs.

3. *Paragonimus kellicotti* is a fluke that infects the lungs of dogs, and more commonly, cats. In North America, infection occurs primarily in areas around the Great Lakes and in the Midwestern and southern United States.

a. Transmission. The life cycle of *P. kellicotti* involves two intermediate hosts, aquatic snails and crayfish. Dog and cats are usually infected by ingesting crayfish. Once ingested, flukes migrate to the lung and form pulmonary cysts, which communicate with bronchioles. Fluke eggs formed within cysts enter the airways and then are coughed or carried up by ciliary action, swallowed, and passed in the feces.

b. Clinical findings

(1) Signs result from a granulomatous reaction to adult flukes, secondary bacterial infection, cyst rupture resulting in pneumothorax or a generalized inflammatory response in the lungs to the eggs, and can include a **chronic cough, audible wheezes** or **crackles,** and **acute respiratory distress** due to pneumothorax from a ruptured cyst.

(2) Some dogs and cats are asymptomatic.

c. Diagnosis is confirmed by finding the large operculated eggs on a fecal examination or transtracheal wash sample.

(1) Radiography. Thoracic radiographs typically reveal solid or cystic mass lesions (usually around 1 cm in diameter) in the caudal (especially right) lung lobes. Bronchial, interstitial, or patchy alveolar patterns can also occur. Pneumothorax may also be detected.

(2) Transtracheal wash cytology usually reveals eosinophilic inflammation.

d. Treatment

(1) Fenbendazole and **praziquantel** have been effective.

(2) Thoracocentesis (with or without the placement of chest tubes) may benefit animals with pneumothorax.

4. *Capillaria (Eucoleus) aerophila* inhabits the large airways of dogs and cats. This parasite may also infect the nasal cavity in dogs.

a. Transmission. Infection results from the ingestion of an embryonated egg or an earthworm paratenic host. The prepatent period is 3–5 weeks.

b. Clinical findings. Most infections are asymptomatic. A chronic cough or nasal discharge may occur.

c. Diagnosis is made by identifying a double operculated egg on **fecal flotation** or transtracheal wash samples. **Transtracheal wash cytology** is typically eosinophilic.

d. Treatment. Fenbendazole is recommended for animals with clinical signs.

5. Other lungworm infections that can occur in dogs include ***Crenosoma vulpis, Filaroides hirthi,*** and **Andersonstrongylus (Filaroides) milksi** infections.
  a. Clinical signs. Infection may not be associated with clinical signs.
  b. Diagnosis is made by identifying larvae or larvated eggs in fecal or transtracheal wash samples.
  c. Treatment. Fenbendazole, albendazole, and ivermectin can be considered for treatment.

E. **Aspiration pneumonia**

1. Etiology. Aspiration pneumonia can result from the inhalation of food and gastric contents (the most common cause), water, hydrocarbons (e.g., gasoline), mineral oil, or foreign bodies. **Predisposing conditions** include esophageal disease (e.g., megaesophagus, esophageal obstruction), congenital defects (e.g., cleft palate, bronchoesophageal fistula), pharyngeal dysfunction (e.g., polyneuropathy), severe protracted vomiting, decreased consciousness (e.g., sedation, general anesthesia, head trauma), and iatrogenic factors (e.g., misplaced stomach tube).

2. Pathogenesis
  a. Mechanisms. Aspiration of food and gastric contents leads to:
    (1) Gastric acid-induced damage, which results in alveolar collapse, bronchoconstriction, pulmonary edema, and systemic hypotension
    (2) Obstruction of airways by food particles, which can result in a granulomatous inflammatory response
    (3) Bacterial infection, which can occur immediately or later
  b. Effects include **ventilation–perfusion mismatching** (possibly marked), **decreased pulmonary compliance,** and **severe** and **fulminant pulmonary edema** that resembles that of acute respiratory distress syndrome (ARDS).

3. Clinical findings. The severity of clinical signs can vary.
  a. Acute, severe respiratory signs are frequently accompanied by shock.
  b. Some animals have a more chronic and progressive course characterized by **coughing** and the development of **dyspnea. Audible crackles** and **wheezes** are common over the ventral lung fields. **Fever, anorexia,** and **lethargy** are frequently present.

4. Diagnosis is based on compatible clinical signs, a suspected or known predisposing cause, and suggestive thoracic radiographic findings.
  a. Radiography. Thoracic radiographs taken 12–24 hours after aspiration typically reveal interstitial densities, an alveolar pattern, and consolidation mostly affecting the dependent lung lobes.
  b. Transtracheal wash cytology usually reveals marked neutrophilic inflammation, which may be septic.
  c. Bronchoscopy is not performed unless obstruction of a large airway by a piece of food is suspected.
  d. Blood gas analysis usually reveals hypoxemia with or without hypercapnia.
  e. Other diagnostic tests should be directed at detecting or characterizing diseases that could predispose to aspiration.

5. Treatment. Patency of the airway should be assured, especially in animals with acute, severe inspiratory dyspnea.
  a. Supplemental oxygen is frequently required. Mechanical ventilatory support may be indicated in animals with ARDS.
  b. Fluid therapy using intravenous crystalloid solutions (e.g., lactated Ringer's solution) is important to combat hypotension, maintain hydration, and encourage clearance of respiratory secretions and foreign material. However, overhydration and exacerbation of the pulmonary edema must be avoided. The placement of a jugular catheter to monitor central venous pressure can help prevent overhydration.
  c. Pharmacologic therapy
    (1) Bronchodilators (e.g., theophylline, terbutaline) may be helpful during the first 1–2 days. Benefit after this period is controversial.

(2) Corticosteroids for up to 24 hours are indicated if shock is present.

(3) Antibiotic therapy with trimethoprim/sulfonamide, cephalosporin, or chloramphenicol should be instituted until culture results from a transtracheal wash are obtained. Antibiotic therapy should continue for at least 3–4 weeks and at least 1 week beyond clinical and radiographic resolution of signs.

d. Physiotherapy using airway humidification and coupage in patients that are stable and have recovered from pulmonary edema can help clear respiratory secretions and hasten recovery.

6. Prognosis. The prognosis is good when pulmonary pathology is mild and a predisposing cause is not present or is correctable. It is poor to guarded in animals with severe pulmonary pathology or irreversible predisposing conditions.

F. **Pulmonary neoplasia** can occur from primary or metastatic disease or as part of a multicentric tumor (e.g., lymphosarcoma).

1. Types

a. Most primary tumors are malignant carcinomas (e.g., adenocarcinoma, bronchoalveolar carcinoma, squamous cell carcinoma).

b. Metastatic disease commonly affects the lungs and can involve many tumor types (e.g., thyroid carcinoma, mammary carcinoma, osteosarcoma, hemangiosarcoma, oral and digital melanomas, transitional cell carcinoma, and squamous cell carcinoma).

2. Clinical findings. Chronic, slowly progressive exercise intolerance and dyspnea are typical, although some animals are asymptomatic.

a. Coughing is heard if the neoplasia involves or compresses airways.

b. Hemorrhage or pneumothorax may follow tumor erosion into a major blood vessel or airway, respectively, causing acute signs.

c. Pulmonary inflammation, edema, or bacterial infection may be associated with tumors. Pleural effusion is not uncommon.

d. Weight loss, anorexia, lethargy, regurgitation or vomiting (in cats), and fever may also occur.

e. Lameness due to hypertrophic osteopathy occurs in some animals.

f. Other organ involvement may accompany metastatic or multicentric disease.

3. Diagnosis is based on cytologic or histologic confirmation of neoplasia. Metastatic pulmonary neoplasia may be highly suspect if malignant neoplasia is found in other organs.

a. Radiography. Thoracic radiographic findings are variable and resemble those of many other conditions [e.g., fungal infection, pulmonary infiltrates with eosinophils (PIE), lung parasites, atypical bacterial infections, lymphomatoid granulomatosis, lipid pneumonia]. Solitary mass lesions, lung lobe consolidation, cavitated mass lesions, diffuse reticular or nodular interstitial pattern, alveolar pattern from inflammation or edema, pleural effusion, pneumothorax, and intrathoracic lymphadenopathy may be seen.

b. Fine-needle lung aspiration, needle biopsy of masses adjacent to the chest wall, **bronchial biopsy** (via bronchoscopy) or **exploratory thoracotomy** can be used to obtain samples of lung tissue.

c. Bronchoalveolar lavage, transtracheal wash, or **pleural fluid analysis** may detect neoplastic cells in some cases.

4. Treatment

a. Excision of solitary lung masses (usually with a lobectomy) is the preferred treatment if primary neoplasia is present. Palliative debulking of nonresectable tumors that are compressing airways or are large and necrotic may be considered.

b. Chemotherapy for diffuse nonresectable tumors using a variety of agents (e.g., cisplatin, doxorubicin, cyclophosphamide, vinblastine, vindesine) has not resulted in marked improvement with most primary or metastatic tumors. However, in animals with lymphosarcoma, combination chemotherapy will usually induce a partial or complete remission and improve clinical signs.

TABLE 40-2. Causes of Pulmonary Edema

Decreased plasma oncotic pressure
  Hypoalbuminemia
Vascular volume overload
  Left-sided heart failure
  Overhydration
Lymphatic obstruction
  Neoplasia
Increased vascular permeability or **Acute respiratory distress syndrome (ARDS)**
  Smoke inhalation
  Aspiration of gastric acid
  Oxygen toxicity
  Cisplatin therapy in cats
  Snake venom
  Electrocution
  Sepsis
  Trauma (pulmonary or multisystemic)
  Pancreatitis
  Uremia
  Disseminated intravascular coagulation (DIC)
Miscellaneous causes
  Near-drowning
  Severe upper respiratory obstruction
  Pulmonary thromboembolism
  Head trauma or seizures leading to neurogenic edema

---

5. **Prognosis.** Although benign neoplasia is associated with a good prognosis, most pulmonary neoplasia is malignant and is associated with a poor long-term prognosis. However, most primary malignant neoplasms grow slowly and may be associated with a relatively long symptom-free period. In dogs that have undergone lobectomy for the excision of a solitary primary lung mass, survival times have ranged from 7–46 months or more.

G. **Pulmonary edema**

1. **Pathogenesis.** Pulmonary edema can result from decreased plasma oncotic pressure, vascular volume overload, lymphatic obstruction, increased vascular permeability, or a combination of these factors (Table 40-2). Once the removal of excess fluid by pulmonary lymphatics is overwhelmed, fluid accumulates in the interstitial compartment, which quickly overflows into the alveoli.
   a. Respiratory dysfunction results from atelectasis, decreased lung compliance, and increased resistance to airflow in edematous small bronchioles.
   b. Hypoxemia results from ventilation–perfusion mismatching.

2. **Clinical findings**
   a. Coughing, varying degrees of respiratory distress, and signs associated with underlying disorders are common. When the edema is very severe, blood-tinged foam may be expectorated.
   b. Lung sounds may be normal when edema is mild, but crackles can be heard as edema worsens.

3. **Diagnosis** is usually established by characteristic radiographic findings and detection of a causative underlying disease.
   a. **Radiography**
      (1) Radiographs in mild or early pulmonary edema reveal an interstitial pattern that progresses to an alveolar pattern as edema worsens.
      (2) Edema due to vascular volume overload (e.g., heart failure) is typically worse in the hilar region in dogs but has a patchy diffuse pattern in cats.

      (3) Edema from increased vascular permeability (e.g., ARDS) tends to be more severe in the dorsocaudal lung areas.

  b. **Arterial blood gas analysis** in animals with moderate to severe pulmonary edema usually reveals hypoxemia, hypocapnia, and an increased A-a gradient.

  c. **Laboratory tests** help rule out hypoalbuminemia as a cause for reduced oncotic pressure. Generally, plasma albumin concentrations must be very low (i.e., < 1g/dl) to be a significant factor in edema formation.

  d. **Echocardiography** can help rule out cardiac disease.

4. Treatment

  a. **General measures**

    (1) **Cage rest** and **oxygen supplementation** is the initial treatment.

    (2) **Sedation** with morphine in dogs or acepromazine in cats can help reduce patient anxiety, oxygen requirements, and cardiac workload.

    (3) **Bronchodilators** may be given.

    (4) **Positive-pressure ventilation** may be required.

    (5) **Intravenous fluids.** To avoid a marked reduction in cardiac output, hypovolemic animals should be cautiously treated with intravenous fluids.

    (6) **Plasma transfusions** can be given to hypoalbuminemic animals.

  b. **Therapy for edema resulting from vascular volume overload.** Animals with myocardial failure may require **positive inotropic support** (i.e., dobutamine). **Diuretic therapy** is more effective when the edema is associated with vascular volume overload (e.g., heart failure) than when the edema results from increased vascular permeability or ARDS.

  c. **Therapy for edema resulting from increased vascular permeability** or **ARDS** is difficult and primarily involves oxygen supplementation. Occasionally positive-pressure ventilation, diuretics (in normovolemic patients), and corticosteroids (for shock) are given.

5. Prognosis depends on the severity of the edema and the underlying cause. Early aggressive therapy will improve the outcome in most animals; however, the prognosis for edema due to increased vascular permeability or ARDS is often poor. The edema is usually severe, rapidly progressive and resistant to therapy.

H. **Pulmonary thromboembolism**

1. Etiology. Pulmonary thromboembolism is usually related to an underlying disease.

  a. The most **common cause in dogs** is **heartworm infection.**

  b. Other causes include hyperadrenocorticism, corticosteroid therapy, nephrotic syndrome, immune-mediated hemolytic anemia or thrombocytopenia, cardiac disease, neoplasia, sepsis, pancreatitis, and disseminated intravascular coagulation (DIC). Many of these diseases are associated with a **hypercoagulable state,** which increases the risk of spontaneous thrombus formation.

2. Pathogenesis. When many thromboemboli or a single large thrombus obstructs a significant number of small or large pulmonary arteries, severe ventilation–perfusion mismatching occurs. Additional factors that can contribute to abnormal respiratory function following thromboembolic events include vasoconstriction and bronchoconstriction from platelet degranulation, pulmonary edema in unaffected lung areas due to overcirculation, and infarction of pulmonary tissue. Pulmonary hypertension can develop and lead to right-sided heart failure.

3. Clinical findings

  a. Most animals with significant thromboembolism develop **peracute dyspnea** and **tachypnea.**

  b. A **cough, hemoptysis, tachycardia,** or **audible crackles** can occur.

  c. A **split second heart sound (S_2)** may be heard if pulmonary hypertension has developed.

4. Diagnosis. The combination of an acute onset of dyspnea, few or no thoracic radiographic abnormalities, and hypoxemia is very suggestive of pulmonary thromboembolism, but definitive diagnosis requires angiography or pulmonary scintigraphy.

a. **Radiography**

(1) The radiographic and diagnostic features of heartworm-induced pulmonary thromboembolism are discussed in Chapter 39 VI A 3.

(2) In other animals with thromboembolism, thoracic radiographic findings can be normal or may reveal hyperlucent areas due to decreased perfusion, lobar or triangular-shaped areas of alveolar infiltrate, a diffuse interstitial pattern, mild pleural effusion, and enlargement of the main pulmonary artery or right side of the heart.

b. **Blood gas analysis** typically reveals hypoxemia, hypocapnia, and an increased A-a gradient.

5. **Treatment.** The underlying disorder (e.g., heartworm-related thromboembolism) should be treated, if possible. General measures for the treatment of pulmonary thromboembolism include the following:

a. **Supplemental oxygen** and treatment for **shock** may be necessary.

b. **Anticoagulant therapy** using heparin will decrease thrombus progression. Dosage is determined by that amount required to prolong the partial thromboplastin time (PTT) to 1.5–2.5 times normal. Warfarin can be considered for long-term therapy.

c. **Thrombolytic drugs** [e.g., streptokinase or recombinant tissue plasminogen activator (TPA)] have not been used to any extent to treat pulmonary thromboembolism in dogs and cats. The body's fibrinolytic system should gradually dissolve formed thrombi.

6. **Prevention.** Prophylactic treatment of high-risk animals with **low-dose heparin** should be considered.

7. **Prognosis** depends on the severity of clinical signs and the nature of the underlying disease. The prognosis is usually poor for animals with severe respiratory signs.

I. **Pulmonary contusions**

1. **Etiology.** Contusions result when blunt trauma to the chest leads to localized hemorrhage into the interstitium and alveoli. Contusions may be associated with other injuries such as pneumothorax, rib fractures, and hemothorax.

2. **Clinical findings** relate to the extent of the trauma. **Increased respiratory effort** and **audible crackles** over contused areas may be present.

3. **Diagnosis.** Radiographic changes may not be evident until 6–24 hours after trauma and will reveal large localized areas of interstitial and alveolar densities.

4. **Treatment.** Contusions are not treated specifically. Instead, the animal is treated for trauma and related injuries.

5. **Prognosis** for resolution of contusions is usually excellent, and complications (e.g., bacterial infection and abscessation, cyst formation) are infrequent.

J. **Pulmonary infiltrates with eosinophils (PIE)** refers to an eosinophilic inflammation within the pulmonary parenchyma. Involvement of the bronchi can also occur. A form of PIE that results in nodular pulmonary densities has been referred to as **eosinophilic pulmonary granulomatosis.**

1. **Etiology.** The eosinophilic inflammatory response is a **hypersensitivity reaction,** which can result from lungworms, heartworm, drugs, inhaled allergens, bacteria, fungi, or neoplasia. Many dogs with PIE are infected with heartworms.

2. **Clinical findings.** Coughing is common, and increased breath sounds and crackles may be heard. Systemic signs of illness (e.g., weight loss, anorexia, lethargy) may be noted.

3. **Diagnosis**

a. **Radiography.** Thoracic radiographic abnormalities can vary from mild interstitial changes with alveolar densities to large nodular masses. Hilar lymphadenopathy can be marked. Radiographic changes can be very similar to those seen with neoplasia, fungal infection, or heartworm infection.

    b. Laboratory studies. A **CBC** commonly reveals eosinophilia and possibly basophilia.

    c. Transtracheal wash. Cytologic examination of transtracheal wash samples reveals eosinophilic inflammation. Samples should be scrutinized for the presence of infectious agents.

    d. Fecal samples should be examined for lungworms, and **heartworm tests** should be performed.

4. Treatment. Current medications should be discontinued. **Corticosteroid therapy** is indicated if an infectious agent has not been identified.

5. Prognosis. Control is usually possible, but many animals require long-term corticosteroid therapy. If eosinophilic granulomatosis is thought to be present, long-term control or remission is less likely.

K. **Lymphomatoid granulomatosis** is a rare disease of dogs that results from cellular infiltration (i.e., lymphoreticular cells, plasmacytoid cells, eosinophils, plasma cells, lymphocytes) of the pulmonary parenchyma directed around and in small blood vessels.

1. Clinical findings

    a. Dogs usually have slowly progressive signs of coughing and increased respiratory effort.

    b. Increased bronchial sounds, wheezes, and crackles may be ausculted.

    c. Fever, weight loss, anorexia, and lethargy can also occur.

2. Diagnosis. Definitive diagnosis requires histopathologic examination of biopsy samples.

    a. Radiographs usually reveal an interstitial pattern with multiple, variably sized nodules, lobar consolidation of one or more lung lobes, and hilar lymphadenopathy.

    b. Laboratory studies. A **CBC** may reveal basophilia with or without eosinophilia.

    c. Transtracheal wash. Cytologic examination of samples reveals a mixture of eosinophilic and neutrophilic inflammation with reactive macrophages. Criteria for malignancy are often present, and regional lymph nodes may be infiltrated. All diagnostic samples from the lungs should be carefully examined for infectious agents.

3. Treatment. If no infectious agents have been identified, **immunosuppressive therapy** using a combination of prednisone and cyclophosphamide is recommended. Animals should be monitored for cyclophosphamide side effects (i.e., bone marrow suppression, hemorrhagic cystitis).

4. Prognosis is difficult to predict due to the small number of animals treated. Long-term remission can occur in some patients.

V. PLEURAL SPACE AND MEDIASTINAL DISORDERS

A. Diagnostic and therapeutic approaches and techniques

1. Radiography (pleural space and mediastinum)

    a. Pleural effusion results from a variety of disease processes and can be detected radiographically when 50–100 ml of fluid have accumulated within the thoracic cavity. Pleural fissure lines, retraction of the lung lobes from the thoracic wall, and an obscured cardiac silhouette and diaphragmatic outline may be observed.

    b. Pneumothorax occurs when air is free within the pleural cavity outside of the lung parenchyma. The heart is usually elevated in relation to the sternum, and the lung tissue appears denser than normal. Lucent areas with an air density but without airway or vascular markings may be visible between lung lobes.

    c. Cranial mediastinal masses appear as a tissue density cranial to the heart, which may displace the trachea dorsally. On a dorsoventral (DV) view, there is widening of the mediastinum cranial to the heart. Many cranial mediastinal masses are accompanied by pleural effusion, which may obscure the presence of a mass.

    d. Other mediastinal abnormalities visible radiographically include pneumomediastinum, megaesophagus, and diaphragmatic hernia. Deviation of the mediastinum may be associated with lung lobe collapse or space-occupying lesions in the pulmonary parenchyma.

2. Ultrasonography is very useful for detecting and evaluating mediastinal, thoracic wall, and pulmonary parenchymal masses. Ultrasound can also help guide biopsy procedures.

3. Thoracocentesis is indicated for the removal of fluid for diagnostic and therapeutic purposes.

4. Chest tubes. The placement of chest tubes is indicated when the rate of air (or, less commonly, fluid) accumulation is too rapid for repeated thoracocentesis to be a feasible option, and for the management of pyothorax, chylothorax, and some effusions associated with intrathoracic neoplasia. The main complication of chest tube placement is the development of pneumothorax from leaks in or around the tubing. Close patient monitoring is a prerequisite when chest tubes are in place.

B. **Pleural space disorders**

1. Pleural effusion is a clinical sign of pleural space and mediastinal disorders. It is a common clinical problem in dogs and cats.
    a. Etiology. Causes of pleural effusion are summarized in Table 40-3.
    b. Clinical signs
        (1) Dyspnea is the main sign of pleural effusion. Inspiration is prolonged and labored and may be accompanied by a marked abdominal component.
        (2) Lung sounds are decreased in the ventral thorax.

TABLE 40-3. Causes of Pleural Effusion

Transudative effusion
  Hypoalbuminemia
  Right-sided heart failure
  Pericardial effusion
Modified transudative effusion
  Right-sided heart failure
  Pericardial effusion
  Neoplasia
  Diaphragmatic hernia
Nonseptic exudative effusion
  Feline infectious peritonitis (FIP)
  Neoplasia
  Diaphragmatic hernia
  Lung lobe torsion
Septic exudative effusion
  Pyothorax
Chylous effusion
  Idiopathic chylothorax
  Right-sided heart failure
  Heartworm infection
  Neoplasia
  Cardiomyopathy
  Trauma (e.g., thoracic duct rupture)
Hemorrhagic effusion
  Coagulopathy
  Trauma
  Neoplasia
  Lung lobe torsion

TABLE 40-4. Fluid Characteristics

	Transudate	Modified Transudate	Nonseptic Exudate	Septic Exudate	Chylous Effusion	Hemorrhagic Effusion
Protein (g/dl)	<2.5–3.0	2.5–5.0	>3.0	>3.0	>2.5	>3.0
Cells (cells/μl)	<500–1000	500–10,000	>5000	>5000 + bacteria	400–10,000	>1000, RBCs predominate

RBCs = red blood cells.

      (3) In cats, a mediastinal mass can be associated with pleural effusion and may result in a noncompressible cranial thorax.

  c. Diagnosis is usually based on the detection of fluid following thoracocentesis or on thoracic radiographs.

    (1) Radiography. Radiographic findings associated with pleural effusion are discussed in V A 1 a.

    (2) Thoracocentesis. Thoracic fluid is classified as a transudate, modified transudate, septic or nonseptic exudate, chylous effusion, or hemorrhagic effusion (Table 40-4).

  d. Treatment and **prognosis** depend on the cause of the effusion.

 2. Pneumothorax

  a. Etiology. Causes of pneumothorax include **chest trauma** (the most common cause), **ruptured cavitary** (e.g., cysts or bullae from congenital or idiopathic causes, past trauma, or *P. kellicotti* infection) or **mass lesions** (e.g., neoplasia, abscess, granuloma).

  b. Pathogenesis. Pneumothorax results when air enters the pleural space from the outside (e.g., chest wound) or from a rent or tear in an airway or the pulmonary parenchyma. **Tension pneumothorax** may occur if a one-way valve forms in the parenchyma, allowing air to escape into the pleural space but preventing it from returning to the parenchyma or an airway. High intrathoracic pressures develop, which lead to severe compression of the lung tissue.

  c. Clinical findings

    (1) Dyspnea is the main sign of pneumothorax.

    (2) Penetrating wounds on the thoracic wall may be detected.

    (3) Lung sounds are **decreased** or **absent** and the **chest cavity** is **resonant** when percussed.

    (4) Tension pneumothorax results in **acute, severe respiratory distress.**

  d. Diagnosis is based on either radiographic findings or thoracocentesis. The radiographic findings associated with pneumothorax are quite distinctive. Cysts or mass lesions may be obscured.

  e. Treatment depends on the severity and rate of air accumulation.

    a. Asymptomatic animals may need no more than observation and repeated radiographs.

    b. Symptomatic animals may require **repeated needle thoracocentesis** or the **placement of chest tubes.** Chest tubes are connected to a water seal drainage system and maintained for several days.

 3. Pyothorax refers to the accumulation of a septic exudate within the pleural space.

  a. Etiology. Pyothorax can develop from penetrating thoracic wall injuries, migrating foreign bodies, perforations in the esophagus or an airway, or a ruptured pulmonary abscess, or it can be idiopathic (especially in cats).

  b. Clinical findings

    (1) Varying degrees of **dyspnea** are present.

    (2) Lung sounds are **reduced in the ventral thorax.**

    (3) Fever, lethargy, anorexia, and **weight loss** are common.

    (4) Signs of septic shock may be present in some animals.

  c. **Diagnosis** is based on the detection of a septic exudate within the pleural cavity.
    (1) **Radiography.** Thoracic radiographic findings are consistent with pleural effusion but may be localized or involve one side of the thorax.
    (2) **Bacterial culture** of the pleural fluid may reveal only one, many, or no pathogens. Anaerobes and *Pasteurella multocida* are commonly isolated in cats. *Nocardia* and *Actinomyces* species are the most common isolates in dogs.
  d. **Treatment** should be prompt and aggressive, especially if septic shock is present.
    (1) **Needle thoracocentesis** may be necessary in severely dyspneic patients.
    (2) **Antibiotic therapy** should be selected on the basis of culture and sensitivity results whenever possible. Ampicillin is a good initial choice. Antibiotic therapy should be given intravenously during the first 3–7 days of therapy. The duration of therapy is 4–6 weeks.
    (3) **Placement of chest tubes.** Drainage of the thoracic cavity is necessary to ensure eradication of the infection. Failure to do so can result in fibrosis, abscessation, and recurrence of infection. Chest tube placement followed by continuous suction drainage or intermittent lavage is recommended. Chest tubes are usually left in place 3–7 days.
    (4) **Exploratory thoracotomy** is rarely necessary but may be indicated if a localized abscess develops or a foreign body is suspected.
    (5) **Supportive care** is often necessary. Animals are frequently dehydrated and require fluid therapy.
  e. **Prognosis**
    (1) In general, the outlook for idiopathic pyothorax in cats is good if prompt and aggressive therapy is undertaken and tests for feline leukemia or immunodeficiency virus are negative.
    (2) Pyothorax from *Nocardia* or *Actinomyces* infection in dogs has a fair prognosis.
    (3) If pyothorax is associated with a migrating foreign body, the prognosis is guarded if the foreign body cannot be retrieved.

4. **Chylothorax** refers to the accumulation of chyle within the thoracic cavity and can affect both dogs and cats of any age. Afghan and possibly Shibu Inu dogs are predisposed.
  a. **Etiology.** Chylothorax has been associated with traumatic damage to the thoracic duct, severe right-sided heart failure, cardiomyopathy, heartworm infection, lymphosarcoma, cranial mediastinal masses, diaphragmatic hernia, pulmonary neoplasia, and idiopathic causes. Chylothorax resulting from anomalous formation of the thoracic duct or its venous connection may also occur in dogs and cats. The exact reason for chyle leakage in nontraumatic disorders is poorly understood. Cranial mediastinal lymphangiectasia accompanies many of these disorders, which suggests a functional or mechanical obstruction to chyle flow.
  b. **Clinical findings** can include **dyspnea, cough, lethargy, anorexia,** and **weight loss. Lung sounds** are **muffled** in the ventral thorax. **Dehydration, cyanosis,** and **emaciation** may occur in animals with long-standing disease.
  c. **Diagnosis** is based on the identification of chylous fluid within the thoracic cavity.
    (1) **Radiography.** Findings include pleural effusion and, in some cases, signs of associated disorders (e.g., heart disease, neoplasia).
    (2) **Thoracocentesis.** Chylous fluid can be difficult to differentiate from other effusions.
      (a) Chylous fluid is usually opaque and pink or white in color. The protein concentration and cell counts are given in Table 40-4. Small lymphocytes predominate early but nondegenerate neutrophils and macrophages increase in number with chronicity.
      (b) The best way to differentiate chylous fluid from other effusions is to determine the triglyceride concentration in the pleural fluid and compare it to the serum triglyceride concentration. In chylous fluid, the triglyceride concentration is at least twice as high as the serum triglyceride concentration.

d. Treatment. Underlying disorders should be treated while symptomatically treating the chylothorax. The more aggressive medical and surgical treatments are usually pursued in animals with idiopathic disease.

    (1) Needle thoracocentesis should be used to remove as much pleural fluid as possible to stabilize severely dyspneic animals.

    (2) Medical treatment entails a **reduced-fat diet, fluid therapy** (if dehydration is present), and **thoracic drainage.**

    (3) Surgical treatments include **thoracic duct ligation, passive drainage** by creating a shunt through the diaphragm, and **active drainage** by implanting a manual pump to move fluid from the pleural to peritoneal cavity.

e. Prognosis

    (1) Overall, the long-term prognosis for idiopathic chylothorax in dogs and cats is fair to poor. Medical therapy with or without thoracic duct ligation will resolve idiopathic chylothorax in 20%–50% of cats, and medical management is successful in approximately 50% of affected dogs.

    (2) Little information is available on the success of pleurodesis or surgical drainage procedures.

    (3) Long-term complications include pleural fibrosis and restrictive lung disease and malnutrition.

5. Diaphragmatic hernia is usually associated with blunt trauma to the abdomen or caudal thorax. The extent of the hernia and the number of abdominal organs that herniate into the thoracic cavity vary.

a. Clinical findings can be extremely variable.

    (1) Typically, dyspnea is observed after a traumatic episode.

    (2) Lung sounds may be absent over the herniated viscera, and gut sounds may be heard within the thoracic cavity.

    (3) Diaphragmatic hernias may be detected months to years after the traumatic episode, producing chronic GI signs, exercise intolerance, or dyspnea (which may be intermittent and follow exercise or recumbency). Asymptomatic patients may develop clinical signs because of intrathoracic gastric dilatation (causing lung compression and dyspnea), intrathoracic splenic torsion, incarceration or obstruction of herniated bowel, or cholangiohepatitis due to liver lobe incarceration.

b. Diagnosis is based on clinical signs and radiographic findings.

    (1) Plain film radiography. Thoracic radiographic findings can include loss of the ventral diaphragmatic outline, cranial displacement of the stomach, loss of the caudal outline of the liver, and gas-filled bowel loops within the thoracic cavity. Pleural effusion is present in 40%–50% of cases and may obscure the presence of a hernia. Other evidence of thoracic trauma may be evident (e.g., fractured ribs, pulmonary contusions).

    (2) Contrast radiography may help outline displaced bowel loops and help confirm a hernia in difficult cases.

c. Treatment consists of surgically closing the hernia; however, stabilization of the patient following acute trauma is a first priority. Rapidly deteriorating respiratory function (e.g., intrathoracic gastric dilatation) may necessitate emergency surgery.

d. Prognosis is good in most cases.

6. Mediastinal disorders

a. Mediastinal masses constitute the most common abnormality of the mediastinum. They occur most often in the cranial mediastinum or over the heart base.

    (1) Types

        (a) The most common mass in the cranial mediastinum in dogs and especially in cats is lymphosarcoma. Other tumors include thymoma and, less frequently, thyroid carcinoma, parathyroid carcinoma, and chemodectoma.

        (b) Nonneoplastic masses include granulomas, abscess, branchial cysts, and hematomas.

    (2) Clinical findings

        (a) Dyspnea is common. **Coughing, regurgitation** (due to esophageal impingement), and **head** and **neck edema** (due to compression of the cranial vena cava) can also occur. In cats, the cranial thorax becomes less compressible when a cranial mediastinal mass is present.

   (b) **Paraneoplastic syndromes** associated with specific tumors may also help identify the mass (e.g., hypercalcemia with lymphosarcoma, myasthenia gravis with thymoma).

  (3) **Diagnosis**

   (a) **Radiography.** Thoracic radiographs often reveal the presence of a mass, but it may be obscured by pleural fluid.

   (b) **Ultrasonography** can help document the presence of a mass and determine its characteristics and what structures it involves or is adjacent to.

   (c) **Pleural fluid analysis** may help identify the mass, especially if it is lymphosarcoma.

   (d) **Fine-needle aspiration** of masses may be also be performed.

   (e) **Exploratory thoracotomy** and **biopsy** can be considered in some cases.

  (4) **Treatment** depends on the nature of the mass.

   (a) **Combination chemotherapy** can be considered if lymphosarcoma is present.

   (b) **Surgical excision** for other tumors can be considered in the absence of significant local infiltration or metastatic disease.

b. **Pneumomediastinum** results from a tear or rent in the esophagus, trachea, bronchi, bronchioles, or alveoli. Subcutaneous air accumulation from a skin wound or tracheal injury in the neck may dissect into the mediastinum.

  (1) **Etiology.** Air leakage from lower airways may result from thoracic trauma, coughing, and respiratory efforts against obstructed airways.

  (2) **Treatment** is focused on the underlying disorder. For animals with leaks in the lower airways, strict cage rest may be adequate.

DIRECTIONS: Each of the numbered items or incomplete statements in this section is followed by answers or by completions of the statement. Select the ONE numbered answer or completion that is BEST in each case.

1. An owner telephones her veterinarian and complains that her cat has started sneezing and has a clear, runny nasal discharge. The cat's symptoms began 3 days after being discharged from the clinic after an elective surgical procedure. The cat is kept exclusively indoors. The veterinarian recalls there was a cat with upper respiratory signs in the clinic at the same time. They were housed in the same ward but at opposite ends of the room (about 20 feet apart). What should the veterinarian do?

(1) Assume responsibility and have the ventilation checked in the ward.
(2) Assume responsibility and discuss procedures for handling animals with potentially infectious disease (e.g., hand washing, cage and dish disinfection) with hospital staff.
(3) Do not assume responsibility. It is probable that the stress of surgery brought a previous infection out of latency.
(4) Do not assume responsibility because the cat could not have developed an upper respiratory infection so soon after discharge. It was likely infected before the visit to the clinic.
(5) Assume responsibility and have the clinic cat food and kitty litter tested for the presence of viruses.

2. A 5-year-old Labrador retriever is presented with a 6-month history of bilateral mucopurulent nasal discharge that is occasionally bloody. Cytologically, abundant neutrophils with moderate numbers of bacteria are observed in the nasal discharge. Nasal radiographs reveal areas of increased lucency and loss of the fine trabecular pattern within both nasal cavities. Rhinoscopic examination reveals marked atrophy and destruction of turbinates bilaterally. Which of the following choices is the most likely cause of the nasal disease?

(1) Nasal aspergillosis
(2) Nasal adenocarcinoma
(3) Lymphosarcoma
(4) Bacterial rhinitis
(5) Allergic rhinitis

3. A veterinarian is presented with a 7-year-old, neutered, male golden retriever. The owner has noticed noisy breathing over the last 3 months, which gets worse during exercise. The owner has also noted that the dog's bark has changed in pitch. On physical examination, mild dyspnea with stridor is observed during inspiration. What is the most likely diagnosis?

(1) Nasopharyngeal polyp
(2) Nasal neoplasia
(3) Pharyngitis
(4) Laryngitis
(5) Laryngeal paralysis

4. What is the best method to distinguish chylous pleural fluid from other types of pleural fluid?

(1) Cytologic examination
(2) Comparison of the concentration of cholesterol in pleural fluid to that in the serum
(3) Thoracic radiographs
(4) Comparison of the concentration of triglyceride in pleural fluid to that in the serum
(5) Visual inspection of the fluid color and turbidity

5. A 1-year-old female fox terrier is presented because of an acute onset of cough. The cough is nonproductive, honking, and frequent. The dog is bright and alert and has a good appetite. The owner attended a dog obedience class 1 week ago. What is the most likely diagnosis?

(1) Canine distemper virus (CDV) infection
(2) Infectious tracheobronchitis
(3) Allergic bronchitis
(4) Collapsing trachea
(5) Lungworm infection

Questions 6–7

A 5-year-old male, neutered, Siamese cat is presented with a 3-month history of progressively worsening cough. The cat is bright and alert and has a good appetite. Physical examination is normal. Thoracic radiographs reveal a mild bronchial pattern. A complete blood count (CBC) and serum biochemical profile reveal no abnormalities. A fecal flotation test and Baermann examination are negative. Cytologic examination of transtracheal wash fluid reveals predominantly eosinophils with a small number of nondegenerate neutrophils.

6. What is the most likely diagnosis?

(1) Infectious tracheobronchitis
(2) Pulmonary infiltrate with eosinophils (PIE)
(3) *Aelurostrongylus abstrusus* infection
(4) Heartworm infection
(5) Allergic bronchitis

7. The initial treatment for this cat should be:

(1) prednisone.
(2) aminophylline.
(3) terbutaline.
(4) butorphanol.
(5) amoxicillin with clavulanic acid.

8. A 6-year-old male Dalmatian is presented because of acute blindness, a chronic cough, and weight loss. On physical examination, the dog is thin and has moderate lymphadenopathy affecting the prescapular and popliteal lymph nodes bilaterally. Ophthalmic examination reveals bilateral retinal detachment. A diffuse, nodular interstitial pattern is observed on thoracic radiographs. Of the diseases listed below, which one would be the most likely cause of the dog's respiratory signs?

(1) Aspiration pneumonia
(2) Bronchoalveolar carcinoma
(3) Fungal pneumonia
(4) Bacterial pneumonia
(5) *Oslerus (Filaroides) osleri* infection

9. A 4-year-old male domestic short-haired cat is presented because of a chronic cough. Mild wheezing is heard over the lung fields. Thoracic radiographs reveal a cystic lesion in the right caudal lung lobe and a mild bronchial pattern. Transtracheal wash reveals eosinophilic inflammation and a few large operculated eggs. What is the most likely diagnosis?

(1) *Aelurostrongylus abstrusus* infection
(2) *Oslerus (Filaroides) osleri* infection
(3) *Capillaria aerophila* infection
(4) *Toxocara cati* infection
(5) *Paragonimus kellicotti* infection

10. Which one of the following conditions would significantly increase the risk of developing aspiration pneumonia?

(1) Pulmonary neoplasia
(2) Megaesophagus
(3) Inflammatory bowel disease
(4) Nasopharyngeal polyp
(5) Collapsing trachea

11. The placement of a chest tube is usually required for the optimal management of:

(1) pneumothorax.
(2) mediastinal lymphosarcoma.
(3) hemothorax.
(4) pyothorax.
(5) pleural effusion associated with feline infectious peritonitis virus (FIP).

1. The answer is 2 [I C 1 b, Table 40-1]. This cat most likely was infected with feline calicivirus (FCV) or feline rhinotracheitis (FRV) during its stay at the clinic. The incubation period for FCV or FRV would be compatible with the time since discharge. The most common mode of infection is by fomites (e.g., food bowls, blankets, human hands) and direct contact between cats; therefore, the veterinarian should review procedures for limiting nosocomial disease with the clinic staff. Aerosol transmission only occurs over very short distances (i.e., less than 4 feet). Although it is possible that the stress of surgery could result in a recrudescent infection, it would be unlikely given the high potential for in-hospital exposure in this case. The heat used to prepare commercial cat foods and litter would destroy any infectious agents.

2. The answer is 1 [I C 2 a]. In dogs, nasal *Aspergillus* infection typically results in turbinate atrophy and destruction, which appears radiographically as areas of radiolucency (in most, but not all, cases). Rhinoscopic examination corroborated this finding and failed to reveal a mass lesion. Although turbinate destruction is common with neoplasia, extensive atrophy is not. Furthermore, tumors are usually associated with an increase in radiodensity due to the tissue mass. Different neoplasias cannot be differentiated based on radiographic or visual assessment. The nasal cytology indicates bacterial infection; however, the majority of bacterial infections in the nose are secondary to an underlying disease and are not usually associated with marked turbinate destruction. Allergic rhinitis would tend to have a serous nasal discharge with little to no abnormal radiographic abnormalities. Rhinoscopic examination would not reveal turbinate destruction, but rather mucosal erythema and edema.

3. The answer is 5 [II A, C 1]. Inspiratory dyspnea and stridor suggest an upper respiratory obstructive disease. The change in bark is specific to laryngeal disease. The chronicity of these signs plus their appearance in a large-breed dog make laryngeal paralysis a good possibility. Although a nasopharyngeal polyp could result in inspiratory dyspnea and stridor, the bark would be unaffected and it is an uncommon disorder in dogs. Nasal neopl may cause inspiratory dyspnea if both na cavities are occluded; however, nasal dis charge is almost always associated with plasia and the bark would be unaffected. yngitis would not affect respiratory effort Laryngitis could alter the bark, but it do(last for months nor does it result in insp dyspnea (unless laryngeal edema develc

4. The answer is 4 [V B 4 c (2) (b)]. Cc son of serum and pleural fluid triglycer els is the most specific test for identifyi chylous effusion. Chyle has a much hi glyceride concentration than serum. Tl fore, chylous effusions have triglyceric centrations that are significantly highe than two times higher) than the serum tration. Visual inspection and cytolog nation may be suggestive but are not atory. Pleural fluid cholesterol conce vary considerably. Thoracic radiogra, be used to detect the presence of an effusion but cannot be used to differentiate fluid types.

5. The answer is 2 [III C 1]. The acute onset of a honking cough shortly after being exposed to other dogs with no signs of systemic illness is highly suggestive of infectious tracheobronchitis (kennel cough). Canine distemper virus (CDV) infection would produce systemic signs of illness in addition to other organ system involvement. Allergic bronchitis and collapsing trachea would not have such an acute history. Lungworm infection cannot be ruled out with the information provided, but it is much less common than infectious tracheobronchitis.

6–7. The answers are 6-5 [III C 3], **7-1** [III C 3 d]. The presence of eosinophilic airway inflammation in the absence of identifiable lungworm (e.g., *Aelurostrongylus abstrusus*) infection makes allergic bronchitis very likely. Infectious tracheobronchitis does not occur in cats. Pulmonary infiltrates with eosinophils (PIE) is predominantly a disease of dogs and would have different radiographic characteristics. Heartworm infection has not been ruled out but is unlikely because of the absence of pulmonary arterial abnormalities on thoracic radiographs.

Allergic bronchitis in cats is best treated with corticosteroids, such as prednisone. The response is usually good. Bronchodilators (e.g., aminophylline, terbutaline) may be used if the response to prednisone is not adequate. Butorphanol can be used to suppress the cough, but this is rarely necessary in cats with allergic bronchitis. The cytology did not indicate active bacterial infection (i.e., degenerate neutrophils with bacteria); therefore, antibiotic therapy with amoxicillin would not be indicated at this time.

8. The answer is 3 [IV C 2]. The combination of retinal detachment, a nodular interstitial pattern on thoracic radiographs, and signs of systemic illness is suggestive of blastomycosis, a fungal infection. Ocular involvement would be unusual in any of the other infections listed [i.e., aspiration pneumonia, bacterial pneumonia, and *Oslerus (Filaroides) osleri* infection]. In addition, a nodular interstitial radiographic pattern would not typically be associated with aspiration or bacterial pneumonia. Pulmonary neoplasia cannot be distinguished from many fungal infections on the basis of radiographs. However, ocular signs would be unusual with most pulmonary neoplasms, especially bronchoalveolar carcinoma (lymphosarcoma would be an exception). Radiographic changes in the pulmonary parenchyma are not a marked feature of *O. osleri* infection.

9. The answer is 5 [IV D 3]. The presence of cystic lesions in the caudal lung fields combined with the detection of operculated eggs on transtracheal wash is very suggestive of infection with the lung fluke *Paragonimus kellicotti. Aelurostrongylus abstrusus* and *Oslerus (Filaroides) osleri* infections are not associated with cystic pulmonary lesions. Also, L$_1$ larvae, not eggs, are usually detected in diagnostic samples. Similarly, *Capillaria aerophila* infection is not associated with cystic lesions but is associated with the detection of an egg on diagnostic samples. However, the egg is double operculated and can be differentiated from that of *P. kellicotti. Toxocara cati* is a gastrointestinal (GI) ascarid that migrates through the lungs during its development. Infection with *T. cati* usually does not produce clinical or radiographic signs of respiratory disease.

10. The answer is 2 [IV E 1]. Megaesophagus is usually associated with frequent and long-standing regurgitation, which predisposes an animal to aspiration of esophageal contents. Aspiration pneumonia is a common cause of death in animals with megaesophagus. Pulmonary neoplasia, nasopharyngeal polyps, and collapsing trachea do not increase the risk of aspiration. Inflammatory bowel disease can be associated with chronic vomiting, but this seldom results in a significant risk of aspiration (unless the vomiting is severe, protracted, and frequent).

11. The answer is 4 [V B 3]. The placement of chest tubes is indicated in all cases of pyothorax. Chest tube placement is the only means of ensuring good drainage of the thoracic cavity in the presence of this disorder. Successful resolution of the infection is much less likely if they are not used. Pneumothorax does not require chest tubes in all cases, only those with rapid reaccumulation of large volumes of air after needle thoracocentesis. Similarly, treatment of hemothorax would not require chest tubes in many cases. The pleural effusion that may accompany feline infectious peritonitis (FIP) or mediastinal lymphosarcoma is not usually treated with chest tube placement.

Chapter 41

Gastrointestinal Diseases

I. **OROPHARYNGEAL DISORDERS**

A. **Clinical evaluation**

1. **Predisposition**
   a. **Species and breed.** All breeds of dogs and cats can develop oropharyngeal problems, but certain breeds are at increased risk. For example, congenital abnormalities of the lips and palate are more common in brachycephalic breeds.
   b. **Age**
      (1) **Young animals.** Congenital problems and viral disease are primary considerations.
      (2) **Middle-aged to older animals.** Neoplasia is more common in middle-aged to older animals.
   c. **Environment.** An animal that has free access to an entire neighborhood is more likely to have been exposed to a toxin or to have chewed plant material than is an indoor animal.
   d. **Vaccination status.** Viral disease is less likely in a vaccinated animal.

2. **Clinical signs**
   a. **Primary signs**
      (1) **Drooling** is a common sign of oropharyngeal disease. Drooling results from excessive secretion of saliva (**ptyalism**) or excessive loss of saliva from the mouth due to the inability or reluctance to swallow (**pseudoptyalism**). Causes include gastrointestinal (GI) disease, metabolic disease (e.g., hepatic encephalopathy, renal disease), viral infection, toxins and drugs, and fear or excitement.
      (2) **Halitosis** may result from abnormal bacterial proliferation in conjunction with decreased clearance of saliva and food particles, from tissue necrosis, or from dental tartar and periodontal disease. GI and respiratory disorders can also cause halitosis.
      (3) **Dysphagia** can result from pain, motility disturbances, or obstruction.
      (4) **Anorexia** may be due to a true lack of appetite or an unwillingness or inability to prehend, chew, or swallow the food as a result of abnormal oropharyngeal function, obstruction, or pain.
      (5) **Weight loss** can occur if anorexia or pseudoanorexia is present.
      (6) **Oral lesions** may include hyperemic mucosa, erosions, ulcers, plaques, proliferative tissue, or a mass.
      (7) **Pain** can result from mucosal lesions, dental disorders, bony lesions, myositis, or an abscess. The animal may paw at the mouth in response to the pain and irritation.
      (8) **Facial swelling**
         (a) **Unilateral swelling** can indicate an abscess, neoplasia, inflammation, a salivary mucocele, or trauma.
         (b) **Bilateral mandibular swelling** can be seen with craniomandibular osteopathy.
      (9) **Gagging** may be seen in animals with pharyngeal irritation.
   b. **Concurrent signs**
      (1) **Sneezing** and **nasal discharge** may be seen with a cleft palate, oronasal fistula, and viral upper respiratory disease.
      (2) **Coughing** may also be seen with a cleft palate.
      (3) **Mucocutaneous** or **cutaneous lesions** in areas other than the oral cavity may be seen in animals with immune-mediated skin disease, contact dermatitis, eosinophilic granuloma complex, trauma, or toxin exposure or ingestion.

(4) Polyuria and **polydipsia** may be present in pets with uremia or diabetes mellitus.

(5) Neurologic signs may be seen with cricopharyngeal achalasia, neuropraxia, rabies, and botulism.

3. Physical examination

a. General appearance. The animal's gait, body symmetry, and skin should be evaluated. Abnormalities may suggest the presence of an underlying systemic disease.

b. Oral cavity. Sedation or general anesthesia may be necessary in order to thoroughly examine the teeth or pharyngeal region or to examine the oropharyngeal cavity in an uncooperative patient. Gloves should always be worn if rabies is a consideration. Examination may reveal:

(1) Foreign bodies, punctures, lacerations, and fractures

(2) Swelling, hyperemia, and ulceration (e.g., as a result of trauma, neoplasia, infection, or inflammation)

(3) Proliferative lesions (neoplastic or inflammatory)

(4) Dental abnormalities

(5) Facial asymmetry, dropped jaw, or dysphagia (e.g., as a result of neuromuscular disorders)

4. Diagnostic studies

a. Complete blood count (CBC) may show anemia (e.g., as a result of chronic disease), inflammation, cyclic neutropenia, or thrombocytopenia (e.g., as a result of reticuloendothelial or hematologic disorders).

b. Serum biochemical profile and **urinalysis** may help identify underlying disorders (e.g., diabetes mellitus in an animal with concurrent polyuria and polydipsia).

c. Serology [e.g., for feline leukemia virus (FeLV) or feline immunodeficiency virus (FIV)] can help identify underlying viral disease.

d. Radiographs may help identify foreign bodies, assess the size and extent of any masses, and assess the teeth and other bony structures. Anesthesia is often needed to properly position the patient for the required views.

e. Fluoroscopic evaluation using a barium swallow may help define the location and type of swallowing disorders.

f. Bacterial and **fungal cultures** are of limited value because of the variety of organisms found as normal flora in the mouth. Culture may be useful if samples are taken from a deeper localized lesion.

g. Biopsy and **histopathology** of oropharyngeal masses or lesions will often yield a diagnosis and allow better determination of a treatment regimen and prognosis.

B. Disorders of the lips, tongue, palate, and oral mucosa

1. Congenital disorders

a. Cleft lip (harelip) is most common in brachycephalic breeds and is caused by incomplete fusion of the maxillary process and the medial nasal process. Cleft lip is easily identified on physical examination and is often surgically repaired for cosmetic reasons.

b. Cleft palate occurs most commonly in brachycephalic breeds.

(1) Diagnosis is readily made with an oral examination. Signs may include difficulty in nursing, sneezing, nasal discharge, coughing, and gagging.

(2) Treatment consists of surgical correction. Tube feeding and antibiotic treatment for secondary rhinitis or aspiration pneumonia may be required until the animal is old enough to undergo surgery to repair the defect (i.e., 6–8 weeks old).

2. Trauma

a. Puncture wounds and **lacerations** require cleaning, and possibly suturing and antibiotic treatment.

b. Foreign bodies may be found in or near a puncture wound or in the absence of a wound. Physical examination will reveal most foreign bodies, but radiographs may be needed. Following removal of the foreign body, antibiotic treatment may be necessary.

    c. Burns may be **thermal, electrical,** or **chemical.**
        (1) Pathology. Burns can result in tissue ischemia, tissue necrosis, and adjacent edema and inflammation. Damage to deeper tissues may result from electrical burns.
        (2) Clinical findings. Concurrent clinical signs may indicate the cause of the burns (e.g., GI damage from ingested chemicals, respiratory signs from electrocution or smoke inhalation).
        (3) Treatment includes patient stabilization, antibiotics, and wound flushing and debridement. In the case of chemical burns, the animal's mouth should be flushed immediately.

3. Acquired disorders
    a. Lip-fold dermatitis is most common in breeds with pendulous lips.
        (1) Etiology. Trapped saliva and debris is the most common cause of this chronic moist dermatitis. Other disorders that cause oral or mucocutaneous lesions should also be considered, especially in atypical breeds.
        (2) Treatment
            (a) Palliative therapy consists of daily lip fold cleansing following treatment of any concurrent periodontal disease.
            (b) Definitive therapy. If the animal's lip configuration is responsible for the lip-fold dermatitis, surgery is required.
    b. Feline eosinophilic granuloma complex includes **eosinophilic plaques, eosinophilic ulcers,** and **linear granulomas.** The latter two conditions more commonly cause oral lesions. The cause of the disease is unknown, although underlying infectious, immune-mediated, or allergic disorders have been proposed.
        (1) Clinical findings may include drooling and dysphagia. On oral examination, one or more firm, raised, hyperemic nodules may be seen. Additional lesions may be seen on other areas of the body.
        (2) Diagnosis is based on biopsy. A CBC may reveal eosinophilia.
        (3) Treatment
            (a) Medical therapy. Corticosteroids are usually effective. Progesterones have also been used, but these agents are not approved for use in cats and have been associated with side effects.
            (b) Other treatments (e.g., cryosurgery) can be tried in patients that fail to respond to medical therapy, but the response is often poor.
        (4) Prognosis. Recurrence is fairly common in cats with chronic lesions or lesions that respond poorly to corticosteroid treatment. The prognosis is poor in patients that fail to respond to medical therapy.
    c. Labial granuloma is seen most often in young Siberian huskies.
        (1) Clinical findings may include halitosis, pain, and the presence of firm, raised, hyperemic nodules on the tongue or palate.
        (2) Diagnosis is based on biopsy results.
        (3) Treatment usually requires glucocorticoid administration.
        (4) Prognosis. Some lesions will regress spontaneously. A higher recurrence rate is seen in dogs with tongue lesions.
    d. Stomatitis and **glossitis.** Stomatitis (i.e., inflammation of the oral mucosa) and glossitis (i.e., inflammation of the tongue) are often seen together. Many local and systemic disorders can cause stomatitis (Table 41-1). Sometimes no cause is found.
        (1) Clinical findings may include halitosis, drooling, and dysphagia resulting from oral pain. Findings on oral examination may be specific to the cause. For example:
            (a) Dental plaque, tartar and periodontal lesions are suggestive of periodontitis.
            (b) Erosions and ulcers are seen in inflammatory stomatitis, infectious stomatitis, uremia, toxicity, and immune-mediated diseases.
            (c) Tissue proliferation is seen in inflammatory stomatitis.
            (d) White, plaque-like lesions are typical of candidiasis.

TABLE 41-1. Stomatitis—Underlying Disorders, Diagnostic Approach, and Treatment

Disorders	Diagnostic Approach	Treatment
Local disorders		
Periodontitis or dental disease	Oral examination, radiographs	Dental prophylaxis, antibiotics
Lymphocytic–plasmacytic stomatitis	Biopsy	Dental prophylaxis, glucocorticoids or other immunosuppressive medications
Feline plasma cell stomatitis	Biopsy	Dental prophylaxis, antibiotics, dental extractions
Contact dermatitis	History	Symptomatic treatment
Foreign objects	Oral examination, scraping (burrs), biopsy	Foreign object removal, antibiotics
Candidiasis	Oral examination, culture	Topical nystatin or oral ketoconazole, treatment for underlying disease
Systemic disorders		
Feline leukemia virus (FeLV) infection	Serology	Symptomatic treatment (i.e., oral rinses, parenteral fluids)
Feline immunodeficiency virus (FIV) infection	Serology	Symptomatic treatment (i.e., oral rinses, parenteral fluids)
Feline calicivirus (FCV) or feline rhinotracheitis	History, physical examination (concurrent naso-ocular signs)	Symptomatic treatment (i.e., oral rinses, parenteral fluids)
Feline herpesvirus infection	History, physical examination	Symptomatic treatment (i.e., oral rinses, parenteral fluids)
Canine distemper virus (CDV) infection	History, physical examination (concurrent respiratory, GI, or neurologic signs)	Symptomatic treatment, control of secondary infections
Feline panleukopenia	History, physical examination (concurrent GI signs), CBC	Symptomatic treatment (i.e., oral rinses, parenteral fluids)
Uremia	Serum biochemical profile, urinalysis	Symptomatic treatment, treatment for uremia
Diabetes mellitus	Serum biochemical profile, urinalysis	Symptomatic treatment, treatment for diabetes mellitus
Cyclic neutropenia	CBC, bone marrow aspirate	Symptomatic treatment
Heavy metal toxicity	History	Symptomatic treatment
Systemic lupus erythematosus (SLE)	ANA test, LE test	Glucocorticoids or other immunosuppressive drugs
Pemphigus	Biopsy with immunofluorescent staining	Glucocorticoids or other immunosuppressive drugs
Idiopathic vasculitis	Biopsy	Glucocorticoids or other immunosuppressive drugs
Toxic epidermal necrolysis (TEN)	Biopsy	Glucocorticoids or other immunosuppressive drugs
Drug reaction	History, biopsy	Removal of offending medication, symptomatic treatment

ANA = antinuclear antibody; CBC = complete blood count; GI = gastrointestinal; LE = lupus erythematosus.

(2) **Diagnosis** is based on the history, physical examination findings, and test results (see Table 41-1).

(3) **Treatment** varies with the cause (see Table 41-1).

(4) **Prognosis** varies with the underlying disorder. Periodontitis can usually be successfully managed.

e. **Benign gingival hyperplasia** is most commonly seen in collies, boxers, and other large-breed dogs and is thought to result from chronic irritation. Biopsy results may be needed to rule out neoplasia. Treatment consists of gingivectomy and gingivoplasty.

f. **Oronasal fistulae.** An abnormal communication between the oral and nasal cavities can result from trauma or tooth root abscess or extraction. Clinical findings include nasal discharge and possibly halitosis and oral pain. Treatment consists of surgical repair of the fistula and antibiotic treatment of the secondary rhinitis.

g. **Neoplasia**

(1) **Benign.** Epulides and papillomas are the most common benign oral neoplasms.

(a) **Epulides,** which may be **fibromatous, ossifying,** or **acanthomatous,** originate from the periodontal tissues. Although benign, the acanthomatous epulis can be locally invasive and can cause bone destruction.

(i) **Clinical findings.** Drooling, dysphagia, and the presence of a single gingival mass, often near the incisors, may be observed.

(ii) **Diagnosis** is based on biopsy, but radiographs may help determine the extent of the mass.

(iii) **Treatment.** Aggressive surgical resection is optimal, but radiation may also prove effective for lesions that recur or that cannot be completely excised.

(b) **Oral papillomatosis** occurs in young dogs and is caused by papillomavirus infection.

(i) **Clinical findings.** Growths begin as smooth, pale plaques, which become lobular and gray, then compact and hyperpigmented. Multiple lesions may occur.

(ii) **Diagnosis** is usually based on oral examination, but biopsy results are useful with atypical lesions.

(iii) **Treatment** is usually unnecessary (unless a mass interferes with eating) because the lesions spontaneously regress.

(2) **Malignant.** Squamous cell carcinomas, malignant melanomas, and fibrosarcomas are the most common malignant oral neoplasms.

(a) **Squamous cell carcinoma** most commonly appears as an eroded or ulcerated gingival lesion medial to the canine teeth in dogs and ventral to the tongue in cats. The tumor is locally invasive and often metastasizes to regional lymph nodes, but pulmonary metastasis does not occur until late in the disease.

(i) **Clinical findings** may include oral pain, dysphagia, drooling, halitosis, and the oral lesion itself.

(ii) **Diagnosis** is based on biopsy results.

(iii) **Treatment** of localized disease consists of aggressive surgical resection with or without radiation. **Prognosis** is usually guarded.

(b) **Malignant melanoma** is most commonly seen as a rapidly growing, pink to black, raised lesion of the gingiva. Invasion of deeper structures and early metastasis are common.

(i) **Clinical findings** may include oral pain, dysphagia, drooling, halitosis, and the oral mass itself.

(ii) **Diagnosis** is based on biopsy results.

(iii) **Treatment** of localized disease consists of aggressive surgical resection, but metastasis still usually occurs. **Prognosis** is usually poor.

(c) **Fibrosarcoma** is most commonly seen as a firm, smooth or ulcerated nodular lesion on the lateral maxillary gingiva. The tumor is locally invasive but metastasis is rare.

(i) **Clinical findings** may include oral pain, dysphagia, drooling, halitosis, and the oral mass itself.

(ii) **Diagnosis** is based on biopsy results.

(iii) **Treatment** involves aggressive surgical resection, but chemotherapy may palliate the disease for a short time. Local recurrence is common.

C. **Disorders of the jaw** and **teeth**

1. **Congenital disorders**
   a. **Brachygnathism (overshot bite)** is characterized by a short mandible relative to the maxilla. Secondary trauma to the palate can occur. Treatment options involve advanced dentistry.
   b. **Prognathism (undershot bite)** is characterized by a long mandible relative to the maxilla. This is considered normal for brachycephalic dogs and cats. Treatment is usually not needed.
   c. **Retained deciduous teeth** remain firmly attached when the permanent teeth erupt. Treatment requires prompt extraction of the retained teeth to prevent malocclusion of the permanent teeth.
   d. **Enamel hypoplasia** is the thinning or absence of the dental enamel. The affected areas are usually relatively soft. If dentin is exposed, disease of the pulp can also occur.

2. **Trauma** can result in fractures of the jaw or teeth. Oral pain is the predominant clinical sign. Discoloration of the affected tooth or teeth (i.e., reddish with inflammation or infection of the pulp; gray with pulp necrosis) may also be seen. Treatment entails surgery, dental extraction, or endodontic therapy.

3. **Acquired disorders**
   a. **Craniomandibular osteopathy** is most commonly seen in young terriers. The cause is unknown.
      (1) **Clinical findings** can include drooling, dysphagia, pain on opening the mouth, bilateral mandibular swelling, and fever. With time, the masticatory muscles may atrophy and jaw motion may be restricted.
      (2) **Radiographic findings.** Bony proliferation along the mandibles and the tympanic bulla-petrous temporal bones is usually seen.
      (3) **Diagnosis** is usually based on the physical findings and skull radiographs. A biopsy may be needed in atypical cases.
      (4) **Treatment.** The disease is self-limiting; palliative relief can be achieved with anti-inflammatory drugs.
      (5) **Prognosis** is usually fair. It is guarded if bony proliferation severely limits movement of the temporomandibular joints.
   b. **"Dropped jaw"** results from trigeminal nerve paralysis, which can be caused by idiopathic neuritis (see Chapter 47 V D), trauma, or infectious disease (e.g., rabies). **Clinical findings** include drooling and an inability to close the mouth.
   c. **Masticatory muscle myositis (eosinophilic myositis, atrophic myositis)** is discussed in more detail in Chapter 47 VI C 2.
      (1) **Clinical findings** include dysphagia, pain when the mouth is opened, and swollen masticatory muscles (in acute disease) or symmetrical atrophy of these muscles (in chronic disease).
      (2) **Diagnosis** is primarily based on muscle biopsy.
      (3) **Treatment** is with glucocorticoids, but underlying disorders should be investigated if other muscles are also affected.
   d. **Retrobulbar abscess**
      (1) **Clinical findings** often include acute dysphagia, severe pain on opening of the mouth, and unilateral exophthalmus. Swelling or hyperemia of the oropharyngeal mucosa caudal to the last upper molar may or may not be noted.
      (2) **Treatment** involves drainage caudal to the last upper molar and subsequent oral antibiotic treatment.

    e. Systemic disease. Both primary and secondary **hyperparathyroidism** can result in bone resorption, jaw swelling, and loose teeth.

    f. Periodontal disease ranges from gingivitis (reversible) to periodontitis (irreversible). Inflammation and infection of any of the periodontal tissues (i.e., the gingiva, periodontal ligament, or alveolar bone) can occur. Small-breed dogs, animals with malocclusions or dental crowding, "mouth breathers," and animals fed soft food are at increased risk for periodontal disease. Periodontal disease affects 60%–80% of all dogs and cats.

        (1) Pathogenesis. Bacteria and cells accumulate as plaque, and the resulting bacterial products cause inflammation in the adjacent gingiva. With time, the bacterial flora changes, more plaque forms, the bacterial products increase, and deeper tissues are affected. Immunocytes infiltrate the periodontal tissues and alveolar bone resorption begins. Local neutrophil numbers also increase.

        (2) Clinical findings

            (a) Initially, halitosis or a change in eating or chewing habits may be reported. Dental calculus (mineralized plaque) and gingival hyperemia may be visible.

            (b) As the disease progresses, inappetence, depression, and weight loss may also occur. Gum recession, purulent exudate, and loose teeth may be seen.

        (3) Diagnosis is based on physical and oral examination findings and periodontal evaluation using a dental probe. Radiographs may be necessary.

        (4) Treatment

            (a) Early disease responds to dental scaling and polishing.

            (b) Advanced disease may require tooth extraction, gingivectomy, surgical removal of periodontal pockets, and antibiotic treatment.

            (c) Antibiotic treatment should be initiated 12 hours prior to any dental procedure.

        (5) Prognosis. Gingivitis is reversible with proper treatment. Advanced disease is irreversible, but the progression may be halted with treatment.

        (6) Prevention. Feeding hard foods, providing firm chew toys, brushing the teeth, using dental rinses, and practicing periodic dental prophylaxis can help prevent disease progression.

    g. Periapical abscesses. The canine and carnassial teeth are most commonly affected.

        (1) Clinical findings usually include pain when chewing. With carnassial involvement, a draining tract or small swelling ventrolateral to the medial canthus of the eye may also be seen.

        (2) Diagnosis is confirmed with radiographs.

        (3) Treatment often requires extraction of the affected tooth.

    h. Caries result from acid demineralization of dental enamel. In cats, subgingival and **cervical erosive lesions** (neck lesions) are more common.

        (1) Diagnosis may require radiography for identification of the associated root resorption.

        (2) Treatment. Early lesions can be restored; more advanced lesions require extraction.

D. **Disorders of the pharynx**

    1. Trauma. Most pharyngeal trauma results from **ingestion of a foreign object.**

      a. Clinical findings. Gagging, drooling, and dysphagia are the most common clinical signs.

      b. Diagnosis is usually based on history, an oropharyngeal examination, and possibly radiographs.

      c. Treatment requires removal of any foreign object, antibiotic treatment, and, possibly, analgesic treatment.

    2. Acquired disorders

      a. Pharyngitis and **tonsillitis** can occur as a primary disease, in association with stomatitis (see I B 3 d) or trauma, or secondary to chronic nasal disease, regurgitation, vomiting, or coughing. Primary pharyngitis or tonsillitis may be seen in young, small-breed dogs.

    (1) Clinical findings may include drooling, gagging, retching, and dysphagia. Pharyngeal hyperemia and swelling may be noted.

    (2) Diagnosis is based on the presence of concurrent clinical signs. Biopsy may be necessary.

    (3) Treatment includes antibiotics, resolution of any underlying disease, and possibly analgesics.

  b. Neoplasia. Tonsillar squamous cell carcinoma (unilateral) and **tonsillar lymphosarcoma** (bilateral) are the most common neoplasms of the pharyngeal region. Diagnosis is based on biopsy.

    (1) Tonsillar squamous cell carcinoma is difficult to impossible to completely excise because of the location. It has a poor prognosis because the neoplasm is aggressive and quickly metastasizes to the regional lymph nodes.

    (2) Lymphosarcoma is usually treated with chemotherapy, but cures are very rare.

  c. Pharyngeal neuromuscular disorders

    (1) Clinical findings. Pharyngeal neuromuscular disorders usually cause dysphagia and drooling.

    (2) Diagnosis is based on concurrent clinical signs, neurologic examination, a barium swallow with fluoroscopy, and possibly specialized tests. **Differential diagnoses** include rabies, other central nervous system (CNS) diseases, neuropathy affecting cranial nerves VII, IX, X, or XII, neuromuscular disease (e.g., myasthenia gravis, botulism), cricopharyngeal achalasia, and pharyngeal incoordination.

    (3) Treatment and **prognosis** vary with the underlying disease.

E. Disorders of the salivary glands

  1. Salivary mucoceles (sialoceles) are an accumulation of saliva in tissue, not true cysts, that result from duct blockage or rupture of the salivary gland. The saliva accumulates as a slowly enlarging swelling ventral to the affected gland. Saliva accumulation under the oral mucosa is termed a **ranula.**

    a. Clinical findings include swelling, drooling, and possible dysphagia or dyspnea if the pharyngeal region is affected.

    b. Diagnosis is based on the clinical signs and a fine-needle aspirate. The aspirated fluid is usually stringy, contains few nucleated cells, and may be blood-tinged.

    c. Treatment consists of surgical removal of the involved gland and drainage of the mucocele. Aspiration of the mucocele will only temporarily relieve the swelling.

  2. Salivary fistulae are uncommon but can occur with traumatic rupture of a duct, a penetrating wound to the salivary gland, or secondary to a sialocele.

    a. Diagnosis is based on the history, physical examination, evaluation of any draining fluid, and a possible contrast study of the fistula.

    b. Treatment consists of surgery.

  3. Sialadenitis (i.e., inflammation or infection of the salivary glands) is a rare cause of clinical disease in the dog and cat. Drooling, fever, pain on opening the mouth, and exophthalmus may be seen, depending on the gland affected. Treatment consists of antibiotics and drainage if the gland is abscessed.

  4. Xerostomia (i.e., decreased salivation) may be seen following radiation therapy of oral or nasal tumors or as part of an immune-mediated syndrome (Sjögren's syndrome).

II. ESOPHAGEAL DISORDERS

A. Clinical evaluation

  1. Predisposition

a. Species and breed. All breeds of dogs and cats can develop an esophageal problem, but certain breeds are at increased risk. For example, Shar peis have a high incidence of abnormal esophageal motility, esophageal redundancy, megaesophagus, and hiatal hernia.

b. Age

(1) Young animals

(a) Clinical signs that first appear at the time of weaning are suggestive of a persistent right aortic arch (PRAA), other vascular ring anomalies, or idiopathic megaesophagus. Although the problem has been present since birth, often liquid is tolerated fairly well. The problem only becomes apparent when the animal regurgitates solid food.

(b) Progressive clinical signs of neurologic dysfunction during the next 10 months are suggestive of a neuronal storage disease, hydrocephalus, or other degenerative neurologic disease.

(c) Foreign bodies are more common in young animals.

(2) Older animals. Neoplasia is more common in older animals.

c. The animal's **environment** and **vaccination status** should also be considered.

2. Clinical signs

a. Primary signs may include **dysphagia, regurgitation, odynophagia,** and **anorexia.**

b. Concurrent signs

(1) Neurologic signs

(a) Weakness may be seen with neuromuscular disorders, hypoadrenocorticism, or hypothyroidism.

(b) Seizures or **abnormal mentation** may be seen with intracranial diseases.

(c) Ataxia may accompany CNS and neuromuscular disorders.

(2) Lameness may be seen with polyarthritis or polymyositis.

(3) Respiratory signs. A chronic or recurrent **cough, dyspnea, mucopurulent nasal discharge,** and **fever** are signs of aspiration pneumonia, which is a common complication of severe obstruction, megaesophagus, and diverticula. If the respiratory symptoms are more prominent than the regurgitation, with or without a history of an esophageal problem (e.g., foreign body), a bronchoesophageal fistula should be considered.

(4) Weight loss or **poor growth** can result from decreased food consumption or decreased volume that reaches the stomach and intestines.

(5) Vomiting may suggest pyloric stenosis. A history of vomiting may support a diagnosis of esophagitis.

(6) Constipation may be seen with dysautonomia.

(7) Truncal alopecia may be seen with hypothyroidism.

3. Physical examination

a. General appearance. The animal may be thin or cachexic.

b. Oral cavity

(1) Mucocutaneous lesions may be seen with systemic lupus erythematosus (SLE) and some toxicities.

(2) Slightly pale mucous membranes may indicate anemia due to chronic metabolic disease or malnutrition.

c. Thorax

(1) Ballooning of the esophagus at the thoracic inlet on expiration suggests esophageal dilatation.

(2) A **noncompressible cranioventral thorax** in a young cat suggests the presence of a cranial mediastinal mass that may be compressing the esophagus.

(3) Crackles may be auscultated in a patient with aspiration pneumonia.

(4) Bradycardia often occurs with dysautonomia and may be present with hypoadrenocorticism.

d. Musculoskeletal system

(1) Pain or **swelling of multiple joints** can occur with SLE-associated polyarthritis.

(2) Muscle pain suggests a myopathy.

e. **Eyes**
(1) **Dilated pupils** in a cat with megaesophagus is suggestive of dysautonomia.
(2) **Retinal lesions** may be present with distemper, other types of meningoencephalitis, and toxoplasmosis.
f. **Nervous system.** Neurologic examination may reveal CNS disease, peripheral neuropathy, or neuromuscular disease.

4. **Diagnostic tests**
a. **Radiography**
(1) **Survey radiographs**
(a) A **radiodense foreign body** may be seen.
(b) **Dilatation of the entire esophagus** suggests but does not confirm megaesophagus; aerophagia, stress, and dyspnea can also dilate the esophagus with air.
(c) **Dilatation of the esophagus cranial to the heart** may be seen with a vascular ring anomaly.
(d) A **soft tissue density** protruding into the esophageal lumen may be seen with granuloma or neoplasia. A **periesophageal mass** may also be visible.
(e) An **interstitial–alveolar pattern** in the cranioventral lung lobes is usually seen with a secondary aspiration pneumonia.
(f) **Focal consolidation** of a lung lobe can be seen with a bronchoesophageal fistula.
(2) **Contrast esophagram** with **fluoroscopy** should be performed if possible. Fluoroscopy will best demonstrate abnormalities in peristalsis (primary or secondary). Aspiration is a risk when administering contrast medium to an animal with a swallowing problem.
(a) A **dilated, hypomotile esophagus** is consistent with megaesophagus.
(b) **Dilatation of the cranial esophagus** with constriction at the heart base is consistent with a vascular ring anomaly.
(c) A **circumferential narrowing of the esophageal lumen** suggests a stricture.
(d) A **soft-tissue narrowing of the lumen** will be seen with a granuloma or neoplasm.
(e) An **intraluminal filling defect** suggests a radiolucent foreign body.
(f) A **contrast-filled outpouching** of the esophagus can be seen with a diverticulum.
(g) **Contrast material in the lungs, pleura,** or **soft tissues** suggests a fistula.
(h) **Roughened esophageal mucosa** may be seen with esophagitis.
b. **CBC.** The CBC is often normal; however it may be useful if an inflammatory, metabolic, or immune-mediated disorder is thought to be present.
(1) Leukocytosis may be seen with severe esophageal inflammation or perforation and with aspiration pneumonia.
(2) Mild nonregenerative anemia can be seen with underlying metabolic disease or malnutrition.
(3) Regenerative anemia in the absence of blood loss can suggest an immune-mediated hemolytic anemia and possible SLE.
c. **Endoscopy** is useful if an intramural or intraluminal obstruction or esophagitis is suspected.
(1) Biopsies can be obtained from abnormal areas.
(2) Many foreign bodies can be removed and the mucosa can be viewed following removal.
(3) Strictures may be lessened using balloon catheter dilatation or bougienage (i.e., gradual distention using rubber or metal bougies).

B. **Specific disorders**

1. **Megaesophagus,** which is characterized by esophageal dilatation and hypomotility, is the most common esophageal disorder in dogs and cats.
a. **Etiology**

TABLE 41-2. Disorders that may Cause Secondary Megaesophagus

Central nervous system (CNS) disorders

Viral meningoencephalitis or encephalitis (e.g., distemper)

Brain stem disease

Hydrocephalus

Neuronal storage disease

CNS depressant drugs

Neuromuscular disorders*

Polyneuropathies (e.g., polyradiculoneuritis, giant axonal neuropathy, heavy metal toxicity, dysautonomia)

Junctionopathies (e.g., myasthenia gravis, botulism, tick paralysis)

Myopathies (e.g., idiopathic polymyositis, toxoplasmosis, dermatomyositis, immune-mediated myopathy, myotonia)

Metabolic disorders

Hypoadrenocorticism

Hypothyroidism

Miscellaneous disorders

Esophageal neoplasia

Esophagitis

Pyloric stenosis†

* Megaesophagus secondary to congenital or acquired neuromuscular disease is more common in Bouviers des Flandres, collies, German shepherds, golden retrievers, Jack Russell terriers, Labrador retrievers, Rottweilers, smooth-coated fox terriers, and springer spaniels.

† Megaesophagus associated with pyloric stenosis has only been reported in cats.

(1) **Idiopathic megaesophagus.** Inadequate peristalsis results in retention of ingesta in the esophagus, which over time progressively dilates the esophagus.

   (a) **Congenital idiopathic megaesophagus** may result from delayed or defective maturation of the neural pathways involved in swallowing. It is inherited in wirehaired fox terriers and miniature schnauzers. A breed predisposition has been shown for German shepherds, golden retrievers, Great Danes, greyhounds, Irish setters, Labrador retrievers, Newfoundlands, Shar peis, and Siamese cats.

   (b) **Acquired idiopathic megaesophagus** in adults may result from a sensory defect in the afferent arm of the swallowing reflex.

(2) **Secondary megaesophagus.** Disorders that cause secondary megaesophagus are summarized in Table 41-2.

b. **Diagnosis**

   (1) **Clinical findings.** Regurgitation is the most common sign. Chronic or recurrent respiratory signs, weight loss or poor growth, and a grossly visible cervical esophageal bulge may also be noted. With secondary megaesophagus, clinical signs related to the underlying disorder may be present.

   (2) **Radiographic findings**

   (a) **Survey radiographs** usually reveal dilatation of the entire esophagus. An interstitial–alveolar pattern in the cranioventral lung lobes consistent with aspiration pneumonia is common.

   (b) A **contrast esophagram** shows dilatation without an obstruction. Fluoroscopy reveals little or no motility. Radiolucent foreign bodies, strictures, or masses causing a secondary megaesophagus will be apparent. In cats, a radiograph should also be taken later to rule out pyloric stenosis.

   (3) **Endoscopic findings.** In an animal with primary megaesophagus, endoscopy will reveal a dilated, hypomotile, noninflamed esophagus.

TABLE 41-3. Diagnostic Tests for Disorders Causing Secondary Megaesophagus

Suspected Disorder	Appropriate Tests
Inflammatory disorders	Complete blood count (CBC)
Metabolic disorders	CBC, serum biochemical profile
Immune-mediated disorders	CBC, serum biochemical profile, urinalysis
Myopathies	Serum biochemical profile, electromyography, muscle biopsy
Obstructive or neoplastic disorders	Cervical and thoracic radiographs, contrast radiographs, endoscopy
Pyloric stenosis	Contrast radiographs
Esophagitis	Endoscopy
Hypoadrenocorticism	Adrenocorticotropic hormone (ACTH)-stimulation test
Hypothyroidism	Thyroid-stimulating hormone (TSH)-stimulation test
Toxoplasmosis	Serologic studies
Meningoencephalitis	Cerebrospinal fluid (CSF) cytology and titers
Hydrocephalus	Computed tomography (CT) scan
Brain stem disease	CSF cytology and titers, CT scan
Myasthenia gravis	Acetylcholine receptor antibody titer
Systemic lupus erythematosus (SLE)	Antinuclear antibody (ANA) titer, lupus erythematosus (LE) test
Polyneuropathies	Nerve conduction studies, nerve biopsy
Intoxication	Assays

(4) **Other findings.** Specific tests may be necessary in order to detect disorders that may cause secondary megaesophagus (Table 41-3). The results of these tests will be normal in animals with idiopathic megaesophagus.

c. **Treatment** is mainly supportive; in the case of secondary megaesophagus, treatment should be aimed at the underlying cause if at all possible.

(1) Retention of ingesta in the esophagus can be minimized by elevating the food and water supply, keeping the animal's upper body raised for 5–10 minutes following a meal, feeding multiple small meals, and feeding a food of optimal consistency (this varies with the individual). Administration of cisapride, a prokinetic agent, 30 minutes prior to feeding may also be considered.

(2) Gastrostomy tube placement is helpful for animals that are debilitated, have severe aspiration pneumonia, or are poorly responsive to medical therapy.

(3) Coupage and antibiotic therapy aimed at Gram-negative bacteria may be indicated in animals with concurrent aspiration pneumonia. Oral antibiotics should be avoided initially if regurgitation is severe.

d. **Prognosis**

(1) **Idiopathic megaesophagus**

(a) In animals with congenital idiopathic megaesophagus, maximal improvement has usually occurred by 6 months of age. If there is minimal esophageal distention and fair esophageal motility, the prognosis is usually good. If esophageal dilatation has occurred or motility is poor or absent, the long-term prognosis is grave.

(b) The long-term prognosis is poor for animals with acquired idiopathic megaesophagus.

(2) **Secondary megaesophagus.** The prognosis varies based on the underlying disease and the extent of secondary esophageal damage.

2. **Esophageal foreign body.** An ingested object may pass into the stomach, but if it is sharp, large, firm, or irregular, it may lodge in the esophagus. The most common sites for esophageal foreign bodies are the thoracic inlet, the heart base, and at the level of the diaphragm. Esophageal foreign bodies are more common in dogs than in cats.

   a. **Pathogenesis.** All foreign bodies damage the esophagus, causing erosion and laceration. The normal peristaltic activity of the esophagus often perpetuates the esophageal trauma, and may lead to perforation. Secondary pneumonia can result from aspiration of regurgitated material.

   b. **Diagnosis**

      (1) **Clinical findings**

         (a) Acute findings may include regurgitation, anorexia, ptyalism, pain, and depression.

         (b) Chronic findings commonly include regurgitation, salivation, depression, and weight loss.

         (c) If perforation has occurred, fever, injected mucous membranes, pain, depression, and shock can be seen. In rare cases where the perforation is small and somewhat contained, odynophagia and weight loss may be the predominant signs.

      (2) **Radiographic findings**

         (a) **Survey radiographs** may reveal a radiodense foreign body and an alveolar or interstitial pattern in the cranioventral lung lobes consistent with aspiration pneumonia.

         (b) **Contrast esophagrams** are necessary for visualization of radiolucent foreign bodies. A water-soluble contrast medium should be used if a perforation is suspected.

      (3) **Endoscopic findings.** Endoscopy allows visualization of the foreign body and the adjacent mucosa, and may permit removal of the object through the mouth.

   c. **Treatment**

      (1) **Definitive therapy** entails **removal of the foreign object.**

         (a) Removal can often be accomplished via **endoscopy** with peroral removal of the object, or by gently pushing the object aborally into the stomach for subsequent digestion and passage or for removal via **gastrotomy.** Care must be taken to avoid causing or exacerbating esophageal perforation. The entire esophagus should be assessed endoscopically for traumatic lesions caused by the foreign body.

         (b) **Esophageal surgery,** which is associated with many peri- and postoperative complications, should be considered only when other methods of foreign body removal are unsuccessful.

      (2) **Supportive therapy**

         (a) **Parenteral fluid administration** is usually required for at least 24 hours because oral intake of food and water can mechanically irritate the damaged esophagus.

         (b) **Gastrostomy tube placement** may be necessary if esophageal damage is so severe as to preclude oral intake for more than 48–72 hours.

         (c) **Treatment for esophagitis** should be carried out as described in II B 4 c.

         (d) **Parenteral antibiotic therapy** is required if perforation has occurred and recommended if the patient has secondary aspiration pneumonia.

   d. **Prognosis** varies with the method of foreign body removal and the degree of esophageal damage. Potential secondary complications from esophageal foreign bodies include ulceration, perforation, and stricture.

3. **Esophageal obstruction,** partial or complete, can disrupt swallowing by narrowing the esophageal lumen or altering esophageal peristalsis.

   a. **Vascular ring anomalies** (e.g., **PRAA**) can lead to constriction of the esophagus and are discussed in Chapter 39 V J.

   b. **Other periesophageal obstructions** include **cervical** and **thoracic masses** and

postoperative or **posttraumatic fibrous tissue.** Diagnosis is based on survey radiographs, a contrast esophagram, endoscopy, and/or exploratory surgery of the affected area. The prognosis varies with the site and the cause of the lesion.

   c. **Esophageal strictures.** Narrowing of the esophagus due to fibrous tissue usually occurs secondary to esophagitis, a previous foreign body, or esophageal surgery. Recent anesthesia and subsequent esophagitis are the most common causes of stricture.

      (1) **Diagnosis**

         (a) **Clinical findings.** Regurgitation, especially of solid foods, is common. Secondary aspiration pneumonia and weight loss may also occur. There is rarely pain, and the appetite usually remains good.

         (b) **Radiographic findings**

            (i) **Survey radiographs** may show a food-filled dilatation of the esophagus proximal to the stricture, or they may be unremarkable.

            (ii) **Contrast esophagram.** A stricture will be seen as a circumferential narrowing of the esophageal lumen with proximal dilatation of the esophagus. **Definitive diagnosis** is usually based on an esophagram, but endoscopy can also be used to identify a stricture.

      (2) **Treatment**

         (a) **Bougienage** or **balloon catheter dilation** can be attempted. Balloon catheter dilation is more effective, but both techniques usually must be repeated several times. **Surgical excision** of the stricture should be considered only if other treatments fail.

            (i) **Stricture recurrence** may follow successful bougienage, balloon dilation, or surgery.

            (ii) **Esophageal tearing** during bougienage or balloon dilatation is also possible.

         (b) **Concurrent medical treatment** for esophagitis (see II B 4 c) is also needed.

      (3) **Prognosis** is fair with balloon dilation of recent strictures but guarded with chronic strictures, bougienage, or surgery.

   d. **Granulomas** form in response to *Spirocerca lupi* infection. Sarcomas can also form secondary to *Spirocerca* infection.

      (1) **Diagnosis**

         (a) **Radiographic findings.** An esophagram will show a mass lesion protruding into the esophageal lumen.

         (b) **Detection of the *Spirocerca ova* in the feces** or a **biopsy sample** is necessary for definitive diagnosis.

      (2) **Treatment** is with **disophenol** or **fenbendazole.**

   e. **Esophageal neoplasms** (e.g., leiomyomas, squamous cell carcinomas, fibrosarcomas, osteosarcomas, undifferentiated carcinomas) are rare. Cranial mediastinal lymphosarcoma is more common in young cats.

  4. Esophagitis

   a. **Etiology.** Inflammation of the esophageal wall is caused by mechanical or chemical irritation of the esophagus due to the ingestion of sharp or rough objects, the ingestion of caustic substances, chronic vomiting (i.e., exposure to gastric contents), or gastroesophageal reflux (i.e., as a result of decreased sphincter pressure from anesthesia, drugs, neuromuscular disease, hiatal hernias, or a high-fat diet). Infection [e.g., feline calicivirus (FCV) infection, *Candida* infection, systemic phycomycoses] is an uncommon cause of esophagitis.

   b. **Diagnosis**

      (1) **Clinical findings** may be acute or chronic and commonly include anorexia, ptyalism, odynophagia, and weight loss. Regurgitation is a less common sign.

      (2) A **contrast esophagram** may be normal or may show decreased or asynchronous esophageal motility. Reflux of contrast media from the stomach into the distal esophagus may be seen with gastrointestinal reflux.

      (3) **Endoscopy** usually reveals roughened hyperemic mucosa and may reveal

erosions or ulcerations, most commonly in the distal esophagus. With gastric reflux, the gastroesophageal sphincter may be dilated and there may be fluid pooling in the distal esophagus. **Endoscopic biopsy** confirms the diagnosis.

  c. Treatment

    (1) Definitive treatment requires **correction of the underlying problem.**

    (2) Supportive treatment

      (a) Nutrition

        (i) Oral food and water should be withheld for at least 24–72 hours. **Parenteral fluid therapy** is needed during this time to maintain hydration.

        (ii) When feeding is resumed, a **low-fat gruel** should be given. If oral intake must be restricted for a longer period of time due to the severity of the esophageal lesions, placement of a gastrostomy tube for nutritional support should be considered.

      (b) Antibiotic therapy may help prevent secondary infection.

      (c) Acid-secretion inhibitors, antacids, and **gastric protective agents** can decrease gastric acid secretion and help protect against additional damage.

        (i) Histamine-2 (H$_2$) antagonists (e.g., cimetidine, ranitidine, famotidine) decrease gastric acid secretion.

        (ii) Antacids decrease gastroesophageal reflux and inactivate pepsin, but to be effective they must be given 4–6 times daily. Side effects include diarrhea, hypophosphatemia, and hypermagnesemia, depending on the compound used.

        (iii) Sucralfate, an aluminum salt that binds injured mucosa, may help protect against further damage from acid, pepsin, and bile salts. It also inhibits pepsin activity and improves prostaglandin synthesis.

      (d) Other agents

        (i) Metoclopramide and a **high-protein, low-fat diet** will help increase lower esophageal sphincter pressure and speed gastric emptying so less material is present to reflux.

        (ii) Cisapride may increase esophageal motility and lessen reflux.

        (iii) Prednisone may decrease inflammation and help decrease the risk of later stricture formation in patients with severe esophagitis. Its effectiveness is unknown.

  d. Prognosis. Esophagitis alone has a good prognosis, but the development of complications (namely, stricture formation), worsens the prognosis to guarded.

5. Hiatal hernia, an uncommon disorder in dogs and cats, may include herniation of the abdominal esophagus, gastroesophageal junction, and stomach.

  a. Diagnosis

    (1) Clinical findings are those of esophagitis [see II B 4 b (1)] or megaesophagus [see II B 1 b (1)]. Concurrent respiratory distress may also be seen.

    (2) Radiographic findings may include esophageal dilatation with a discrete soft-tissue density in the caudal esophagus. **Contrast radiographs** may be necessary for definitive diagnosis.

  b. Treatment involves surgical correction. Medical treatment with H$_2$ antagonists, sucralfate, and a high-protein, low-fat diet may be attempted first.

6. Esophageal diverticulum (i.e., a congenital or acquired outpouching of the esophagus) is rare in dogs and cats.

  a. Diagnosis

    (1) Clinical findings include regurgitation, odynophagia, inappetence, gagging, and retching in an attempt to empty the diverticulum. Respiratory signs due to secondary aspiration pneumonia may be present.

    (2) A **contrast esophagram** will reveal the diverticulum and will identify any concurrent esophageal constriction or motility defect.

  b. Treatment. Large diverticula usually require surgical excision, whereas small diverticula can often be managed medically (see II B 1 c).

7. Esophageal fistulae can form between the esophagus and the airways, pleura, or skin as a congenital malformation or as a result of the chronic presence of a foreign body, chronic inflammation, or neoplasia.

  a. Diagnosis

  (1) **Clinical findings** usually include coughing and respiratory distress after eating, anorexia, weight loss, and pyrexia. Regurgitation is uncommon.

  (2) **Radiographic findings**

  (a) **Survey radiographs** may show a radiopaque foreign body with or without pulmonary consolidation.

  (b) **Contrast radiographs** will identify the site of the fistula.

  b. Treatment consists of surgical closure of the fistula and resection of the infected tissues.

III. GASTRIC DISORDERS

A. Clinical evaluation

  1. Predisposition

  a. Species and breed. All breeds of dogs and cats can develop a gastric problem, but certain breeds are at increased risk. For example, gastric–dilatation volvulus (GDV) occurs primarily in large- and giant-breed dogs.

  b. Age

  (1) **Young animals.** Viral disease, parasitic diseases, foreign bodies, pyloric stenosis, and benign gastric antral hyperplasia are more common in younger animals.

  (2) **Older animals.** Neoplasia is more common in older animals.

  c. The animal's **environment** and **vaccination status** should also be considered.

  2. History. Acute signs of gastric disease are more common with simple gastritis, hemorrhagic gastroenteritis, GDV, some systemic disorders, and during the early phase of a chronic disorder.

  3. Clinical signs

  a. Primary signs

  (1) **Vomiting** is the most common sign of gastric disease (see Chapter 3).

  (2) **Nausea** (evidenced by hypersalivation, frequent swallowing, and restlessness) may precede retching (ineffective vomiting) or vomiting.

  (3) **Hematemesis** is usually caused by gastric or duodenal erosions or ulcers but can also be seen with a systemic coagulopathy or ingestion of blood from another site.

  (4) **Anorexia** can result from gastric pain or nausea.

  (5) **Abdominal pain** may be manifested as restlessness, shivering, or anorexia.

  (6) **Melena** can occur if upper GI hemorrhage is present (see Chapter 5). Ulcers and erosions are the most common cause of melena, but melena can also occur with neoplasia and coagulopathies.

  (7) **Bloating** may result from gastric distention with food, liquid, or air.

  b. Concurrent signs

  (1) **Diarrhea** suggests a disorder that also affects the small intestine, such as infection, dietary indiscretion, toxin ingestion, inflammatory disease, neoplasia, hemorrhagic gastroenteritis (HGE), or a systemic disease.

  (2) **Weight loss** can result if food consumption is decreased or if frequent vomiting results in reduced amounts of food reaching the intestines.

  4. Physical examination

  a. General appearance. The animal may be thin or cachexic. Increased salivation and frequent swallowing may be noted. The abdomen may be distended.

  b. Oral cavity

  (1) Mucous membranes may be slightly pale (as a result of anemia from

chronic metabolic disease or gastric hemorrhage), tacky (as a result of dehydration), or demonstrate a slow capillary refill time (a sign of shock).

    (2) String foreign bodies may be found at the frenulum in vomiting cats.

  c. Abdomen

    (1) The stomach is extremely distended in animals with GDV; gastric retention produces moderate distention.

    (2) Inflammatory gastric disease may cause mild discomfort on cranial abdominal palpation.

    (3) A gastric mass or gastric wall thickening may not be palpable because of the normal location of the stomach relative to the ribs.

5. Diagnostic tests

  a. Radiography

    (1) Survey radiographs

      (a) A **radiodense foreign body** may be seen.

      (b) Dilatation of the stomach with gas can occur with aerophagia, GDV, foreign body ingestion, or hypomotility. With GDV, the stomach is often also in an abnormal orientation or is compartmentalized (i.e., a "double bubble" or a "shelf" of tissue can be seen in the gastric lumen).

      (c) A **food-filled stomach** is a normal finding postprandially, but suggests hypomotility or a pyloric obstruction if the animal has not recently eaten.

      (d) An **irregular gastric shape** can be seen with neoplasia or a foreign body.

      (e) Pneumoperitoneum may be seen if gastric perforation has occurred.

    (2) Contrast radiographs (with fluoroscopy if possible). Barium should be used unless a perforation is suspected.

      (a) An **intragastric filling defect** suggests a radiolucent foreign body, food, or a tumor or granuloma.

      (b) Irregular gastric mucosa, abnormal rugal folds, or a **nondistensible gastric wall** can be seen with inflammatory disease or diffuse neoplasia.

      (c) Contrast material in the gastric wall or **focal retention of contrast** is suggestive of an ulcer.

      (d) Delayed gastric emptying

        (i) Delayed gastric emptying (i.e., longer than 3–4 hours in dogs or 1 hour in cats) in association with a **narrowed pyloric outflow tract** can be seen with pyloric stenosis, benign gastric antral mucosal hypertrophy, foreign body ingestion, neoplasia, inflammatory disease, phycomycosis, a partial volvulus, or pylorospasm due to irritative disease. If the narrowed region fails to enlarge when viewed with fluoroscopy or the narrowing is visible on several repeat films, an anatomical stenosis is present.

        (ii) Delayed gastric emptying with a **normal width pyloric outflow tract** suggests a motility disorder.

      (e) A **dilated stomach** with delayed emptying and poor peristalsis is suggestive of gastric hypomotility.

  b. Laboratory studies

    (1) CBC. In many cases, the CBC is normal.

      (a) Leukocytosis may be seen with severe gastric inflammation or perforation.

      (b) Nonregenerative anemia can be seen with chronic disease, peracute or chronic blood loss, or malnutrition.

      (c) Regenerative anemia may be seen with subacute gastric hemorrhage.

      (d) Eosinophilia can be seen with some parasitic infections and with eosinophilic gastritis.

(2) Serum biochemical profile
 (a) Hypochloremic metabolic alkalosis suggests loss of gastric acid because of gastric or high duodenal vomiting.
 (b) Hypercalcemia is most commonly caused by lymphosarcoma.
 (c) Hypoglycemia may occur in young animals because of inadequate food intake or retention.
 (d) Hypoproteinemia may result from blood loss or severe inflammation.
 (e) Electrolyte abnormalities (e.g., hypokalemia, hyponatremia) may be seen.
(3) Fecal flotation can be used to identify some parasitic infections.
 c. **Endoscopy** allows for evaluation, biopsy sampling, and possibly, retrieval of gastric foreign bodies.
 (1) An intraluminal mass, erosions or ulcers, hyperemia, or irregular mucosa may be seen with inflammation or neoplasia.
 (2) Food or fluid pooling after a fast of 10 hours or more suggests the possibility of a motility abnormality.
 (3) Gastric wall thickening suggests inflammation, neoplasia, or pyloric stenosis).
 (4) The mucosa can be grossly normal with some inflammatory conditions and with submucosal diseases. Multiple biopsies should be taken even if the mucosa is grossly normal.
 d. **Ultrasonography** may reveal a radiolucent gastric foreign body, a mass lesion, or gastric wall thickening.
 e. **Exploratory laparotomy** allows for full-thickness biopsies and may be therapeutic in the case of some foreign bodies, some types of neoplasia, pyloric obstruction, gastric perforation, and ulcers that do not respond to medication.

B. **Specific gastric disorders**

1. **Acute gastritis**
 a. **Etiology.** Acute gastritis is most commonly caused by **dietary indiscretion** or **intolerance, drugs** (e.g., aspirin), **parasitic infection** (e.g., ascariasis), **toxins** (e.g., bacterial enterotoxins, plant toxins, chemicals) and **foreign bodies.** Gastritis may also occur with enteritis in canine parvoviral infection and canine distemper virus (CDV) infection, but usually the vomiting is due to duodenal involvement.
 b. **Clinical findings** may include vomiting (food or bile), anorexia, and diarrhea (with intestinal involvement).
 c. **Diagnosis.** Acute gastritis due to dietary indiscretion, toxins, and drugs is usually a diagnosis of exclusion based on the history and physical examination.
 (1) Ascariasis is detected on fecal examination or response to treatment with pyrantel pamoate.
 (2) Foreign body ingestion is diagnosed radiographically.
 (3) In the case of acute gastritis as a result of viral disease or acute gastritis that fails to respond to conservative therapy, additional testing may be required.
 d. **Treatment** entails resting the GI tract, and possibly, the administration of parenteral fluids and antiemetics (see Chapter 3 V A, B 3). The underlying disorder should be treated.
 e. **Prognosis** is usually excellent with appropriate treatment.

2. **HGE** is primarily an intestinal disorder (see IV B 7), but may produce hematemesis.

3. **GDV.** Large- and giant-breed dogs with deep chests are most commonly affected. Often, there is a history of exercise following ingestion of a large meal, although the relationship between this and GDV has not been proven in research studies.
 a. **Pathogenesis.** The cause of GDV is unknown, but altered gastric motility is thought to play a major role. Initially, gas or food causes gastric dilatation. The stomach may remain in its normal position (dilatation) or twist (volvulus) so that the pylorus lies dorsal to the stomach on the left side).

(1) With volvulus, gastric outflow is often obstructed and progressive dilatation occurs. Splenic torsion may also occur as the stomach twists. Venous return from the abdomen is compromised, causing shock.

(2) Gastric wall ischemia can result from the marked gastric distention and compromise of gastric blood supply.

(3) Endotoxins and other inflammatory mediators can lead to disseminated intravascular coagulation (DIC) and other complications.

(4) Complications (e.g., cardiac arrhythmias, respiratory compromise, electrolyte and acid–base abnormalities, and septic peritonitis) may also occur.

b. Diagnosis

  (1) Clinical findings. Early signs may include nonproductive retching and anxiety or discomfort, progressing to abdominal distention (which may be externally subtle), abdominal pain, shock, and collapse. A presumptive diagnosis can often be based on the history of nonproductive retching and the presence of marked cranial abdominal distention with tympany.

  (2) Radiographic findings. Radiographs will usually allow differentiation of simple dilation from dilatation--volvulus. A right lateral radiograph of an animal with dilatation–volvulus may reveal pyloric displacement to the left with or without compartmentalization of the stomach.

c. Treatment

  (1) Acute therapy

    (a) Shock correction is the first priority. **Aggressive parenteral fluid therapy** with possible concurrent administration of hypertonic saline solution should be instituted immediately. A **rapid-acting glucocorticoid** may also be considered for its proposed stabilization of lysosomal membranes, inhibition of endotoxin, antagonism of vasoactive substances, and positive effects on cardiac function. Following resolution of the shock, parenteral fluid therapy should be continued at a more moderate administration rate.

    (b) Gastric decompression via orogastric tube, needle gastrocentesis, or temporary gastrostomy should be performed.

  (2) Definitive therapy is achieved through **laparotomy.** Surgery should be performed as soon as possible to minimize damage to the stomach and adjacent structures. The stomach should be repositioned, damaged tissue (e.g., splenic tissue or portions of gastric tissue) should be removed, and the stomach should be fixed in normal position using gastropexy.

  (3) Supportive therapy

    (a) Correction of electrolyte abnormalities (e.g., hypokalemia) will facilitate treatment of other complications (e.g., arrhythmias).

    (b) Antibiotics are given intravenously for bacteremia or sepsis.

d. Prognosis varies with the severity of the distention and the speed of diagnosis and treatment.

4. Gastric erosions and **ulcers.** Ulcers extend through the mucosa; erosions are more superficial. The primary complication of gastric ulceration is perforation and subsequent septic peritonitis. The antrum, lesser curvature, and pylorus are the most common sites for gastric ulceration.

a. Etiology

  (1) Iatrogenic. Nonsteroidal anti-inflammatory drugs (NSAIDs) decrease local prostaglandin production and other gastric protection mechanisms, causing gastric erosions and ulcers, usually in the gastric antrum. Concurrent corticosteroid treatment can enhance the development of the erosions by decreasing cell renewal and mucus production and increasing acid secretion.

  (2) Inflammatory gastric disorders are an infrequent cause.

  (3) Metabolic diseases such as renal or hepatic failure can cause erosions or ulcers. In the case of renal failure, uremic toxins and hypergastrinemia due to decreased renal clearance are the responsible mechanisms. In the case of hepatic failure, hypergastrinemia, decreased blood flow, and decreased mucus production are responsible.

(4) Stress caused by trauma, shock, hypotension, or severe illness can result in erosions and ulceration in the stomach and duodenum via ischemia and increased endogenous steroids, catecholamines, and serotonin.

(5) Neoplasia. Mast cell tumors may release histamine, causing hypergastrinemia and hyperacidity. A gastrinoma, usually found in the pancreas, can also cause hyperacidity and ulceration, although the ulcers are more common in the duodenum. Ulceration can also occur secondary to primary gastric neoplasms (see III B 13).

(6) Foreign bodies rarely cause an ulcer, but they may exacerbate an existing lesion.

(7) Neurologic disease and the associated disruption of parasympathetic and sympathetic neural pathways can cause ischemia and hyperacidity, leading to ulceration. This effect may be accentuated by glucocorticoids used in treating the neurologic disease.

b. Diagnosis. Definitive diagnosis is based on contrast radiographs, endoscopy, or surgery.

(1) Clinical findings may include vomiting (the vomitus may contain fresh or digested blood), anorexia, pale mucous membranes (a sign of anemia), peripheral edema (a sign of hypoproteinemia), pain on abdominal palpation, and (if perforation has occurred) depression and shock. **Presumptive diagnosis** is suggested by hematemesis without coagulopathy or by vomiting in an animal with a clinical condition known to predispose to ulcer formation.

(2) Radiographic findings are frequently normal, but **contrast radiographs** sometimes show contrast entering the gastric mucosa or a persistent spot of barium after the remainder of the stomach has emptied. A **contrast gastrogram** can also help rule out the presence of a foreign body.

(3) Endoscopic findings. Endoscopy is the optimal way to diagnose gastric erosions or ulcerations as well as some underlying causes (e.g., neoplasia, inflammatory disease, foreign body ingestion).

(4) Laboratory findings

(a) A **fine-needle aspirate** and **cytology** may identify cutaneous masses as mast cell tumors.

(b) A **CBC** and **serum biochemical profile** may help identify renal, hepatic, or other metabolic disease. Serum gastrin concentrations can be evaluated to check for a gastrinoma if no other cause is found.

c. Treatment. Underlying disorders should be treated.

(1) Supportive therapy. Food should be withheld to minimize mechanical irritation to the stomach and stimulation of additional acid and pepsin secretion. **Parenteral fluids** should be administered to treat or prevent dehydration.

(2) Medical therapy is indicated if the signs are not life-threatening.

(a) H_2 **antagonists** decrease gastric acid secretion.

(b) Sucralfate adheres to the base of the ulcer.

(c) Oral antacids help neutralize gastric acidity.

(d) Misoprostol, a prostaglandin analogue, may also help resolve gastroduodenal ulceration, especially that caused by NSAIDs. Prostaglandin analogues help prevent NSAID-induced ulceration, decrease gastric acid secretion, and may speed ulcer healing.

(e) Omeprazole, a proton pump inhibitor, is the most potent inhibitor of gastric acid secretion, but it is not known if it has any clinical advantages over the H_2 antagonists. It may be useful in patients that respond poorly to other treatment.

(3) Surgical ulcer excision is indicated in the presence of severe bleeding, perforation, or failure to respond to medical treatment within several days.

d. Prognosis is good if treatment prevents gastric perforation and if the underlying cause can be resolved or controlled.

5. Chronic inflammatory gastritis
  a. Etiology. The cause of chronic inflammatory gastritis is poorly defined.
    (1) Immune mechanisms or responses to dietary antigens, parasites, other infectious agents, or chemicals may occur. The trigger may be an initial transient disorder that disrupts the mucosal barrier and exposes mucosal antigens to the immune system.
    (2) Eosinophilic gastritis in cats may be a part of the hypereosinophilic syndrome.
    (3) Infection with *Helicobacter* species may or may not play a role.
  b. Diagnosis. Concurrent disease that may cause nonspecific gastric inflammation should be ruled out.
    (1) Clinical findings may include chronic intermittent (occasionally frequent) vomiting, anorexia, weight loss, abdominal pain, and borborygmus. The affected animal is usually clinically normal between episodes.
    (2) Laboratory findings. Peripheral eosinophilia may be present with eosinophilic gastritis or the hypereosinophilic syndrome.
    (3) Endoscopy findings. Diagnosis is based on gastric biopsy because grossly, the gastric mucosa may appear normal. An eosinophilic, lymphocytic–plasmacytic, or granulomatous infiltrate may be seen.
  c. Treatment. If the underlying disorder can be identified, it should be treated.
    (1) Diet. An **elimination (hypoallergenic) diet** should be fed to all dogs and cats with **chronic idiopathic gastritis.** Ingredients in the diet should be ones that the pet has not eaten before or ones that are unlikely to cause a reaction.
      (a) For dogs, commercial diets or one part cottage cheese or boiled lamb or mutton mixed with two parts boiled rice or potatoes or pasta can be used. Venison, duck, and rabbit are other novel protein sources.
      (b) For cats, commercial diets or boiled turkey, duck, fish, lamb, or rabbit can be used.
    (2) Medical therapy
      (a) Corticosteroids can be added if diet alone is ineffective. Steroid treatment can eventually be discontinued in some patients; others require chronic low-dose therapy.
      (b) H$_2$-receptor antagonists may be helpful.
      (c) Metoclopramide or another prokinetic agent may be useful if a secondary motility disorder has developed.
      (d) Antimicrobials (e.g., amoxicillin, omeprazole, or a combination of metronidazole, tetracycline, and bismuth subsalicylate) may be used to treat *Helicobacter* infection.
  d. Prognosis
    (1) The prognosis is good for dogs and cats with lymphocytic–plasmacytic gastritis, although some patients may later develop lymphosarcoma.
    (2) Dogs with eosinophilic gastritis usually respond well to treatment, but cats with eosinophilic or granulomatous gastritis often fail to respond fully to treatment.

6. Atrophic gastritis is a rare condition that may result from immune mechanisms or from chronic inflammatory gastritis.
  a. Diagnosis is based on finding mucosal thinning and a decrease in gastric gland size on **biopsy.** Clinical findings are similar to those of chronic inflammatory gastritis [see III B 5 b (1)].
  b. Treatment with a high-carbohydrate, low-fat, low-fiber diet, corticosteroids, and metoclopramide can be used, but the response is usually poor.

7. Phycomycosis
  a. Etiology. *Pythium* species or *Zygomycetes* can infect the skin and GI tract of dogs but most commonly causes diffuse or multifocal deep granulomatous inflammation of the stomach, duodenum, and colon.
  b. Diagnosis is based on **biopsy.** Clinical findings may include vomiting, anorexia, and large or small bowel diarrhea.

    c. Treatment and **prognosis.** Treatment consists of surgical excision and the concurrent administration of ketoconazole. The prognosis for cure is guarded to poor despite treatment.

  8. Pyloric stenosis (benign muscular hypertrophy of the pylorus). Pyloric stenosis is most common in male brachycephalic or small-breed dogs and Siamese cats.

    a. Etiology. The cause is unknown, but gastrin may be involved.

    b. Diagnosis

      (1) Clinical findings. Vomiting that occurs for several hours after eating is common. No other clinical signs are seen.

      (2) Radiographic findings. Contrast radiographs reveal gastric outflow obstruction.

      (3) Endoscopic findings may include a few extra folds of normal mucosa at the pylorus. In some cases, there are no endoscopic findings.

      (4) Surgical findings include a normal mucosa with a thickened pyloric wall and narrow lumen.

    c. Treatment and **prognosis.** Treatment entails surgical correction of the stenosis, usually with a pyloroplasty. The prognosis is good following surgery.

  9. Mucosal hypertrophy

    a. Gastric antral mucosal hypertrophy is most common in male, small-breed dogs.

      (1) Etiology. The cause is unknown, but chronic irritation, inflammation, drugs, stress, or increased gastrin concentrations may be involved.

      (2) Diagnosis

        (a) Clinical findings. Vomiting that occurs for several hours after eating is common. Other signs are uncommon.

        (b) Radiographic findings. Contrast radiographs reveal gastric outflow obstruction.

        (c) Endoscopic findings include increased folds of mucosa in the pyloric antrum.

        (d) Surgical findings include increased mucosal folds without thickening of the underlying tissue.

      (3) Treatment and **prognosis.** Treatment consists of surgical resection of the redundant mucosa, often with concurrent pyloroplasty. The prognosis is good following surgery.

    b. Other forms of mucosal hypertrophy (e.g., hypertrophic glandular gastritis, focal cystic hypertrophic gastropathy, hypertrophic gastritis of Basenjis) are less common.

 10. Partial gastric volvulus is similar to classic GDV but is less severe. **Clinical findings** may include chronic, intermittent, nonproductive retching (as opposed to acute, progressive, nonproductive retching) and cranial abdominal distention.

    a. Diagnosis is the same as for GDV (see III B 3 b) but can be complicated by the intermittent nature of the problem. Repeated radiographic studies may be necessary.

    b. Treatment and **prognosis.** Treatment consists of surgical repositioning of the stomach and a gastropexy. The prognosis is good for treatment.

 11. Idiopathic gastric hypomotility. No anatomic, histologic, or metabolic abnormalities are found, despite the fact that various infiltrative and metabolic diseases can cause hypomotility.

    a. Diagnosis is based on finding decreased gastric motility in the absence of any histologic or metabolic abnormalities.

      (1) Clinical findings are primarily the occurrence of vomiting several hours after eating.

      (2) Differential diagnoses. Hypokalemia, acidosis, uremia, hepatic disease, pain, inflammation, hypoadrenocorticism, and hypothyroidism should be ruled out.

    b. Treatment. A **moist, low-fat diet** can be helpful. **Metoclopramide** is often also used to increase gastric tone and contractions and promote gastric emptying. **Ci-**

sapride increases gastric activity by increasing acetylcholine release. It can be used for those pets that do not respond to metoclopramide.

    c. Prognosis for control of the disorder is good if the animal responds to the diet and metoclopramide, but guarded if cisapride therapy is needed.

12. **Enterogastric reflux** is thought to be the cause of the **"bilious vomiting syndrome"** seen in young, small-breed dogs. Probably caused by abnormal motility, the reflux causes gastric mucosal irritation and nausea, especially when the stomach is empty. Affected dogs typically vomit bile-stained fluid in the early mornings but are otherwise clinically normal. **Treatment** includes feeding **multiple small meals** (with one at bedtime), **metoclopramide,** and possibly **H$_2$-receptor antagonists** and **sucralfate.**

13. **Gastric neoplasia.** The cause of gastric neoplasia is unknown. **Adenocarcinoma** is most common in dogs. **Lymphosarcoma** is more common in cats. Other gastric neoplasms are uncommon.

    a. Diagnosis

        (1) Clinical findings can be acute or insidious and may include vomiting, weight loss, anorexia, and, occasionally, hematemesis (if tumors ulcerate).

        (2) Imaging studies

            (a) Radiographic findings. Contrast radiographs may show mucosal irregularity, abnormal gastric motility, a thickened gastric wall, a mass lesion, delayed gastric emptying, or any combination thereof.

            (b) Ultrasonographic findings may include a mass lesion or diffuse wall thickening.

            (c) Endoscopic findings may show ulceration, a firm nondistensible area of the stomach, or a mass lesion.

        (3) Biopsy is necessary for **definitive diagnosis.** Endoscopic biopsies may yield a diagnosis, but with submucosal neoplasia, a surgical biopsy is needed.

    b. Treatment

        (1) Lymphosarcoma is most responsive to chemotherapy. Treatment options are discussed in Chapter 48 IV A 6 e, 7 d.

        (2) Other types of gastric neoplasms have limited treatment options. They are poorly responsive to chemotherapy, and surgical excision is often not possible because of metastasis or the extent of the local lesions.

    c. Prognosis

        (1) Lymphosarcoma. The prognosis for short-term remission is fair, but the prognosis for cure is poor.

        (2) Other gastric neoplasms generally have a poor prognosis.

IV. INTESTINAL DISORDERS

A. Clinical evaluation

1. **Predisposition**

    a. Species and breed. All breeds of dogs and cats can develop intestinal disorders, but certain breeds are at increased risk for some disorders. For example, German shepherds are more prone to exocrine pancreatic insufficiency (EPI), bacterial overgrowth, and inflammatory bowel disease.

    b. Age

        (1) Young animals. Viral disease, parasitic diseases, and foreign bodies are more common causes of enteritis in young animals.

        (2) Older animals. Neoplasia is more common in older animals.

    c. The animal's **environment** and **vaccination status** should also be considered.

2. **History.** Acute signs are more likely in the presence of viral, bacterial, or rickettsial disease; dietary indiscretion; toxin or foreign body ingestion; intussusception; HGE; and some systemic disorders. Acute signs may also be seen during the early phase of a more chronic disorder.

3. **Clinical signs**
   a. **Small intestinal disease**
      (1) **Diarrhea** is one of the most common signs of both small and large bowel disease (see Table 4-5). The diarrhea can be secretory, osmotic, or exudative. Abnormal motility may also play a role.
      (2) **Vomiting** can occur with small bowel disease as a result of stimulation of the vomiting center by neural input from the intestines. Vomiting in association with small bowel disease is most common when the duodenum is involved.
      (3) **Weight loss** can be the primary clinical sign in some animals.
      (4) **Anorexia** can occur due to abdominal pain or nausea.
      (5) **Polyphagia** is most common with EPI (see Chapter 42 II B 4) in dogs and hyperthyroidism (see Chapter 44 III B) and early lymphosarcoma in cats.
      (6) **Abdominal pain** may be manifested as restlessness, shivering, or anorexia.
      (7) **Melena** can occur if upper GI hemorrhage is present.
      (8) **Borborygmus** (i.e., increased GI sounds) can be normal or can occur with numerous small intestinal disorders.
      (9) **Flatulence** can result from aerophagia or various small intestinal disorders as a result of bacterial fermentation of malassimilated food products.
      (10) **Associated clinical syndromes** include **malassimilation (maldigestion, malabsorption)** and **protein-losing enteropathy (PLE)** and are discussed in Chapter 4 II.
   b. **Large intestinal disease**
      (1) **Diarrhea** is one of the most common signs of colonic disease.
      (2) **Tenesmus** is common with large intestinal disease. Irritation of the colon may cause the animal to attempt to defecate despite the absence of feces in the colon. Tenesmus can also occur with colonic obstruction and constipation.
      (3) **Dyschezia** (i.e., difficult or painful defecation) can occur with colonic disease, anal disease, or perianal disease.
      (4) **Increased fecal mucus** can be seen with any irritation of the colon.
      (5) **Frank fecal blood** can result from colonic erosions, ulcerations, or mucosal friability.
      (6) **Constipation** and **obstipation** may occur with retention of feces in the colon.
      (7) **Vomiting** occurs in approximately 30% of dogs and cats with large bowel diarrhea or constipation and results from stimulation of the vomiting center by neural input from the colon.
      (8) **Weight loss** is rare with large bowel disorders and only occurs with severe diseases such as neoplasia and fungal disease.

4. **Physical examination**
   a. **General appearance.** The animal may be thin or cachexic. The haircoat may be dull. Peripheral or ventral edema (as a result of severe hypoproteinemia) may be noted.
   b. **Oral cavity.** Mucous membranes may be slightly pale (a sign of anemia), tacky (a sign of dehydration), or they may have a slow capillary refill time (a sign of shock). String foreign bodies may be seen.
   c. **Abdomen**
      (1) **Mild discomfort** may be evident on palpation and may occur with inflammatory or infectious bowel disease.
      (2) **Moderate** to **severe abdominal pain** may be found with intestinal perforation and peritonitis.
      (3) The intestines may be **fluid-filled, gas-filled,** or have **thickened walls** (suggestive of inflammatory or neoplastic disease).
      (4) **Bunched intestines** (as a result of a linear foreign body), **intestinal masses** or **foreign bodies,** or a **firm, tubular intestinal structure** (a sign of intussusception) may be palpated.

(5) Ascites may be detected in animals with hypoproteinemia, lymphangiectasia, or neoplasia.

(6) A **large, dilated colon** filled **with firm feces** is diagnostic for constipation.

  d. Rectum. A distal colonic mass, foreign body, or stricture may be palpable. The perineal region should be checked for anal gland abnormalities, fistulae, or herniation.

5. Diagnostic tests

  a. Laboratory studies

    (1) CBC

      (a) An increased hematocrit and serum total solids may occur with dehydration. An increased hematocrit with normal serum total solids will occur with HGE.

      (b) Lymphopenia may occur with stress or lymphangiectasia.

      (c) Leukopenia may be seen with parvoviral infection or sepsis.

      (d) Leukocytosis may be seen with severe intestinal inflammation or perforation.

      (e) Nonregenerative anemia can be seen with peracute or chronic hemorrhage, chronic disease, or malnutrition.

      (f) Regenerative anemia may be seen with subacute intestinal hemorrhage caused by ulceration, inflammation, or neoplasia.

      (g) Eosinophila can be seen with some parasitic and fungal infections and eosinophilic enteritis or colitis.

    (2) Serum biochemical profile

      (a) Electrolyte abnormalities, especially hypokalemia, may be detected.

      (b) Panhypoproteinemia is typically seen in patients with PLE, although globulin concentrations may be normal or increased if concurrent inflammation is present.

      (c) Lymphosarcoma is the most common cause of hypercalcemia.

      (d) Hypoglycemia may occur with sepsis or as a result of inadequate food intake or malassimilation in young animals.

      (e) A serum biochemical profile also helps rule out extraintestinal causes of diarrhea.

      (f) In most cases of colonic disease, a biochemical profile is unremarkable.

    (3) Urinalysis is needed to rule out proteinuria as a cause of hypoproteinemia or hypoalbuminemia.

    (4) Fecal examinations

      (a) Flotation tests may aid in the identification of parasites. Multiple samples may be required because some parasites may produce ova or cysts only episodically, and some parasites (e.g., *Giardia*) can be difficult to detect with conventional tests.

      (b) Fecal cytology

        (i) Small bowel disease. Fecal cytology is of limited value in small bowel disease. The presence of leukocytes indicates deep inflammation of the intestinal wall but is not specific for one disease. If spore-forming bacteria are also seen, clostridial infection should be suspected. The presence of W-shaped bacteria suggests campylobacteriosis.

        (ii) Large bowel disease. With colonic disease, leukocytes, fungal organisms, *Clostridium* species or *Campylobacter* species may be visible.

      (c) Enzyme-linked immunosorbent assay (ELISA) is available for parvoviral antigen and *Giardia*.

      (d) Electron microscopy can be used to detect viral infections caused by agents for which no ELISA is available. Electron microscopy is most useful in the early stages of the infection when higher numbers of virus are being shed.

      (e) Fecal cultures are not often needed in dogs and cats with diarrhea but can be useful if bacterial enteritis is suspected or other test results are negative. Because most fecal pathogens require specialized culture techniques, the laboratory should be told which pathogens are of concern. *Salmonella* species, *Campylobacter jejuni, Clostridium perfringens*, and *Yersinia enterocolitica* are the most common enteric pathogens in dogs and cats.

(f) **Fecal occult blood tests.** Meat and meat products in many commercial foods, medications, and some vegetables can cause false–positive test results and should therefore be withheld 3–4 days before testing.

(5) **Tests for malassimilation** are useful in dogs with suspected maldigestion due to EPI (see Chapter 42 II), in dogs and cats with chronic diarrhea, and in dogs and cats with weight loss of unknown cause.

(a) **Fecal microscopy.** Examining feces for undigested starch (using an iodine stain), fat (using a Sudan stain), or protein is a crude test of digestion and absorption. Both false–positive and false–negative results are common, so these tests are now rarely used.

(b) **Fat absorption test.** This test is an indirect indicator of the presence of pancreatic lipase and the ability of the small intestine to absorb fats. If lipemia occurs following oil ingestion, EPI or severe malabsorption is unlikely. Absence of lipemia after oil ingestion but lipemia following ingestion of oil plus pancreatic enzymes suggests fat maldigestion and EPI. Absence of lipemia after ingestion of both oil and oil plus enzymes suggests malabsorption.

(c) **Serum trypsin-like immunoreactivity (STLI) test.** STLI is currently the optimal test for maldigestion due to EPI. Decreased STLI is seen with EPI. A normal value does not rule out maldigestion due to obstruction of the pancreatic duct, a defect in enterokinase, or a deficiency of an enzyme other than trypsin. Increased STLI can be seen with pancreatitis, renal failure, or severe malnutrition.

(d) **BT-PABA (n-benzoyl-1-tyrosyl-*p*-aminobenzoic acid/ bentiromide) digestion test.** This test is an older test of digestion that uses plasma or urine concentrations of PABA as an indicator of the presence of pancreatic chymotrypsin.

　(i) A marked decrease in peak plasma or urine PABA is seen with EPI, pancreatic duct obstruction, or lack of activation of chymotrypsin. A mild decrease in peak plasma or urine PABA can be seen with decreased chymotrypsin or malabsorption. A delay in peak plasma PABA can be seen with delayed gastric emptying or malabsorption.

　(ii) The BT-PABA digestion test is more expensive and cumbersome than STLI and is of questionable use in cats.

(e) **Serum cobalamin (vitamin B$_{12}$)** and **folate concentrations** are indicators of small intestinal absorption capability in dogs and cats. Cobalamin is primarily absorbed in the ileum; folate is absorbed in the proximal small intestine. Bacteria can also bind cobalamin, thus preventing its absorption, and can synthesize folate.

　(i) Decreased serum cobalamin and folate suggests malabsorption due to generalized small intestinal disease. Decreased serum cobalamin and increased folate suggests bacterial overgrowth (often seen with EPI).

　(ii) Normal results do not rule out small intestinal disease.

(f) **D-Xylose absorption test.** This test is an older test for malabsorption in dogs and is of little use in cats. D-xylose does not require digestion prior to absorption. A marked decrease in xylose absorption suggests delayed gastric emptying, bacterial overgrowth, or primary malabsorption; however, ascites, renal failure, and delayed gastric emptying can falsely alter the results. If a repeat test is normal after a 72-hour treatment with antibiotics, bacterial overgrowth is suggested.

(g) **Fecal trypsin measurement, 24-hour fecal fat excretion, intestinal permeability studies,** and **breath hydrogen excretion tests** are not widely available.

b. Radiography

(1) Survey radiographs

(a) A **mass** or a radiodense **foreign body** may be seen.

(b) **Distention** of the small intestine with gas, fluid, or food can occur. Distention is indicated by an intestinal diameter greater than the height of the lumbar vertebral bodies.

(i) **Mechanical** or **anatomic ileus** (i.e., obstruction) produces marked, irregular distention with sharp bends or stacking of the distended intestines.

(ii) **Physiologic ileus** (as a result of inflammation or metabolic abnormalities) produces less distention.

(iii) **Mesenteric torsion** causes distention in all the intestines.

(iv) **Strangulated intestinal obstruction** causes marked distention of only a small segment of intestine.

(c) **Linear foreign bodies** produce bunched or plicated intestines containing only small bubbles of gas.

(d) **Abdominal masses** may displace the intestines.

(e) **Organomegaly** may be apparent with extra-gastrointestinal disease.

(f) **Free abdominal gas, generalized ileus,** and **loss of abdominal detail** may be apparent with intestinal perforation and peritonitis.

(g) **Colonic distention** with feces is suggestive of constipation. With megacolon, the colon may remain somewhat distended following removal of the fecal material.

(2) Contrast radiographs

(a) If both vomiting and diarrhea are present, contrast studies may reveal an obstruction due to a radiolucent or linear foreign body or a mass. Barium will not pass beyond a complete intestinal obstruction. A partial obstruction will appear as a narrowed lumen or a delay of passage of contrast beyond a certain point. Bunching or plication of the intestine will be seen with a linear foreign body. Contrast extending beyond the lumen is suggestive of an ulcer.

(b) With diarrhea only, contrast radiographs of the small bowel are often normal, but they may show a partial obstruction, scalloping of the intestinal margins (suggestive of infection, inflammation, or neoplasia), or a focal dilatation (suggestive of neoplasia).

(c) Barium enemas are not often done because colonoscopy is usually more diagnostic. A contrast enema can reveal irregular mucosa (inflammation or neoplasia), a mass lesion, a radiolucent foreign body, or an ileocecocolic intussusception.

c. Ultrasonography

(1) **Intestinal wall thickening, irregular mucosa,** or a **mass** may be apparent with inflammatory disease or neoplasia.

(2) A **double concentric ring** with a **hyperechoic center** is seen with intussusception.

(3) A **foreign body** may be visible.

(4) **Free abdominal fluid** or **gas** may accompany perforation.

d. Endoscopy

(1) **Intraluminal masses** may be seen with neoplasia or granuloma.

(2) **Erosions** or **ulcers, hyperemia,** or **irregular mucosa** may be seen with inflammation or neoplasia. The mucosa can also be grossly normal with some inflammatory conditions and with submucosal diseases. In this case, multiple biopsies should be taken.

(3) **Foreign bodies, parasites, strictures,** or **polyps** may be seen endoscopically.

e. Exploratory laparotomy permits full-thickness biopsies to be obtained. Surgery may also be therapeutic in the case of obstructive disease (e.g., foreign body, granuloma, torsion) and localized nonlymphoma neoplasia.

B. **Disorders of the small intestine**

1. **Acute simple enteritis** is most commonly caused by a change in diet, dietary indiscretion, drugs or toxins, parasitic infection (see IV B 2), or other infections.
   a. **Diagnosis.** Acute simple enteritis from diet change or dietary indiscretion is usually diagnosed by exclusion and the history and physical examination.
      (1) **Clinical findings** may include diarrhea (most common), vomiting, anorexia, dehydration, and depression.
      (2) **Laboratory findings.** A fecal flotation test and direct fecal examination can help identify parasitism.
      (3) **Radiographic findings.** Radiographs may be needed if a foreign body, mass, or peritonitis is suspected.
      (4) **Additional tests** may be needed if the animal has hemorrhagic diarrhea, is systemically ill, or fails to respond to symptomatic therapy.
   b. **Treatment** of acute diarrhea is given in Chapter 4 VI A.
   c. **Prognosis** varies with the patient's age, body condition, and the underlying disorder.

2. **Parasitic enteritis**
   a. **Roundworm infection (ascariasis)**
      (1) **Etiology**
         (a) *Toxocara canis* causes ascariasis in dogs. Transmission is by ingestion of parasitic ova or transplacental.
         (b) *Toxocara cati* is a common cause of ascariasis in cats. Transmission is by ingestion of parasitic ova or transmammary.
         (c) *Toxocara leonina* causes ascariasis in dogs and cats. Transmission is by ingestion of parasitic ova.
      (2) **Pathogenesis.** Migrating larva of *T. canis* or *T. cati* may cause pulmonary or hepatic lesions. The adult parasites live in the small intestine and may cause intestinal distention or even obstruction.
      (3) **Diagnosis**
         (a) **Clinical findings.** Diarrhea, poor growth, a dull hair coat, and a potbelly are common in young animals with ascarids. With severe infestations, vomiting and intestinal obstruction may also occur.
         (b) **Laboratory findings.** Diagnosis is based on **fecal flotation** results; however, ova may not be found in neonates that have acquired the infection via the transplacental route.
      (4) **Treatment**
         (a) **Pyrantel pamoate** is the most common treatment. Treatment should be repeated in 2 weeks because pyrantel will not kill migrating larva.
         (b) **Fenbendazole** administered for 2 weeks or more to pregnant bitches decreases the risk of transplacental infection.
      (5) **Prognosis** is good, although stunted growth may be permanent with severe infection.
      (6) **Zoonotic potential.** *T. canis* and *T. cati* can cause visceral and ocular larval migrans in humans.
   b. **Hookworm infection**
      (1) **Etiology.** Infection with *Ancylostoma* species and *Uncinaria* species is common in dogs but uncommon in cats. Animals can be infected prenatally, transcolostrally, by ingestion of parasitic ova, or by percutaneous larval infection.
      (2) **Pathogenesis.** The adults live in the small intestine attached to the mucosa and will occasionally infect the colon.
      (3) **Diagnosis**
         (a) **Clinical findings.** Hookworms alone rarely cause a clinical problem in adult animals. In young animals, poor growth, diarrhea, anemia, melena or frank fecal blood, and vomiting are not uncommon.
         (b) **Laboratory findings.** Diagnosis is based on fecal flotation results. In ne-

onates with transcolostral infection, ova may not be found because the worms have not yet reached maturity.

  (4) Treatment

    (a) Pyrantel pamoate is administered as described in IV B 2 a (4) (a).

    (b) Fenbendazole administered for 2 weeks or more to pregnant bitches decreases the risk of transcolostral infection.

    (c) Blood transfusions may be needed with severe infection.

  (5) Prognosis is good in adults and nonanemic young animals but guarded in severely anemic puppies and kittens. Stunted growth may occur with severe infection.

  (6) Zoonotic potential. Hookworms can cause cutaneous larval migrans in humans.

c. Giardiasis. Infection with *Giardia intestinalis* is more common in dogs than it is in cats.

  (1) Pathogenesis. Animals are infected by ingesting parasitic cysts in food or water. The trophozoites attach to the brush border of the intestinal villi and can cause malassimilation.

  (2) Diagnosis

    (a) Clinical findings include mild to severe, intermittent to persistent diarrhea with steatorrhea, weight loss (chronic infection), and, occasionally, large bowel diarrhea.

    (b) Laboratory findings. Diagnosis is based on **fecal examination** results. Because *Giardia* organisms can be difficult to find and may be shed episodically, multiple samples should be examined for cysts or parasites and it may be useful to empirically treat for giardiasis prior to pursuing further diagnostic tests.

      (i) The zinc sulfate fecal flotation test may reveal cysts.

      (ii) Direct fecal examination or examination of duodenal washes and aspirates may reveal parasites.

      (iii) ELISA to detect *Giardia* is also available.

  (3) Treatment. Metronidazole, quinacrine, furazolidone, or **fenbendazole** may be effective. The kennel and other contaminated areas should be cleaned with steam or a quaternary ammonia compound.

  (4) Prognosis is good, although some infections can be difficult to clear.

  (5) Zoonotic potential. It is unknown if humans can be infected with *Giardia* from dogs.

d. Coccidiosis

  (1) Etiology

    (a) *Cytoisospora* species. Infection mainly occurs in puppies and kittens.

    (b) *Cryptosporidia* species. Neonates and immunosuppressed animals are most commonly affected.

  (2) Pathogenesis. After an animal ingests infective (sporulated) oocysts, the coccidia invade the epithelium of the small intestinal villi.

  (3) Diagnosis

    (a) Clinical findings. The animal may be asymptomatic. Bloody diarrhea may be seen.

    (b) Laboratory findings

      (i) *Cytoisospora* infection is diagnosed by finding oocysts on a **fecal flotation.** Because the oocysts may be shed periodically, multiple fecal samples should be examined.

      (ii) *Cryptosporidia* infection is more commonly diagnosed on **intestinal biopsies.**

  (4) Treatment

    (a) *Cytoisospora* infection. There is no treatment to eliminate the coccidia, but **sulfadimethoxine** or **trimethoprim/sulfonamide** will inhibit the organisms so that the animal's own defenses can clear the infection.

    (b) *Cryptosporidia* infection. There is no proven treatment, but **clindamycin** or **tylosin** can be tried.

(5) **Prognosis** is good with *Cytoisospora* infection but guarded with *Cryptosporidia* infection.

(6) **Zoonotic potential.** Cryptosporidiosis is a risk for immunosuppressed humans.

e. *Strongyloides* infection (strongyloidiasis). Puppies can be infected with *Strongyloides stercoralis* via larval migration through the skin or oral mucous membranes.

(1) **Diagnosis**

(a) **Clinical findings** include diarrhea (most common), lethargy, inappetence, and possibly respiratory signs (if larval migration through the lungs has occurred).

(b) **Laboratory findings.** Diagnosis is made by finding larvae on direct fecal examination or on a Baermann test.

(2) **Treatment. Fenbendazole** is the most common treatment.

(3) **Prognosis** is guarded if the animal is very young or if pneumonia is present.

(4) **Zoonotic potential.** Humans, especially those that are immunocompromised, can be infected.

f. **Tapeworm infection.** *Dipylidium caninum* infection is most common in dogs and is transmitted by fleas and lice. Infection by *Taenia* species is common in dogs and cats; transmission is by the ingestion of infected tissues of rodents, rabbits, and other intermediate hosts. Clinical signs are uncommon. **Treatment** most commonly includes **praziquantel** and flea control (for *Dipylidium*).

g. **Other parasitic infections** (e.g., trichinosis, schistosomiasis, macracanthorhynchiasis) are rare.

3. **Viral enteritis**

a. **Canine parvoviral enteritis**

(1) **Pathogenesis**

(a) Transmission is via the fecal-oral route. The disease is highly contagious, especially among young, unvaccinated dogs.

(b) In the host, the virus has a predilection for rapidly dividing cells (e.g., intestinal crypt cells, lymph cells, bone marrow cells). The myocardium can also be affected in puppies 2–4 weeks of age.

(c) Secondary sepsis can occur because of absorption of bacterial toxins and translocation of bacteria across the damaged mucosa.

(2) **Diagnosis.** A presumptive diagnosis can often be based on the history and clinical signs, especially if laboratory findings are supportive.

(a) **Clinical findings.** The severity of the clinical signs will vary with the animal's age, the maternal antibody titer, the immune response, and the viral strain and dose. Rottweilers and Doberman pinschers are often more severely affected.

(i) **After 6 weeks of age,** anorexia, vomiting, diarrhea (often hemorrhagic), and lethargy are common. Dehydration, fever, and pale mucous membranes may also be seen.

(ii) **Before 4–6 weeks of age,** dyspnea or sudden death due to myocarditis is more common than enteritis.

(b) **Laboratory findings** may include leukopenia, anemia, panhypoproteinemia, and hypoglycemia. A positive ELISA test for parvovirus will confirm the diagnosis, although the virus may not be shed later in the course of the disease.

(3) **Treatment.** Isolation from other dogs for 2–3 weeks is recommended, and the animal's environment should be disinfected with a dilute bleach solution.

(a) **Treatment** for **vomiting and diarrhea** is discussed in Chapter 3 V B and Chapter 4 VI B, respectively. The animal can be permitted to take food and water orally when there has been no vomiting for 24 hours and the frequency of diarrhea is decreasing.

(b) **Correction of electrolyte disturbances** may be necessary.

(c) **Plasma transfusions** may be needed if severe hypoproteinemia occurs.

(d) **Antibiotic therapy** is indicated if the patient is febrile, neutropenic, or septic. Ampicillin, amoxicillin, or cefazolin is a common choice with mild to moderate disease; more broad-spectrum antibiotic therapy (e.g., ampicillin or cefazolin plus an aminoglycoside or cefoxitin alone) may be needed with severe disease or sepsis.

(e) **Flunixin meglumine** in a single injection or a **glucocorticoid** may be helpful in the treatment of secondary septic shock, but repeated doses or use of both medications can produce gastric ulceration.

(f) **Metoclopramide** or other anti-emetic therapy may be needed if vomiting persists despite resolution of the other clinical signs. **Ondansetron,** a serotonin-3 receptor antagonist, may be useful in patients that fail to respond to metoclopramide.

(4) **Complications.** Intussusception is a potential complication of parvoviral and other types of enteritis.

(5) **Prognosis** is usually good with sufficient supportive care; however, young puppies, dogs that have developed sepsis, and certain breeds (i.e., Doberman pinschers, Rottweilers) have a more guarded prognosis.

(6) **Prevention.** Puppies should be vaccinated approximately once every 4 weeks from 6–8 weeks of age up to 18–20 weeks of age and then annually thereafter. Until vaccination is complete, exposure to other dogs and public areas potentially contaminated with parvovirus should be avoided. Although helpful in preventing infection, the vaccine does not confer full immunity in all dogs.

b. **Canine coronaviral enteritis.** The coronavirus affects the mature epithelial cells of the intestinal villi rather than the crypts; therefore, coronavirus enteritis is less severe than parvovirus enteritis. Diagnosis can be confirmed by electron microscopy, but most dogs respond to symptomatic treatment. Treatment is the same as that for parvoviral enteritis [see IV B 3 a (3)], and the prognosis is usually good. A vaccine is available for high-risk dogs.

c. **Canine rotaviral enteritis.** This rotavirus affects only cells on the tips of the intestinal villi. Clinical findings are often absent, although mild transient diarrhea can be seen. Definitive diagnosis is rarely made because of the mild, transient nature of the clinical signs. Treatment is symptomatic at most.

d. **CDV infection** can cause enteritis in dogs, but respiratory or neurologic signs are often also present (see Chapter 49 V B).

e. **Feline parvoviral enteritis (feline panleukopenia).** The pathogenesis, clinical features, diagnosis, and prognosis are similar to those discussed for canine parvoviral enteritis (see IV B 3 a). Some canine parvovirus ELISA tests will detect feline parvovirus. A highly effective vaccine is available; cats should be vaccinated at 8 and 12 weeks of age and yearly thereafter. The virus is very stable in the environment, so contaminated areas should be thoroughly disinfected.

f. **Feline coronaviral enteritis** is similar to canine coronaviral enteritis with regard to the pathogenesis, clinical features, diagnosis, and prognosis (see IV B 3 b). Antibodies formed in response to this infection may later cross-react and produce positive results on some serologic tests, particularly for feline infectious peritonitis (FIP) virus. Feline coronavirus may also cause chronic diarrhea in cats infected with FIV. No vaccine is available.

g. **FeLV infection** (see also Chapter 49 V D). Clinical findings resemble those of feline panleukopenia (see IV B 3 e), but the disease is more chronic with weight loss, chronic diarrhea, and vomiting. Diagnosis is presumptive based on the clinical signs and a positive FeLV test and definitive based on the elimination of other disorders. Treatment is symptomatic. The prognosis is poor because of the development of other FeLV-associated disorders.

4. **Bacterial enteritis** is uncommon in dogs and cats. It should be considered in cases of diarrhea because of the zoonotic potential of many of the pathogens.

a. **Salmonellosis.** *Salmonella* species, Gram-negative bacilli, can be isolated from the feces of normal dogs and cats, but they can also cause clinical disease, especially in young or debilitated animals.

    (1) Pathogenesis. The bacteria are transmitted by the fecal-oral route or through ingestion of contaminated foods. The bacteria then invade the mucosa of the distal small bowel, colon, or both.

    (2) Diagnosis is based on fecal culture and clinical findings. *Salmonella* infection is often asymptomatic but can cause acute or chronic diarrhea, fever, vomiting, depression, inappetence, and possibly septicemia and shock. If the large bowel is involved, mucus and frank blood may be present in the diarrhea and tenesmus may be seen. In cats, fever and anorexia are the most common signs.

    (3) Treatment

        (a) Antibacterial treatment. Asymptomatic patients or those with mild diarrhea should not be treated because treatment may promote a carrier state. Antibiotic treatment for patients with moderate to severe clinical signs should be based on results of culture and sensitivity tests. **Ampicillin, enrofloxacin, trimethoprim/sulfonamide,** or **cephalothin** can be used while awaiting culture results.

        (b) Supportive care similar to that for simple enteritis (see Chapter 4 VI A) may also be needed.

    (4) Prognosis is guarded if septicemia occurs but is good for those animals with primarily GI involvement.

    (5) Zoonotic potential. Salmonellosis is a zoonotic disease.

  b. Campylobacteriosis is caused by ***Campylobacter jejuni,*** a Gram-negative curved bacillus. *Campylobacter* species can be isolated from the feces of normal dogs and cats but may also cause clinical disease or exacerbate a preexisting disorder. Campylobacteriosis is most common in young, debilitated, or ill animals.

    (1) Diagnosis

        (a) Clinical findings are often absent, but acute diarrhea (possibly with tenesmus, mucus, or blood) and vomiting can be seen. Chronic or intermittent diarrhea is less common.

        (b) Laboratory findings. Gram-negative, slender, W-shaped rods may be seen on a stained fecal smear, but fecal culture is needed to confirm the diagnosis.

    (2) Treatment. The antibiotic of choice is **erythromycin.** Enrofloxacin, doxycycline, clindamycin, and chloramphenicol are usually also effective.

    (3) Prognosis is excellent unless septicemia has developed; however, the development of septicemia is rare.

    (4) Zoonotic potential. Campylobacteriosis can be transmitted to humans and other animals.

  c. Clostridial disease. *Clostridium* species— Gram-positive, spore-forming bacilli— are normally present in dogs and cats, but toxigenic strains of ***Clostridium perfringens*** and ***Clostridium difficile*** may cause clinical disease in some individuals. Antibiotic treatment may be a predisposing factor in *C. difficile* infection. *C. perfringens* has been reported as a nosocomial infection.

    (1) Diagnosis

        (a) Clinical findings commonly include acute to peracute, hemorrhagic diarrhea or (less often) chronic or intermittent, mucoid diarrhea.

        (b) Laboratory findings

            (i) *C. perfringens* infection is diagnosed presumptively based on the presence of large numbers of leukocytes and spore-forming bacteria on a fecal smear. Subsequent culture of large numbers of organisms can support the diagnosis. Definitive diagnosis requires detection of enterotoxin in the feces.

            (ii) *C. difficile* is diagnosed based on assay of cytotoxin in the feces.

    (2) Treatment

        (a) *C. perfringens* infection can be treated with **ampicillin, amoxicillin, metronidazole, tylosin,** or **another antibiotic effective against anaerobes.** A high-fiber diet may also be useful, especially in chronic cases.

(b) *C. difficile* infection can be treated with **supportive care** and **metronidazole.** Vancomycin is commonly used to treat humans with this disease.

(3) **Prognosis** is generally good for mild cases but is guarded for those animals with severe clinical signs.

d. **Yersiniosis**

(1) **Etiology** and **pathogenesis**

(a) *Yersinia pseudotuberculosis* can infect cats that eat contaminated rodents or birds. Disseminated pyogranulomatous lesions develop. GI and hepatic involvement is most common.

(b) *Yersinia enterocolitica.* Infection with *Y. enterocolitica* is uncommon in dogs and cats. This human pathogen has mainly been isolated from normal dogs and cats.

(2) **Diagnosis**

(a) *Y. pseudotuberculosis* can produce diarrhea, weight loss, vomiting, lethargy, fever, and icterus. Diagnosis is based on biopsy or culture of affected tissues.

(b) *Y. enterocolitica* can produce a bloody mucoid diarrhea and tenesmus in young dogs. Systemic signs of illness are uncommon. The organism has not been associated with clinical disease in cats. Diagnosis is based on fecal culture results.

(3) **Treatment**

(a) *Y. pseudotuberculosis* **infection** requires long-term treatment with **trimethoprim/sulfonamide, tetracycline,** or **chloramphenicol.**

(b) *Y. enterocolitica* **infection** should be treated according to bacterial sensitivity results, but trimethoprim/sulfonamide, tetracycline, or chloramphenicol is usually effective.

(4) **Prognosis** for animals with *Y. enterocolitica* infection is usually good; however, the prognosis for cats with *Y. pseudotuberculosis* infection is guarded because the disease is usually progressive.

e. *Bacillus piliformis infection* is a rare cause of hemorrhagic enterocolitis in dogs and cats. Puppies and kittens are most commonly affected, and concurrent disease (e.g., parasitic or viral infection) is usually present. Acute anorexia, diarrhea, and lethargy are usually seen. The disease is difficult to diagnose antemortem, and there is no treatment. Most affected animals die within 48 hours.

5. **Rickettsial enteritis (salmon poisoning)** is caused by *Neorickettsia helmintheca* or *Neorickettsia elokominica.* Cats are not affected.

a. **Pathogenesis.** Dogs are infected by eating fish carrying an infected fluke (*Nanophyetus salmincola*). The rickettsial organisms become widespread in infected dogs and cause severe clinical disease. The disease is usually seen in the Pacific Northwest of the United States because the intermediate hosts for the flukes (snails) are found in that region.

b. **Diagnosis.** The diagnosis is suggested by the history and clinical signs.

(1) **Clinical findings** resemble those of parvoviral enteritis [see IV B 3 a (2)] and may include high fever, anorexia, hemorrhagic small bowel diarrhea, vomiting, and lymphadenopathy.

(2) **Laboratory findings.** The diagnosis is confirmed by finding operculated fluke ova in the feces or rickettsia in lymph node aspirates.

c. **Treatment**

(1) **Antimicrobial therapy**

(a) **Tetracycline, doxycycline, trimethoprim/sulfonamide,** or **chloramphenicol** can be used to eliminate the rickettsia.

(b) **Fenbendazole** or **praziquantel** should be used to eliminate the fluke.

(2) **Supportive care** as for simple enteritis (see Chapter 4 VI B) may also be needed.

d. **Prognosis** is good if the disease is treated promptly, and poor if the animal is not treated.

6. **Fungal enteritis**

    a. Histoplasmosis is discussed in Chapter 49 II F.

    b. Phycomycosis is discussed in III B 7.

7. **HGE** is most common in young to middle-aged small-breed dogs and has not been reported in cats. Acute hematemesis and hematochezia are the most common clinical signs. The disease can progress very rapidly to a life-threatening illness and shock.

    a. Etiology. The etiology is unknown, although immune-mediated mechanisms and clostridial or other bacterial enterotoxins have been proposed.

    b. Diagnosis is presumptive based on the history, clinical signs, and an increased hematocrit (e.g., 55%–60%) with relatively normal serum protein concentrations. If no improvement has occurred after 24 hours of treatment, then another disorder should be considered.

    c. Treatment

        (1) Intravenous fluid therapy is needed immediately, especially if shock or severe hemoconcentration is present.

        (2) Diet. Food and water should be withheld until there has been no vomiting for 24 hours.

        (3) Antibiotics (e.g., ampicillin, amoxicillin, metronidazole, cephalexin) are often administered, although their value is unknown.

        (4) Transfusions (whole blood or **plasma)** may be needed in very severe cases.

    d. Prognosis. Terminal shock and DIC can occur if treatment is not prompt and aggressive, but the prognosis is good with appropriate therapy.

8. **Small intestinal obstruction**

    a. Simple obstruction

        (1) Etiology. Foreign body ingestion is the most common cause of anatomic or mechanical intestinal obstructions. Other causes include **intussusception, granuloma,** or **neoplasia.** Intussusception (telescoping of one segment of intestine into the adjacent segment of intestine) usually occurs secondary to another disease that has altered intestinal motility and, in dogs, usually involves the ileocolic junction.

        (2) Pathogenesis. Obstruction causes proximal intestinal distention and malabsorption, eventually leading to hypersecretion and bacterial overgrowth. Intestinal perforation and subsequent septic peritonitis can occur.

        (3) Diagnosis of intestinal obstruction is based on the history, physical findings, and radiographs.

            (a) Clinical findings

                (i) With a severe or complete intestinal obstruction, vomiting is the most common sign; diarrhea, anorexia, abdominal discomfort, depression, and shock may also be seen.

                (ii) With a chronic or relapsing intussusception, chronic diarrhea, weight loss, and intermittent vomiting are common. Chronic signs can also be seen with a partial intestinal obstruction.

                (iii) Abdominal distention and severe abdominal pain are uncommon unless devitalization, perforation, and peritonitis have occurred.

                (iv) A mass, foreign object, intussusception, or dilated bowel loops may be palpable.

            (b) Radiographic findings

                (i) Survey films may reveal a radiodense foreign object, an obvious obstructive pattern (see IV A 5 b), or free peritoneal fluid or air (if perforation has occurred).

                (ii) Contrast films will show any obstruction.

            (c) Ultrasonographic findings may include a mass, focal bowel wall thickening, a radiolucent foreign body, a "double-walled" segment of bowel (i.e., intussusception), or free peritoneal fluid or air.

            (d) Laboratory findings

                (i) Serum sodium, potassium, and chloride may be decreased due to the vomiting or diarrhea.

       (ii) Alkalosis (high duodenal obstruction) or acidosis (lower intestinal obstruction) may result from vomiting.

       (iii) Leukocytosis may result from inflammation; a degenerative left shift may occur with perforation and peritonitis.

       (iv) Panhypoproteinemia may also be seen with a chronic partial obstruction.

    (e) **Abdominocentesis** or **abdominal lavage** can be used to diagnose perforation and peritonitis if the clinical findings and other test results are suggestive.

  (4) **Treatment**

    (a) **Surgery** is needed to relieve the obstruction. With septic peritonitis, immediate surgery is needed to remove the obstruction, close or resect the perforated area, and lavage the abdomen. If an intussusception is reduced rather than resected in an acute case, plicating the intestines may help prevent recurrence. The intestine should also be biopsied to identify any underlying disease, which should then be treated.

    (b) **Supportive treatment** entails the administration of **parenteral fluids** (pre-, intra-, and postoperatively), and possibly **antibiotic therapy.**

  (5) **Prognosis** is usually good unless extensive resection is needed or perforation and peritonitis have occurred.

b. **Linear foreign body obstruction.** Cats are more likely than dogs to ingest linear foreign bodies (e.g., string, thread, cloth).

  (1) **Pathogenesis.** The linear foreign body aligns itself in the GI tract. If the object is caught at some point in the tract (usually the base of the tongue or the pylorus), the intestine will bunch up as it tries to pass the portion of the foreign body that extends into the intestines. If untreated, peristalsis can cause the linear object to perforate the intestinal wall, causing peritonitis.

  (2) **Diagnosis**

    (a) **Clinical findings.** Vomiting, anorexia, and depression are most commonly seen. The end of the object may be visible under the tongue or in the oral cavity. Bunched intestines may be palpable.

    (b) **Radiographic findings**

       (i) **Survey films** may show bunching of intestines containing small gas bubbles.

       (ii) **Contrast radiographs** will show bunched or pleated intestines.

    (c) **Laboratory findings.** Alkalosis (high duodenal obstruction) or acidosis (lower intestinal obstruction) may result from vomiting. A CBC may show a leukocytosis or may be normal.

  (3) **Treatment** and **prognosis.** The treatment is the same as that for a simple intestinal obstruction [see IV B 8 a (4)]. The prognosis is generally good unless intestinal perforation and peritonitis has occurred.

c. **Strangulated intestinal obstruction** can occur with intussusception, an incarcerated hernia, or intestinal or mesenteric volvulus. In addition to occlusion of the bowel lumen, the vascular supply to the involved bowel is compromised. The clinical findings, diagnosis, and treatment are similar to those of a simple obstruction with perforation (see IV B 8 a). The prognosis is guarded to poor with a volvulus or incarcerated hernia, even with aggressive treatment.

d. **Physiologic obstruction** can result from segmental devitalization or ileus caused by peritonitis, surgery, metabolic disorders, or neurologic disease. Diagnosis is based on finding distended bowel loops on survey radiographs but no obstruction on contrast radiographs. Cats are more likely to ingest linear foreign bodies than are dogs. Treatment requires identification and treatment of the underlying disease; the prognosis varies with the cause of the ileus.

9. Inflammatory small bowel disease

  a. **Lymphocytic–plasmacytic enteritis** is the most common type of inflammatory bowel disease in dogs and the most common cause of chronic vomiting and diarrhea in dogs and cats. German shepherds may be at increased risk.

(1) **Etiology.** The cause of lymphocytic–plasmacytic enteritis is unknown. Immune mechanisms and a response to dietary, parasitic, or intestinal cell wall antigens have been proposed. In rare cases, lymphocytic–plasmacytic enteritis has been thought, but not proven, to be a premalignant condition.

(2) **Diagnosis**

   (a) **Clinical findings.** Thickened bowel loops may be palpable. No clinical signs are present between episodes, but the episodes progressively become more severe and more frequent. Response to symptomatic treatment is temporary.

      (i) In dogs, chronic intermittent diarrhea is the most common clinical sign. Vomiting, anorexia, weight loss, and lethargy may also be seen.

      (ii) In cats, chronic intermittent vomiting is the most common clinical sign. Diarrhea is also frequently seen, and the appetite may be decreased or increased.

   (b) **Laboratory findings** may include panhypoproteinemia or hypoalbuminemia and hyperglobulinemia (in cats) in the presence of severe disease.

   (c) **Biopsy findings.** Diagnosis is based on intestinal biopsy and ruling out other diseases that could cause a secondary inflammatory infiltrate. Biopsies are necessary because grossly, the intestinal mucosa may be hyperemic, roughened, and eroded, or it may appear normal. In some patients, endoscopic biopsies may be consistent with lymphocytic--plasmacytic enteritis yet lymphosarcoma is actually present deeper in the intestinal wall.

(3) **Treatment.** If the patient fails to respond to therapy, the diagnosis should be reevaluated.

   (a) **Elimination diets,** as described in III B 5 c (1), should be instituted.

   (b) **Immunosuppressive agents.** If diet alone does not control the clinical signs, or the clinical signs or histologic lesions are severe, then **corticosteroid therapy** (e.g., **prednisone**) should be added to the treatment regimen. High-dose therapy should be used initially, and then the dosage should be slowly decreased while monitoring the clinical signs. Steroid treatment can eventually be discontinued in some patients while others will require chronic low-dose therapy to control the signs. **Other immunosuppressive drugs** (e.g., azathioprine) may also be needed if the disease is severe, unresponsive to prednisone and dietary therapy, or the prednisone therapy is poorly tolerated by the patient.

   (c) **Metronidazole** at low doses may be used in conjunction with other treatments for its proposed inhibitory effects on cell-mediated immune responses in addition to its antibacterial and antiprotozoal activity.

   (d) **Antibiotics** (e.g., ampicillin, metronidazole, tylosin) should be considered if concurrent bacterial overgrowth is present.

(4) **Prognosis** varies with the disease severity and the animal's condition at the time of diagnosis. Most animals require lifelong dietary treatment; some also require life-long medication.

b. **Eosinophilic enteritis**

(1) **Etiology.** Eosinophilic enteritis is thought to be a type I hypersensitivity reaction to dietary or parasitic antigens in dogs and some cats. In other cats, eosinophilic enteritis is part of feline hypereosinophilic syndrome, which is thought to be neoplastic or immune-mediated in origin.

(2) **Diagnosis** is based on intestinal mucosal biopsies.

   (a) **Clinical findings.** Chronic small bowel diarrhea, vomiting, and weight loss are the most common signs. Coughing or tachypnea may be seen in dogs if concurrent eosinophilic respiratory disease is present. If feline hypereosinophilic syndrome is present, eosinophilic infiltration of extra-GI tissues can cause a variety of signs.

   (b) **Laboratory findings.** A peripheral eosinophilia is often seen.

(3) **Treatment**

(a) In dogs, the treatment for eosinophilic enteritis is similar to that for lymphocytic–plasmacytic enteritis [see IV B 9 a (3)]. Fenbendazole should also be administered to eliminate any underlying occult parasitism.

(b) In cats with concurrent feline hypereosinophilic syndrome, prednisone therapy alone is not usually effective, but improvement has been reported with concurrent prednisone, azathioprine, and metronidazole therapy. Cats without hypereosinophilic syndrome will usually respond well to diet and glucocorticoid treatment [see IV B 9 a (3)].

(4) Prognosis is generally good for animals with eosinophilic enteritis but more guarded for cats with feline hypereosinophilic syndrome.

c. **Granulomatous enteritis** is rare. The causes and clinical findings are similar to those of lymphocytic–plasmacytic enteritis (see IV B 9 a). Diagnosis is based on intestinal biopsies. In dogs, the optimal treatment is unknown. In cats, high doses of glucocorticoids provide control, but the disease may not remain controlled when the dosage is decreased. The prognosis is poor for dogs and guarded for cats.

d. **Chronic enteropathy in Shar peis** is a severe form of inflammatory bowel disease and bacterial overgrowth.

(1) Diagnosis is based on intestinal biopsies.

(a) Clinical findings include small bowel diarrhea, weight loss, and possibly polyphagia and large bowel diarrhea. Concurrent esophagitis, gastric hypomotility, and colitis may be seen.

(b) Laboratory findings may include panhypoproteinemia, decreased serum cobalamin, and normal or increased serum folate.

(2) Treatment includes prednisone, metronidazole, and amoxicillin.

e. **Lymphocytic–plasmacytic enteritis of Basenjis** is a severe form of inflammatory bowel disease that is thought to occur as a result of a genetic defect in immune regulation.

(1) Diagnosis is by biopsy.

(a) Clinical findings of diarrhea, vomiting, or inappetence are usually first seen by 3–4 years of age and become progressively worse.

(b) Laboratory findings commonly include hypoalbuminemia and hyperglobulinemia.

(2) Treatment and **prognosis.** The treatment is the same as that for lymphocytic–plasmacytic enteritis [IV B 9 a (3)], but despite treatment, most affected dogs die within 2–3 years of diagnosis.

10. Duodenal ulcers are uncommon but can occur with mast cell tumors, NSAID administration, and neoplasia (see III B 4).

11. Bacterial overgrowth is the excessive growth (i.e., $> 10^5$/ml) of bacteria in the small intestine. Bacterial overgrowth is seen mainly in the dog, although cats can also be affected. German shepherds and Shar peis may be at increased risk.

a. **Etiology.** Bacterial overgrowth can result from segmental intestinal stasis, other intestinal disease (e.g., lymphocytic–plasmacytic enteritis), immunodeficiency, or EPI. Less commonly, it can occur as a primary disease.

b. **Diagnosis**

(1) Clinical findings result from the intestinal damage wrought by bacteria and their metabolic products. Chronic intermittent small bowel diarrhea and weight loss may be present along with signs of another intestinal disorder.

(2) Laboratory findings

(a) Quantitative culture of duodenal fluid is the optimal method for diagnosing bacterial overgrowth.

(b) Screening tests include the evaluation of serum cobalamin levels (which would be decreased) and serum folate levels (which would be increased), or duodenal mucosal biopsies. The sensitivity of the serum tests is low.

(3) Treatment. A therapeutic trial may sometimes be diagnostic. Usually mixed bacteria are present, so a broad-spectrum antibiotic also effective against anaerobes (e.g., amoxicillin, metronidazole, oxytetracycline, tylosin) should be used. Any underlying disease should also be identified and treated.

   (a) If predominately one organism is identified, the antibiotic can be selected according to sensitivity.

   (b) Depending on the severity and chronicity of the case, treatment for a few weeks to a few months may be needed.

   (4) Prognosis is good for treatment of the bacterial overgrowth, but the underlying disease may alter the overall prognosis.

12. **Lymphangiectasia** results from lymphatic obstruction. Yorkshire terriers, soft-coated Wheaten terriers, and rottweilers may be at increased risk. The disorder has not been seen in cats.

   a. Etiology. In many cases, lymphangiectasia is idiopathic in origin, but it can also occur as a congenital malformation or secondary to pericardial disease, intestinal mucosal disease, or infiltrative lymphatic or lymph node disease.

   b. Pathogenesis. The obstruction causes the intestinal lacteals to rupture and leak lymph into the lamina propria, where it causes inflammation and granulomas. This in turn causes further lymphatic obstruction. Protein, lymphocytes, and chylomicrons are lost with the fluid, and malabsorption and PLE result.

   c. Diagnosis

   (1) Clinical findings. Small bowel diarrhea and weight loss are common; vomiting is not. Diarrhea may not occur until late in the course of the disease, and the animal may instead exhibit ascites, hydrothorax, or pitting edema as a result of the hypoproteinemia.

   (2) Laboratory findings typically include hypoalbuminemia, hypocalcemia, hypocholesterolemia, lymphopenia, and possibly hypoglobulinemia.

   (3) Endoscopic findings may include multifocal, pale lesions. Diagnosis is based on intestinal biopsies. Because the lesions may be deeper or may be localized to only the jejunum, endoscopic biopsies are occasionally not diagnostic.

   (4) Surgery often reveals dilated intestinal lymphatics and multifocal lipogranulomas.

   d. Treatment. Unless an underlying cause can be identified, treatment is only symptomatic.

   (1) Diet. A very low-fat diet (e.g., low-fat cottage cheese or yogurt mixed with rice or potatoes or pasta plus fat-soluble vitamins; a commercial low-fat diet) should be fed to minimize intestinal lymph formation and subsequent loss. Medium-chain triglycerides, which do not require lymphatics for absorption, can be added if more calories are needed.

   (2) Glucocorticoids may also be helpful in decreasing inflammation and granuloma formation.

   e. Prognosis is variable.

13. **Short bowel syndrome**

   a. Etiology. Short bowel syndrome is usually the result of surgical resection of 75%–90% of the small intestine. Congenital short bowel syndrome is rare.

   b. Pathogenesis. The remaining intestine is insufficient to digest and absorb adequate nutrients, and malnutrition can result. Concurrent bacterial overgrowth may also be present, especially if the ileocolic junction was resected. Clinical findings are commonly diarrhea and weight loss.

   c. Diagnosis is usually based on the patient history, but contrast radiographs can be used to obtain an objective measure of the remaining intestine.

   d. Treatment

   (1) Fluid and **electrolytes.** It is important to maintain fluid and electrolyte balance following surgery.

   (2) Diet. A low-fat, highly digestible diet should be fed. Oral feeding should be initiated and maintained even if diarrhea occurs, because nutrients must be present in the small intestine to aid adaptation. Concurrent total parenteral nutrition may be needed initially if the animal cannot maintain its weight.

    (3) Pharmacologic therapy

        (a) Antibiotics may be helpful against secondary bacterial overgrowth.

        (b) H$_2$ antagonists can decrease the secretion of gastric acid, which may irritate the duodenal mucosa.

        (c) Opiate antidiarrheals may also be used.

  e. Prognosis. In many patients, the remaining intestine adapts with time and treatment and the clinical signs lessen or resolve. Some animals may eventually be able to return to a normal diet once the intestines adapt; others may require a special diet indefinitely. Some animals die despite therapy. Animals that are debilitated at the time of the surgery have a poorer prognosis.

14. Intestinal neoplasia

  a. Lymphosarcoma (see also Chapter 48 IV A 6, 7)

    (1) Clinical findings. Thickened bowel loops, an intestinal mass, or intra-abdominal lymphadenopathy may be palpable. Signs may also be specific to the site of the neoplasm:

        (a) Small intestine. With small intestinal disease, small bowel diarrhea, weight loss, vomiting, and lethargy are most common. Melena, hematemesis, abdominal effusion, or transient polyphagia (in cats) may also be seen.

        (b) Large intestine. Bloody mucoid diarrhea may be seen with colonic disease.

        (c) Extraintestinal sites. The most common signs of extraintestinal involvement are peripheral lymphadenopathy, hepatomegaly, and, possibly, icterus.

    (2) Diagnosis is based on intestinal biopsy or cytology or lymph node aspirates if lymphadenopathy is also present. Radiographs and ultrasound may show the lesion, but the image changes are not pathognomonic.

    (3) Treatment and **prognosis** are discussed in Chapter 48 IV A 6 e–f and 7 d.

  b. Adenocarcinoma. Intestinal adenocarcinomas are more common in dogs than in cats. In dogs, the duodenum and colon are the most common sites; in cats, a jejunal or ileal mass is more common.

    (1) Clinical findings are usually those of small bowel obstruction (see IV B 8) or are nonspecific (e.g., inappetence, weight loss).

    (2) Diagnosis is based on a surgical biopsy or a fine-needle aspirate if the mass is palpable.

    (3) Treatment and **prognosis.** Treatment requires surgery, although many animals have metastasis at the time of surgery. The prognosis is good if the mass can be completely excised but poor if metastasis has occurred.

C. | **Disorders of the large intestine characterized by diarrhea**

  1. Acute colitis

    a. Etiology. Diet change, dietary indiscretion, or parasitic infection account for at least 50% of the cases of acute colitis, and it is more common in dogs. The exact cause is often not determined because the problem usually resolves with symptomatic therapy.

    b. Clinical findings include bloody mucoid diarrhea and tenesmus. Less frequently, vomiting, lethargy, and dyschezia are seen.

    c. Diagnosis. A presumptive diagnosis is usually based on response to symptomatic therapy. Common causes should be ruled out based on fecal examinations and history. Proctoscopy or colonoscopy and biopsy can confirm the diagnosis but are rarely performed. If the signs fail to resolve with simple therapy, then alternative diagnoses should be considered and further tests pursued.

    d. Treatment. Dietary recommendations are given in Chapter 4 VI A 1. A diet with increased fiber is also helpful in some patients. Fenbendazole treatment should be considered to definitively rule out underlying whipworms or other helminths.

    e. Prognosis is good if no other underlying disease is present.

2. Parasitic colitis

a. Whipworm infection (trichuriasis). Infection with **Trichuris vulpis** is a common cause of colitis in dogs, but whipworm infection (with *Trichuris vulpis* or *Trichuris serrata*) is rare in cats.

    (1) Pathogenesis. The ova are ingested and the adults attach to the colon and cecum, leading to inflammation and bleeding.

    (2) Diagnosis

        (a) Clinical findings. Large bowel diarrhea and hematochezia are most common, although more severe disease can also cause hypoproteinemia and pseudohypoadrenocorticism (i.e., hyponatremia and hyperkalemia).

        (b) Laboratory findings. Diagnosis is based on finding ova on a fecal flotation test (multiple tests may be necessary) or seeing adult worms on colonoscopy. Because the ova are only shed intermittently, multiple fecal samples should be evaluated or the animal should be treated prior to eliminating trichuriasis as a cause of large bowel diarrhea.

    (3) Treatment. Fenbendazole is the most commonly used drug to treat trichuriasis. Administration should be repeated in 3 weeks and in 3 months in order to kill parasites that were not in the intestines at the time of the initial treatment.

    (4) Prognosis is very good, but reinfection from contaminated soil is common.

b. Hookworm infection (with *Ancylostoma* species; see IV B 2 b) can cause colonic disease in addition to small bowel disease if the infestation is heavy.

c. *Strongyloides* infection (strongyloidiasis). *Strongyloides tumefaciens* infection is seen in cats in warm humid regions. The parasites burrow into the colonic mucosa and form small nodules. Diarrhea may be the only clinical sign; some animals are asymptomatic. Diagnosis is based on fecal flotation or Baermann test results or biopsy of the colonic nodules. Treatment is with fenbendazole.

d. Trichomoniasis. *Pentatrichomonas hominis* infection can be seen in young puppies and kittens housed in close conditions. Concurrent infection with another intestinal pathogen is common. Large bowel diarrhea may be the only clinical sign; some animals are asymptomatic. Diagnosis is made by direct examination of a fecal smear, and treatment is with metronidazole.

e. Amebic colitis, which results from **Entamoeba histolytica** infection, is rare in dogs and cats. Pets may ingest trophozoites or cysts in contaminated water. Clinical findings include bloody, mucoid diarrhea. Diagnosis is made by examination of a fecal smear, zinc sulfate flotation, or by biopsy. Treatment is with metronidazole or furazolidone. *Ertamoeba* is a human pathogen.

f. Balantidiasis is caused by **Balantidium coli,** an uncommon cause of colitis in dogs. The organisms are ingested in water contaminated by swine feces. Diagnosis is by direct examination, zinc sulfate flotation, or fecal sedimentation. Treatment is with metronidazole or oxytetracycline. *B. coli* is a human pathogen.

3. Viral colitis is uncommon. Canine and feline parvovirus and CDV can cause signs of colitis, but signs of small bowel disease are much more common and typically more severe. FeLV, FIV, and FIP virus can also cause enterocolitis, but signs of small bowel disease or extraintestinal signs are more common.

4. Bacterial colitis is uncommon in dogs and cats but can occur. It should be considered in cases of diarrhea because of the zoonotic potential of many of the pathogens. Causes are the same as those described in IV B 4 a–e.

5. Fungal and **algal colitis**

a. Histoplasmosis is discussed in Chapter 49 II F. When there is large bowel involvement, sulfasalazine may be used early in the course of treatment for symptomatic relief of diarrhea and tenesmus.

b. Phycomycosis is discussed in III B 7.

c. Protothecosis is caused by **Prototheca zopfii** and **Prototheca wickerhamii.** These organisms are found in the environment, but clinical disease in dogs and cats is rare. Immune dysfunction may be needed before clinical disease can result.

(1) Diagnosis
  (a) Clinical findings. Large bowel diarrhea is the most common sign in affected dogs; GI involvement is less common in cats. Weight loss or other organ system involvement (e.g., skin, eyes) can occur in either species.
  (b) Laboratory findings. Diagnosis is based on finding the organisms in a colonic scraping or biopsy.
(2) Treatment and **prognosis.** The response to treatment with amphotericin B is variable. The prognosis is guarded, even with treatment.
d. Other mycotic infections (e.g., candidiasis, aspergillosis) are rare as a cause of colonic disease.

6. Inflammatory large bowel disease
  a. Lymphocytic–plasmacytic colitis is one of the most common causes of chronic large bowel diarrhea in dogs and cats.
    (1) Etiology. The cause of lymphocytic–plasmacytic colitis is unknown. Immune mechanisms and a response to dietary, parasitic, bacterial, or intestinal cell wall antigens have been proposed.
    (2) Pathogenesis. The inflammation alters colonic permeability and motility, resulting in diarrhea.
    (3) Diagnosis
      (a) Clinical findings include chronic intermittent diarrhea (most common), vomiting, anorexia, and lethargy. Affected animals are usually clinically normal between episodes, but the episodes progressively become more severe and more frequent. The dog or cat will often seem to respond to symptomatic treatment but then the signs recur.
      (b) Laboratory findings. Panhypoproteinemia is occasionally seen if the disease is severe. Diagnosis is based on colonic biopsy. Biopsies are always needed because grossly, the intestinal mucosa may be hyperemic, roughened, or eroded, or it may appear normal.
    (4) Treatment
      (a) Diet. The animal should be placed on an **elimination diet** [see III B 5 c (1)]. **High-fiber** or **low-residue diets** may work better for some patients.
      (b) Pharmacologic therapy
        (i) A **5-aminosalicylate drug** (e.g., sulfasalazine, olsalazine, mesalamine) should be added to the treatment regimen in dogs not responsive to diet alone. These drugs inhibit local leukotrienes and other cell-mediated inflammatory effects. They are available in oral preparations, in which the active compound, mesalamine, is bound to another compound so that the drug is only released in the colon. Retention enema preparations are also available.
        (ii) Immunosuppressive agents. Corticosteroids may be added to the regimen for cats with severe or diet-unresponsive disease or in dogs that fail to respond to diet and 5-aminosalicylates. Steroid treatment can eventually be discontinued in some patients; others require chronic low-dose therapy to control the clinical signs. **Other immunosuppressive drugs** (e.g., azathioprine) may also be needed if the disease is unresponsive to other treatment or if the prednisone therapy is poorly tolerated.
        (iii) Metronidazole may be used in low doses in conjunction with other treatments for its proposed inhibitory effects on cell-mediated immune responses in addition to its antibacterial and antiprotozoal activity.
        (iv) Tylosin is also helpful in some cases when the disease is poorly controlled by diet alone. The observed improvement may result from its antibacterial activity or an as-yet undetermined mechanism.

    (5) Prognosis for control is good. Many animals will require life-long dietary treatment; some also require life-long medication.

  b. Eosinophilic colitis is thought to be an allergic response to parasitic or dietary antigens in dogs and some cats. In other cats, eosinophilic enteritis is part of the feline hypereosinophilic syndrome.

    (1) Diagnosis

      (a) Clinical findings. Bloody mucoid diarrhea is the most common clinical sign. If feline hypereosinophilic syndrome is present, eosinophilic infiltration of various tissues may be seen.

      (b) Laboratory findings. A peripheral eosinophilia is often seen. Diagnosis is based on colonic mucosal biopsies. The possibility of underlying parasitism should be thoroughly investigated.

    (2) Treatment

      (a) Dietary recommendations are the same as those for lymphocytic–plasmacytic colitis [see III B 5 c (1); IV C 6 a (4)].

      (b) Immunosuppressive agents. Concurrent prednisone therapy is usually required. If feline hypereosinophilic syndrome is present, better response has been reported with concurrent prednisone, azathioprine, and metronidazole therapy.

      (c) Antiparasitic agents. Fenbendazole treatment helps rule out underlying parasitism.

    (3) Prognosis is generally good for animals with eosinophilic colitis but more guarded for cats with feline hypereosinophilic syndrome.

  c. Neutrophilic colitis is uncommon in dogs and cats. An infectious agent is suspected, but no pathogens have been identified. Diagnosis is based on biopsy. Infectious agents, especially bacterial pathogens, should be ruled out. Treatment is with antibiotics and a regimen similar to that for lymphocytic–plasmacytic colitis [see IV C 6 a (4)].

  d. Regional granulomatous colitis is a rare cause of colitis in dogs and cats. Mass-like thickening of the ileus and colon develops and can cause obstruction. Clinical findings include large bowel diarrhea, possibly with pain and tenesmus. A mass or thickened intestine may be palpable. Diagnosis is by biopsy. Treatment is similar to that for lymphocytic–plasmacytic colitis [see IV C 6 a (4)]. Surgical resection may be required if obstruction has occurred.

  e. Histiocytic ulcerative colitis is primarily seen in young boxers. Severe, bloody diarrhea is the primary clinical sign. Diagnosis is based on biopsy. Treatment is similar to that for lymphocytic–plasmacytic colitis [see IV C 6 a (4)], except high-fiber diets should be avoided. The prognosis for good control of the disease is poor.

7. Colonic obstruction

  a. Cecocolic intussusception/cecal inversion is an uncommon cause of large bowel disease.

    (1) Etiology. The cause of cecal invagination into the colon is unknown in most cases, but trichuriasis or another primary colonic disease may contribute.

    (2) Clinical findings. If a partial obstruction occurs, mucoid diarrhea and tenesmus may be the primary signs. If a complete obstruction occurs, anorexia, vomiting, and lethargy may be seen.

    (3) Diagnosis is based on endoscopy or a barium enema.

    (4) Treatment and **prognosis.** The obstruction is treated surgically; the prognosis is generally good with treatment.

  b. Colonic foreign body. Most ingested foreign bodies either pass without irritation or become lodged higher in the GI tract. Occasionally, however, a foreign body will pass to the colon before causing problems. Foreign objects can also be placed in the colon per rectum by malicious individuals.

    (1) Clinical findings depend on the foreign object and may include large bowel diarrhea, normal feces streaked with fresh blood, or constipation.

(2) Diagnosis is based on the history, abdominal palpation and rectal examination, and abdominal radiographs.

(3) Treatment depends on the foreign body and the degree of obstruction. Methods of removal include enemas, endoscopy, or surgery. Concurrent antibiotic therapy should be considered if there is significant mucosal damage.

(4) Prognosis is good if colonic perforation or prolonged severe colonic distention have not occurred.

c. **Colonic strictures** usually occur secondary to colonic trauma (e.g., foreign body, surgery) but can also be congenital.

(1) Clinical findings. Constipation is the most common clinical sign, although large bowel diarrhea and tenesmus can occur.

(2) Diagnosis is based on the history and colonoscopy or a barium enema.

(3) Treatment

(a) Surgical excision of the stricture is often required, but recurrence at the surgical site is possible. **Balloon catheter dilation** may be helpful with more caudal strictures.

(b) Symptomatic treatment [i.e., with diet modification, stool softeners, and laxatives, as described in Chapter 7 V] may be helpful if the stricture is not severe.

8. **Colonic perforation** can occur as a result of trauma, surgery or biopsy, foreign body, corticosteroid treatment of spinal cord disease, or neoplasia. The clinical signs, diagnosis, and treatment are similar to those of perforation caused by small intestinal obstruction [see IV B 8 a (4)]. The prognosis is grave.

9. **Colonic neoplasia**
   a. **Benign colonic neoplasms** include colonic or rectal polyps, adenomas, and leiomyomas. Diarrhea is uncommon, but streaks of fresh blood may be seen on formed stools as a result of fecal material abrading the surface of the masses. Tenesmus or constipation may also be seen. Diagnosis is based on biopsy. Treatment is by surgical excision of the masses; the prognosis is good.
   b. **Malignant neoplasms** include adenocarcinoma and lymphosarcoma (the two most common), leiomyosarcoma, carcinoid, fibrosarcoma, anaplastic sarcoma, and hemangiosarcoma.
      (1) Adenocarcinomas are most common in older animals. Clinical findings may include blood on the feces, diarrhea, tenesmus, or constipation. Endoscopy may reveal a tumor that is ulcerated, infiltrative, or proliferative.
         (a) Diagnosis is by biopsy.
         (b) Treatment and **prognosis.** Surgery is the treatment of choice if no metastasis is present. The prognosis is guarded unless surgery allows complete excision of the neoplasm.
      (2) Lymphosarcoma of the colon most commonly is seen as a diffuse infiltration of the colonic wall. Clinical findings include mucoid or bloody mucoid diarrhea. Diagnosis, treatment, and prognosis are discussed in Chapter 48 IV A 6, 7.

10. **Short colon** is a rare developmental defect characterized by absence of the ascending and transverse colon. The animal is usually asymptomatic; diagnosis is often made radiographically as an incidental finding during evaluation for colitis or another clinical problem. Treatment, if needed, is with a low-residue diet.

11. **Stress colitis (irritable colon).** The exact cause is unknown, but the clinical signs result from abnormal colonic motility. Stress, either physical or psychological, seems to play a significant role in many cases.
    a. **Diagnosis** is based on clinical signs (i.e., episodic mucoid or bloody diarrhea) and the exclusion of all other causes of colonic inflammation or irritation.
    b. **Treatment** entails avoidance of stress-producing situations and a high-fiber diet. Antidiarrheal medications such as opioids (e.g., diphenoxylate, loperamide) or anticholinergics (e.g., propantheline, clidinium, dicyclomine) may be used.

Mood-altering drugs (e.g., acepromazine, chlorpromazine, phenobarbital) are helpful if the clinical signs commonly accompany stressful situations.

c. **Prognosis.** The response to treatment is variable.

D. Disorders of the large intestine associated with constipation

1. **Colonic obstruction**
   a. **Etiology**
      (1) **Intraluminal** or **intramural obstruction** can occur with a rectal foreign body, neoplasia, granuloma, stricture, or perineal hernia.
      (2) **Extraluminal obstruction** can occur as a result of prostatic disease, neoplasia, granuloma, pelvic fractures, sublumbar lymphadenopathy, or pseudo-coprostasis (i.e., matted hair covering the anus).
   b. **Diagnosis** of colonic obstruction is based on the history and the presence of a distended feces-filled colon on physical examination. Radiographs and ultrasound can identify extraluminal causes of obstruction and radiodense foreign bodies. Colonoscopy and possibly biopsy can identify other intraluminal or intramural causes of obstruction.
   c. **Treatment.** Initial treatment is symptomatic (see Chapter 7 V). The underlying problem should then be corrected if possible.
   d. **Prognosis** varies with the underlying problem and the degree and duration of colonic distention. Bacteremia and septicemia can result from severe obstipation. Prolonged severe distention of the colon can cause irreversible dysfunction of the colonic wall (see IV D 2).

2. **Colonic weakness**
   a. **Etiology**
      (1) **Neuromuscular disease** (e.g., lumbosacral spinal cord disease, dysautonomia, bilateral pelvic nerve damage) can disrupt normal colonic contraction.
      (2) **Systemic diseases** (e.g., hypokalemia, hypercalcemia, hypothyroidism) can disrupt colonic neuromuscular function.
      (3) **Prolonged severe colonic distention** can cause colonic weakness.
   b. **Clinical findings.** Constipation or obstipation is the most consistent sign. Anorexia, lethargy, dehydration, and possible concurrent diarrhea may also be seen. Other clinical signs will vary with the underlying problem.
   c. **Diagnosis** of colonic weakness is based on the history and the presence of a distended feces-filled colon. Results of a neurologic examination can help localize a neurologic problem, and a serum biochemical profile will identify electrolyte disturbances. Thyroid testing should be done if other signs of hypothyroidism are present.
   d. **Treatment.** Initial treatment is symptomatic (see Chapter 7 V). The underlying problem should then be corrected if possible.
   e. **Prognosis** varies with the underlying problem. Bacteremia and septicemia can result from severe obstipation, and prolonged severe distention of the colon can cause irreversible dysfunction of the colonic wall.

3. **Idiopathic megacolon**
   a. **Etiology.** The cause of idiopathic megacolon is not well understood, but colonic neuromuscular dysfunction is involved.
   b. **Clinical findings.** The primary clinical sign is constipation or obstipation. If the constipation is severe or prolonged, anorexia, lethargy, dehydration, and vomiting may also be seen. On physical examination, a firm, distended colon is palpable.
   c. **Diagnosis.** Idiopathic megacolon is diagnosed if the colon is very distended and no other cause for the constipation can be identified.
   d. **Treatment.** Most therapy for megacolon is symptomatic or aimed at preventing recurrent constipation.
      (1) **Symptomatic treatment** is described in Chapter 7 V.
      (2) **Prevention**
         (a) **Diet.** A moist, high-fiber diet should be fed. Commercial diets contain-

ing increased fiber are available; alternatively, bran, canned pumpkin, or psyllium can be added to the normal diet.

(b) Oral laxatives can be added if dietary changes alone are unsuccessful.

    (i) Emollient laxatives (e.g., dioctyl sodium sulfosuccinate, dioctyl calcium sulfosuccinate) work by increasing water penetration of feces. They should not be used in dehydrated animals.

    (ii) Osmotic laxatives (e.g., milk, lactulose, magnesium hydroxide) work by retaining water in the bowel lumen. Magnesium hydroxide should not be used in animals with renal failure, and care should be taken to avoid overdosage with lactulose because hypernatremic dehydration can result.

    (iii) Stimulant or **irritative laxatives** (e.g., bisacodyl) stimulate defecation but do not change the consistency of the feces. They should not be used on a long-term basis or if an obstruction is present.

    (iv) Lubricant laxatives (e.g., mineral oil, white petrolatum) lubricate feces but do not change fecal consistency. These can alter absorption of fat-soluble vitamins and aspiration pneumonia is a risk with use of unflavored mineral oil.

(c) Cisapride, a prokinetic drug, can increase colonic motility in many dogs and cats with idiopathic megacolon. It should be used in conjunction with dietary therapy and a stool softener (e.g., an osmotic laxative).

(d) Colectomy (subtotal or total) can prevent recurrence of constipation and obstipation if medical management is unsuccessful.

    (i) In cats, postoperative diarrhea is common but usually lessens after several weeks.

    (ii) In dogs, persistent diarrhea and tenesmus more commonly follow colectomy.

E. **Disorders of the anus and perineum**

1. Rectal prolapse is more common in young animals and in Manx cats.

    a. Etiology. Rectal prolapse usually occurs secondary to colitis and repeated straining. The exposed mucosa becomes more irritated and more straining occurs. Straining associated with stranguria and dystocias can also initiate the prolapse.

    b. Clinical findings. Tenesmus is common, and the prolapsed mucosa is seen protruding from the anus. The tissue may be dry and black if it is necrotic.

    c. Diagnosis is based on physical examination. A careful rectal examination should be done to rule out ileal or colonic intussusception. With rectal prolapse, a fornix is present between the prolapsed mucosa and the anus.

    d. Treatment

        (1) Prolapse reduction may be **digital** (if the tissue is not necrotic), by placing a **purse-string suture** in the anus for 24–72 hours (if the prolapse recurs), or by **colopexy** (if the prolapse repeatedly recurs despite other therapy).

        (2) Surgical resection may be needed if the tissue is necrotic or the prolapse is very large.

        (3) Prevention of additional straining entails treatment of the underlying problem. An epidural anesthetic, anti-inflammatory enemas, anticholinergic drugs, antispasmodic drugs, or sedation may also help.

    e. Prognosis is usually good, although the problem may recur.

2. Atresia ani is the congenital absence of an anal opening. Clinical findings include tenesmus, abdominal distention, and abdominal discomfort. Diagnosis is based on physical examination and radiographs. The defect is corrected surgically; the prognosis is good if no concurrent congenital malformations are present.

3. Perineal hernias result from weakening of the muscles of the pelvic diaphragm and are most common in older male dogs.

    a. Pathogenesis. Rectal sacculation or distention occurs along with possible lateral deviation of the rectum, formation of a rectal diverticulum, or prolapse of fat,

the prostate, or bladder into the hernia. The cause of the initial muscle weakening is unknown.
   b. **Clinical findings** are most commonly constipation or obstipation, tenesmus, and dyschezia. Other signs may be seen if a portion of the urogenital tract is trapped in the herniation. On physical examination, a reducible swelling is seen ventrolateral to the anus. The weakened pelvic muscles and abnormal rectal shape can be palpated rectally.
   c. **Diagnosis** is based on physical findings.
   d. **Treatment**
      (1) If the bladder is trapped in the defect, the urine should be removed and the bladder returned to its normal position. Parenteral fluid therapy and other therapy for postrenal uremia should be instituted.
      (2) If the urinary tract is not involved, retained feces should be evacuated [see Chapter 7 V A]. In some dogs, diet and laxative treatment will prevent recurrence of clinical signs. However, surgical reconstruction of the pelvic diaphragm is usually needed.
   e. **Prognosis** is good but the problem may recur.

4. **Perianal fistulae.** The cause of perianal fistulae is unknown, but infection and abscessation of glands near the anus is suspected. Dogs with a broad tail base (e.g., German shepherds, Irish setters, Labrador retrievers) are more commonly affected.
   a. **Clinical findings.** Dyschezia is the most common clinical sign. Hematochezia, constipation, and a foul-smelling discharge are sometimes also seen. One or more draining tracts are usually seen near the anus.
   b. **Diagnosis** is based on physical and rectal examination.
   c. **Treatment** consists of surgery and possibly antibiotics and stool softeners.
   d. **Prognosis** is guarded because of the risk of recurrence, a common complication. Postoperative stenosis or fecal incontinence are uncommon complications.

5. **Anal sac infection** or **abscessation** is rare in cats.
   a. **Pathogenesis.** Inadequate emptying of the anal sacs can cause impaction. Subsequent inflammation and infection can lead to cellulitis or abscessation.
   b. **Clinical findings.** "Scooting" and licking or biting at the area are the most common signs. Hematochezia, dyschezia, and constipation are usually only seen in severe cases. The anal sacs are usually painful and may be enlarged. The anal sac contents may be yellow, bloody, or purulent. If an infected sac has ruptured, a fistulous tract may be present.
   c. **Diagnosis** is based on physical and rectal examination.
   d. **Treatment**
      (1) In mild cases, the anal sacs should be expressed and the animal reevaluated in 1 week.
      (2) With a moderate infection or if the problem recurs, the anal sac should be flushed with a povidone–iodine solution, infused with an antibiotic ointment, or both.
      (3) Abscesses should be lanced, drained, and flushed. Concurrent systemic antibiotic therapy is indicated.
      (4) If medical therapy is ineffective or the problem repeatedly recurs, surgical removal of the anal sacs can be considered.
   e. **Prognosis** is usually good.

6. **Perianal neoplasia**
   a. **Perianal gland adenomas** originate from glands near the anus and tail base. Because androgens stimulate growth of these tumors, older male dogs are most commonly affected.
      (1) **Clinical findings.** The animal may be asymptomatic or may scoot and lick at the anal area. One or more small, firm nodules are seen near the anus. The masses may be ulcerated due to self-trauma.
      (2) **Diagnosis** is based on biopsy results.
      (3) **Treatment** and **prognosis.** Surgical excision and concurrent castration (to decrease the risk of recurrence) is the optimal treatment. Castration alone

will cause regression of the tumor, but excisional biopsy is often needed to rule out malignancy. The prognosis is good.

b. Perianal gland adenocarcinomas resemble perianal gland adenomas except that they are locally invasive and eventually metastasize to the sublumbar lymph nodes and lungs. Treatment may include repeated partial surgical resections, chemotherapy, radiation therapy, or combination therapy, but the prognosis is generally poor.

c. Anal sac (apocrine gland) adenocarcinomas arise from the apocrine glands and often produce a parathyroid hormone (PTH)-like substance that causes hypercalcemia. Older spayed female dogs are most commonly affected.

   (1) Clinical findings. Signs of hypercalcemia of malignancy (e.g., anorexia, polyuria, polydipsia, vomiting, weakness) are most common. Constipation is occasionally seen. An anal sac mass can usually be palpated but may be quite small.

   (2) Diagnosis. A presumptive diagnosis is often based on the concurrent presence of an anal sac mass and hypercalcemia. A biopsy will confirm the diagnosis.

   (3) Treatment. Hypercalcemia, if present, must be treated. Surgical excision is recommended if no evidence of metastasis is found. Chemotherapy is recommended if metastasis has occurred or is later found.

   (4) Prognosis is poor because metastasis has usually occurred by the time of diagnosis.

d. Other perianal tumors include lipomas, leiomyomas, melanomas, mast cell tumors, and squamous cell carcinomas.

STUDY QUESTIONS

DIRECTIONS: Each of the numbered items or incomplete statements in this section is followed by answers or by completions of the statement. Select the ONE numbered answer or completion that is BEST in each case.

1. The optimal treatment for an eosinophilic ulcer in a cat is:

(1) antibiotics.
(2) glucocorticoids.
(3) surgical excision.
(4) progesterone.
(5) oral chlorhexidine rinses.

2. Which one of the following canine oral tumors often metastasizes to the lungs and other tissues early in the course of the disease?

(1) Nontonsillar squamous cell carcinoma
(2) Malignant melanoma
(3) Fibrosarcoma
(4) Tonsillar squamous cell carcinoma
(5) Chrondrosarcoma

3. A 4-year-old neutered male mixed-breed dog is brought to the veterinarian because the owners have noticed that over the last day or so, the dog has been unable or unwilling to open his mouth. On physical examination, the dog exhibits extreme pain when the veterinarian tries to open his mouth, and his left eye seems slightly exophthalmic. The veterinarian anesthetizes the dog so she is able to examine his mouth. The most likely diagnosis is:

(1) retrobulbar abscess.
(2) masseter myositis.
(3) craniomandibular osteopathy.
(4) sialocele.
(5) neuropathy.

4. A 2-year-old domestic shorthair cat is presented with regurgitation and constipation. The most likely diagnosis is:

(1) multifocal lymphosarcoma.
(2) feline immunodeficiency virus (FIV) infection.
(3) feline leukemia virus (FeLV) infection.
(4) dysautonomia.
(5) hypothyroidism.

5. Aspiration pneumonia, a common sequelae to esophageal problems, most commonly affects:

(1) the caudodorsal lung lobes.
(2) the accessory lung lobe.
(3) the cranioventral lung lobes.
(4) the left lung lobes.
(5) the right lung lobes.

6. In which one of the following disorders is acute odynophagia likely to be an early clinical sign?

(1) Idiopathic megaesophagus
(2) Persistent right aortic arch (PRAA)
(3) Esophageal neoplasm
(4) Congenital diverticulum
(5) Esophageal foreign body

7. The most likely cause of hematemesis in a 10-year-old, spayed female collie with no other clinical signs is:

(1) a coagulopathy.
(2) hemorrhagic gastroenteritis (HGE).
(3) gastric ulcers.
(4) chronic esophagitis.
(5) dietary intolerance.

8. A 3-year-old spayed female miniature poodle is presented with a 4-month history of intermittent vomiting. The vomiting occurs only in the morning and only yellow froth is vomited. The dog's appetite, attitude, and other activities are normal. No abnormalities are found on physical examination. The most likely diagnosis is:

(1) lymphocytic–plasmacytic gastritis.
(2) pyloric stenosis.
(3) chronic renal failure.
(4) enterogastric reflux.
(5) gastric foreign body.

9. Small bowel disease is associated with:

(1) mucus and blood in the feces.
(2) tenesmus.
(3) weight loss and flatulence.
(4) weight gain and tenesmus.
(5) tenesmus and mucus in the feces.

10. The antibiotic of choice for treatment of campylobacteriosis is:

(1) ampicillin.
(2) erythromycin.
(3) trimethoprim/sulfonamide.
(4) cephalexin.
(5) neomycin.

11. A 6-year-old neutered male Yorkshire terrier has chronic small bowel diarrhea. On physical examination, the dog is very thin, but no other abnormalities are detected. A complete blood count (CBC) shows a mild nonregenerative anemia and a marked lymphopenia. A serum biochemical profile reveals mild hypocalcemia, hypocholesterolemia, and a moderate panhypoproteinemia. The most likely diagnosis is:

(1) histoplasmosis.
(2) salmonellosis.
(3) lymphosarcoma.
(4) ascariasis.
(5) lymphangiectasia.

12. The most common cause of streaks of fresh blood on formed feces is:

(1) colonic lymphosarcoma.
(2) histiocytic ulcerative colitis.
(3) lymphocytic–plasmacytic colitis.
(4) cecal inversion.
(5) colonic polyps.

DIRECTIONS: Each of the numbered items or incomplete statements in this section is negatively phrased, as indicated by a capitalized word such as NOT, LEAST, or EXCEPT. Select the ONE numbered answer or completion that is BEST in each case.

---

13. For stomatitis, which of the following cause-and-treatment pairs is INCORRECT?

(1) Candidiasis— topical nystatin
(2) Feline plasma cell stomatitis— dental prophylaxis
(3) Lymphocytic–plasmacytic stomatitis— glucocorticoids
(4) Periodontal disease— glucocorticoids
(5) Pemphigus— azathioprine

14. Management of a dog with idiopathic megaesophagus should include all of the following measures EXCEPT:

(1) always having the animal take food and water in an upright position.
(2) always feeding a food with a gruel-like consistency.
(3) always feeding several small meals a day.
(4) initiating antibiotic treatment if secondary aspiration pneumonia is present.

15. Which one of the following is NOT a cause of delayed gastric emptying?

(1) Pyloric hypertrophy
(2) Ileal adenocarcinoma
(3) Hypokalemia
(4) Gastric antral mucosal hypertrophy
(5) Chronic renal failure

16. Which one of the following is NOT a zoonotic disease?

(1) Trichuriasis
(2) Ancylostomiasis
(3) Ascariasis
(4) Campylobacteriosis
(5) Salmonellosis

17. Which one of the following treatments would NOT be indicated in treatment of a dog with severe parvoviral enteritis?

(1) Oral neomycin
(2) Parenteral fluids
(3) Potassium supplementation
(4) Injectable broad-spectrum antibiotics
(5) Withholding of food and water

18. Which one of the following substances should NOT be given to a dehydrated animal?

(1) Dioctyl sodium sulfosuccinate
(2) Bisacodyl
(3) Mineral oil
(4) Cisapride

19. Anal sacculectomy may be indicated for an animal with any of the following conditions EXCEPT:

(1) anal sacculitis with a draining tract.
(2) chronic recurrent anal sacculitis.
(3) anal sac adenocarcinoma.
(4) acute sacculitis and perirectal cellulitis.
(5) chronic anal sac impaction.

ANSWERS AND EXPLANATIONS

1. The answer is 2 [I B 3 b (3)]. Glucocorticoids are the treatment of choice based on the proposed etiology of feline eosinophilic granuloma complex (i.e., immune-mediated or allergic disease). Antibiotics and oral chlorhexidine rinses, while not harmful, are usually of little use in a cat with an eosinophilic ulcer because bacteria are not involved in development of the lesion. Progesterone compounds are effective in some animals, but these compounds are a second choice because they have more potential serious side effects. Surgical excision should be considered only if all medical treatments have failed, because the lesions often recur despite resection of the initial lesion.

2. The answer is 2 [I B 3 g (2) (b)]. Malignant melanomas are aggressive, and metastatic disease is often present at the time of initial diagnosis. Nontonsillar and tonsillar squamous cell carcinomas usually quickly metastasize to regional lymph nodes but do not metastasize to the lungs until later in the course of the disease. Fibrosarcomas and chondrosarcomas are locally invasive but tend to be slow to metastasize.

3. The answer is 1 [IC 3 d]. Masseter myositis, a retrobulbar abscess, and craniomandibular osteopathy can all cause pain on manipulation of the jaw. Of these three disorders, only a retrobulbar abscess would also cause unilateral exophthalmus. With craniomandibular osteopathy, mandibular swelling would often also be seen. Muscle swelling or atrophy may be seen with myositis. With a sialocele, there is often no significant pain, but a fluctuant soft-tissue swelling is usually present. Neuropathies are also not painful; instead, cranial nerve dysfunction (e.g., dropped jaw, facial droop, abnormal tongue motility) would be seen.

4. The answer is 4 [II A 2 b (5), B 1 b (1); Table 41-2]. Megaesophagus (causing regurgitation) and constipation are often both seen with dysautonomia. Lymphosarcoma can cause secondary esophageal dilatation if a mass or enlarged lymph node causes extraesophageal compression, but colonic lymphosar-

coma usually causes diarrhea, not constipation. Feline leukemia virus (FeLV) and feline immunodeficiency virus (FIV) infection can both cause a myriad of clinical signs, but neither regurgitation nor constipation is common. Hypothyroidism can cause constipation and may cause megaesophagus (and regurgitation), but naturally occurring hypothyroidism is extremely rare in cats and no other signs of hypothyroidism are present.

5. The answer is 3 [II A 4 a (1) (e)]. Aspiration pneumonia most commonly affects the cranioventral lung lobes. When gastric or esophageal contents are aspirated, they will usually come to rest in the upper part of the airway system (the mainstem bronchi to the cranial lung lobes are located most cranial) and gravity will tend to pull the material ventral. Other lung lobes are occasionally affected. For example, if an animal is in lateral recumbency when regurgitation and aspiration occur, one side of the lungs may be more affected.

6. The answer is 5 [II B 2 b]. The lacerations, erosions, ulcerations, and pressure necrosis associated with foreign bodies commonly cause acute esophageal pain. Idiopathic megaesophagus, congenital diverticulum, and persistent right aortic arch (PRAA) may cause discomfort as esophageal distention progresses, but the pain is usually chronic and other clinical signs are seen first.

7. The answer is 3 [III B 4]. In the absence of other clinical signs, gastric ulcers are the most common cause of hematemesis in an older dog. A coagulopathy can result in hematemesis, but commonly bleeding from or into other tissues is also seen. Hematemesis is also often seen with hemorrhagic gastroenteritis (HGE), but this syndrome is more common in younger, small-breed dogs, and hemorrhagic diarrhea is usually the overriding clinical sign. Hemorrhage, even subclinical amounts, rarely occurs with chronic esophagitis; in addition, esophagitis results in regurgitation rather than vomiting. Dietary intolerance can cause vomiting, diarrhea, or both, but hematemesis is not typically seen.

8. The answer is 4 [III B 12]. Enterogastric reflux is most common in young, small-breed dogs and is usually characterized by vomiting of bile-stained fluid, primarily in the morning. Lymphocytic–plasmacytic gastritis usually causes vomiting at variable times during the day and food is sometimes vomited. With pyloric stenosis, food is commonly vomited several hours after eating and vomiting of just liquid is rare. Dogs that are vomiting due to chronic renal failure do not have a good appetite but instead are often inappetent or anorexic and weight loss is also often observed. A gastric foreign body usually causes more acute and persistent vomiting and would not cause clinical signs only in the mornings.

9. The answer is 3 [IV A 3 a]. Weight loss and flatulence can occur with small bowel disease. Weight loss occurs as a result of anorexia or malassimilation. Flatulence can occur in healthy dogs as a result of aerophagia but may also be seen in small bowel disease as a result of altered intestinal motility and bacterial fermentation of malabsorbed food products. Tenesmus and mucus and fresh blood in the feces suggest large bowel disease. Weight gain does not occur with either small or large bowel disease.

10. The answer is 2 [IV B 4 b (2)]. Erythromycin is the treatment of choice for campylobacteriosis, although enrofloxacin, doxycycline, clindamycin, and chloramphenicol are also often effective.

11. The answer is 5 [IV B 12]. Severe lymphopenia, mild hypocalcemia, hypocholesterolemia, and moderate panhypoproteinemia are typical clinical pathologic abnormalities seen in dogs with lymphangiectasia, in which there is loss of lymphocytes, lipids, and proteins from the lymphatics and concurrent malabsorption. Histoplasmosis, chronic salmonellosis, and lymphosarcoma may cause panhypoproteinemia, but an inflammatory leukogram, fever, and melena are also often seen. It would be rare for ascarids to cause any clinical signs (especially a moderate panhypoproteinemia) in an adult dog.

12. The answer is 5 [IV C 9 a]. With colonic polyps, streaks of fresh blood on the feces are often the only clinical sign of disease; because the polyps are sometimes friable, the fecal material may abrade the surface of the polyps and cause a small amount of bleeding.

Colonic lymphosarcoma, histiocytic ulcerative colitis, and lymphocytic colitis can cause bloody feces but the feces are usually soft or liquid (i.e., diarrheic) rather than formed. With a cecal inversion, mucoid diarrhea and tenesmus may be seen if a partial obstruction has resulted, or anorexia, vomiting, and lethargy may be seen if the inversion causes a complete obstruction.

13. The answer is 4 [I B 3 d; Table 41-1]. Glucocorticoids are not indicated in the treatment of periodontal disease because bacteria and bacterial products are the cause of the inflammation and can result in abscessation and deep infection. Oral antibiotics are useful in the treatment of periodontal disease, plasma cell stomatitis, and nocardiosis. Dental prophylaxis should be a component of treatment for periodontal disease, lymphocytic–plasmacytic stomatitis, and feline plasma cell stomatitis. Glucocorticoids with or without other immunosuppressive drugs are indicated for treatment of lymphocytic–plasmacytic stomatitis and pemphigus because both are characterized by immunocyte infiltration of the oral tissue. Topical nystatin or oral ketoconazole is used to treat oral candidiasis.

14. The answer is 2 [II B 1 c]. Feeding a food with a gruel-like consistency is not always the best option for dogs or cats with megaesophagus. Some animals do well with a gruel, but others have less regurgitation and esophageal food retention when food with a paste-like consistency, canned food, or dry kibble is used. Short trials should be performed to determine which food consistency works best for the affected individual. Regardless of the food used, the animal should always eat and drink in an upright position to allow gravity to assist with food passage, and several small meals a day should be given to minimize possible accumulation of food in the esophagus. Antibiotic treatment is indicated if an aspiration pneumonia is present.

15. The answer is 2 [IV B 14 b]. An ileal tumor is unlikely to have an effect on the pyloric outflow tract or gastric motility unless it has caused a complete intestinal obstruction or perforation and periodontitis; more commonly, weight loss and chronic diarrhea are seen with eventual identification of the lesion based on a gastrointestinal (GI) contrast study, which will reveal focal luminal narrowing, or at exploratory laparotomy. Delayed gastric emptying is a hallmark of pyloric hypertrophy and gastric antral mucosal hypertrophy. Hypokalemia and the uremia and acidosis of renal failure can cause GI hypomotility and may thus delay gastric emptying; gastric hypomotility will be seen with fluoroscopy.

16. The answer is 1 [IV C 2 a]. Infection with *Trichuris vulpis* does not cause disease in humans. *Ancylostoma* species can cause cutaneous larval migrans in humans and ascarids can cause visceral and ocular larval migrans. In the case of salmonellosis and campylobacteriosis, special attention to cleanliness and disinfection is necessary because these bacterial infections can be readily transmitted to humans.

17. The answer is 1 [IV B 3 a (3)]. In a dog with parvoviral enteritis, all oral intake should be withheld in order to avoid exacerbating the vomiting and diarrhea and to rest the gastrointestinal (GI) tract. Intravenous fluids are initially required to correct any dehydration and to maintain hydration. Hypokalemia is often present because of decreased intake and increased losses in the vomitus and diarrhea, so potassium supplementation is often required. Although antibiotic therapy is indicated for the bacteremia or septicemia that commonly results secondary to intestinal mucosal compromise, parenteral administration is required in a vomiting animal. In addition, oral neomycin is poorly absorbed even in an animal with intact intestinal mucosa and so would be of little use for systemic infection.

18. The answer is 1 [IV D 3 d (2) (b)]. Dioctyl sodium sulfosuccinate should not be used in a dehydrated animal because it increases water penetration of the feces, making the dehydration worse. Bisacodyl does not change the water content of the feces but rather stimulates defecation; therefore, the animal's hydration status is not affected. Mineral oil and cisapride do not alter the fecal water content.

19. The answer is 4 [IV E 5]. Although anal sacculitis and anal sac impaction are usually treated medically, if the infection or impaction is recurrent, anal sacculectomy may definitively resolve the problem. Surgical treatment may also be needed if a draining tract has formed. However, in the case of acute sacculitis, medical treatment alone will often resolve the problem and should be attempted first because anal sacculectomy is not without potential complications. Because anal sac adenocarcinomas readily metastasize, surgical excision of the primary tumor should be performed as soon as the mass is identified.

Chapter 42

Hepatobiliary and Exocrine Pancreatic Diseases

I. HEPATOBILIARY DISORDERS

A. Clinical evaluation

1. **Predisposition**
   a. **Species and breed.** All breeds of dogs and cats can develop hepatobiliary diseases, but certain breeds are at increased risk. For example:
      (1) **Bedlington terriers, cocker spaniels, Doberman pinschers, Skye terriers, standard poodles, West Highland White terriers,** and, possibly, **Labrador retrievers** are more prone to chronic hepatic disease.
      (2) **Cats.** Biliary disorders are more common than hepatic parenchymal disorders in cats.
   b. **Age**
      (1) **Young animals.** Congenital disorders (e.g., portosystemic shunts) occur more often in young dogs or cats.
      (2) **Middle-aged to older animals.** Neoplasia is more common in older animals.
   c. **Environment.** An animal with free access to an entire neighborhood is more likely to have been exposed to a toxin than a more confined animal.
   d. **Vaccination status.** Viral disease is less likely in a vaccinated animal.

2. **Patient history**
   a. **Medication history**
      (1) Glucocorticoids, anticonvulsants, thiacetarsamide, mebendazole, acetaminophen, and many other medications can cause hepatic disease.
      (2) A history of intolerance to drugs normally metabolized by the liver (e.g., sedatives, anticonvulsants, anesthetics) can also be suggestive of hepatic dysfunction.
   b. **Chronicity of signs.** Acute signs of disease may occur with hepatic necrosis, some drug-induced hepatopathies, some types of infectious hepatitis, or the early phase of a chronic disorder.

3. **Clinical signs**
   a. **Neurologic signs** (e.g., abnormal behavior, depression, coma, anorexia, aggression, central blindness, seizures) may be seen with **hepatic encephalopathy.** The signs often wax and wane and may be exacerbated by a high-protein meal, medications, gastrointestinal (GI) hemorrhage, uremia, infection, constipation, and large intestinal bacterial overgrowth. Underlying causes include:
      (1) Accumulation of neurotoxins (e.g., ammonia, amino acids, mercaptans, fatty acids)
      (2) Altered neurotransmitter balance [e.g., γ-aminobutyric acid (GABA)]
      (3) Changes in the blood–brain barrier
      (4) Abnormal cerebral metabolism
      (5) Other contributing factors, such as azotemia, electrolyte abnormalities (especially hypokalemia), hypoglycemia, alkalosis, hypoxia, or hypovolemia
   b. **Icterus (jaundice)** may be prehepatic, hepatic, or posthepatic (see Chapter 9 II). Jaundice is not clinically visible until serum bilirubin concentrations are 1.5–3 times normal, and it will persist for several days following resolution of the hyperbilirubinemia because of tissue staining.
   c. **GI signs.** Altered GI bacterial flora, hypergastrinemia, or altered gastric blood flow due to portal hypertension may lead to small intestinal irritation, GI ulceration and hemorrhage, or both. As a result:
      (1) **Vomiting** and **diarrhea** are common with many acute and chronic hepatic diseases.
      (2) **Hematemesis** or **melena** may be seen.

(3) **Exacerbation of neurologic signs** may occur as a result of GI hemorrhage because blood is a nitrogen source for ammonia production in the colon.

d. **Ptyalism** is a common sign in cats with hepatic disease. Ptyalism may result from nausea and GI irritation or hepatic encephalopathy.

e. **Ascites.** Hepatic disease can produce free abdominal fluid as a result of increased salt and water retention, chronic portal hypertension, or hypoalbuminemia. The fluid may be a transudate or a modified transudate (as is the case with posthepatic portal hypertension). Loss of albumin to the ascitic fluid further lowers serum albumin concentrations. Ascites is usually suggestive of chronic hepatic dysfunction, although it can also result from rupture of the biliary tract and resulting bile peritonitis.

f. **Acholic feces** result from the absence of intestinal bile. This only occurs with complete extrahepatic bile duct or bile duct transection.

g. **Dark** or **orange urine** can be seen as a result of increased urine bilirubin. Hemoglobinuria or myoglobinuria should also be considered.

h. **Polyuria** and **polydipsia** can occur with hepatobiliary disease as a result of hepatic encephalopathy, decreased availability of urea for the renal medullary concentrating gradient, secondary hyperaldosteronism, and other mechanisms.

i. **Fever** can occur with hepatic inflammation or infection, or it may occur as a result of bacteremia or infection secondary to hepatic disease as a result of decreased hepatic reticuloendothelial system function.

j. **Hemorrhage** or **petechiae.** The liver produces nearly all of the coagulation factors as well as activators and inhibitors of fibrinolysis. Spontaneous hemorrhage is rare, but significant hemorrhage can occur from GI lesions, venipuncture, surgery, or hepatic biopsy. Hepatobiliary disease may cause abnormal coagulation as a result of:

(1) Decreased synthesis of coagulation factors
(2) Disseminated intravascular coagulation (DIC)
(3) Platelet dysfunction
(4) Decreased vitamin K absorption due to chronic bile duct obstruction with a subsequent decrease in vitamin-K dependent coagulation factors (i.e., factors II, VII, IX, X)

k. **Anorexia** is a common nonspecific sign of hepatobiliary disease. **Weight loss** usually follows prolonged anorexia, thereby suggesting a chronic hepatic disorder.

l. **Poor growth** is often seen with congenital hepatic disorders such as portosystemic vascular anomalies. Growth may be inhibited as a result of decreased hepatic production of proteins and other substances and possible concurrent anorexia, vomiting, or diarrhea.

m. **Hepatomegaly** due to congestion, inflammation, steroid hepatopathy, lipidosis, neoplasia, glycogen storage disease, or a cyst or abscess may be palpable.

n. **Cranial abdominal pain** may be detected in the animal with pancreatitis, cholangiohepatitis, an abscess, or peritonitis.

o. **Extrahepatic masses** with possible metastasis to the liver may be detected.

p. **Other signs**
(1) **Ocular lesions** can occur with fungal disease, toxoplasmosis, and feline infectious peritonitis (FIP).
(2) **Abnormal lung sounds** may be ausculted in animals with systemic infectious diseases (e.g., fungal infection, heartworm disease).

4. **Diagnostic tests**
a. **Complete blood count (CBC)**
(1) A nonregenerative anemia is consistent with chronic disease.
(2) A regenerative anemia may be seen if GI hemorrhage has occurred secondary to the hepatic disease.
(3) Target cells and poikilocytosis are often seen.
(4) A microcytosis without anemia may be seen with a portosystemic shunt.
b. **Serum biochemical profile**
(1) **Bilirubin.** An increase in total bilirubin can be seen with prehepatic, hepatic, or posthepatic disorders (see Table 9-1).

(2) Albumin
  (a) Hypoalbuminemia can occur with severe subacute to chronic liver disease as a result of decreased synthesis, inhibition of albumin release, and an increased volume of distribution with ascites.
  (b) Hyperalbuminemia may be seen as a result of dehydration and hyperproteinemia in acute disease.
(3) Glucose
  (a) Hypoglycemia can occur with severe hepatic dysfunction as a result of decreased gluconeogenesis, decreased glycogen storage, and decreased hepatic degradation of insulin.
  (b) Hyperglycemia, although less common, can also occur with hepatic disease as a result of decreased glycogenesis and decreased glucocorticoid clearance.
(4) Hyperglobulinemia can result from decreased reticuloendothelial function and increased exposure to GI antigens.
(5) Serum alanine aminotransferase (ALT) concentrations are increased when this cytoplasmic enzyme leaks into the circulation through damaged hepatocyte membranes.
  (a) The greatest increases are seen with hepatic necrosis and inflammatory hepatitis.
  (b) Lesser increases can be seen with pancreatitis, sepsis, biliary obstruction, hypoxia, hyperadrenocorticism, and anticonvulsant therapy.
  (c) Normal values are often seen with portosystemic shunts and cirrhosis.
(6) Serum aspartate aminotransferase (AST) concentrations often parallel those of ALT, but AST concentrations can also increase as a result of muscle damage.
(7) Serum alkaline phosphatase (ALP) concentrations may be elevated. ALP is found in hepatic, bone, intestinal, renal, and placental tissue, but only the isoenzymes from the liver and bone are clinically important. ALP elevations result from increased production by cells of the bile canaliculi rather than from leakage.
  (a) Increased production occurs in response to intrahepatic or extrahepatic cholestasis, steroid therapy, and anticonvulsant therapy. The bone isoenzyme can increase with growth, bone tumors, bone destruction, and hyperparathyroidism.
  (b) In cats, the half-life of ALP is much shorter than in dogs (6 hours versus 3 days), and less ALP is produced in response to cholestasis. Therefore, any increase in ALP is clinically significant in cats. Cats are also resistant to steroid or drug induction of ALP.
(8) Serum γ-glutamyl transpeptidase (GGT) concentrations usually parallel ALP concentrations. Although also found in renal, intestinal, and pancreatic tissue, only hepatic GGT is clinically significant. Anticonvulsant therapy may also increase GGT concentrations in dogs.
(9) Cholesterol
  (a) Hypocholesterolemia. Portosystemic shunts and hepatic failure may cause decreased production of cholesterol.
  (b) Hypercholesterolemia. Serum cholesterol concentrations may be increased with cholestasis.
(10) Blood urea nitrogen (BUN) may be decreased with liver failure because less urea is produced from ammonia. However, many other factors also influence BUN concentrations.
(11) Serum thyroxine (T_4) levels should be evaluated in any middle-aged to older cat with increased serum hepatic enzyme concentrations because hepatic disease may occur secondary to hyperthyroidism.

c. Urinalysis
  (1) Urine bilirubin
    (a) In dogs, the renal threshold for bilirubin is low; therefore, urine bilirubin up to 2 + in the urine can be normal and only large amounts suggest pathologic hyperbilirubinemia.

(b) In cats, the renal threshold for bilirubin is high; therefore, any amount of bilirubinuria suggests hyperbilirubinemia.

(2) Urobilinogen is normally present in urine. Its absence in an icteric patient is suggestive of a complete bile duct obstruction. Urobilinogen levels are also influenced by many other factors.

(3) Urate crystals may be seen in dogs or cats with chronic hepatic dysfunction, especially as a result of a portosystemic shunt.

(4) Glucosuria. If glucosuria and hyperglycemia (i.e., diabetes mellitus) are found in an animal with hepatic disease, secondary hepatic lipidosis should be considered as the cause of the hepatic disease.

(5) Dilute or **isosthenuric urine** may be seen in animals with portosystemic shunts or severe hepatic disease.

d. Diagnostic imaging

(1) Radiography

(a) Abdominal radiographs

(i) Hepatomegaly can occur with inflammation, steroid hepatopathy, hepatic lipidosis, neoplasia, portal vein obstruction, and bile duct obstruction. Young animals also have relative hepatomegaly.

(ii) Microhepatica may be seen with a portosystemic shunt, arteriovenous fistula, or cirrhosis. Microhepatica may be a normal finding in some animals.

(iii) Irregular liver margins may be seen with neoplasia, cysts, abscesses, cirrhosis, and nodular hyperplasia.

(iv) Ascites can occur with chronic hepatitis, cirrhosis, venous outflow obstruction, and neoplasia.

(v) Gall bladder. The gall bladder is only visible if the wall is mineralized or emphysematous or if radiodense choleliths are present.

(vi) Renal or **cystic calculi** (i.e., urate calculi) are sometimes seen in dogs or cats with a portosystemic shunt or hepatic failure.

(b) Thoracic radiographs may help identify fungal or other systemic infections, heartworm disease, or metastatic neoplasia.

(2) Angiography or **portography (contrast radiography)** may be used to identify vascular anomalies such as portosystemic shunts and arteriovenous fistulae. **Scintigraphy** can also be used to check for vascular anomalies, but this technique does not always allow localization of the shunt, so subsequent contrast radiographs may still be needed.

(3) Ultrasonography of the liver can differentiate diffuse disease from focal or multifocal disease and can reveal biliary obstruction. It is useful in the presence of increased hepatic enzyme concentrations, ascites, icterus, or radiographic hepatic abnormalities, and when gall bladder or metastatic hepatic disease is suspected.

(a) A **hyperechoic liver** may be seen with steroid hepatopathy, lipidosis, fibrosis, cirrhosis, and some neoplasms.

(b) A **hypoechoic liver** may be seen with some neoplasms, inflammatory hepatopathies, and congestion.

e. Liver function tests are indicated for animals with suspected hepatic disease but normal serum hepatic enzyme concentrations, animals with increased serum enzyme concentrations but no clinical signs of hepatic disease, and evaluation of disease progression or response to treatment.

(1) Serum bile acid concentrations are the most useful measure of liver function in dogs and cats. Bile acids are synthesized in the liver and are normally secreted into the intestines (in bile), where they stimulate pancreatic enzymes and aid in lipid absorption. The majority are then reabsorbed in the ileum and are removed and recirculated by the liver (enterohepatic cycle). Abnormal hepatobiliary function and abnormal portal blood flow can disrupt the cycle of bile acid synthesis, secretion, and absorption. Evaluation of both **fasting** and **postprandial** serum bile acid concentrations is recommended.

(2) Plasma ammonia concentrations are a sensitive indicator of liver function.

    (a) Nitrogenous materials (e.g., dietary proteins, blood, intestinal cells, urea) are converted to ammonia by colonic bacteria and the ammonia is absorbed. Normally, the ammonia is then removed from the circulation by the liver and converted to urea. With liver dysfunction or portosystemic shunting, ammonia is not removed from the blood by the liver.

    (b) Although fasting ammonia concentrations are often increased with hepatic dysfunction, the sensitivity of the test can be increased by also evaluating a postprandial plasma ammonia level or performing an oral ammonia tolerance test.

    (c) Samples for ammonia determination require special handling, and the ammonia challenge may exacerbate clinical signs.

(3) Sulfobromophthalein (BSP) or **indocyanine green (ICG) clearance tests** have been used to assess hepatic function and perfusion, but they are rarely used because of many potential problems.

(4) Evaluation of serum albumin, glucose, BUN, and **cholesterol concentrations.** Albumin, glucose, BUN, and cholesterol are all produced by the liver. Although evaluation of serum levels of these markers of liver function is not used on its own to evaluate liver function, low values, especially of several of the markers, suggests a need to consider liver disease.

f. Coagulation tests

  (1) Prothrombin time (PT), partial thromboplastin time (PTT), and **activated clotting time (ACT)** may be increased if severe hepatic failure has caused decreased synthesis of clotting factors. Routine coagulation tests will not detect all coagulopathies, and a marked reduction in coagulation factor concentration (i.e., to less than 30% of normal) is needed before coagulation test results will be abnormal.

  (2) DIC, the most common coagulopathy seen with hepatic disease, is characterized by a prolonged PT, prolonged PTT, prolonged thrombin time, increased fibrin degradation products, thrombocytopenia, and hypofibrinogenemia.

  (3) With disorders that cause a decrease in the vitamin K–dependent clotting factors, the PT and PTT may be prolonged but will normalize with parenteral vitamin K administration.

g. Abdominocentesis should be performed if ascites is detected (see Table 10-1).

  (1) A transudate may be seen with severe hypoalbuminemia (i.e., albumin less than 1.5 mg/dl) and disorders causing hepatic or prehepatic portal hypertension.

  (2) A modified transudate is more common with posthepatic portal hypertension.

  (3) Other potential findings in the animal with primary or secondary hepatic disease include neoplastic cells, intracellular and extracellular bacteria (suggestive of septic peritonitis), hemorrhage (suggestive of hemangiosarcoma), bile (suggestive of bile peritonitis from biliary rupture), neutrophils in the absence of bacteria (suggestive of sterile peritonitis), or the fluid of FIP.

h. Fine-needle liver aspirate may identify lymphosarcoma, carcinoma, lipidosis, or fungal organisms.

i. Biopsy is needed to establish a definitive diagnosis with most hepatic diseases. An appropriate evaluation (e.g., laboratory tests, radiographs, coagulation tests) should be done prior to biopsy. Before the biopsy, a transfusion with fresh whole blood may be needed if coagulation is abnormal, and after the biopsy, the patient should be closely monitored for hemorrhage.

  (1) Percutaneous biopsy methods (e.g., blind percutaneous biopsy, keyhole percutaneous biopsy) are useful when diffuse hepatic disease is suspected.

  (2) Biopsy with ultrasound guidance is useful with diffuse, focal, or multifocal hepatic disease.

  (3) Laparoscopy or **laparotomy** is useful with microhepatica, focal or multifocal disease, or ascites. Laparotomy is most useful when posthepatic biliary disease is suspected.

    j. **Bacterial culture** should be obtained from any biopsy or bile aspirate.

    k. **Serology** may be useful if toxoplasmosis or leptospirosis is suspected.

B. **Specific hepatobiliary disorders**

  1. **Hepatic necrosis**

    a. **Etiology.** Causes of hepatic necrosis include chemicals, drugs (see I B 2), infection (see I B 3), inflammation, pancreatitis (see II B 1), trauma, and ischemia. In animals with acute, severe hepatic failure, the cause may not be identified because the animal either markedly improves or dies before a biopsy is possible.

    b. **Diagnosis**

      (1) **History.** The history may disclose exogenous toxins, extrahepatic disease, or trauma.

      (2) **Clinical findings**

        (a) Affected animals may exhibit acute anorexia, vomiting, diarrhea, depression or coma, fever, dehydration, polyuria and polydipsia, neurologic signs (i.e., hepatic encephalopathy), icterus, and, possibly, hemorrhage caused by DIC.

        (b) Some affected animals are asymptomatic.

      (3) **Laboratory findings**

        (a) **Serum biochemical profile.** Serum biochemistry usually reveals markedly increased ALT and AST concentrations with smaller increases in ALP, GGT, and bilirubin levels. Hypoglycemia may be seen, depending on the cause of the necrosis.

        (b) **Hepatic function test results** are usually normal.

      (4) **Hepatic biopsy** usually shows lobular necrosis and a neutrophilic infiltrate. Other changes may be seen if another primary hepatic disease (e.g., viral hepatitis, idiopathic chronic hepatitis) is the cause of the necrosis.

    c. **Treatment**

      (1) **The inciting cause should be removed and the underlying disease treated, if possible.**

      (2) **Dehydration and any electrolyte or acid–base abnormalities should be treated.** Overaggressive fluid therapy should be avoided because animals in acute hepatic failure may be unable to handle excess sodium and water.

        (a) In most cases, 0.45% saline with 2.5% dextrose and potassium supplementation is a good choice.

        (b) Even in the absence of hypoglycemia, low-level glucose supplementation may decrease catabolism and help decrease ammonia concentrations.

      (3) **Clinical signs of hepatic encephalopathy should be treated.**

        (a) **Withholding food** decreases the proteins in the colon that can form ammonia and other toxins. A **high-quality, restricted-protein diet** [see I B 5 a (3) (b)] is recommended when feeding is resumed.

        (b) **Cleansing enemas** of saline with povidone iodine or saline with neomycin physically remove nitrogenous wastes from the colon and decrease colonic bacterial numbers and the colonic pH so that less ammonia is formed and absorbed.

        (c) **Lactulose** or **lactitol** can be given orally or as an enema. These agents decrease colonic bacterial numbers (via their laxative effects) and acidify the colon so that less ammonia is formed and absorbed. Lactulose or lactitol can be used orally on a long-term basis, if needed.

        (d) **Oral nonabsorbable antibiotics** (e.g., aminoglycosides) or **metronidazole** also reduce colonic bacterial numbers.

        (e) **Mannitol** and **furosemide** may be given to counteract possible secondary cerebral edema if neurologic signs persist after blood ammonia concentrations have returned to normal.

      (4) **Drugs metabolized by the liver** (e.g., many analgesics, anesthetics, barbiturates, sedatives, tranquilizers) **should be avoided, if possible.**

(5) **GI hemorrhage should be controlled** with a bland, easily digestible diet, a histamine-2 (H_2) antagonist (e.g., cimetidine, ranitidine, famotidine), sucralfate, and possibly misoprostol.

(6) **Antibiotic therapy may be warranted if the animal is at risk for sepsis or endotoxemia.** The choice of antibiotics should be based on results of blood or hepatic biopsy cultures. If cultures are not available or the results are negative, antibiotic therapy should be aimed at Gram-negative anaerobes. Metronidazole, enrofloxacin, or an aminoglycoside with a penicillin or cephalosporin should be considered, based on the severity of the disease.

(7) **Coagulopathies should be treated** if hemorrhage is seen or if an invasive procedure is being considered.

    (a) **DIC** is treated with intravenous fluid administration, a transfusion of fresh whole blood (to replace coagulation factors and antithrombin III), and possible low doses of heparin and aspirin.

    (b) **Coagulation factor deficiency** requires a fresh whole blood transfusion. Animals with hepatic disease should not be given stored blood because it contains high concentrations of ammonia.

    (c) **Vitamin K deficiency** (and the subsequent low levels of vitamin K–dependent coagulation factors) requires parenteral administration of vitamin K.

2. **Drug-induced hepatic disease** can be predictable and dose-dependent, or the reaction can be idiosyncratic.

  a. **Anticonvulsants** (i.e., primidone, phenytoin, phenobarbital). Hepatic disease is more common with chronic primidone or primidone and phenytoin therapy.

    (1) **Clinical findings.** Clinical signs (e.g., anorexia, depression, weight loss, icterus, hepatic encephalopathy) and abnormal hepatic function test results occur in 6%–15% of dogs receiving chronic anticonvulsant therapy. The signs may be acute, or they may not occur until after months or years of treatment. Increased serum hepatic enzyme concentrations with no clinical signs of hepatic disease and normal hepatic function test results are often seen.

    (2) **Treatment**

      (a) If abnormal function is found in the absence of clinical signs, the anticonvulsant dose should be decreased and the liver reevaluated with laboratory tests and possibly a biopsy.

      (b) If abnormal liver function is found in the presence of clinical signs, medication should be withdrawn if possible and a liver biopsy taken. Other treatment should be based on results of the biopsy.

    (3) **Prognosis** is poor if abnormal hepatic function and clinical signs are present.

  b. **Acetaminophen** can cause methemoglobinemia and hepatic necrosis. **Clinical findings** may include dyspnea, cyanosis, depression, and vomiting. **Treatment** includes supportive care and the oral administration of n-acetylcysteine and vitamin C.

  c. **Thiacetarsamide** toxicity, if seen, usually occurs within 1 week of administration.

    (1) **Clinical findings.** Signs of hepatic disease (e.g., depression, anorexia, vomiting, icterus, diarrhea) or renal failure may be seen. Increased serum hepatic enzymes will occur with or without clinical signs, and bilirubinuria may be found.

    (2) **Treatment.** If icterus, persistent vomiting, or any two other clinical signs are present, thiacetarsamide treatment should be discontinued and resumed later. Treatment of the hepatopathy is supportive.

  d. **Glucocorticoids** (either endogenous, as a result of **hyperadrenocorticism,** or exogenous, as a result of **glucocorticoid administration)** can result in **steroid hepatopathy.** This disorder is very common in dogs but rare in cats. Regardless of the source, excess glucocorticoids can cause hepatic glycogen accumulation. In the case of iatrogenic glucocorticoid excess, there is great individual variability.

Some dogs develop a steroid hepatopathy after one dose of a short-acting gluco-corticoid; other dogs show no changes despite prolonged high-dose therapy.

   (1) **Diagnosis** is usually based on the history, results of the biochemical profile, and results of tests for hyperadrenocorticism. If the diagnosis remains in question, a liver biopsy will show vacuolization of hepatocytes.

   (a) **Clinical findings.** There are usually no signs of liver disease. Signs of glucocorticoid excess (e.g., polyuria and polydipsia, polyphagia, bilaterally symmetrical alopecia, abdominal distention) may be seen, or the animal may be clinically normal.

   (b) **Laboratory findings**

   (i) ALP and GGT concentrations are usually markedly increased; smaller increases in ALT and AST concentrations may be observed. Bilirubin is usually normal.

   (ii) Serum bile acid concentrations are usually normal to slightly increased, but ammonia concentrations are usually normal.

   (c) **Diagnostic imaging findings.** Radiographs reveal hepatomegaly. Ultrasonography usually shows increased echogenicity.

   (2) **Treatment** requires discontinuation of exogenous glucocorticoid administration or treatment of the spontaneous hyperadrenocorticism.

   e. **Mebendazole** can cause acute hepatic necrosis. The reaction is believed to be idiosyncratic; however, use of other, safer anthelminthics is preferred.

   f. **Methimazole** will cause hepatic disease in some cats being treated medically for hyperthyroidism.

   (1) **Clinical findings.** If toxicity is going to occur, clinical signs (e.g., anorexia, vomiting, depression, icterus) will usually be seen within the first 2 months of therapy. Serum hepatic enzymes are usually increased.

   (2) **Treatment** and **prognosis.** Supportive care and withdrawal of the medication enable a good prognosis.

3. **Infection**

   a. **Viral hepatitis** is rare in dogs and cats. Treatment is supportive.

   (1) **Canine adenovirus-1 infection** causes **infectious canine hepatitis,** but this disease has nearly been eliminated through vaccination.

   (2) **Canine herpesvirus infection** can cause acute, severe hepatitis and rapid death in neonates.

   (3) **FIP virus infection** can cause hepatic disease along with the pyogranulomatous vasculitis of other organs (see Chapter 49 V F).

   b. **Bacterial cholangiohepatitis.** Primary bacterial cholangiohepatitis is uncommon, but secondary bacterial infection is common, often as a result of ascending biliary or hematogenous infection. Chronic hepatitis, diabetes mellitus, hyperadrenocorticism, enteritis, hypoxia, necrosis, and immunosuppressive drug therapy may increase the risk of infection.

   (1) **Etiology.** GI bacteria (i.e., anaerobes such as *Bacteroides, Clostridium, Fusobacterium*) are the most common pathogens. Systemic infection with organisms such as *Leptospira* can also cause hepatitis.

   (2) **Diagnosis**

   (a) **Clinical findings** may include anorexia, fever, and, possibly, hepatomegaly and hepatic pain. If systemic infection is present, lymphadenopathy and signs of pneumonia, urinary tract infection, or bacterial endocarditis may also be seen.

   (b) **Laboratory findings.** ALT and AST concentrations are usually increased. ALP, GGT, and bilirubin levels may be increased. Neutrophilia and hyperglobulinemia may be noted.

   (c) **Diagnostic imaging findings.** Radiographs are usually unremarkable unless gas-forming organisms are responsible for the infection. Ultrasonography may reveal an echolucent area (i.e., abscess) or a thickened gall bladder (i.e., cholecystitis).

   (d) **Biopsy** and **culture** are necessary for definitive diagnosis.

(3) Treatment

    (a) Antibiotics are selected according to culture results. If the culture is negative, one of the following regimens is usually effective: an aminoglycoside and ampicillin, or cephalosporin and metronidazole, or enrofloxacin.

    (b) Surgery may be necessary to treat an abscess or severe cholecystitis.

  (4) Prognosis is variable.

c. Extrahepatic bacterial infection. Hepatic invasion by circulating bacteria, or endotoxins, fever, malnutrition, or hypoxia resulting from extrahepatic bacterial infection, can cause hepatic disease. **Clinical findings** include shock, thermoregulatory problems (fever or hypothermia), hypoglycemia, neutrophilia, and hyperbilirubinemia. **Treatment** is aimed at the primary infection.

d. Fungal hepatitis

  (1) Etiology. Histoplasmosis and coccidioidomycosis are the most common causes.

  (2) Diagnosis

    (a) Clinical findings may include icterus, hepatomegaly, and, possibly, ascites. Respiratory signs, vomiting and diarrhea, lymphadenopathy, and bone pain may also be present.

    (b) Laboratory findings. Serum hepatic enzyme concentrations are often increased. Diagnosis is based on finding fungal organisms on a fine-needle aspirate or biopsy.

  (3) Treatment. See Chapter 49.

e. Parasitic hepatitis is uncommon.

  (1) Etiology. Liver flukes (*Platynosomum* species), toxoplasmosis, and other systemic parasitic infections can cause hepatic disease.

  (2) Diagnosis

    (a) Clinical findings. With liver fluke infestation, there may be no clinical signs, or there may be signs of extrahepatic biliary obstruction (e.g., icterus, anorexia, vomiting).

    (b) Laboratory findings. Diagnosis is based on the presence of fluke ova in feces or liver biopsy.

  (3) Treatment is with praziquantel. Glucocorticoids may also be needed if concurrent eosinophilic cholangiohepatitis is present.

4. Hepatocutaneous syndrome (superficial necrolytic dermatitis) is characterized by a crusting, ulcerative dermatitis of the foot pads, mucocutaneous junctions, and pressure points in conjunction with a severe vacuolar hepatopathy. ALP and ALT levels are usually increased, and hepatic biopsy shows severe vacuolation and nodular regeneration but no necrosis or inflammation. Although some affected animals also have diabetes mellitus, the cause of this rare disorder is unknown, and the prognosis is usually poor.

5. Chronic hepatitis

a. Idiopathic chronic hepatitis is most common in middle-aged dogs but can occur at any age. The familial chronic hepatopathies may be forms of idiopathic chronic hepatitis, but these disorders are discussed in II B 5 b and c.

  (1) Etiology. No underlying cause has been identified. Idiopathic chronic hepatitis may be a specific disorder or a general immune-mediated reaction to many types of hepatic irritation and damage. Continuous hepatic damage leads to chronic inflammation.

  (2) Diagnosis

    (a) Clinical findings are generally those of chronic hepatic disease (i.e., anorexia, depression, weight loss, icterus, ascites, polyuria and polydipsia, neurologic signs). The signs may wax and wane or they may be acute. They are always progressive. Subclinical disease may be an incidental finding discovered while testing for another problem.

    (b) Laboratory findings. Serum hepatic enzyme and bilirubin concentrations are usually increased, especially ALT and AST. Liver function is abnormal.

(c) **Diagnostic imaging findings.** Radiographically, the liver is normal to small. Ascites may be present.

(d) **Biopsy findings** form the basis for diagnosis. Grossly, the liver may be normal or it may be small, firm, and irregular. Histopathologically, piecemeal and bridging necrosis, lymphocytic–plasmacytic infiltrate, and variable cirrhosis may be seen. Underlying diseases should also be ruled out. Biopsies should be repeated after therapy is initiated to assess the efficacy of the therapy.

(3) **Treatment**

(a) **Anti-inflammatory drugs.** Glucocorticoids alone or glucocorticoids and azathioprine are most commonly used. In theory, prednisolone rather than prednisone should be used because prednisolone does not require hepatic activation, but clinically there is no difference. If a positive response is seen, then the dose is slowly tapered.

(b) **Diet**

(i) **High-quality, restricted-protein food** should be given in frequent meals. The diet should contain sufficient protein to meet metabolic needs and prevent catabolism but not so much that it provides increased substrate for ammonia production. Use of a high-quality protein will also reduce the amount of nitrogenous wastes. Because increased aromatic amino acid concentrations play a role in hepatic encephalopathy, it is preferable to feed a protein source that is high in **branched-chain amino acids** (e.g., milk proteins and vegetable proteins, although some vegetable proteins are also less digestible).

(ii) **Moderate carbohydrate** and **fiber** should be included.

(iii) **Sodium** and **copper** should be minimized.

(iv) **Supplementation with B vitamins** (normally activated and stored in the liver), **vitamin C** (which increases urinary excretion of copper and is normally made by the liver), and **zinc** (which inhibits copper absorption) may also be useful. Fat-soluble vitamins, including vitamin K, are rarely needed.

(c) **Resolution of concurrent problems.** Concurrent problems, such as hepatic encephalopathy [see I B 1 c (3)], GI hemorrhage [see I B 1 c (5)], and coagulopathy [see I B 1 c (7)], should be treated.

(d) **Colchicine therapy** may help decrease collagen production and increase removal of fibrous tissue. It also has some anti-inflammatory effects. Vomiting and diarrhea may result but usually resolve with a temporary reduction in the dosage.

(e) **Reduction of ascites**

(i) **Paracentesis** should only be used if the ascites is compromising respiration or if removal of some of the fluid is needed prior to a diagnostic test. Fluid should be removed slowly while supporting the animal with parenteral fluids.

(ii) **Dietary salt restriction** should be initiated.

(iii) **Diuretics.** An **aldosterone inhibitor** (e.g., spironolactone) will minimize renal resorption of sodium. Other diuretics may be useful if other measures fail; however, care must be taken not to cause dehydration.

(f) **Ursodeoxycholic acid** may help decrease cholestasis and minimize hepatic damage by altering bile acids.

(g) **Antibiotics** may be helpful in treating any secondary infection.

b. **Chronic hepatitis in Doberman pinschers** is most common in female dogs and may actually be idiopathic chronic hepatitis, but a genetic component to the disease is suspected. The disease often progresses to cirrhosis.

(1) **Diagnosis**

(a) **Clinical findings.** The signs are those of chronic hepatitis.

(b) **Laboratory findings.** Serum hepatic enzymes and bilirubin levels are usually increased before clinical signs are seen.

(c) **Biopsy findings.** Diagnosis is based on biopsy results. Inflammation, piecemeal and bridging necrosis, varying amounts of cirrhosis, and possibly increased hepatic copper levels (whether the increase is primary or secondary is not known) are seen. Grossly, the liver is often small and nodular by the time of biopsy.

(2) **Treatment** is aimed at decreasing ongoing inflammation, preventing further copper accumulation (if present), preventing further fibrosis, and minimizing clinical signs [see I B 5 a (3)].

(3) **Prognosis** is usually poor because of the advanced stage of disease at the time of diagnosis. Yearly or twice yearly evaluation of serum hepatic enzymes in young Dobermans will help with early diagnosis and, therefore, early treatment.

c. **Chronic hepatitis in cocker spaniels** occurs mostly in young male dogs.

(1) **Diagnosis.** Clinical signs are usually of short duration, but the signs and test results are usually those seen with chronic hepatic disease. Ascites and hypoalbuminemia are very common. Serum bilirubin concentrations are usually normal. The liver is often small. Biopsies reveal chronic periportal inflammation and portal fibrosis.

(2) **Treatment** includes prednisone and supportive treatment based on the clinical signs.

(3) **Prognosis** is poor due to the severity of disease at the time of diagnosis.

d. **Copper storage disease**

(1) **Pathogenesis.** With copper storage disease, increased hepatic copper accumulation causes hepatocyte destruction. Note that this mechanism is different from those of other hepatobiliary disorders, such as idiopathic chronic hepatitis and cirrhosis, which cause primary hepatic damage with secondary copper accumulation. A hemolytic crisis can also occur if the excess copper is suddenly released into the circulation.

(a) **Bedlington terriers.** Copper storage disease is an autosomal recessive disorder; 66%–80% of Bedlington terriers are affected. Copper accumulates in hepatocyte lysosomes, which eventually become overloaded so that copper is released into the cytoplasm. When free in the cytoplasm, copper is toxic to the hepatocyte and alters cell permeability and function. Excess copper can be detected in affected dogs at a few months of age, and the accumulation continues until a peak level is reached at 5–6 years of age, after which copper levels decline.

(b) **West Highland White terriers.** There is no age-related increase in copper concentrations. Peak concentrations are usually seen at 6 months of age and then decrease.

(c) **Skye terriers.** Abnormal bile secretion occurs first, followed by copper accumulation later.

(d) **Doberman pinschers.** It is not known if excess copper accumulation is primary or secondary to the breed-associated chronic hepatitis.

(2) **Clinical findings.** Three clinical scenarios are seen in **Bedlington terriers:**

(a) Some dogs are asymptomatic but have increased ALT levels and excess copper in a hepatic biopsy.

(b) Some dogs show slowly progressive clinical signs beginning at middle-age. Anorexia, intermittent vomiting, weight loss, poor body condition, and ascites may be seen.

(c) Some young adults present with acute progressive signs of hepatic failure (e.g., anorexia, vomiting, icterus, possible hemolytic crisis). Serum hepatic enzyme and bilirubin concentrations are increased. Most affected dogs die despite aggressive supportive care.

(3) **Diagnosis**

(a) **Laboratory findings.** ALT concentrations are increased, and ALP and bilirubin may also be increased.

(b) **Biopsy findings.** Definitive diagnosis is based on copper quantitation or copper staining of a hepatic biopsy. A biopsy will also help rule out primary hepatic diseases with secondary copper accumulation. Because of the high incidence of the disease in Bedlington terriers, twice yearly evaluation of serum hepatic enzyme concentrations or hepatic biopsy at approximately 6 and 14 months of age will allow early diagnosis.

  (4) Treatment
- **(a) Reduction of hepatic copper accumulation** is accomplished through the administration of D-**penicillamine** or **2,2,2-tetramine** (to chelate copper), **zinc gluconate** or **zinc sulfate supplementation** (to help decrease copper absorption from the intestines), **vitamin C supplementation** (to increase urine copper excretion), and feeding of a **low-copper diet.**
- **(b) Symptomatic therapy** addresses clinical signs, which are similar to those of idiopathic chronic hepatitis [see I B 5 a (3)].

  (5) Prognosis varies with the severity of hepatic damage at the time of diagnosis.

6. Idiopathic hepatic fibrosis occurs most often in young dogs, especially German shepherds. The cause is unknown, and the clinical signs are similar to those of chronic hepatic disease. Diagnosis is made based on finding fibrosis without inflammation on biopsy.

7. Cirrhosis
  a. Etiology. The causes of cirrhosis are variable. Cirrhosis can occur as the end result of many chronic hepatic disorders.
  b. Diagnosis
- **(1) Clinical findings** are those of chronic hepatic disease (i.e., anorexia, depression, vomiting, weight loss, polyuria and polydipsia with later icterus, ascites, and neurologic signs).
- **(2) Laboratory findings** usually reveal normal to mildly increased serum hepatic enzymes and bilirubin. Liver function is abnormal.
- **(3) Biopsy findings.** Definitive diagnosis is based on finding fibrosis and regenerative nodules on biopsy. Grossly, the liver is often small, firm, and irregular.

  c. Treatment is similar to that discussed for idiopathic chronic hepatitis [see I B 5 a (3)].

8. Nodular hyperplasia causes no clinical signs but may be detected as an incidental finding when evaluating the liver for other possible hepatic disease. Because of the nodular appearance, a biopsy may be needed to differentiate nodular hyperplasia from hepatic adenoma or adenocarcinoma.

9. Feline cholangiohepatitis is a complex of diseases and is one of the most common hepatobiliary disorders of cats. The cause is unknown. Concurrent inflammatory bowel disease, pancreatitis, or extrahepatic bile duct obstruction is not uncommon.
  a. Forms. Three forms occur:
- **(1) Nonsuppurative or lymphocytic cholangiohepatitis,** the most common form, may be caused by an immune-mediated process, although toxins and concurrent disorders may also trigger the inflammation. It is most common in young to middle-aged cats.
- **(2) Suppurative or neutrophilic cholangiohepatitis** is most likely caused by bacterial infection. It is most common in older cats.
- **(3) Biliary cirrhosis** may be a late stage of the other two forms of the disease.

  b. Diagnosis
- **(1) Clinical findings** are those of hepatic disease (e.g., anorexia, vomiting, weight loss, depression). Fever may also be seen with the suppurative form.
- **(2) Laboratory findings** usually include marked increases in ALT concentrations, moderate increases in GGT concentrations, and elevations in the ALP and conjugated bilirubin levels.
- **(3) Biopsy findings.** Definitive diagnosis is based on finding predominately lymphocytic (nonsuppurative form) or neutrophilic (suppurative form) inflammation on a biopsy. Grossly, the liver is often large and rounded and may be smooth or irregular or nodular.

c. Treatment

(1) **Prednisone** is used to treat lymphocytic–plasmacytic cholangiohepatitis. Concurrent antibiotic treatment is often used.

(2) **Antibiotics** are used for 1–2 months to treat suppurative cholangiohepatitis. In the absence of culture results, ampicillin, cephalothin, or metronidazole can be used. Glucocorticoid therapy may also be needed later to fully resolve the disease.

(3) **Ursodeoxycholic acid** may help decrease cholestasis and minimize hepatic damage by altering bile composition.

(4) A **high-quality, restricted-protein diet** should be fed, to minimize ammonia and toxin production.

(5) **Symptomatic treatment** may be needed if hepatic encephalopathy develops [see I B 1 c (3)].

d. Prognosis

is guarded for cats with suppurative cholangitis/cholangiohepatitis, fair for cats with the lymphocytic form of the disease, and guarded for cats with the biliary form.

10. Hepatic lipidosis

a. **Secondary hepatic lipidosis** can be a sequelae to overnutrition, malnutrition, endocrine disorders (e.g., diabetes mellitus, hypothyroidism, "puppy hypoglycemia"), drugs, exogenous and endogenous toxins, hypoxia, and many other disorders. Diagnosis is usually based on identification of the primary disorder.

b. **Idiopathic hepatic lipidosis** is one of the most common hepatic disorders in cats.

(1) **Etiology.** The etiology is unknown. Historically, most affected cats have been obese and then became anorexic. Suggested mechanisms include increased mobilization of fatty acids, impaired fatty acid oxidation, impaired fatty acid transport, and altered nutritional status (e.g., protein, arginine, carnitine deficiencies).

(2) **Diagnosis**

(a) **Clinical findings** usually include anorexia, weight loss, vomiting, and icterus. Hepatomegaly may be palpable. Muscle wasting may be seen despite continued obesity.

(b) **Laboratory findings.** Serum bilirubin and all the hepatic enzyme concentrations are usually increased, ALP most markedly.

(c) **Diagnostic imaging findings.** Radiographs confirm hepatomegaly, and the liver is usually hyperechoic on ultrasound evaluation.

(d) **Biopsy findings** form the basis for definitive diagnosis. Grossly, the liver is often yellow and friable. Extrahepatic causes of secondary hepatic lipidosis should be ruled out.

(3) **Treatment**

(a) **Intravenous fluids** and correction of electrolyte abnormalities may be needed initially.

(b) **Aggressive feeding** of a high-quality food is the primary treatment, once a diagnosis is established. Tube feeding through a nasoesophageal or, optimally, a gastrostomy tube, may be necessary and should be continued until the cat resumes voluntary eating, which may take 2–8 weeks. **Metoclopramide** can be administered 30 minutes prior to feeding to control vomiting.

(4) **Prognosis** is guarded to fair, with 50%–75% of affected cats showing full recovery.

11. Vascular anomalies

a. **Portosystemic shunts** are abnormal vascular connections between the portal and systemic circulation that bypass the liver. Normally, hepatic blood flow brings nutrients and trophic hormones to the liver, and the liver removes bacterial products and toxins before the blood from the intestines reaches the general circulation. In animals with a shunt, hepatic nutrients are deficient or absent, so hepatic atrophy and dysfunction result. Because the blood bypasses the liver, toxins are not removed. Portosystemic shunts may be **acquired** (occurring secondary to chronic hepatic disease and portal hypertension) or **congenital.** Because treatment of acquired shunts is primarily aimed at treatment of the primary disease, the remainder of the discussion focuses on congenital shunts.

- **(1) Predisposition**
  - **(a) Dogs.** All breeds can be affected, but congenital shunts are more common in purebred than in mixed-breed dogs. A familial predisposition for single extrahepatic shunts is suspected in Lhasa apsos, miniature schnauzers, Shih Tzus, and Yorkshire terriers. Irish setters, Labrador retrievers, and other large-breed dogs are predisposed to intrahepatic shunts. Affected male dogs are also frequently cryptorchid. Most shunts are diagnosed in dogs younger than 1 year of age.
  - **(b) Cats.** Shunts are rare in cats, but when they do occur, they are seen more in mixed-breed cats. Left gastric vein shunts are most common. Most shunts are diagnosed in cats younger than 3 years of age.
- **(2) Diagnosis**
  - **(a) Clinical findings** are often intermittent and may be exacerbated by feeding. There may be a history of poor tolerance for anesthesia or of a prolonged recovery time.
    - **(i) Dogs.** Clinical signs may include depression, weight loss or poor growth, inappetence, vomiting and diarrhea, polyuria and polydipsia, and signs of hepatic encephalopathy. Ascites is rare.
    - **(ii) Cats.** Ptyalism, vomiting and diarrhea, and signs of hepatic encephalopathy are most common. Urate cystic calculi in a cat or a dog (other than a dalmatian) should also lead to a suspicion of hepatic dysfunction and the possibility of a shunt.
  - **(b) Laboratory findings.** A CBC is often normal or may show a mild nonregenerative anemia with microcytosis and target cells. Hepatic serum enzyme concentrations and bilirubin levels are usually normal, but BUN, albumin, glucose, and cholesterol levels may be low. Urate crystals may be seen on a urinalysis. Liver function is abnormal.
  - **(c) Diagnostic imaging findings.** The liver is usually small on radiographs. **Definitive diagnosis** is based on ultrasonography (occasionally), a contrast portogram (more common), or rectal scintigraphy.
  - **(d) Biopsy findings.** A hepatic biopsy will show hepatic atrophy, lobular collapse, and no inflammation if possible.
- **(3) Treatment** is by **surgical ligation.** Care must be taken to avoid causing excessive portal vein pressure. The liver should also be biopsied.
  - **(a)** Prior to surgery, the animal should receive supportive care (e.g., antibiotics, fluid and electrolyte therapy) and treatment for hepatic encephalopathy [see I B 1 c (3)].
  - **(b)** Following surgery, the animal should be monitored for signs of portal hypertension (e.g., endotoxic shock, abdominal pain, hemorrhagic diarrhea), which can be life-threatening. If these signs are seen, the ligature should be removed. Supportive care should be continued for 2–4 weeks postoperatively.
  - **(c) Complications** include severe portal hypertension, mild ascites (which usually resolves after a short time), and seizures (which are occasionally seen during the first few days following surgery and have an unknown pathogenesis).
- **(4) Prognosis**
  - **(a)** Medical treatment provides a poor long-term prognosis; therefore, the prognosis for animals with multiple or noncorrectable intrahepatic shunts is generally poor.
  - **(b)** Surgical treatment of dogs with a single extrahepatic shunt is generally very good if the animal survives the first few postoperative days. Surgical treatment of cats provides a fair prognosis.
  - **(c)** The prognosis is generally poor if seizures occur following surgery.
- **b. Microvascular dysplasia** is a congenital abnormality that results in microvascular shunting in the liver. Small-breed dogs and mixed-breed cats are most commonly affected.

(1) **Diagnosis.** Clinical signs and laboratory test results are similar to those of portosystemic shunts [see I B 11 a (2)]; however, the signs are milder, affected animals are usually older, and serum bile acid concentrations are only mildly increased. Diagnosis is based on hepatic biopsy findings after the possibility of a gross portosystemic shunt has been ruled out.

(2) **Treatment** is aimed at preventing or minimizing the signs of hepatic encephalopathy [see I B 1 c (3)].

c. **Arteriovenous fistulae** are rare connections between the hepatic artery and the portal vein, which cause portal hypertension and multiple acquired portosystemic shunts.

(1) **Diagnosis** is based on results of angiography or scintigraphy, or exploratory laparotomy.

(a) **Clinical findings** usually include the acute onset of ascites, vomiting and diarrhea, and depression in a young animal. Less common are neurologic signs, poor growth, polyuria and polydipsia, and abdominal pain. A continuous murmur (bruit) may be auscultable over the affected liver lobe.

(b) **Laboratory findings** are similar to those found with a portosystemic shunt [see I B 11 a (2)].

(2) **Treatment.** Surgical removal of the affected lobe and possible banding of the caudal vena cava is necessary. Medical treatment for hepatic encephalopathy [see I B 1 c (3)] may also be needed.

d. **Hepatic venous outflow obstruction** most commonly results from right-sided heart failure (e.g., congestive heart failure, pericardial disease, some congenital defects, cardiac neoplasia), but can also occur with caudal vena cava or hepatic vein compression. This obstruction can cause passive hepatic congestion and portal hypertension.

(1) **Diagnosis**

(a) **Clinical findings** include ascites (a modified transudate) and signs of the primary disease but no signs of hepatic disease.

(b) **Laboratory findings** usually reveal normal or slightly increased serum hepatic enzyme concentrations and normal serum bile acid concentrations.

(c) **Diagnostic imaging findings** via thoracic and abdominal radiographs, cardiac and abdominal ultrasound, and possibly contrast radiographs will identify the primary disease.

(2) **Treatment** is aimed at resolution or control of the primary disease.

12. **Hepatobiliary neoplasia** accounts for 1% of all canine neoplasms and 1%–3% of feline neoplasms, with metastatic lesions occurring twice as often as primary neoplasms. With the exception of lymphosarcoma, neoplasia is more common in older animals.

a. **Types**

(1) **Dogs. Hepatocellular adenomas** and **carcinomas** are the most common primary neoplasms. Lymphosarcoma and hemangiosarcoma are the most common metastatic lesions.

(2) **Cats. Bile duct carcinomas** and **adenomas** are the most common primary neoplasms. Lymphosarcoma is the most common metastatic neoplasm.

b. **Diagnosis**

(1) **Clinical findings.** Often the disease is advanced before clinical signs of hepatobiliary disease (e.g., anorexia, depression, vomiting, icterus) occur. If the liver lesions are metastatic, the clinical signs may result from the primary tumor.

(2) **Laboratory findings**

(a) With primary hepatocellular neoplasms, ALT, AST, and ALP levels are often markedly increased. Hyperbilirubinemia, hypoalbuminemia, and hypoglycemia may also be seen.

   (b) With bile duct neoplasia, ALP and GGT concentrations are usually increased more than ALT and AST concentrations. Hyperbilirubinemia is also seen.

   (c) With metastatic disease, serum hepatic enzyme concentrations are usually normal to slightly increased.

  (3) Diagnostic imaging findings. The liver may be enlarged or may have irregular margins on radiographs. One or more nodules or diffuse disease may be seen on ultrasonograms.

  (4) Biopsy findings. Definitive diagnosis is based on a needle aspirate or biopsy.

 c. Treatment

  (1) Localized hepatomas or **hepatocellular carcinomas** should be surgically resected.

  (2) Biliary carcinomas should be resected, if possible, but resection is often difficult.

  (3) Metastatic lymphosarcoma or **hemangiosarcoma** may be treated with chemotherapy (see Chapter 48 IV A 6 e, 7 d, C 3 f). Chemotherapy for metastatic disease is only palliative.

 d. Prognosis is good following resection of a local hepatoma or hepatocellular carcinoma and guarded with multiple lesions or biliary carcinoma.

13. Extrahepatic bile duct obstruction

 a. Etiology. Extrahepatic bile duct obstruction can result from disorders of the pancreas, duodenum, or the bile duct itself. Inflammation, neoplasia, choleliths, fluke infestation in cats (see I B 3 e), foreign bodies, or trauma can cause the obstruction. Pancreatitis is the most common cause of extrahepatic bile duct obstruction.

 b. Diagnosis

  (1) Clinical findings. The primary clinical signs are usually those of the underlying disorder. In addition, clinical signs referable to the bile duct obstruction may include depression, vomiting, diarrhea, anorexia, weight loss, icterus, abdominal pain, and acholic feces.

  (2) Laboratory findings. SAP and SGGT concentrations are usually increased to a greater extent than the SALT and SAST concentrations. Bilirubin is often also increased, and hypercholesterolemia may be seen in cats. Other findings vary with the underlying disorder.

  (3) Diagnostic imaging findings by hepatic ultrasound include enlargement of the gall bladder and bile duct distention. The cause of the obstruction may also be seen (i.e., choleliths, flukes, mass).

 c. Treatment

  (1) Surgery is usually necessary, except in cases of pancreatitis, liver flukes, and some cases of cholecystitis.

  (2) Medical therapy

   (a) Pancreatitis usually responds to medical therapy (see II B 1 c).

   (b) Flukes may be eliminated with praziquantel treatment.

   (c) Mild cases of cholecystitis (see I B 14) may respond to antibiotics.

  (3) Supportive care is also needed.

 d. Prognosis varies with the underlying disease and the severity of the obstruction. The prognosis is guarded if **bile peritonitis** occurs following rupture of the gall bladder or bile duct. Progressive clinical signs, ascites, and shock may be seen. A diagnostic abdominocentesis can be helpful if bile peritonitis is suspected.

14. Cholecystitis is uncommon in dogs and cats.

 a. Etiology. Cholecystitis can result from an ascending biliary infection or bacteremia/septicemia. *Escherichia coli* is the most common pathogen.

 b. Diagnosis

  (1) Clinical findings vary with the severity of the disease. With mild cholecystitis, fever, intermittent vomiting, and mild abdominal pain may occur. With acute severe disease, anorexia, fever, vomiting, diarrhea, severe abdominal pain, icterus, and shock can be seen. Choleliths and bile stasis may also be present.

(2) **Laboratory findings** commonly include neutrophilia with a shift toward immaturity, hypoproteinemia, azotemia, increased serum hepatic enzymes, and hyperbilirubinemia. Diagnosis is confirmed by bacterial culture of bile. Bile peritonitis indicates biliary rupture.

(3) **Diagnostic imaging findings**

(a) Radiographs may show loss of abdominal detail, an emphysematous gall bladder, or radiodense choleliths.

(b) Ultrasound often shows an enlarged gall bladder and distended bile ducts, thickening of the gall bladder wall, and bile sludging. Choleliths may also be seen.

c. **Treatment**

(1) Mild disease can be treated with antibiotics (e.g., a cephalosporin and an aminoglycoside, ampicillin and enrofloxacin) and supportive care. The animal should be closely monitored, and surgery should be considered if improvement is not seen.

(2) Severe disease requires supportive care and prompt surgery to remove the gall bladder and obtain bile cultures. Postoperative antibiotic therapy should be based on the culture results.

d. **Prognosis** is fair with mild disease but guarded to poor with severe disease. **Complications** can include biliary rupture with subsequent bile and septic peritonitis.

15. **Choleliths** are rare in dogs and cats. They are most common in older, female, small-breed dogs.

a. **Etiology.** The cause of choleliths is often unknown, but they may result from infection, bile stasis, or altered bile composition.

b. **Diagnosis**

(1) **Clinical findings.** If the choleliths are sterile and are not obstructing bile flow, there may be no clinical signs. If there is infection, then vomiting, fever, and abdominal pain may be seen. If there is biliary obstruction, the animal will be icteric. Acholic feces are suggestive of complete bile duct obstruction.

(2) **Laboratory findings** are usually similar to those of extrahepatic bile duct obstruction [see I B 13 b (2)].

(3) **Diagnostic imaging findings.** Diagnosis is based on finding choleliths on abdominal radiographs or ultrasonograms. Radiodense choleliths will be apparent radiographically; ultrasonography is necessary to detect radiopaque choleliths, which are hyperechoic with a hypoechoic shadow.

c. **Treatment** requires surgery, especially if the animal is showing clinical signs of disease. A bile sample should be cultured.

d. **Prognosis** is usually good.

II. EXOCRINE PANCREATIC DISORDERS

A. Clinical evaluation

1. **Predisposition**

a. **Species and breed.** All breeds of dogs and cats can develop pancreatic disease, but certain breeds are at increased risk. For example:

(1) Exocrine pancreatic insufficiency (EPI) is more common in German shepherds.

(2) Pancreatic neoplasia and EPI are rare in cats.

b. **Age.** Middle-aged to older dogs and older cats are more prone to pancreatitis and pancreatic neoplasia.

c. **Diet.** A high-fat diet may contribute to the development of pancreatitis.

d. **Medications.** Azathioprine, furosemide, L-asparaginase, sulfa drugs, tetracycline, possibly glucocorticoids, and others may play a role in the development of pancreatitis.

2. Clinical signs

a. Vomiting may occur with pancreatitis or pancreatic neoplasia (as a result of pancreatic, hepatic, and duodenal irritation or secondary bile duct obstruction).

b. Anorexia and **abdominal pain** are also common with pancreatitis and pancreatic neoplasia.

c. Fever may be seen with pancreatitis because of pancreatic inflammation or secondary bacteremia/septicemia.

d. Diarrhea may be seen with EPI or pancreatitis.

    (1) In the case of EPI, the diarrhea originates in the small bowel as a result of maldigestion and possible secondary bacterial overgrowth.

    (2) In the case of pancreatitis, colitis can result from the anatomical proximity of the transverse colon to the pancreas, but small bowel diarrhea can also result from duodenal irritation.

e. Weight loss may be seen with EPI (because of the resulting maldigestion) or pancreatic neoplasia (because of anorexia or cancer cachexia).

f. Polyphagia may occur with EPI as an attempt to compensate for lost nutrients and calories.

g. Icterus can be a complication of pancreatitis if extrahepatic bile duct obstruction occurs.

h. Petechiae can be a complication of pancreatitis if DIC occurs.

3. Physical examination

a. Animals with EPI are often thin, alert, and active. They may have a dull haircoat.

b. Animals with pancreatitis are usually of normal weight or obese. They are lethargic or depressed.

4. Diagnostic tests

a. Laboratory studies

    (1) A **CBC** may show neutrophilia with a shift toward immaturity in an animal with severe pancreatitis, or it may be normal in milder cases.

    (2) A **serum biochemical profile** may show increased amylase, lipase, or both (suggestive of pancreatitis or neoplasm) or it may be normal. Other biochemical abnormalities may also be seen with pancreatitis [see II B 1 b (2) (a)].

    (3) Serum trypsin-like immunoreactivity (STLI) test. The STLI test, discussed in Chapter 41 IV A 5 a (5) (c), uses serum trypsinogen and trypsin concentration as an indicator of functional pancreatic exocrine tissue. STLI will be low in dogs affected with EPI and high in dogs with pancreatitis.

b. Imaging studies

    (1) Radiography. Abdominal radiographs may be normal or they may reveal:

        (a) Widening of the angle between the pylorus and the duodenum (suggestive of pancreatitis)

        (b) Duodenal gas pockets (suggestive of pancreatitis)

        (c) Loss of detail in the cranial abdomen (as a result of focal peritonitis caused by pancreatitis)

        (d) Poor abdominal contrast (as a result of loss of intra-abdominal fat in animals with EPI)

    (2) Ultrasonography may show an enlarged nonhomogeneous or hypoechoic pancreas (suggestive of acute pancreatitis or neoplasia) and, in the case of acute pancreatitis, a small amount of free fluid in the cranial abdomen.

c. Biopsy and histopathology may be needed to differentiate pancreatic neoplasia from chronic pancreatitis and fibrosis.

B. | Specific disorders

1. Pancreatitis is most common in overweight, middle-aged to older dogs. Females may be somewhat predisposed. Pancreatitis is uncommon in cats, but it may be seen in older animals, often in conjunction with cholangiohepatitis.

a. Etiology. Acute pancreatitis occurs when digestive enzymes are activated within the pancreas and overwhelm enzyme inhibitors (e.g., α_1-macroglobulin, α_1-antitrypsin, trypsin inhibitor). Local autodigestion occurs, and additional enzymes are released into the circulation where they can damage other tissues (e.g., heart, lungs). Pancreatitis may be initiated by obesity, a high-fat diet, hyperlipidemia, medications (see II A 1 d), ischemia, trauma, bile reflux, pancreatic duct obstruction, or infection. Often the initiating cause is not known.

b. Diagnosis of pancreatitis can be difficult, especially in cats. A presumptive diagnosis of pancreatitis may be made if there are appropriate clinical signs in conjunction with leukocytosis, an increase in serum lipase or amylase (two times normal in cats, three times normal in dogs), loss of cranial abdominal detail and widening of the pyloroduodenal angle on radiographs, or an enlarged nonhomogenous or hypoechogenic pancreas on ultrasonograms.

(1) Clinical signs

(a) Dogs may exhibit vomiting, anorexia, depression, fever, and diarrhea. Shock may be seen in severe cases.

(b) Cats most commonly exhibit lethargy and anorexia. Vomiting is uncommon. Concurrent cholangiohepatitis is often seen.

(c) Fever, dehydration, and cranial abdominal pain (common in dogs, uncommon in cats) may be found. Icterus, petechiae, cardiac arrhythmias, or respiratory distress may be seen as complications of severe cases.

(2) Laboratory findings

(a) In addition to increased serum lipase or amylase levels, azotemia, hypo- or hyperglycemia, hypoalbuminemia, mild hypocalcemia, increased serum hepatic enzyme concentrations, and hyperbilirubinemia may be seen.

(b) A CBC commonly reveals hemoconcentration and a neutrophilia with a possible shift toward immaturity.

(c) STLI concentrations are increased early in the course of pancreatitis.

(d) If abdominocentesis is performed in the patient with localized loss of abdominal detail, cytologic evaluation is usually consistent with a chemical (sterile) peritonitis.

c. Treatment

(1) Mild pancreatitis

(a) During the first 48–72 hours, oral food and water should be withheld to minimize additional pancreatic secretion. Fluids should be administered intravenously to correct dehydration, maintain hydration and electrolyte balance, and to facilitate excretion of circulating enzymes.

(b) When there has been no vomiting for 24–48 hours, small amounts of water can be given orally. The following day, small amounts of a high-carbohydrate, low-fat, low-protein diet can be given if the animal does well with the oral water. Diets that are high in fat or protein should be avoided because they increase pancreatic secretion.

(c) Long-term feeding of a high-carbohydrate, low-fat, moderate-protein diet may be needed to prevent recurrence.

(2) Severe pancreatitis. If the clinical signs fail to resolve with treatment for severe pancreatitis or keep recurring when food is reintroduced, then a pancreatic abscess or neoplasm should be considered.

(a) Food and water should be withheld for up to 5 days. Fluids should be administered intravenously during this time.

(b) When the clinical signs have resolved and there has been no vomiting for 24–48 hours, oral water and food are then slowly reintroduced as discussed for mild pancreatitis. If oral feeding cannot be resumed after 5 days, total parenteral nutrition or enteral nutrition should be considered.

(c) If hypoproteinemia becomes severe, plasma or dextran administration may be needed. Plasma will provide added enzyme inhibitors to help inactivate circulating enzymes.

(d) If the abdominal pain is severe, analgesics that have minimal effects on the pancreas (e.g., meperidine or butorphanol) may be helpful.

(e) Secondary bacterial infection of the damaged pancreas should be treated with parenteral antibiotics (e.g., ampicillin, cephalothin, trimethoprim/sulfonamide).

    (f) If hyperglycemia is accompanied by persistent glucosuria, treatment with regular (crystalline) insulin may be needed on a short-term basis.

    (g) Antiemetics should be avoided, if possible. If severe vomiting necessitates their use, a centrally acting antiemetic (e.g., chlorpromazine, prochlorperazine) should be used.

    (h) Glucocorticoids should be used only on an acute basis when shock accompanies severe pancreatitis.

  d. Prognosis

    (1) Mild pancreatitis. The prognosis is generally good, although recurrence is possible.

    (2) Severe pancreatitis or **pancreatitis with complications.** The prognosis is guarded. **Complications** of severe pancreatitis may include transient or severe enterohepatic bile duct obstruction, DIC, cardiac arrhythmias, pulmonary edema, acute renal failure, sepsis, permanent diabetes mellitus, and EPI.

2. Pancreatic abscesses are rare but can develop as a sequela to severe pancreatitis. Clinical findings and initial treatment are the same as those discussed for pancreatitis (see II B 1), but the signs fail to resolve with treatment or recur whenever oral feeding is reintroduced. Ultrasound may show a pancreatic mass or a focal hypoechoic area in the pancreas. Definitive diagnosis is usually made at surgery or on the basis of a pancreatic biopsy. Treatment usually requires surgical drainage of the abscess and continued antibiotic therapy. The prognosis is guarded, even with surgery.

3. Pancreatic adenocarcinomas are rare in dogs and cats. They are seen more commonly in older animals and Airedale terriers.

  a. Diagnosis. Clinical, laboratory, and radiographic findings are similar to those of pancreatitis (see II B 1) or extrahepatic bile duct obstruction (see I B 13). Ultrasound may show a mass if the tumor is large. Definitive diagnosis requires biopsy because grossly, chronic pancreatitis and pancreatic neoplasia can look similar.

  b. Treatment. Surgical excision is required but complete resection is usually difficult, due to the location, extent of local invasion, and high incidence of metastasis.

  c. Prognosis is poor because extensive local invasion or metastasis has usually occurred by the time diagnosis is made.

4. EPI is heritable in German shepherds, but an idiopathic form can occur in any breed. Affected German shepherds are usually diagnosed by 2 years of age. Affected dogs of other breeds are usually middle aged at the time of diagnosis. EPI is rare in cats.

  a. Etiology. EPI most commonly results from pancreatic acinar atrophy, but the cause of the atrophy is unknown. Congenital abnormalities, nutritional abnormalities, ischemia, duct obstruction, and immune-mediated mechanisms have all been proposed. Uncommon causes of EPI are congenital pancreatic hypoplasia and chronic recurrent pancreatitis.

  b. Pathogenesis. The deficiency of pancreatic enzymes in animals with EPI results in maldigestion and secondary small intestinal mucosal abnormalities. Small intestinal bacterial overgrowth (see Chapter 41 IV B 11) is also common secondary to EPI.

  c. Diagnosis

    (1) Clinical findings include weight loss despite a good or ravenous appetite. Small bowel diarrhea or soft feces, flatulence, borborygmus, coprophagy, pica, and a dull haircoat may also be seen. Lethargy, depression, anorexia, and fever are not typically seen.

    (2) Laboratory findings. Results of a CBC, serum biochemical profile, urinalysis, and fecal tests for parasites will be normal. Diagnosis is based on finding a **low STLI concentration.** Other tests of GI function [see Chapter 41 IV A 5 a (5)] may also be used to document maldigestion but are less accurate or more cumbersome or costly.

    (3) Diagnostic imaging findings. Radiographs will be normal or will only show poor abdominal detail because of loss of intraabdominal fat.

d. Treatment

    (1) Pancreatic enzyme supplementation. In dogs, powdered enzymes administered in the food or in gelatin capsules are more effective than tablet forms.

    (2) Maintenance diet. If clinical signs persist despite enzyme supplementation, then a highly digestible or a low-fat diet should be fed. High-fat diets should be avoided. If a treated dog fails to gain weight, considerations should be given to caloric supplementation with medium-chain triglyceride oil.

    (3) Metronidazole or **tylosin** treatment should be instituted if small intestinal bacterial overgrowth is present.

e. Prognosis is very good with treatment. A small intestinal biopsy should be obtained to rule out concurrent intestinal disease if the clinical signs do not promptly resolve with treatment.

DIRECTIONS: Each of the numbered items or incomplete statements in this section is followed by answers or by completions of the statement. Select the ONE numbered answer or completion that is BEST in each case.

1. Which one of the following statements regarding exocrine pancreatic insufficiency (EPI) due to pancreatic atrophy is true?

(1) It occurs mostly in German Shepherds.
(2) It is associated with diabetes mellitus.
(3) It is most common in older dogs.
(4) It results in diarrhea and inappetence.
(5) It is usually the result of chronic recurrent pancreatitis.

2. The most common clinical coagulopathy seen in dogs and cats with hepatic disease is:

(1) vitamin K deficiency.
(2) disseminated intravascular coagulation (DIC).
(3) decreased coagulation factor concentrations.
(4) thrombocytopenia.
(5) platelet dysfunction.

3. A dog has a mild increase in serum alanine aminotransferase (ALT) and serum alkaline phosphatase (ALP) levels, hepatomegaly, and ascites. The ascitic fluid has 2.9 g/dl of protein and 2400 cells/μl. The most likely cause of the ascites is:

(1) hypoalbuminemia.
(2) prehepatic portal hypertension.
(3) hepatic portal hypertension.
(4) posthepatic portal hypertension.

4. Which set of findings is most characteristic of severe cirrhosis?

(1) Markedly increased serum alanine aminotransferase (ALT) levels, mildly increased serum alkaline phosphatase (ALP) and bilirubin levels, and normal serum bile acid concentrations
(2) Mildly increased ALT levels, markedly increased ALP levels, moderately increased bilirubin levels, and normal serum bile acid concentrations
(3) Markedly increased ALT levels, mildly increased ALP and bilirubin levels, and mildly increased serum bile acid concentrations
(4) Normal ALT, ALP, and bilirubin levels and mildly increased serum bile acid concentrations
(5) Normal ALT, ALP, bilirubin, and serum bile acid concentrations

5. A 5-year-old, obese, domestic shorthair cat is brought to the clinic. The owner reports that the cat's appetite rapidly decreased approximately 2 weeks ago. On physical examination, the only abnormalities found are icterus and hepatomegaly. The most likely diagnosis is:

(1) steroid hepatopathy.
(2) hepatic necrosis.
(3) copper storage disease.
(4) hepatic lipidosis.
(5) cirrhosis.

DIRECTIONS: Each of the numbered items or incomplete statements in this section is negatively phrased, as indicated by a capitalized word such as NOT, LEAST, or EXCEPT. Select the ONE numbered answer or completion that is BEST in each case.

6. Which of the following is NOT commonly used in the treatment of hepatic encephalopathy?

(1) Withholding of food
(2) Oral dextrose
(3) Cleansing enemas
(4) Oral lactulose
(5) Neomycin

7. All of the following statements regarding steroid hepatopathy are true EXCEPT:

(1) It can occur after only one dose of glucocorticoids.
(2) It often results in vomiting.
(3) It is rare in cats.
(4) It often causes hepatomegaly.
(5) It does not usually cause significant hepatic dysfunction.

8. Clinical signs of a congenital portosystemic shunt may include all of the following EXCEPT:

(1) seizures.
(2) polyuria and polydipsia.
(3) icterus.
(4) depression.
(5) poor growth.

9. All of the following statements regarding pancreatitis are true EXCEPT:

(1) A high-fat diet and certain medications may initiate pancreatitis.
(2) The disease is most common in older female dogs.
(3) Common clinical signs in dogs include anorexia, vomiting, and diarrhea.
(4) Common clinical signs in cats include anorexia and vomiting.
(5) Treatment of pancreatitis includes withholding oral food and water, intravenous fluid therapy, and, possibly, antibiotic therapy.

1. The answer is 1 [II B 4]. Exocrine pancreatic insufficiency (EPI) due to pancreatic atrophy is most common in German Shepherds as a heritable disorder. Although chronic recurrent pancreatitis and fibrosis can also be a cause of EPI, this occurrence is rare. Clinical signs of pancreatic atrophy are usually seen by 1 year of age and often include weight loss, a ravenous appetite, and diarrhea or soft feces. Concurrent diabetes mellitus is not usually seen.

2. The answer is 2 [I A 4 f]. Vitamin K deficiency, disseminated intravascular coagulation (DIC), decreased coagulation factor concentrations, and platelet dysfunction can all occur with hepatobiliary disease, but DIC is the most common coagulopathy seen in dogs and cats.

3. The answer is 4 [I A 4 g;Table 10-1]. Ascitic fluid with 2.9 g/dl of protein and 2400 cells/μl is a modified transudate. Modified transudates are most common with posthepatic portal hypertension. In dogs and cats, right-sided heart failure is the most common cause of posthepatic portal hypertension. If ascites is present as a result of hypoalbuminemia or prehepatic portal hypertension, the fluid is usually a transudate (i.e., it has a lower protein concentration and fewer cells). Hepatic portal hypertension will occasionally cause a modified transudate, but then greater increases in serum alanine aminotransferase (ALT) and serum alkaline phosphatase (ALP) levels (as a result of inflammation or neoplasia) or a small liver (as a result of cirrhosis) would be expected.

4. The answer is 4 [I B 7 b]. Severe cirrhosis results in liver dysfunction, so bile acid concentrations will always be increased. However, serum alanine aminotransferase (ALT), serum alkaline phosphatase (ALP), and bilirubin levels are often normal or only mildly increased because many of the hepatocytes (which would leak ALT) and bile ducts (which would produce ALP) have been replaced with fibrous tissue.

5. The answer is 4 [I B 10 b]. Cats with hepatic lipidosis are often obese, have a history of inappetence and anorexia followed by icterus, and have hepatomegaly. Steroid hepatopathy is rare in cats. Hepatic necrosis would cause more acute clinical signs. Copper storage disease has not been reported in cats. Cirrhosis could cause anorexia and icterus, but the liver is usually small, not enlarged.

6. The answer is 2 [I B 1 c (3)]. Food should be withheld in an animal with acute hepatic encephalopathy to minimize the amount of protein presented to the colon. Metabolism of proteins in the colon can lead to the formation of ammonia and other toxins, which animals with impaired liver function are unable to handle. Cleansing enemas help remove bacteria and proteins that are present in the colon. Neomycin also helps reduce bacterial numbers. Lactulose acidifies the colon so that ammonia stays in the form of ammonium, which is nonabsorbable. Dextrose may be administered in an animal with hepatic encephalopathy if the animal is also hypoglycemic, but dextrose is usually given parenterally to these patients.

7. The answer is 2 [I B 2 d]. Steroid hepatopathy, a fairly common disorder in dogs and a rare disorder in cats, can occur as a result of exogenous glucocorticoid administration (as little as one dose in some dogs) or with spontaneous hyperadrenocorticism. Although hepatomegaly and increased serum alkaline phosphatase (ALP) levels are common, significant liver dysfunction and clinical signs of hepatic disease are rare. Vomiting is not a clinical finding in animals with steroid hepatopathy.

8. The answer is 3 [I B 11 a (2) (a)]. Icterus does not occur with a congenital portosystemic shunt. Instead, most clinical signs seen in animals with a shunt occur as a result of hepatic dysfunction. Seizures and depression (i.e., hepatic encephalopathy) occur because of decreased hepatic removal of ammonia and other toxins; polyuria and polydipsia occur because of hepatic encephalopathy or because of decreased hepatic production of urea for the renal medullary concentration gradient; and poor growth occurs because of decreased hepatic production of proteins and other substances and possible concurrent anorexia, vomiting, or diarrhea.

9. The answer is 4 [II B 1]. Although vomiting can occur with pancreatitis in cats, it is a rare occurrence. Anorexia and lethargy are more commonly seen in cats. Pancreatitis can be caused by many things, including consumption of a high-fat diet or administration of certain medications. The disease is most common in older dogs, and females may have a slightly increased incidence. Anorexia, vomiting, and diarrhea are common signs of pancreatitis in dogs. Treatment of pancreatitis in both species includes withholding oral food and water, intravenous fluid therapy, and possibly antibiotic administration.

Chapter 43

Urinary Tract Diseases and Fluid and Electrolyte Disorders

PART I: URINARY TRACT DISEASES

I. INTRODUCTION

A. Definitions

1. **Renal failure** is the clinical syndrome that results when excretory and renal endocrine function cannot maintain homeostasis; that is, the glomerular filtration rate (GFR) is less than or equal to 25% of normal.

2. **Azotemia** is an **increased concentration of nonprotein nitrogenous wastes** (i.e., urea, creatinine) **in the blood.** In addition to renal failure, azotemia can result from nonrenal and nonurinary influences. Localizing the source of the azotemia is critical in formulating appropriate diagnostic and therapeutic plans. In order for the following guidelines to apply, urine specific gravity [see Part I: I B 3 c (1)] must be measured before fluid therapy is initiated.

   a. **Prerenal azotemia** occurs when renal blood flow is reduced (e.g., as a result of dehydration, hemorrhage, heart failure, hypoadrenocorticism). If the decrease in renal blood flow is not severe or prolonged, the azotemia is rapidly reversible with fluid therapy. Prerenal azotemia may be superimposed on renal or postrenal azotemia. The **key diagnostic feature** is the presence of azotemia with a urine specific gravity that is greater than or equal to 1.030 in dogs or greater than or equal to 1.035 in cats.

   b. **Renal azotemia** occurs when primary (parenchymal) renal disease has reduced the GFR to less than or equal to 25% of normal (i.e., chronic or acute renal failure is present). The **key diagnostic feature** is the presence of mild to marked azotemia with a urine specific gravity that is less than 1.030 in dogs and less than 1.035 in cats. Often, the urine specific gravity is in the isosthenuric range (i.e., 1.007–1.015).

   c. **Postrenal azotemia** results from lower urinary tract obstruction or a rent or rupture of the urinary tract. The **key diagnostic feature** is the presence of a mild to marked azotemia, a variable urine specific gravity, and clinical signs of obstruction (e.g., a distended, turgid urinary bladder) or urine leakage (e.g., a distended, fluid-filled abdomen or lack of bladder filling or urination following fluid therapy).

3. **Uremia** is azotemia accompanied by the systemic signs of renal failure.

B. Clinical evaluation

1. **Clinical signs**

   a. **Urinary tract dysfunction.** Specific signs of urinary tract dysfunction include polyuria, polydipsia, hematuria, dysuria, pollakiuria, stranguria, and urinary incontinence. Nonspecific signs may include anorexia, lethargy, weakness, and weight loss.

   b. **Renal disease** is more likely than lower urinary tract (i.e., bladder, urethra) disease to result in systemic signs.

      (1) Signs include anemia (advanced chronic renal failure), polyuria and polydipsia (which usually develop when two-thirds of the nephrons are nonfunctional), subcutaneous edema or body cavity effusions resulting from hypoalbuminemia (due to glomerular disease), and ophthalmologic signs secondary to hypertension (e.g., retinal edema, detachment, hemorrhage, and vessel tortuosity).

(2) Uremia may result in gastrointestinal (GI) signs (e.g., vomiting, diarrhea, melena), halitosis, oral and lingual ulcers, and (rarely) tongue tip necrosis.

(3) Fibrous osteodystrophy (rubber jaw) may develop in juvenile dogs.

2. Physical examination

a. Renal palpation may reveal small and irregular kidneys (e.g., chronic renal failure) or enlarged and sometimes painful kidneys (e.g., acute renal failure, pyelonephritis, neoplasia, hydronephrosis).

b. Bladder palpation may reveal turgid distention, uroliths, or wall thickening.

c. Rectal palpation of the prostate and pelvic urethra can detect pain and abnormalities in size and shape.

3. Laboratory studies

a. Complete blood count (CBC)

(1) **Anemia** (normocytic, normochromic nonregenerative) frequently accompanies advanced chronic renal failure (CRF).

(2) **Leukocytosis** can be associated with pyelonephritis and acute prostatitis.

b. Serum biochemical profile

(1) **Urea** and **creatinine levels** are elevated (i.e., azotemia is present) if the GFR is less than or equal to 25% of normal.

(a) Urea levels can also be increased by high-protein diets, tissue catabolism, GI hemorrhage, and drugs (e.g., corticosteroids) and decreased by low-protein diets, hepatic failure, and drugs (e.g., anabolic steroids).

(b) Creatinine is minimally affected by nonrenal variables and is a more reliable estimate of GFR.

(2) **Phosphorus, potassium,** and **amylase elevations** can result from decreased renal excretion.

(3) **Hypoalbuminemia** may result from urine protein loss associated with glomerular disease.

c. Urinalysis

(1) **Specific gravity.** Urine specific gravity can range from 1.001–1.070 in dogs and 1.001–1.080 in cats. There is no normal urine specific gravity; it is influenced by renal function, diet, and drinking habits. The ability to dilute (< 1.007) or concentrate (> 1.030 in dogs; > 1.035 in cats) requires normal tubular function.

(2) **Dipstick analysis**

(a) **Color.** Yellow to amber and clear is normal urine color.

(i) Red or red-brown urine can result from erythrocytes, hemoglobin, or myoglobin.

(ii) Yellow-brown urine can be caused by bilirubinuria.

(b) **Turbidity.** Increased turbidity can be associated with cells, crystals, mucus, or debris.

(c) **pH.** Normal canine and feline urine is acidic with a pH of 5.0–7.5. Urine pH can be altered by diet, drugs, acid–base status, and urinary tract infections (UTIs) caused by urease-producing bacteria.

(d) **Glucose** is not normally present in urine. Glucosuria is associated with diabetes mellitus, stress hyperglycemia in cats, glucose-containing intravenous fluid therapy, and (rarely) primary renal glucosuria.

(e) **Ketones** are not normally present in urine. Ketonuria is associated with diabetic ketoacidosis, prolonged fasting or starvation, a low-carbohydrate diet, persistent fever, and persistent hypoglycemia. Urine dipsticks react mostly with the ketone acetoacetate and, to a lesser extent, acetate. They do not detect β-hydroxybutyrate.

(f) **Bilirubin.** Small amounts of bilirubin may be present in the urine of normal dogs but not cats. Significant amounts of bilirubin in canine urine and any bilirubin in feline urine can be associated with liver disease or excessive erythrocyte degradation.

(g) **Urobilinogen.** Small amounts of urobilinogen are normally present in the urine. Complete absence of urobilinogen on repeat testing can be associated with biliary duct obstruction.

(h) Occult blood. The urine dipstick reacts with erythrocytes, hemoglobin, and myoglobin. Differentiation is based on a urine sediment examination, discoloration of plasma, and clinical signs. (See Chapter 33.)

(i) Leukocytes. The urine dipstick is relatively insensitive to the presence of leukocytes.

(3) Sediment examination

(a) Red blood cells (RBCs). Low numbers of erythrocytes are normal and depend on the method of collection. Free-flow (voiding) may result in 0–8 erythrocytes per high-power field; catheterization, 0–5 erythrocytes per high-power field; and cystocentesis, 0–3 erythrocytes per high-power field. **Hematuria** (i.e., excessive numbers of RBCs in urine) may be microscopic (not grossly visible) or macroscopic (grossly visible).

(b) White blood cells (WBCs). Small numbers of neutrophils are normal (0–5 WBC per high-power field). **Pyuria** (i.e., increased numbers of WBCs in urine) can be associated with infection, hemorrhage, urolithiasis, and urinary tract neoplasia. Increased WBCs in the absence of urinary tract disease can occur with genital tract contamination of voided samples.

(c) Epithelial cells. Normal urine can contain transitional cells (from the renal pelvis, urinary bladder, proximal urethra) and squamous epithelial cells (arising from the distal urethra or genital tract). Any disease process that disrupts mucosal surfaces (e.g., inflammation, trauma, neoplasia) may increase the number of cells in the urine. Rarely, neoplastic epithelial cells are detected.

(d) Bacteria. No bacteria should be visible in a sample collected by cystocentesis. Variable numbers may be present when samples are collected with a catheter or by voiding.

(e) Casts are cylindric molds of renal tubules that may be composed of protein or cells (intact or degenerating). **Cylinduria** refers to the presence of casts in the urine. An occasional hyaline or granular cast is normal.

(i) Hyaline casts (clear and composed of pure protein) may be observed with heavy proteinuria.

(ii) Granular casts (aggregates of protein and degenerating cells) indicate acute tubular necrosis due to ischemic or toxic injury.

(iii) Cellular casts of any type (i.e., epithelial, RBC, WBC) or large numbers of granular casts indicate renal disease (usually acute).

(f) Crystals are dependent on urine specific gravity, temperature, and pH. **Crystalluria** is not usually of great diagnostic significance but there are exceptions.

(i) Cystine crystals indicate cystinuria (see Part I:VI C).

(ii) Urate (ammonium biurate) crystals indicate a portosystemic shunt. In Dalmatians, this can be a normal finding.

(iii) Calcium oxalate crystals in large numbers associated with renal failure indicate ethylene glycol intoxication.

4. Special assessments

a. Protein assessment. Normally, protein is excreted in minimal amounts (usually undetectable by dipstick analysis). Significant or abnormal urinary protein excretion with an inactive urinary sediment (i.e., no casts, hematuria, or pyuria) indicates glomerular disease. Other causes of proteinuria are summarized in Table 43-1.

(1) 24-Hour urine protein excretion is the most accurate method of quantification. Excretion of less than 20 mg/kg/day of protein is normal.

(2) Urine protein:urine creatinine ratio ($U_{Pr}:U_{Cr}$). Calculating the $U_{Pr}:U_{Cr}$ is a more practical test because it is done on a single randomly collected sample and does not require a 24-hour urine collection. A $U_{Pr}:U_{Cr}$ ratio less than 1.0 is normal.

b. Urine culture. The kidneys, ureters, bladder, and proximal urethra are normally sterile. The distal urethra, vagina, and vulva have a normal bacterial flora. Collection methods influence results.

TABLE 43-1. Causes of Proteinuria

Physiologic*
Strenuous exercise
Seizures
Fever
Extreme heat or cold
Stress
Pathologic
Nonurinary
Bence-Jones proteinuria
Hemoglobin/myoglobin
Genital tract inflammation (free-flow urine sample)
Urinary
Nonrenal
Urinary tract inflammation (e.g., from urolithiasis, neoplasia, urinary tract infection, trauma)
Renal[†]
Glomerular disease
Tubular disorders
Renal parenchymal inflammation

* Physiologic causes of proteinuria are usually mild and transient
† Proteinuria with an inactive urinary sediment and no nonurinary factors is almost pathognomonic for glomerular disease. Tubular disorders usually result in only mild proteinuria.

    (1) Cystocentesis. Bacterial growth of any degree (more than 10^2 colony-forming units per ml) is significant.
    (2) Catheterization. Bacterial growth greater than 10^5 colony-forming units/ml in female dogs or greater than 10^3 colony-forming units per ml in male dogs or cats is significant.
    (3) Voiding. Bacterial growth is highly variable and should not be relied upon.
  c. Renal tubular function assessment
    (1) Specific gravity is an indicator of renal tubular function [see Part I: I B 3 c (1)].
    (2) Water deprivation testing can be performed when diabetes insipidus or psychogenic polydipsia is suspected and after other causes of polyuria and polydipsia (e.g., renal failure, hyperadrenocorticism) have been ruled out. Following water deprivation sufficient to cause a 5% decrease in body weight:
      (a) Psychogenic polydipsia will be associated with a urine specific gravity greater than 1.025 –1.045 and a urine osmolality greater than 900 mmol/kg.
      (b) Diabetes insipidus will be associated with little or no increase in urine specific gravity. Aqueous antidiuretic hormone (ADH or vasopressin) is administered to differentiate central diabetes insipidus (i.e., ADH deficiency) from nephrogenic diabetes insipidus (i.e., kidneys unresponsive to ADH).
  d. Fractional clearance of electrolytes refers to the percentage of the filtered load of a specific electrolyte that is actually excreted in the urine.
    (1) Sodium (Na^+), chloride (Cl^-), and **calcium (Ca^{2+})** have fractional clearances of less than 1% in normal dogs and cats.
    (2) Potassium (K^+). The fractional clearance of potassium is usually less than 20% in dogs and less than 24% in cats.

(3) **Phosphorus.** The fractional clearance of phosphorus is usually less than 39% in dogs and less than 73% in cats.

e. **GFR assessment.** The GFR is usually measured if renal failure is suspected but azotemia has not yet developed. Tests include the endogenous and exogenous creatinine clearance test, the use of radioisotopes, and others.

f. **Calculation of the osmolal gap** requires access to a laboratory with an osmometer. The osmolal gap equals the measured osmolality minus the calculated osmolality. The normal osmolal gap for dogs and cats is less than 10 mOsm/kg.

g. **Urodynamic testing** is used in the evaluation of urinary incontinence and includes techniques such as **cystometrography** (assessment of bladder contractile function) and **urethral pressure profilometry** (assessment of urethral sphincter function).

5. **Diagnostic imaging studies**
   a. **Radiography**
      (1) **Survey films** can evaluate renal, bladder, and prostatic size and shape and detect the presence of radiopaque uroliths.
      (2) **Contrast procedures** [e.g., **intravenous pyelography (IVP), urethrocystography**) can be used to evaluate renal, bladder, and urethral size and shape and to help detect mass lesions, uroliths, obstructions, urinary tract rupture, and congenital defects (e.g., unilateral renal agenesis).
   b. **Ultrasonography** is an excellent noninvasive imaging technique that can assess renal and prostatic size, shape, and tissue architecture (e.g., mass lesions, cysts, hydronephrosis), as well as bladder masses and uroliths.

6. **Cytologic and histopathologic studies**
   a. **Needle aspirate cytology.** The kidneys of dogs are usually not accessible for aspiration, but those of cats frequently are.
      (1) **Indications.** Kidney and prostate cytology is very useful when neoplastic disease is suspected.
      (2) **Contraindications.** Needle aspirates should not be performed in the presence of a cyst, abscess, or bleeding tendency.
   b. **Suction aspiration** of a urethral or bladder trigone mass with a urinary catheter may provide samples for cytology.
   c. **Renal biopsy** is considered when the result will alter patient management. Methods include blind percutaneous biopsy, keyhole biopsy, laparoscopy, open biopsy (via laparotomy), and ultrasound-guided techniques.
      (1) **Indications** include glomerular disease (i.e., glomerulonephritis, amyloidosis), differentiation of acute and chronic renal failure, assessment of tubular basement membrane integrity (following acute renal failure), and the monitoring of disease progression.
      (2) **Complications** include minor and major hemorrhage, transient hematuria, linear renal infarcts, infection, and hydronephrosis (related to blood clots in the renal pelvis). Complications are reduced if biopsies are confined to the renal cortex and if fluid diuresis is instituted following the procedure.

II. ACUTE RENAL FAILURE (ARF) is an acute and sustained reduction in GFR that results in azotemia.

A. **Etiology.** An acute reduction in GFR can be associated with prerenal, renal, or postrenal causes. However, in this discussion, ARF will refer to a reduction in GFR associated with direct injury (usually ischemic or toxic) to the kidney (i.e., acute intrinsic renal failure). The most common causes of ARF in dogs and cats are ethylene glycol intoxication (see Part I:III), gentamicin administration, and prolonged anesthesia and surgery.

1. **Ischemia** can be associated with any condition that results in a severe and prolonged reduction in renal perfusion [e.g., shock, cardiac arrest, trauma, deep anes-

thesia, prolonged surgery, hyperthermia, hypothermia, nonsteroidal anti-inflammatory drugs (NSAIDs)].

2. **Toxic injury** to the renal tubular epithelium can be caused by antimicrobials (e.g., gentamicin, amikacin), amphotericin B, chemotherapeutic agents (e.g., cisplatin), intravenous contrast agents, heavy metals (e.g., lead), myoglobin, hemoglobin, and ethylene glycol.

3. **Other disease states** that may cause ARF include hypercalcemia (e.g., malignancy, cholecalciferol rodenticides), infection (e.g., pyelonephritis, leptospirosis), and immune-mediated disease (e.g., glomerulonephritis, amyloidosis).

B. **Risk factors** include preexisting renal disease, dehydration, decreased cardiac output, sepsis, trauma, hyperviscosity syndromes, advanced age, hypotension, nephrotoxic drugs, multiple organ disease, and electrolyte and acid–base abnormalities.

C. **Diagnosis.** The key diagnostic feature of ARF is the identification of an acute onset of renal azotemia in the absence of prerenal and postrenal causes. Occasionally, a renal biopsy may be required to differentiate ARF from chronic renal failure (CRF; see Part I: IV).

1. **Clinical findings**
   a. The **history** often reveals an acute onset of lethargy, anorexia, vomiting, and diarrhea. Polyuria and polydipsia are usually absent.
   b. **Physical examination** reveals uremia-related signs (Part I:I B 6), dehydration, and weakness. Marked weight loss, poor body condition, and pale mucous membranes are notably absent in most cases. Renomegaly and pain on renal palpation may be evident with intoxication or pyelonephritis.
   c. **Urine volume** may be decreased, usually in proportion to the severity of the renal insult. Normal urine output is 1–2 ml/kg/hour.
      (1) **Anuria** is a urine output of less than 0.08 ml/kg/hour.
      (2) **Oliguria** is a urine output of less than 0.27 ml/kg/hour.

2. **Laboratory findings**
   a. **CBC.** Leukocytosis may accompany pyelonephritis. Anemia is usually absent.
   b. **Serum biochemical profile.** Azotemia is usually moderate to marked with variable elevations in phosphorus and potassium. A moderate to marked increased anion gap metabolic acidosis is usually present [see Part II:V B 1 b (1); Table 43-9].
   c. **Urinalysis**
      (1) **Urine specific gravity.** The urine specific gravity is less than 1.030 in dogs and less than 1.035 in cats. Often it is **isosthenuric** (i.e., similar to the plasma specific gravity, 1.007–1.015).
      (2) **Mild proteinuria** and **glucosuria** may be present with acute tubular injury.
      (3) **Casts** (epithelial or granular) may be observed.
      (4) **Crystals.** A large number of calcium oxalate monohydrate crystals, dihydrate crystals, or both commonly occur with ethylene glycol intoxication.

3. **Diagnostic imaging findings**
   a. **Radiographic findings.** Renomegaly may be seen in acute toxic nephrosis.
   b. **Ultrasonographic findings.** Increased echogenicity of the renal cortex and a "halo sign" (i.e., decreased echogenicity at the corticomedullary junction) may be seen in patients with ethylene glycol intoxication; however, these changes are not pathognomonic.

D. **Treatment**

1. **Correct underlying causes.**
   a. Nephrotoxic drugs should be discontinued.
   b. Ethylene glycol intoxication of less than 24 hours should be treated with 4-methylpyrazole or ethanol (see Part I:III E 1 c).
   c. Dehydration should be corrected to maintain renal blood flow.

2. **Correct extracellular fluid volume.** The **estimated fluid deficit** should be corrected over the first 4–6 hours with normal (0.9%) saline, lactated Ringer's solution if marked hyperkalemia is absent, or a solution of 2.5% dextrose/0.45% saline if hypernatremia is present. Overhydration should be avoided.
   a. Urine production should be monitored via free-catch samples, the use of a metabolic cage, weighing of litter pans, intermittent urinary catheterization, or the use of an indwelling urinary catheter with a closed collection system.
   b. The daily fluid requirement can be matched to urine output via weighing the animal twice daily. A small daily loss of body weight is to be expected from anorexia and tissue catabolism.

3. **Correct hyperkalemia.** The potassium level should be kept below 6.5–7.0 mEq/L (cardiotoxic levels). The therapies below can rapidly lower serum potassium concentrations.
   a. **Intravenous fluids with no potassium** have a dilutional effect and will increase renal potassium excretion if urine flow can be reestablished.
   b. **Sodium bicarbonate** will reverse acidemia and encourage the intracellular shift of potassium.
   c. **Calcium salts** (e.g., calcium gluconate, calcium chloride) given intravenously will not reduce serum potassium but will counteract the cardiotoxic effects of potassium. The therapeutic effect is seen within minutes but is transient (about 1 hour). The patient should be monitored with electrocardiograms (ECGs) at regular intervals.
   d. **Glucose** or a combination of **glucose** and **insulin** given intravenously promotes the intracellular shift of potassium. Careful monitoring of blood glucose is required when using insulin.

4. **Correct acid-base disturbances.** Guidelines for the treatment of metabolic acidosis are given in Part II: V B 4.

5. **Restore urine output.** Urine output should be restored if it is less than 1–2 ml/kg/hour following fluid therapy. Diuretics (mannitol or furosemide), renal vasodilators (dopamine), or both, may be used to increase urine output and reduce the risk of overhydration and help control hyperkalemia and acid–base disturbances.

6. **Control vomiting.**
   a. Gastric acid secretion can be reduced with histamine-2 (H_2) antagonists (e.g., cimetidine, ranitidine) or proton pump blockers (e.g., omeprazole). Mucosal protectants (e.g., sucralfate) may aid healing of gastric ulcers or intestinal ulcers.
   b. Antiemetics include metoclopramide (a dopamine antagonist; therefore, it should not be used concurrently with dopamine) and chlorpromazine (if hydration and blood pressure are adequate).

7. **Provide nutritional support.** The use of enteral feeding techniques (e.g., nasogastric or gastrostomy tube feeding) or total parenteral nutrition may be required.

8. **Dialysis.** Peritoneal dialysis may be considered when fluid and diuretic therapy has failed to reverse oliguria or alleviate uremia. Consideration must be given to the long-term prognosis (i.e., the reversibility of the renal disease) and whether the high cost and labor involved are justified.

E. **Prognosis** depends on several factors:

1. **Urine output.** Oliguria is usually associated with more severe renal damage.

2. **Cause.** Toxin-induced ARF may carry a better prognosis than ischemic ARF because tubular basement membranes remain intact, facilitating tubular regeneration. However, ethylene glycol toxicity is typically severe and has a poor prognosis.

3. The presence of **concomitant organ failure** or **disease,** the animal's **age,** the **severity of the renal failure** (i.e., the degree of azotemia or histologic damage), the **response to treatment,** and the **ability to manage uremic signs** also affect the prognosis.

III. **ETHYLENE GLYCOL INTOXICATION** is seen equally in dogs and cats, more commonly in males, usually in the fall and spring when antifreeze (which is approximately 95% ethylene glycol) is changed in vehicles. **The minimum lethal dose** is 4.2–6.6 ml/kg for dogs and 1.5 ml/kg for cats; **oliguric ARF** is usually the cause of death.

A. **Pharmacokinetics.** Ethylene glycol is rapidly absorbed from the GI tract and rapidly metabolized by the liver via a number of oxidation reactions to organic acids (e.g., glycolate, glyoxylate, oxalate). Alcohol dehydrogenase is responsible for the initial oxidation of ethylene glycol to glycoaldehyde. More than half is excreted unchanged in the urine, with peak urine concentrations occurring approximately 6 hours after ingestion. Ethylene glycol is usually not detectable in serum or urine 76 hours following ingestion.

B. **Pathophysiology.** The toxicity of unmetabolized ethylene glycol is mild to moderate. Metabolites are responsible for the most significant toxic effects. Severe renal tubular damage (acute tubular necrosis and renal failure) is primarily due to the cytotoxic effects of oxalate and glycolate.

1. **Glycolate** is the primary toxic metabolite, producing severe metabolic acidosis, renal tubular cell injury, and central nervous system (CNS) dysfunction.

2. **Oxalate** results in renal tubular cell injury, tubular obstruction (secondary to precipitation of oxalate crystals within the tubular lumen), and metabolic acidosis.

C. **Clinical findings** occur in three stages.

1. **Stage 1** (30 minutes to 12 hours after ingestion). CNS signs (e.g., ataxia, lethargy, knuckling, nausea, vomiting, polyuria, and polydipsia) occur. Seizures, coma, and death can also occur.
   a. Polydipsia and polyuria are noted within the first hours following ingestion (i.e., before metabolism and excretion) because ethylene glycol is osmotically active and induces serum hyperosmolality.
   b. Vomiting may occur as a result of gastric irritation or stimulation of the chemoreceptor trigger zone.

2. **Stage 2** (12–24 hours after ingestion). Cardiopulmonary signs (e.g., tachypnea, tachycardia) occur but are often mild or absent in dogs and cats.

3. **Stage 3** (24–72 hours in dogs, 12–24 hours in cats). Signs of ARF are related to severe uremia and metabolic acidosis (e.g., vomiting, diarrhea, lethargy, weakness, anorexia, oliguria).

D. **Diagnosis.** The nonspecific nature of the signs makes early diagnosis difficult. Intoxication should be considered in a young dog or cat with access to the outdoors showing clinical signs of depression, vomiting, ataxia, or polyuria and polydipsia.

1. **Laboratory findings.** Important clues include:
   a. Large numbers of calcium oxalate monohydrate or dihydrate crystals in the urine as early as 3--5 hours after ingestion
   b. Hyperosmolality and an increased serum osmolal gap (greater than 25 mOsm/kg) up to 12 hours after ingestion, after which time the osmolal gap decreases
   c. Severe increased anion gap metabolic acidosis within 3 hours of ingestion
   d. Ethylene glycol detected in the serum or urine
   e. Other abnormalities, such as a stress leukogram, hypocalcemia, hyperphosphatemia (secondary to renal failure or the ingestion of a phosphate-containing rust inhibitor in the antifreeze solution), and hyperglycemia

2. **Diagnostic imaging findings.** A "halo sign" on ultrasound examination of the kidneys is suggestive but not pathognomonic.

E. **Treatment**

1. **Acute treatment** entails limiting the absorption of ethylene glycol and minimizing the generation of toxic metabolites.

    a. Absorption should be limited by induction of emesis unless the animal is severely depressed and there is a danger of aspiration. Gastric lavage with activated charcoal is indicated if the animal is seen within 2–3 hours of ingestion.

    b. Excretion of unmetabolized ethylene glycol in the urine can be maximized by administering isotonic intravenous fluids at 2–3 times a maintenance rate.

    c. Toxic metabolite generation should be prevented with ethanol or 4-methylpyrazole (fomepizole). These agents block the metabolism of ethylene glycol by inhibiting alcohol dehydrogenase. If more than 24 hours have passed since ingestion, these agents are of little benefit. The main advantage of 4-methylpyrazole is that it does not cause CNS depression; however, it does not work well in cats.

  2. Supportive treatment. The treatment for ARF and metabolic acidosis is discussed in Part I: II D.

IV. CHRONIC RENAL FAILURE (CRF)

CHRONIC RENAL FAILURE (CRF) is the most common renal disorder in dogs and cats. It is defined as long-standing primary renal failure (i.e., renal failure that has been present for months to years) and is associated with irreversible structural lesions within the kidney. Renal function remains relatively stable for weeks to months but has a tendency to deteriorate over time; hence, it is usually a progressive and irreversible disease.

A. Etiology. CRF is an endpoint to many diseases, such as chronic tubulointerstitial nephritis, chronic glomerulonephritis, amyloidosis, pyelonephritis, ARF, hypercalcemia, leptospirosis, neoplasia (e.g., renal lymphoma in cats), pyogranulomatous nephritis [i.e., feline infectious peritonitis (FIP)], chronic urinary tract obstruction (leading to hydronephrosis), congenital disorders (e.g., polycystic kidney disease), and familial renal disease.

B. Predisposition

  1. Dogs. The mean age of dogs with CRF is 6.5–7 years. Familial renal diseases have been recognized in Norwegian elkhounds, Lhasa apsos, Shih Tzus, Samoyeds, cocker spaniels, Doberman pinschers, standard poodles, soft-coated wheaten terriers, Shar peis, beagles, chow chows, basenjis, golden retrievers, and schnauzers.

  2. Cats. The mean age of cats with CRF is 7.4 years with a range of 9 months to 22 years. CRF is more common in cats than in dogs. There is an increased frequency in Maine coon, Abyssinian, Siamese, Russian blue, and Burmese cats.

C. Diagnosis is based on the identification of renal azotemia with historical and physical signs that suggest chronic versus acute disease (Table 43-2). Rarely, a renal biopsy may be needed to confirm the presence of CRF.

TABLE 43-2. Differentiation between Acute and Chronic Renal Failure

Sign	Acute Renal Failure	Chronic Renal Failure
Polydipsia	No	Yes
Urine volume	Variable	Increased
Ischemic or toxic precipitating event	Yes	No
Weight loss	No	Yes
Kidney size/shape	Normal/smooth	Small/irregular
Osteodystrophy	No	Occasionally
Nonregenerative anemia	No	Common
Active urinary sediment	Yes	No
Serum potassium level	Normal to high	Normal to low
Metabolic acidosis	Moderate to severe	Mild to moderate

1. **Clinical findings** often reflect the uremic state.
   a. **Historical signs** may include polyuria, polydipsia, weight loss, anorexia, lethargy, nausea, vomiting, diarrhea, and weakness.
   b. **Physical signs** may include halitosis, oral or lingual ulcers, poor body condition, pale mucous membranes, dehydration, depression, lethargy, and signs related to hypertension (e.g., retinal edema, vessel tortuosity, or detachment). Abdominal palpation may reveal small, irregular kidneys.

2. **Laboratory findings**
   a. **CBC.** A normocytic, normochromic nonregenerative anemia commonly occurs when CRF is advanced.
   b. **Serum biochemical profile**
      (1) **Azotemia** is a consistent feature of CRF and varies from mild to severe.
      (2) **Hyperphosphatemia** is common and indicates the onset of renal secondary hyperparathyroidism.
      (3) **Hypokalemia** (defined as a serum potassium level less than 3.5 mEq/L) occurs in approximately 20% of cats with CRF. It varies from mild to severe. Clinical signs of muscle weakness develop when potassium levels fall below 2.5 mEq/L.
      (4) **Hyperamylasemia** is common and related to the reduction in GFR.
      (5) **Hyper- and hypocalcemia** are infrequent abnormalities and reflect derangements of calcium metabolism associated with renal secondary hyperparathyroidism.
      (6) **Acidosis** (mild to moderate increased anion gap metabolic acidosis) is common.
   c. **Urinalysis.** Variable degrees of proteinuria accompany CRF, depending on the underlying disease process (e.g., amyloidosis). The urine specific gravity is less than 1.030 in dogs and less than 1.035 in cats and is frequently isosthenuric (1.007– 1.015).

3. **Diagnostic imaging findings**
   a. **Radiographic findings.** Survey abdominal radiographs frequently reveal small, irregularly shaped kidneys. However, normal or increased renal size may be observed depending on the cause of the CRF (e.g., neoplasia, amyloidosis). Renal mineralization, osteomalacia, or fibrous osteodystrophy may be observed.
   b. **Ultrasonographic findings.** The most common finding is reduced renal size and increased echogenicity of the renal tissue.

D. **Treatment**

1. **Treatment for dehydration** is with a balanced replacement fluid, given subcutaneously or intravenously. Due to the obligatory polyuria associated with CRF, plenty of fresh water should be available at all times.

2. **Dietary protein restriction** (to 13% of gross energy in dogs and 21% of gross energy in cats) reduces the severity of uremic symptoms and may also slow the rate of progression of CRF.

3. **Treatment for hyperphosphatemia** (see Part II: IV C 3). Dietary phosphorus restriction (i.e., with the reduced protein diet, which is phophorus restricted) should be attempted first. If the serum phosphorus level is still elevated, oral phosphorus-binding agents (e.g., aluminum hydroxide) should be used. Treating hyperphosphatemia will slow the development of renal secondary hyperparathyroidism, osteodystrophy, soft-tissue mineralization, and perhaps the progression of CRF. Serum phosphorus concentration should be monitored every 10–14 days until it is normal, and then at 4- to 6-week intervals as needed.

4. **Treatment for hypokalemia** is necessary if the potassium level is less than 4.0 mEq/L (see Part II: II B 3).

5. **Treatment for acidosis** is necessary if the blood bicarbonate concentration is less than 17 mEq/L (see Part II:V B 4).

6. **Treatment for anemia**
   a. **Blood transfusions** will often ameliorate most of the signs associated with anemia (i.e., weakness, lethargy); however, the chronic use of blood transfusions is problematic due to cost, risk of transfusion reactions, and the continued need for blood products.
   b. **Recombinant human erythropoietin (rHuEPO)** can reverse the anemia associated with CRF in dogs and cats. Initially, injections are given subcutaneously 3 times weekly until a satisfactory hematocrit is reached (33%–40% in dogs, 30%–35% in cats). The dose is then usually reduced and individualized.
      (1) Oral iron supplementation is recommended when using rHuEPO.
      (2) Adverse effects associated with rHuEPO include refractory anemia, polycythemia, vomiting, seizures, discomfort at the injection site, transient cutaneous and mucocutaneous reactions, and decreased effectiveness as anti-rHuEPO antibodies develop.

7. **Treatment for hypertension,** which is present in 60% of dogs with CRF and 80% of dogs with glomerular disease, will reduce ocular damage or the risk of damage. Gradual dietary sodium restriction (to 0.1%–0.3% of diet on a dry matter basis or 10–40 mg/kg/day) can be followed by drug treatment with angiotensin-converting enzyme (ACE) inhibitors (e.g., captopril, enalapril), calcium channel blockers (e.g., diltiazem), adrenergic receptor blockers (e.g., propranolol, atenolol, prazosin), arteriolar vasodilators (e.g., hydralazine), and diuretics (e.g., furosemide), if required.

8. **Treatment for nausea** and **vomiting.** Reducing the severity of the uremia (e.g., by administering intravenous fluids and putting the animal on a reduced-protein diet) often alleviates these symptoms. However, antiemetics (e.g., metoclopramide), gastric mucosal protectants (e.g., sucralfate), and drugs to reduce gastric hyperacidity (e.g., cimetidine, ranitidine) may also be necessary.

9. **Treatment for anorexia.** Anorexia is also often alleviated by reducing uremia. Additional measures include the administration of vitamin B, enhancing the palatability of food (e.g., warming food to body temperature, the use of flavor enhancers (e.g., clam juice, tuna juice, chicken broth), gradually introducing new foods, paying careful attention to preferred texture, frequent feeding of small meals and hand feeding, or the administration of diazepam and oxazepam.

10. **Calcitriol therapy** in low doses may be needed to control renal secondary hyperparathyroidism. If serum parathyroid hormone (PTH) concentrations remain elevated after the use of a reduced phosphorus diet and oral phosphorus binders, calcitriol therapy can be considered.
    a. Calcitriol is the vitamin D product of choice because it does not require metabolic activation by the kidney and it has a rapid onset and short duration of action.
    b. The maintenance dose is established by serial serum calcium, phosphorus, and PTH determinations.
    c. Hypercalcemia is the main adverse effect and occurs more frequently if calcium-based phosphorus binding agents are used concomitantly.

E. **Prognosis.** The long-term prognosis is poor. With conservative intervention, dogs and cats may achieve a good quality of life for a few months to years.

V. GLOMERULAR DISEASE (NEPHROTIC SYNDROME)

A. **Etiology** and **pathophysiology.** Most glomerular disease in dogs and cats is caused by **glomerulonephritis** or **amyloidosis.** Damage to the glomeruli results in proteinuria, a hallmark sign of glomerular disease. Severe glomerular damage can result in the development of nephrotic syndrome (i.e., proteinuria, hypoalbuminemia, hypercholesterolemia, edema, and effusion), and, possibly, CRF.

1. **Glomerulonephritis** can be associated with infection [e.g., dirofilariasis, feline leukemia virus (FeLV) infection], chronic inflammation [e.g., systemic lupus erythematosus (SLE), chronic skin disease], neoplasia (e.g., lymphosarcoma), idiopathic causes, metabolic disease (e.g., hyperadrenocorticism), and familial disease. It is caused by immune-mediated processes in which glomerular deposition of antigen is followed by deposition of antibody or preformed circulating immune (antigen–antibody) complexes. Following deposition of antibody within the glomerulus, activation of the complement cascade and other inflammatory processes results in damage to the filtration apparatus, resulting in proteinuria. Complete destruction of the glomerulus can occur and, if widespread, CRF can develop.

2. **Amyloidosis** results from the renal deposition of polymerized protein subunits. In most instances, these protein subunits are considered to be fragments of serum amyloid A protein. Sustained elevations in serum amyloid A protein result from chronic inflammation. Tissue deposition of amyloid A protein combined with the decreased degradation and removal of amyloid A protein are required for amyloidosis to develop. Underlying (chronic inflammatory) disease is not found in the majority of dogs and cats with amyloidosis.

B. **Predisposition**

1. **Glomerulonephritis**
   a. **Age.** The mean age of animals with glomerulonephritis is 7 years in dogs and 4 years in cats.
   b. **Sex and breed.** There is no sex or breed predilection in dogs. There is no breed predilection in cats, but 75% of cases of glomerulonephritis are diagnosed in males. Familial glomerulopathies have been described in cats, Samoyeds, Doberman pinschers, greyhounds, rottweilers, Bernese mountain dogs, and soft-coated wheaten terriers.

2. **Amyloidosis**
   a. **Age.** Dogs and cats with renal amyloidosis are usually older than 5 years; however, familial amyloidosis is usually diagnosed before the animal reaches 6 years of age.
   b. **Sex and breed.** Beagles, collies, and Walker hounds may be at increased risk, and German shepherds and mixed-breed dogs may be at decreased risk for amyloidosis. Familial amyloidosis occurs in Abyssinian cats and Shar pei dogs and has been reported in Oriental shorthair and Siamese cats.

C. **Diagnosis**

1. **Clinical findings.** Mild glomerular disease may be associated with no clinical signs other than proteinuria.
   a. **Uremia-related signs** are seen if CRF has developed.
   b. **Subcutaneous edema, dyspnea** (from pleural effusion), and **ascites** are seen if hypoalbuminemia is severe. Occasionally, dyspnea results from thromboembolism of the pulmonary artery as a result of a hypercoagulable state induced by the urinary loss of anticoagulant proteins (e.g., antithrombin III).
   c. **Lameness** or **paresis** may be seen if thromboembolism of the arterial supply to a limb occurs. Shar peis with familial amyloidosis have bouts of fever and lameness (unilateral, painful swelling of the hock joint).
   d. **Clinical findings associated with an underlying inflammatory** or **neoplastic disorder** may be present.
   e. **Acute blindness** may result from hypertension-induced ocular abnormalities.

2. **Laboratory findings**
   a. **CBC.** Nonregenerative anemia may be seen with CRF. Leukocytosis may be seen with underlying inflammatory disorders or neoplasia.
   b. **Serum biochemical profile**
      (1) Hypercholesterolemia is a common finding when hypoalbuminemia is moderate to severe.

(2) Azotemia, hyperphosphatemia, and hyperamylasemia will be detected if CRF has developed.

(3) Familial amyloidosis in dogs and cats may affect other organs, particularly the liver, causing elevations in serum alanine transferase (ALT), serum γ-glutamyl transpeptidase (GGT), and serum alkaline phosphatase (ALP).

  c. Urinalysis

    (1) Proteinuria in the absence of an active urinary sediment (i.e., no pyuria, hematuria, cellular casts) is the **hallmark sign** of glomerular disease. It is produced when the glomerular filtration barrier is disrupted. Other causes of proteinuria are listed in Table 43-1. **Quantification of urine protein** excretion (see Part I: I B 4 a) is necessary to determine if the glomerular origin proteinuria is significant.

    (2) Hyaline casts may be increased because of excessive protein excretion.

    (3) Isosthenuria may be present if CRF has developed or significant medullary amyloid deposition has occurred. The amyloid in Abyssinian cats and some Shar pei dogs is deposited primarily in the renal medulla (as opposed to glomeruli), resulting in isosthenuria and minimal proteinuria.

3. Renal biopsy is the only way to differentiate glomerulonephritis from amyloidosis. Cortical biopsies may not detect medullary amyloid deposition in cats and some dogs with familial forms of amyloidosis.

D. **Treatment**

1. Glomerulonephritis

  a. Underlying conditions should be treated.

  b. Immunosuppressive drugs, (e.g., corticosteroids, azathioprine, cyclophosphamide, chlorambucil, cyclosporine) have been used in dogs and cats with glomerulonephritis, although their effectiveness has not been studied (except cyclosporine, which showed no benefit). Unless there is a specific steroid-responsive underlying disease (e.g., SLE), corticosteroids should be avoided.

  c. Anti-inflammatory therapy with **aspirin** and **omega-3 fatty acids** (e.g., the fish oils eicosapentaenoic and docasahexanoic acid) may be beneficial. These agents interfere with platelet function.

2. Amyloidosis

  a. Underlying conditions should be treated.

  b. Treatment for CRF may be necessary.

  c. Dimethylsulfoxide may help solubilize tissue deposits of amyloid; however, its beneficial effect is primarily related to a reduction in renal interstitial inflammation and fibrosis in animals with amyloidosis and CRF. It is administered subcutaneously as a diluted solution. Its effectiveness in dogs with amyloidosis is controversial.

  d. Colchicine may prevent the deposition of amyloid in Shar pei dogs with relapsing fever and lameness but has no effect on amyloid once it has been deposited.

3. Associated disorders

  a. Treatment for hypertension, sodium retention, and **edema**

    (1) Diet

      (a) Sodium-restricted diets should be gradually introduced with the objective of reducing the dietary sodium content to 0.1%–0.3% on a dry matter basis.

      (b) Reduced-protein diets may help reduce glomerular hyperfiltration and progressive injury. Sufficient protein should be provided to avoid protein malnutrition.

    (2) Antihypertensive drugs such as ACE inhibitors and diuretics may be necessary to normalize blood pressure if dietary sodium restriction is inadequate.

    (3) Plasma transfusion may be considered if hypoalbuminemia is marked and edema or body cavity effusions (especially pleural) are severe.

    (4) Fluid removal may be necessary for animals in severe respiratory distress due to pleural effusion or in discomfort from marked abdominal effusion.

Diuretics may help reduce body cavity effusions, but their effectiveness is variable and dehydration is a risk.

b. Treatment for hypercoagulable states. Hypercoagulable states may respond to prophylactic anticoagulant therapy. Aspirin, heparin, or warfarin should be considered for animals at increased risk for thrombosis (i.e., those with blood antithrombin III concentrations that are less than 70% of normal and fibrinogen concentrations that are greater than 300 mg/dl). Heparin may be less effective because adequate concentrations of antithrombin III are necessary in order for the drug to be effective.

c. Treatment for thromboembolism consists of supportive care (see Chapter 39 XIII A, Chapter 40 IV H 5).

E. **Prognosis**

1. Glomerulonephritis. Animals with glomerulonephritis may remain stable for long periods, spontaneously regress, or progress to CRF. CRF, underlying disease, and thromboembolism worsen the prognosis.

2. Amyloidosis is associated with a poor prognosis in both dogs and cats. The disease is progressive, and many animals are in CRF at the time of diagnosis. Survival times are short (weeks to months).

VI. RENAL TUBULAR DISORDERS

A. **Fanconi's syndrome** is characterized by diminished tubular reabsorption of water, sodium, potassium, glucose, phosphorus, bicarbonate, and amino acids. Most cases of Fanconi's syndrome are inherited; approximately 75% of the reported cases have occurred in basenjis. Prevalence within the basenji breed in North America is estimated at 10%–30%. There is no sex predilection, and Fanconi's syndrome has not been reported in cats.

1. Diagnosis. The average age at the time of diagnosis is 1–8 years; most patients are diagnosed between the ages of 2 and 4 years.
   a. Clinical findings
      (1) Polyuria, polydipsia, and **weight loss** are common.
      (2) CRF with clinical **signs of uremia** develops in many basenjis.
      (3) Muscle weakness (due to hypokalemia from renal potassium wasting) and **osteomalacia** (due to calcium and phosphorus loss) may also be observed.
   b. Laboratory findings
      (1) Serum biochemical profile. Hypokalemia is present in about one-third of cases. **Azotemia** will be present if CRF has developed.
      (2) Blood gas analysis usually reveals a **normal anion gap metabolic acidosis,** which results from urinary bicarbonate loss.
      (3) Urinalysis. The **urine specific gravity** is low (1.001–1.018), and **mild proteinuria** is common. **Glucosuria** in the absence of hyperglycemia is common, and is a strong indicator of disease in basenjis.
   c. Bicarbonate loading to demonstrate diminished bicarbonate reabsorption or clearance studies involving amino acids may be necessary to confirm the presence of the disease.

2. Treatment. Because there is marked variability in the number and severity of transport defects, therapy will need to be individualized. Abnormalities that may require treatment include hypokalemia, metabolic acidosis, and CRF. Because of renal bicarbonate wasting, large doses of bicarbonate may be needed.

3. Prognosis. Some dogs remain stable for years; others develop rapidly progressive renal failure. Death often results from ARF accompanied by severe metabolic acidosis. Renal papillary necrosis is a common postmortem finding.

B. **Primary renal glucosuria** is a rare disorder characterized by glucosuria in the absence of hyperglycemia. It is not associated with other tubular transport defects or diminished renal function. Primary renal glucosuria has been reported in Scottish terriers, mixed-breed dogs, and as a familial disorder in Norwegian elkhounds. Dogs are at increased risk for UTI.

1. **Diagnosis** is based on the presence of glucosuria and the absence of hyperglycemia, reduced renal function, or other solute transport defects. Clinical findings include polyuria and polydipsia, caused by the osmotic diuresis induced by the glucosuria.

2. **Treatment.** There is no treatment that will improve tubular reabsorption of glucose.

3. **Prognosis.** The long-term prognosis is usually good.

C. **Cystinuria** results from defective renal tubular reabsorption of the amino acid cystine. Occasionally, diminished reabsorption of other amino acids such as lysine will occur. Cystinuria occurs in many breeds, but English bulldogs and dachshunds are most often affected. It occurs almost exclusively in male dogs.

1. **Etiology.** Cystinuria is an inherited defect in most dogs and may represent a sex-linked or autosomal recessive disorder.

2. **Diagnosis**
   a. **Clinical findings.** Cystinuria is asymptomatic unless urolithiasis develops. Urolithiasis may be associated with dysuria, hematuria, pollakiuria, and urinary tract obstruction and is usually diagnosed in young to middle-aged dogs.
   b. **Laboratory findings.** Flat, hexagonal cystine crystals are usually observed in acidic urine; the presence of **cystine crystalluria** is the basis for diagnosis.

3. **Treatment** is focused on reducing the risk of or preventing the recurrence of urolithiasis (see Part I:VIII).

4. **Prognosis.** The long-term prognosis depends on whether or not urolithiasis develops and how successfully it is managed.

D. **Abnormal urate transport in Dalmatians.** Urate is derived from purine metabolism. In breeds other than Dalmatians, it is converted to allantoin in the liver by the enzyme uricase. In Dalmatians, a genetic breed-specific alteration in urate transport occurs, leading to reduced urate transport into hepatocytes for metabolism to allantoin and increased renal tubular secretion of urate into the urine. As a result, blood and urine urate concentrations are elevated. Urate crystalluria is asymptomatic, but it is a risk factor for the development of urate urolithiasis (see Part I: VIII). The metabolic defect in urate transport cannot be reversed; therefore, the long-term prognosis depends on the occurrence of and complications associated with urolithiasis.

E. **Renal tubular acidosis** is a rare disorder characterized by reduced renal acid excretion and the development of a normal anion gap metabolic acidosis [see Part II:V B 1 b (2)].

1. **Types.** Reduced acid excretion can occur as a result of reduced bicarbonate reabsorption in the proximal tubule (proximal renal tubular acidosis) or reduced hydrogen ion secretion in the distal nephron (distal renal tubular acidosis).
   a. **Proximal renal tubular acidosis** in dogs has not been reported as an isolated entity, but it may occur as part of Fanconi's syndrome and cause the metabolic acidosis associated with that disorder. Proximal renal tubular acidosis is usually seen in basenjis because of the association with Fanconi's syndrome.
   b. **Distal renal tubular acidosis** has been reported in dogs and cats as an isolated disorder or associated with other diseases (e.g., hepatic lipidosis, pyelonephritis, calcium phosphate urolithiasis). Distal renal tubular acidosis has no breed or sex predilection and has been reported in dogs and cats ranging in age from 1 to 8 years.

2. **Diagnosis**
   a. **Clinical findings.** In animals with distal renal tubular acidosis, anorexia and lethargy are common and muscle weakness due to hypokalemia has been observed.

  b. Laboratory findings vary depending on associated diseases.

   (1) Distal renal tubular acidosis is associated with a normal anion gap metabolic acidosis and an inappropriately alkaline urine (pH > 6.0). Diagnosis is based on finding a normal anion gap metabolic acidosis and an alkaline urine pH, assuming UTI is absent. If the urine pH is equivocal (i.e., 5.5–6.0) and a nonrenal cause for the normal anion gap metabolic acidosis cannot be found (e.g., diarrhea), then an acid load (i.e., oral ammonium chloride) may be required to demonstrate inadequate hydrogen ion secretion by the distal nephron.

   (2) Proximal renal tubular acidosis is also associated with a normal anion gap metabolic acidosis, but the urine is usually acidic. Abnormal bicarbonate reabsorption and resultant bicarbonaturia are only observed when an oral bicarbonate load is administered. A fractional excretion of bicarbonate exceeding 15% following the administration of an oral bicarbonate load is consistent with proximal renal tubular acidosis.

   (3) Hypokalemia may accompany both proximal and distal renal tubular acidosis and results from renal potassium wasting.

 3. Treatment

  a. Oral bicarbonate therapy is used to treat both proximal and distal renal tubular acidosis. Large doses may be required with proximal renal tubular acidosis because of renal bicarbonate wasting.

  b. Potassium supplementation may be required.

 4. Prognosis depends on the associated disorders. Untreated renal tubular acidosis can be associated with hypokalemia, unthriftiness, and bone demineralization. Little information is available on the long-term course of either proximal or distal renal tubular acidosis.

F. **Nephrogenic diabetes insipidus** refers to a state where the distal nephron is unresponsive to ADH (vasopressin), resulting in the excretion of dilute urine (often with a specific gravity below 1.007).

 1. Etiology

  a. Nephrogenic diabetes insipidus can be **idiopathic** or **congenital.**

  b. Acquired causes include **drug therapy** (e.g., furosemide, glucocorticoids), *Escherichia coli* **endotoxin, hypokalemia, hypercalcemia,** and **chronic tubulointerstitial disease** (e.g., medullary amyloidosis, pyelonephritis, chronic interstitial nephritis).

 2. Diagnosis

  a. Clinical findings. Marked polyuria with compensatory polydipsia develops. Other signs vary depending on associated diseases, but polyuria and polydipsia are consistent.

  b. Laboratory findings. Specific diagnosis of nephrogenic diabetes insipidus requires a **water deprivation test.** Inadequate urinary concentration followed by a lack of response to ADH administration is indicative of nephrogenic diabetes insipidus.

 3. Treatment

  a. Suspect medications should be discontinued, and underlying conditions corrected.

  b. Gradual dietary sodium restriction may help decrease the polyuria, if no drugs or diseases are associated with the nephrogenic diabetes insipidus. Free access to large volumes of fresh water will help prevent severe dehydration.

  c. Thiazide diuretics may paradoxically reduce urine output (by 20%–50%) by inducing mild dehydration and enhanced proximal tubular fluid reabsorption.

 4. Prognosis depends on the cause of the nephrogenic diabetes insipidus. Congenital or idiopathic disease may be associated with a good quality of life as long as the animal has free access to water.

TABLE 43-3. Risk Factors Associated with the Development of Urinary Tract Infections (UTIs)

Urine stasis or retention
   Urinary tract obstruction
   Neurogenic disorders of micturition (e.g., reflex dyssynergia)
Urinary incontinence
Mucosal damage to the urinary tract
   Urolithiasis
   Neoplasia
Urethral catheterization
Altered urinary tract anatomy
   Ectopic ureters
   Surgery (i.e., perineal urethrostomy)
   Urachal diverticulum
Decreased immune system function
   Hyperadrenocorticism
   Diabetes mellitus
   Renal failure
   Cancer chemotherapy
   Corticosteroid therapy
   Feline leukemia virus (FeLV) or feline immunodeficiency virus (FIV) infection

VII. **URINARY TRACT INFECTION (UTI)** is microbial colonization of the urinary tract. It is common in dogs and uncommon in cats. It is categorized according to the site of involvement: **cystitis** is colonization of the bladder, **urethritis** is colonization of the urethra, **pyelonephritis** is colonization of the kidney, and **prostatitis** is colonization of the prostate. Uropathogens colonize areas with normal bacterial flora (i.e., distal urethra, vagina, vulva, prepuce) before ascending into the proximal urethra, bladder, or kidney. Hematogenous infection of the urinary tract is rare. Risk factors are listed in Table 43-3.

A. **Etiology.** Bacteria cause the vast majority of UTIs (Table 43-4). Fungal causes (e.g., *Candida albicans*) are rare.

B. **Diagnosis**

  1. Clinical findings

    a. Lower UTI . Clinical signs include hematuria, dysuria, pollakiuria, and stranguria. Systemic signs of illness are uncommon (except with acute prostatitis). Asymptomatic lower UTI can occur and is most often associated with diseases and drugs that suppress inflammation (e.g., glucocorticoid therapy, hyperadrenocorticism).

TABLE 43-4. Bacterial Pathogens and their Frequency of Isolation in Urinary Tract Infections (UTIs)

Bacterial Pathogen	Frequency of Isolation (%)
Escherichia coli	40
Staphylococcus species	15
Proteus species	12
Streptococcus species	10
Enterobacter species	10
Klebsiella species	8
Pseudomonas species	2
Other	3

TABLE 43-5. Interpretation of Bacterial Culture Results Based on Method of Collection

Method of Urine Collection	Colony Count Indicative of Urinary Tract Infection (UTI)
Cystocentesis	$>10^2$ CFU/ml
Catheterization—male dogs	$>10^3$ CFU/ml
Catheterization—female dogs	$>10^5$ CFU/ml
Catheterization—cats	$>10^3$ CFU/ml
Voided (free-flow) sample	Unreliable

CFU = colony-forming units.

b. Upper UTI. Acute pyelonephritis may be associated with systemic illness (e.g., fever, lethargy, anorexia, lumbar pain, polydipsia, polyuria, signs of renal failure). Chronic pyelonephritis may be asymptomatic.

2. **Laboratory findings**
   a. **Lower UTI**
      (1) **Hemogram** or **serum biochemical profiles** are usually unchanged.
      (2) **Urinalysis** usually reveals pyuria, hematuria, proteinuria (related to urinary tract inflammation), and bacteriuria. Urine may be alkaline if infection is caused by a urease-producing bacteria (e.g., *Staphylococcus, Proteus*). Occasionally, bacteriuria is the only abnormality.
      (3) **Urine culture** is necessary for definitive diagnosis. Results are affected by the method of urine collection; cystocentesis is the preferred method. Quantitative culture will aid in interpretation (Table 43-5).
   b. **Upper UTI.** Pyelonephritis may be associated with leukocytosis, renal failure, hematuria, pyuria, cylinduria (especially increased numbers of WBC casts), and bacteriuria. A positive urine culture is required for the diagnosis of UTI.

3. **Diagnostic imaging findings.** Excretory urography and ultrasonography may help localize the infection to the upper urinary tract if there are changes in the renal size, shape, or pelvis (e.g., dilation, asymmetry). Alterations in prostate size or shape and a thickened bladder wall may also be detected.

C. Treatment is with **antimicrobial agents.**

1. **Selection of agents.** Antimicrobial agents should be selected on the basis of culture and sensitivity results (Table 43-6).

TABLE 43-6. Suggested Antimicrobial Choices for Bacterial Pathogens Causing Urinary Tract Infections (UTIs)

Bacterial Pathogen	Antimicrobial Agents
Escherichia coli	Trimethoprim/sulfa, cephalexin, amoxicillin/clavulanic acid
Staphylococcus species	Amoxicillin, trimethoprim/sulfa, cephalexin
Streptococcus species	Amoxicillin, trimethoprim/sulfa, penicillin
Enterobacter species	Trimethoprim/sulfa
Proteus species	Amoxicillin, trimethoprim/sulfa, cephalexin, amoxicillin/clavulanic acid
Klebsiella species	Cephalexin, trimethoprim/sulfa
Pseudomonas species	Tetracycline, gentamicin, enrofloxacin

a. The Kirby-Bauer disk diffusion method is the most commonly used method. It is based on expected serum drug concentrations, not urine concentrations (much higher for many drugs), and tends to underestimate the effectiveness of some drugs for the treatment of lower UTI.

b. If sensitivities are established by determining the minimum inhibitory concentration (MIC), an antibiotic that reaches a urine concentration four times the MIC should be selected.

2. Specific treatment regimens

a. Urethrocystitis

(1) Uncomplicated urethrocystitis should be treated with antimicrobials for 10–14 days. A second urinalysis and culture should be performed 4–7 days following cessation of treatment.

(2) Complicated urethrocystitis. A UTI is complicated if it is recurrent or associated with an identified risk factor (see Table 43-3). All UTIs in cats (usually resistant to UTI) and male dogs (due to the risk of occult prostatitis) should be considered complicated and treated accordingly.

(a) Antimicrobial therapy should be given for 3–4 weeks and followed by a urine culture 3–5 days after beginning therapy to ensure bacterial eradication. A second urine culture should be performed 4–7 days after cessation of therapy to detect relapse or reinfection. Reevaluation on a regular basis may be needed.

(b) Risk factors should be identified and corrected, if possible.

b. Pyelonephritis is a complicated UTI that requires prolonged antimicrobial therapy (i.e., for 4–6 weeks) as well as supportive care and treatment for renal failure or other complications. Rigorous follow-up is essential.

c. Recurrent infection

(1) Relapses (i.e., recurrence with the same bacteria following eradication) require reassessment of antimicrobial choice based on sensitivity testing and treatment for any complicating risk factors. A deep-seated infection could require a second, longer course of therapy (i.e., for 4–6 weeks).

(2) Reinfection (i.e., recurrence with a different organism within a few weeks to months following eradication) requires evaluation and treatment for complicating risk factors. Each episode should be treated according to culture and sensitivity results for 3 weeks and followed up like a complicated UTI.

d. Catheter-induced infection. Urine should be cultured and treatment initiated following urinary catheter removal (unless systemic signs are noted) with an appropriate antimicrobial. Antimicrobial treatment while a catheter is in place encourages colonization and infection by antimicrobial resistant bacterial species.

3. Prophylactic therapy for animals with frequent relapses or reinfection consists of long-term, low-dose antimicrobial therapy.

D. Prognosis

1. Uncomplicated urethrocystitis carries an excellent prognosis and rarely recurs.

2. Complicated urethrocystitis carries a fair to good prognosis, depending on underlying conditions. Risk of recurrent infection may be high.

3. Pyelonephritis carries a fair to poor prognosis, depending on the extent of renal damage at the time of diagnosis. If renal failure has developed, the long-term prognosis is poor.

VIII. UROLITHIASIS. Uroliths are mineral concretions within the urinary tract. **Urocystoliths** (concretions within the urinary bladder) and **urethroliths** (concretions within the urethra) are common. **Nephroliths** (concretions within the kidney) account for less than 4% of uroliths.

A. Etiology. Uroliths are thought to form from precipitation–crystallization (supersaturation of mineral components in the urine), matrix–nucleation (precipitation of minerals around a preformed organic nidus), or crystallization–inhibition (the absence of inhibitors in the urine leading to mineral precipitation).

TABLE 43-7. The Radiodensity of Uroliths

Mineral Type	Radiodensity
Struvite (magnesium ammonium phosphate)	$++$ to $++++$
Calcium oxalate	$++++$
Ammonium urate	$-$ to $++$
Cystine	$+$ to $++$
Silica	$++$ to $++++$
Calcium phosphate	$++++$

B. **Types and incidence.** Uroliths are named according to which mineral type makes up more than 80% of the composition.

1. **Struvite (magnesium ammonium phosphate)—** 54% (dogs and cats) of uroliths

2. **Calcium oxalate—** 28% (dogs) and 37% (cats) of uroliths

3. **Urate—** 7% (dogs and cats) of uroliths

4. **Cystine—** 1.3% (dogs) and 0.3% (cats) of uroliths

5. **Silica—** less than 1% of uroliths

6. **Mixed mineral composition—** 2% of uroliths

7. **Calcium phosphate—** less than 1% (dogs and cats)

C. **Diagnosis**

1. **Clinical findings**
   a. **Upper urinary tract (nephrolithiasis).** Signs may include hematuria, lumbar or abdominal pain, and signs of renal failure. Nephrolithiasis may be asymptomatic for long periods of time.
   b. **Lower urinary tract.** Signs may include dysuria, hematuria, pollakiuria, and stranguria. Partial or complete urinary obstruction may result in systemic signs of illness (e.g., lethargy, anorexia, vomiting).
      (1) Abdominal palpation may reveal uroliths in the bladder. If urinary tract obstruction occurs, a distended, turgid, and painful bladder will be palpated.
      (2) Rectal palpation may reveal uroliths lodged in the proximal urethra.

2. **Laboratory findings**
   a. **CBC** and **serum biochemical profile.** Abnormalities may help determine a metabolic basis for urolith formation (e.g., a portosystemic shunt).
   b. **Urinalysis**
      (1) **Hematuria, pyuria,** and **bacteriuria** may be present. A UTI may induce struvite stone formation or occur after the development of urolithiasis and mucosal damage.
      (2) **Crystalluria** does not indicate the presence of urolithiasis; however, it may aid in the identification of any urolith present.
      (3) **Urine pH** affects the solubility of many minerals and can influence urolith formation or dissolution.

3. **Diagnostic imaging findings**
   a. **Survey abdominal radiographs** are a cost-effective method of determining presence of uroliths; however, the radiodensity of uroliths differs (Table 43-7).
   b. **Contrast urethrocystography, excretory urography,** or **ultrasound** may be needed to rule out urolithiasis or identify the presence of urate or cystine stones.

4. **Quantitative analysis** of the mineral content of uroliths is very reliable. Uroliths may be obtained for analysis by surgical removal, bladder catheterization, voiding urohydropropulsion, and, occasionally, by spontaneous voiding. **Subjective assess-**

TABLE 43-8. Clinical Associations that Aid in the Subjective Assessment of Urolith Composition

Typical Clinical Features

Urine pH	Predisposition	Clinical Conditions or Signs	Radiographic Appearance of Urolith	Probable Urolith Composition
Alkaline	Female dog	UTI with urease-producing bacteria (e.g., *Staphylococcus, Proteus*)	Radiodense	Struvite
Acidic to neutral	Middle-aged to older male miniature schnauzer, Lhasa apso, or Yorkshire terrier	Hypercalcemia, hyperadrenocorticism	Radiodense	Calcium oxalate
Acidic to neutral	Dalmatian	Portosystemic shunt	Radiolucent	Ammonium urate
Acidic to neutral	Young to middle-aged male English bulldog or dachshund	Cystine crystalluria	Radiolucent	Cystine
Acidic to neutral	Middle-aged to older male German shepherd, golden retriever, or Labrador retriever	. . .	Radiodense, jackstone shape	Silica

UTI = urinary tract infection.

ment of urolith composition in the absence of quantitative analysis can be based on various clinicopathologic findings (Table 43-8).

D. Treatment

1. **Medical dissolution.** Nephroliths should be treated medically if possible, except in immature patients, in which the safety of protein- and mineral-restricted diets has not been established. Indications for medical dissolution include:
   a. A urolith amenable to dissolution (e.g., struvite)
   b. A patient that is a poor anesthetic or surgical candidate
   c. An owner unwilling to consider surgery
   d. Frequent urolith recurrence following surgery
   e. Patients in which surgery may be detrimental (e.g., those with bilateral nephroliths)

2. **Surgical removal.** Indications include:
   a. Patients with uroliths not amenable to medical dissolution (e.g., calcium oxalate)
   b. Patients at high risk for urinary tract obstruction (i.e., male dogs)
   c. An owner unwilling to comply with dietary or medical measures
   d. Anatomic defects of the urinary tract amenable to correction (e.g., urachal diverticulum)
   e. Urinary tract obstruction that cannot be corrected medically
   f. Nephroliths, when:

(1) Renal function is declining rapidly

(2) Calcium-based uroliths are suspected (because these stones typically respond poorly to medical dissolution)

(3) Partial or complete urinary obstruction is present

(4) The animal is young and growing (i.e., a poor candidate for dietary restriction)

3. Nonsurgical removal (urethral catheters and bladder lavage, voiding urohydropropulsion) may remove all or part of a urolith load if the diameter of the urolith is small.

E. **Specific syndromes**

1. Struvite (magnesium ammonium phosphate) urolithiasis can occur at any age in all breeds of dogs, but female dogs, miniature schnauzers, dachshunds, and poodles are predisposed.

a. Etiology. In dogs, struvite uroliths are usually induced by **UTI with urease-producing bacteria** (i.e., *Staphylococcus, Proteus*). Urease degrades urea, releasing ammonia that alkalinizes the urine and leads to struvite precipitation and urolith formation. In cats, struvite uroliths are not usually associated with UTI.

b. Treatment

(1) Medical dissolution. Struvite uroliths are the uroliths most amenable to medical dissolution. Treatment should be continued for 4 weeks after no radiographically detectable uroliths remain (on average, 12 weeks in dogs and 4 weeks in cats). If uroliths do not (or only partially) dissolve, then a nonstruvite urolith, poor dietary compliance, or recurrent UTI should be considered.

(a) Calculolytic diets are restricted in protein, phosphorus, and magnesium, but they have a high sodium content. They acidify the urine and promote diuresis.

(b) Appropriate antimicrobial therapy should be initiated.

(2) Surgical removal may be necessary.

c. Prevention of recurrence. Early identification and appropriate antimicrobial therapy for UTI will prevent urolith formation. Moderately protein- and mineral-restricted diets that are acidifying may help.

2. Calcium oxalate urolithiasis occurs more often in middle-aged to older male miniature schnauzers, Lhasa apsos, and Yorkshire terriers. Many nephroliths are composed of calcium oxalate.

a. Etiology. Increased urinary calcium excretion is a predisposing factor and may be due to absorptive hypercalciuria (i.e., increased GI calcium absorption), renal-leak hypercalciuria (i.e., a primary increase in renal calcium excretion), or hypercalcemia (a rare cause). Calcium oxalate uroliths have been associated with hyperadrenocorticism in dogs (presumably due to a cortisol-induced increase in renal calcium excretion).

b. Treatment. Medical dissolution is unsuccessful; therefore, **surgical removal** is indicated. **Prophylactic measures** include:

(1) Correction of hypercalcemia, if present

(2) A reduced protein, calcium, and oxalate diet

(3) Urine alkalinization using potassium citrate (included in some specially formulated commercial diets)

(4) Vitamin B_6 supplementation (helps reduce oxalate formation)

c. Prognosis. Recurrence is common despite prophylactic measures.

3. Ammonium urate urolithiasis. Dogs of any breed with portosystemic shunts and Dalmatians (see Part I:VI D) are predisposed to urate urolithiasis. Uroliths tend to form in acidic urine.

a. Treatment

(1) Dogs without portosystemic shunts

(a) Medical dissolution can take from 4–40 weeks.

(i) Calculolytic diets are reduced in protein and designed to augment urine flow.

(ii) Urine alkalinization can be achieved using sodium bicarbonate or potassium citrate.

   (iii) Allopurinol can be used to reduce uric acid production and uri-
       nary excretion by inhibiting the enzyme xanthine oxidase, thereby
       reducing the conversion of hypoxanthine and xanthine to uric acid.
 (b) Surgery. If no improvement is noted after 8 weeks of medical therapy,
     surgical removal is indicated. Surgery may be preferred for male dogs
     because small urate uroliths tend to cause urethral obstruction.
 (2) Dogs with portosystemic shunts. Medical dissolution has not been evalu-
     ated. **Surgical removal** is indicated.
 b. Prophylactic measures
   (1) In Dalmatians, life-long therapy with diet, urine alkalinization, and allopuri-
       nol (to achieve a urine urate:urine creatinine ratio of about 50% of the pre-
       treatment level) are usually necessary. Long-term allopurinol administration
       has been associated with the formation of xanthine uroliths.
   (2) Surgical correction of congenital portosystemic shunts will decrease urine
       urate excretion and urolith recurrence.
 4. Cystine urolithiasis can occur in any breed but is most prevalent in young to mid-
     dle-aged male dachshunds and English bulldogs. Acidic urine encourages cystine
     urolith formation.
   a. Treatment
     (1) Medical dissolution with protein-restricted diets, urine alkalinization, and
         administration of N-2-mercaptopropionylglycine (2-MPG) can be effective.
         D-Penicillamine is not tolerated as well as 2-MPG but may also be used.
     (2) Surgical removal is effective.
   b. Prophylactic measures include life-long dietary and 2-MPG therapy.
 5. Silicate urolithiasis occurs most often in middle-aged to older male German shep-
     herds, golden retrievers, and Labrador retrievers. Diets high in plant protein (e.g.,
     corn gluten feed, soybean hulls) are thought to predispose to silica urolith forma-
     tion. **Surgical removal** is indicated; medical dissolution protocols have not been de-
     veloped. The diet should be changed to reduce plant protein and increase urine
     output.

IX. PROSTATIC DISEASE affects intact, older male dogs (the mean age at diagnosis is
8–9 years). It is more prevalent in large-breed dogs, especially Doberman pinschers
and German shepherds. It is very rare in cats.

 A. Diagnosis
   1. Clinical findings. The prostate gland should be palpated per rectum and assessed
       for symmetry, size, surface contour, and pain.
     a. The history may include dysuria, hematuria, stranguria, preputial discharge, and
         tenesmus (from prostatic enlargement and impingement on the rectum). Pros-
         tatic disease can be associated with a purulent or serosanguineous urethral dis-
         charge.
     b. Lethargy, depression, anorexia, and vomiting may accompany bacterial infec-
         tion, prostatic abscess rupture, neoplasia, or urethral obstruction. Caudal ab-
         dominal pain is often present with acute bacterial infections or urinary tract ob-
         struction.
     c. Hindlimb stiffness may result from prostatic pain or metastasis of prostatic neo-
         plasia to the lumbar vertebrae.
     d. Fever and dehydration may be present.
   2. Laboratory findings
     a. CBC. Leukocytosis may accompany acute or chronic bacterial infection.
     b. Serum biochemical profile. Azotemia may result from urinary tract obstruction.
     c. Urinalysis. Pyuria, hematuria, and bacteriuria are present in most cases of acute
         and chronic bacterial infection or abscessation.
     d. Prostatic fluid analysis. Prostatic fluid should be evaluated to localize hematu-
         ria, pyuria, or bacteriuria to the prostate gland. Cytology and quantitative bacte-
         rial culture (considered significant if it yields more than 10^5 colony-forming
         units/ml) will help characterize inflammatory disease or infection.

3. **Diagnostic imaging findings**
   a. **Radiographic findings**
      (1) **Survey films**
         (a) Marked prostatic enlargement suggests an abscess, cyst, or neoplasia.
         (b) Bony reaction involving the ventral aspect of the caudal lumbar vertebrae suggests metastatic prostatic neoplasia.
         (c) Mineralization of the prostate can been observed with inflammation or neoplasia.
      (2) **Retrograde urethrography**
         (a) Evidence of urethral narrowing can be associated with neoplasia, abscessation, large parenchymal cysts, or hyperplasia.
         (b) Irregularity of the urethral mucosa occurs most often with neoplasia.
      (3) **Excretory urography** may be necessary to document ureteral obstruction causing hydronephrosis.
   b. **Ultrasonographic findings** can be used to guide needle aspiration or biopsy procedures.
      (1) Inflammation and neoplasia can cause focal, multifocal, or diffuse increases in echogenicity.
      (2) Cysts and abscesses appear hypoechoic to anechoic.

4. **Needle aspiration** of the prostate by a perirectal or transabdominal approach is performed when neoplasia is suspected or when other noninvasive tests are not diagnostic. It should not be performed in dogs who may have prostatic abscesses.

5. **Prostatic biopsy** is considered when neoplasia is suspected, response to therapy has been poor, or less invasive procedures are not diagnostic. Percutaneous needle biopsy can be performed using a perirectal or transabdominal approach. A needle or a wedge biopsy may be obtained during a laparotomy.

B. **Specific disorders**

1. **Benign prostatic hyperplasia** is a common condition in intact male dogs, thought to result from an altered androgen-to-estrogen ratio that develops with advancing age. It may begin as early as 2.5 years of age and has a tendency to become cystic after 4 years of age.
   a. **Pathology.** Intraparenchymal cysts may form, which often communicate with the urethra and are filled with a thin, clear amber fluid. On cross-section, cystic change gives a honeycomb appearance to the prostatic parenchyma.
   b. **Diagnosis** is usually based on compatible clinicopathologic signs. Histopathology is the only way to definitively diagnose benign prostatic hyperplasia, but it is rarely needed.
      (1) **Clinical findings.** Benign prostatic hyperplasia results in symmetric, firm, nonpainful enlargement of the prostate gland. Most dogs show no symptoms, but a large gland may impinge on the rectum dorsally and result in tenesmus. Occasionally, hyperplasia is associated with an intermittent hemorrhagic or clear, yellow urethral discharge, and possibly intermittent or persistent hematuria. Systemic signs of illness are absent.
      (2) **Laboratory findings.** No hematologic or serum biochemical abnormalities are present. Urinalysis is usually unremarkable, and signs of UTI are typically absent.
      (3) **Diagnostic imaging findings**
         (a) Abdominal radiographs may reveal uniform prostatic enlargement.
         (b) Ultrasound examination reveals a diffuse increase in echogenicity. Cystic areas will appear hypoechoic to anechoic.
   c. **Treatment** is not needed in asymptomatic animals. If symptoms are present, castration and medical therapy are the therapeutic options.
      (1) **Castration,** the most effective treatment, usually reduces prostatic size by 70%. A decrease in prostatic size following castration will help confirm the diagnosis.
      (2) **Medical therapy.** If castration is not possible, then various drugs can be considered.

(a) **Low-dose estrogen therapy** using diethylstilbestrol is effective at reducing glandular size but will not alter cysts. Potential side effects of estrogen include bone marrow suppression and prostatic enlargement. Prolonged or high doses of estrogen may result in the growth of fibromuscular stroma, squamous metaplasia of glandular epithelium, and secretory stasis, all of which can increase prostatic size.

(b) **Other drugs** that may reduce gland size include **flutamide** (an antiandrogen), **megestrol acetate, medroxyprogesterone acetate,** and **ketoconazole.**

2. **Bacterial prostatitis** can be acute or chronic. It may be associated with abscessation. Urethral diseases such as urolithiasis, UTI, strictures, or neoplasia can predispose to prostatic infection. Causative bacteria are similar to those responsible for UTI, with *E. coli* being the most common isolate. *Brucella canis* is a rare cause of prostatitis.

   a. **Acute bacterial prostatitis**

      (1) **Diagnosis** is usually based on compatible clinicopathologic findings.

         (a) **Clinical findings** may include systemic signs of illness (i.e., fever, depression, anorexia), septicemia, caudal abdominal pain localized to the prostate gland, and an intermittent or constant urethral discharge. Rectal palpation of the prostate gland usually reveals a normal to modestly enlarged gland that is symmetric, firm, and painful.

         (b) **Laboratory findings**

            (i) **CBC.** A neutrophilic leukocytosis with a variable left shift is common.

            (ii) **Serum biochemical profile.** Findings may include prerenal azotemia, hyperbilirubinemia, and an increased ALP level.

            (iii) **Urinalysis.** Hematuria, pyuria, and bacteriuria are usually present; urine cultures are positive.

            (iv) **Prostate fluid analysis** is contraindicated. In dogs, the prostate is usually too painful to allow ejaculate collection. Prostatic massage may increase the risk of septicemia, and the results would be difficult to interpret in the presence of a UTI.

         (c) **Diagnostic imaging findings**

            (i) Radiographs may reveal prostatomegaly.

            (ii) Ultrasound examination may reveal focal or diffuse increases in echogenicity.

      (2) **Treatment**

         (a) **Antimicrobials** should be chosen on the basis of urine culture and sensitivity testing and administered for 4 weeks. The blood–prostate barrier is not intact in acute inflammation; however, an antimicrobial that achieves good prostatic concentrations regardless of inflammation is a superior choice [see Part I:IX B 2 b (2)]. Reevaluation (i.e., urinalysis, urine culture, prostatic fluid examination) should be performed 3–7 days after antibiotic therapy has ceased.

         (b) Supportive care, intravenous fluids, and intravenous antibiotics may be required.

   b. **Chronic bacterial prostatitis**

      (1) **Diagnosis** is based on consistent physical and laboratory findings. Definitive diagnosis is based on histopathology and tissue culture but is rarely necessary.

         (a) **Clinical findings** can include dysuria, hematuria, and intermittent or persistent urethral discharge. Systemic signs of illness are infrequent. Some dogs may be asymptomatic. Rectal palpation of the prostate gland usually reveals an absence of pain, and variable alterations in symmetry, size, and texture (resulting from fibrosis associated with chronic inflammation).

         (b) **Laboratory findings**

        (i) **CBC** and **serum biochemical profile** abnormalities are infrequent unless abscessation has occurred.

        (ii) **Urinalysis** usually reveals UTI associated with hematuria, pyuria, and bacteriuria.

        (iii) **Prostatic fluid analysis** reveals inflammatory cells, and a quantitative bacterial culture is significant.

    (c) **Diagnostic imaging findings.** There are no radiographic or ultrasonographic findings specific for chronic bacterial prostatitis. Occasionally, diffuse mineralization of the prostatic parenchyma is observed. A diffuse or multifocal increase in echogenicity is observed on ultrasound examination.

(2) Treatment

    (a) **Antimicrobial therapy** based on sensitivity results should be administered for a minimum of 6 weeks. Urine and prostatic fluid should be recultured 3–7 days after antibiotic therapy has ceased and at monthly intervals for 6 months. The ability of antimicrobials to penetrate the prostate gland in the absence of acute inflammation is limited. Drug properties that enhance penetration include a basic (versus acidic) nature, high lipid solubility, and a low degree of plasma protein binding. Because prolonged therapy is required, pertinent drug side-effects should be considered.

        (i) **Gram-positive infections** may be treated with erythromycin, clindamycin, oleandomycin, chloramphenicol, or trimethoprim/sulfonamide.

        (ii) **Gram-negative infections** may be treated with chloramphenicol, trimethoprim/sulfonamide, or enrofloxacin.

    (b) **Castration** may aid in resolution.

    (c) **Prostatectomy** or low-dose daily antibiotic therapy (to suppress clinical signs but not cure) may be considered if antibiotic therapy and castration fail to resolve the infection. Prostatectomy is a difficult surgical procedure, and postoperative urinary incontinence is a common complication.

(3) Prognosis. The chances of successfully resolving chronic bacterial prostatitis are fair. Many dogs will have persistent or relapsing infection despite appropriate antibiotic therapy.

3. Prostatic abscessation is a severe form of chronic bacterial prostatitis that is associated with variably sized intraparenchymal abscesses.

  a. Diagnosis

    (1) **Clinical findings** are variable and related to prostatic enlargement, UTI, or bacterial peritonitis.

      (a) Large abscesses may impinge on the rectum, resulting in tenesmus, or on the urethra, resulting in dysuria or obstruction.

      (b) Infection may result in persistent or intermittent fever or purulent/hemorrhagic urethral discharge.

      (c) In approximately 20% of dogs, abscesses rupture into the peritoneal space, resulting in acute diffuse bacterial peritonitis with associated systemic signs.

      (d) Occasionally, prostatic abscessation has been associated with edema of the hindlimbs, scrotum, and prepuce, and caudal abdominal pain.

      (e) Rectal palpation of the prostate gland often reveals asymmetric enlargement. Fluctuant areas may be detected.

    (2) **Laboratory findings**

      (a) **CBC.** A neutrophilic leukocytosis with a variable left shift is present in many dogs, especially those with local or diffuse peritonitis.

      (b) **Serum biochemical profile.** Elevations in serum bilirubin and liver enzymes may occur due to sepsis-related alterations in hepatobiliary function. Hypoglycemia and azotemia (prerenal, renal, postrenal) can also occur.

(c) **Urinalysis.** Hematuria, pyuria, and bacteriuria are usually present.
(d) **Prostatic fluid analysis** reveals inflammation and positive bacterial cultures.
(3) **Diagnostic imaging findings**
   (a) **Radiographic findings.** Abdominal radiographs reveal asymmetric prostatic enlargement.
   (b) **Ultrasonographic findings** usually include hyperechoic prostatic parenchyma with variably sized hypoechoic cavities (with or without septae). Cystic hyperplasia may appear similar.
   b. **Treatment. Surgical drainage** is the treatment of choice.
      (1) Antibiotic therapy (similar to the treatment for chronic bacterial prostatitis) and castration are recommended.
      (2) Shock therapy, prompt surgical intervention (i.e., peritoneal lavage and drainage), and extensive supportive care are necessary for animals with diffuse peritonitis or endotoxic shock.
   c. **Prognosis.** The prognosis for complete resolution is poor to fair. Prostatic abscesses are usually expensive and difficult to treat. Survival is approximately 50% after 1 year.

4. **Paraprostatic cysts** usually occur as single or multiple large cysts adjacent to the prostate and connected to it by either a stalk or adhesions. They may communicate with the urethra. Large cysts may be located in the caudal abdomen cranial to the prostate or in the pelvic canal caudal to the prostate and may result in perineal swelling.
   a. **Etiology.** Paraprostatic cysts are thought to develop from congenital remnants of the uterus masculinus or from the prostate. Occasionally, they have been associated with hyperestrogenism (e.g., Sertoli cell tumors).
   b. **Diagnosis**
      (1) **Clinical findings** include tenesmus, dysuria, or urinary obstruction (related to a large cyst impinging on the rectum or urethra), hematuria, or intermittent hemorrhagic, serosanguineous, or yellow urethral discharge.
      (2) **Laboratory findings.** Hematology, serum biochemistry, and urinalysis are typically normal. Cystic fluid is usually yellow, serosanguineous, or brown, containing low numbers of WBCs, RBCs, and epithelial cells. It is sterile.
      (3) **Diagnostic imaging findings.** The presence of one or more large, fluid-filled structures closely associated with the prostate gland with no UTI or systemic signs of illness is suggestive of a paraprostatic cyst.
         (a) **Radiographic findings.** Abdominal radiographs may show an enlarged, irregular shape in the region of the prostate. With large cysts in the caudal abdomen, it may appear as if two urinary bladders are present.
         (b) **Ultrasonographic findings.** Ultrasonographic examination reveals large hypoechoic to anechoic structures with smooth internal margins.
   c. **Treatment.** Surgical drainage and excision accompanied by castration is recommended.

5. **Prostatic neoplasia** is discussed in Part I: XII D.

X. DISORDERS OF MICTURITION

A. **Clinical evaluation.** Age of onset, neuter status, drug administration, and previously diagnosed diseases should be considered.

1. **Clinical findings**
   a. **Incontinence** (involuntary urination) is the most common clinical sign associated with micturition disorders. Incontinence must be differentiated from polyuria, dysuria, pollakiuria, behavioral problems, and urethral or vulvar discharges.
   b. **Increased bladder size** and **increased residual urine volume** following urination

can be associated with neurogenic (upper or lower motor neuron) abnormalities, bladder obstruction, or bladder atony.

c. **Lack of bladder distention** and **no residual volume** suggests urethral sphincter incompetence (common) or reduced bladder storage (uncommon).

2. **Laboratory findings**
   a. **CBC** and **serum biochemical profile.** Hematologic or serum biochemical abnormalities are usually absent (unless urinary obstruction is present).
   b. **Urinalysis.** Low urine specific gravity may indicate polyuria. UTI or inflammation can mimic urinary incontinence.

3. **Diagnostic imaging findings.** Survey abdominal radiographs, urethrocystography, and ultrasound examination can help evaluate the lower urinary tract for diseases that may result in incontinence (e.g., obstruction, prostatic disease, neoplasia).

4. **Urodynamic assessment** can help identify and characterize functional abnormalities of the bladder detrusor muscle (cystometrogram) or urethral sphincter (urethral pressure profile).

B. **Specific disorders**

1. **Neurogenic disorders of micturition.** Cerebral disease may result in loss of conscious control, and cerebellar disease may result in loss of inhibition. However, most neurologic abnormalities that affect micturition involve upper or lower motor neuron lesions affecting the spinal cord or peripheral nerves.
   a. **Upper motor neuron (UMN) disease** results from spinal cord lesions cranial to the sacral spinal cord segments. Loss of conscious perception of bladder filling allows the bladder to remain in the storage phase indefinitely. Clinically, this results in a "spastic bladder"— that is, a moderately full bladder that is very difficult to manually express (due to high urethral sphincter tone). With time, a local reflex arc develops, which initiates bladder contraction and results in involuntary, intermittent, and incomplete bladder emptying.
   b. **Lower motor neuron (LMN) disease** results from either a lesion in the sacral spinal cord segments (S1–S3) or bilateral peripheral nerve (e.g., pudendal nerve) injury. Conscious perception of bladder filling as well as the contractile function of the detrusor muscle and urethral sphincter are absent, resulting in a moderately full bladder that is flaccid and easy to express.
   c. **Detrusor–urethral (reflex) dyssynergia** is a loss of coordination in the transition from storage to emptying and is thought to be due to a UMN lesion. A normal urine stream is initiated, followed by an abrupt cessation of urination resulting in inadequate bladder emptying. This may be occur several times over a few minutes.

2. **Non-neurogenic disorders of micturition** are usually caused by reduced function of the detrusor muscle or urethral sphincter or by a functional or partial physical obstruction to urine flow.
   a. **Incontinence with bladder distention**
      (1) **Causes**
          (a) **Detrusor atony** is characterized by a distended, flaccid urinary bladder that may or may not be easy to express, depending on resting urethral sphincter tone. It can occur from dysautonomia or detrusor muscle damage resulting from long-standing overdistention of the bladder. It is difficult to confirm the diagnosis without a cystometrogram.
          (b) **Partial physical obstruction** can be due to urolithiasis, neoplasia, urethral fibrosis or stricture, prostatic disease, or granulomatous urethritis. It is usually characterized by dysuria and stranguria. Only a small volume of urine is passed as a small, thin stream or dribbling.
          (c) **Functional obstruction** is related to increased urethral sphincter tone from irritation or inflammation, neurogenic abnormalities, idiopathic causes, or detrusor–urethral dyssynergia. Dyssynergia often results in a normal urine stream that abruptly tapers off or terminates prior to complete bladder emptying.

(2) Diagnosis. Physical obstruction can be ruled out by urethral catheterization, survey radiography, urethrocystography, or ultrasound. If no physical obstruction is found, then functional obstruction or detrusor atony must be considered.

b. Incontinence with no bladder distention is caused by detrusor dysfunction (hypercontractility, reduced storage) or in most cases, by reduced urethral sphincter tone. Intermittent or continual leakage of small amounts of urine (especially when sleeping) may be noted. Urination is otherwise normal.

(1) Causes

(a) Bladder hypercontractility can be caused by bladder inflammation, neoplasia, chronic partial obstruction, or it can be idiopathic (detrusor instability). It has been associated with FeLV infection in cats.

(b) Reduced bladder storage can be congenital or can result from bladder fibrosis or neoplasia.

(c) Urethral sphincter incompetence is one of the most common causes of incontinence. Reproductive hormone–responsive incontinence (common) is typically observed in large-breed, spayed female dogs. Other causes include urethral inflammation, UTI, prostatic disease, and congenital causes.

(d) Ectopic ureters are the most common cause of incontinence in juvenile dogs. Females are affected most often, and ectopic ureters are more prevalent in Siberian huskies. The ectopic ureter bypasses the bladder and enters the urethra distal to the sphincter. In some dogs, the ectopic ureter enters the vagina or vulva. Unilateral or bilateral ectopic ureters can occur, and this condition can be associated with other urinary tract abnormalities. Reduced urethral sphincter function is common and may result in persistent incontinence after successful surgical correction.

(2) Diagnosis

(a) Urinalysis and **culture** will help rule out UTI or inflammation.

(b) Radiography and **ultrasound** can help detect prostatic disease, urethral obstruction, or abnormalities of the bladder wall (i.e., neoplasia, thickening).

(c) Cystometrograms and **urethral pressure profiles** can characterize bladder and urethral sphincter dysfunction.

(d) Excretory urography is usually necessary to detect ectopic ureters.

3. Incontinence in cats may be associated with trauma to the sacrococcygeal area, complications associated with urinary tract obstruction (e.g., detrusor atony, increased urethral tone, detrusor hypercontractility), congenital malformation of the sacrococcygeal area in Manx cats, dysautonomia, and FeLV infection. Anisocoria is common in FeLV-positive incontinent cats.

C. **Treatment.** Underlying diseases (e.g., obstruction, ectopic ureters, UTI) should be treated. Drug therapy to correct bladder or urethral dysfunction (neurogenic and non-neurogenic) may be indicated.

1. Treatment for bladder (detrusor) atony or **hypocontractility.** Detrusor atony or bladder hypocontractility can be treated with parasympathomimetic agents (e.g., bethanechol), which stimulate detrusor muscle contraction. Physical obstructions should be relieved and functional obstructions pharmacologically treated before using parasympathomimetics. Bladder volume should be kept to a minimum. Intact neurologic function aids response.

2. Treatment for bladder hypercontractility. Parasympatholytic (anticholinergic) drugs (e.g., oxybutynin, propantheline) reduce detrusor muscle contractility.

3. Treatment for urethral sphincter incompetence. α-Adrenergic receptor agonists (e.g., phenylpropanolamine, ephedrine) and reproductive hormones (i.e., diethylstilbestrol in females, testosterone in males) can be used to increase urethral sphincter tone. α-Adrenergic agonists may be used alone or in combination with hormonal therapy. Dogs may become refractory.

4. **Treatment for increased urethral resistance.** Functional obstruction can be treated with α-adrenergic receptor antagonists (e.g., phenoxybenzamine), which decrease urethral sphincter tone. Diazepam may relax the striated muscle portion of the urethral sphincter.

XI. FELINE LOWER URINARY TRACT DISEASE (FLUTD)

A. **Etiology.** The cause of FLUTD is often unknown (idiopathic). Other causes include uroliths, infection (e.g., bacteria, viruses), neoplasia, trauma, urethral disease (e.g., stricture, inflammation), and iatrogenic causes (e.g., urethral catheterization). Urethral obstruction is caused most often by urethral plugs, which are composed of a proteinaceous matrix and crystalline material, but also by uroliths, tissue debris, edema, inflammation, stricture, neoplasia, blood clots, and functional obstruction.

B. **Predisposition**

1. **Age.** Young adult cats, 2–6 years old (range: 1–10 years) are most commonly affected, except when congenital malformation or neoplasia is the cause.

2. **Sex.** Males and females are affected equally, but males are most prone to urethral obstruction. Neutered cats (both sexes) are affected more often than non-neutered cats.

3. **Breed.** There may be an increased frequency in Persians and a decreased frequency in Siamese cats.

4. **Lifestyle.** Overweight, sedentary indoor cats are at increased risk. An increased occurrence in the late fall and winter has been reported. Stress may be a factor in some cats, especially if it alters their food and water intake.

5. **Diet.** Dry cat food seems to increase risk, possibly because of the higher magnesium content, increased food intake due to lower caloric density and digestibility, or decreased urine volume (because of increased fecal water loss). Concentrated urine favors supersaturation of minerals and subsequent precipitation.

6. **Frequency of feeding.** Frequent or ad lib feeding results in more frequent postprandial alkaline tides, which may cause a sustained increase in urine pH and resultant struvite crystal precipitation. Struvite crystals can lead to urethral plug formation or uroliths.

7. **Vesicourachal remnants** or **diverticula** may encourage the development and persistence of UTI.

C. **Diagnosis.** All cats with FLUTD exhibit an acute dysuria, stranguria, hematuria, and pollakiuria; however, signs and management differ if urinary obstruction has developed.

1. **Cats with no urethral obstruction**
   a. **Clinical findings.** No systemic signs of illness are present. Physical examination is often unremarkable, and the bladder is normal to small in size.
   b. **Laboratory findings.** In idiopathic cases, hematuria in the absence of pyuria is a common finding. Urine culture is usually negative.
   c. **Diagnostic imaging findings.** Survey abdominal radiographs are usually unremarkable unless urolithiasis is present. Cystograms or ultrasound examinations (rarely performed in cats with no signs of urethral obstruction) may reveal irregular bladder mucosa, a thickened bladder wall, urocystolithiasis, neoplasia, or sand-like sediment in the bladder.

2. **Cats with urethral obstruction**
   a. **Clinical findings**

(1) Signs of systemic illness (e.g., lethargy, anorexia, vomiting) are common. Following complete obstruction, signs of lethargy and anorexia develop within 12 hours and, without treatment, will progress to coma and death in 48–72 hours.

(2) Specific signs include a turgid, distended urinary bladder, which may be accompanied by varying degrees of depression and dehydration. Hyperkalemia may result in bradycardia and pulse deficits. The tip of the penis may be protruded and congested.

b. Laboratory findings

(1) Urinary tract obstruction results in metabolic acidosis and mild to severe elevations in urea, creatinine, phosphorus, and potassium.

(2) Urine parameters are similar to those of nonobstructed cats.

c. Diagnostic imaging findings. Abdominal radiographs reveal a markedly enlarged urinary bladder and occasionally a radiodense urethral plug. Urethrocystography may reveal a urethral plug, urolith, or urethral stricture or narrowing.

D. **Treatment**

1. Cats with no urethral obstruction. Idiopathic FLUTD will resolve spontaneously in most cats in 5–7 days. Antimicrobials are not indicated unless a UTI is present.

2. Cats with urethral obstruction. Aggressive therapy is required in cats that are very depressed or moribund. Life-threatening hyperkalemia should be treated with intravenous saline, followed by an ECG to assess cardiotoxicity. Potassium-induced cardiac abnormalities may need to be controlled before relieving the urethral obstruction.

a. Treatment for metabolic abnormalities

(1) Dehydration or **azotemia.** Before relieving the obstruction in systemically ill cats, administration of intravenous fluids such as 0.9% saline (potassium-free) or lactated Ringer's solution (low potassium) should be initiated. Over the first 2–4 hours, estimated fluid deficits are replaced. Intravenous fluid therapy is continued until the cat can eat and drink normally. After relieving the obstruction, fluid and potassium losses from postobstructive diuresis need to be monitored and corrected as needed.

(2) Hyperkalemia (see Part II:II C 3). Prompt and aggressive intravenous fluid therapy (which has a dilutional effect) and relief of the obstruction (to restore urinary potassium excretion) will usually correct serum potassium concentration within 3–5 hours. Significant cardiotoxicity may necessitate additional measures to reduce serum potassium (e.g., sodium bicarbonate, insulin, glucose) or to protect the myocardium (i.e., calcium gluconate).

(3) Metabolic acidosis (see Part II:V B 3). Alkalinizing solutions (e.g., lactated Ringer's solution) and relief of the obstruction will usually correct the acidosis when it is mild to moderate. Severe acidosis (pH < 7.15) should be treated with sufficient sodium bicarbonate to raise the pH to 7.2.

b. Relief of urinary obstruction

(1) Occasionally, urethral plugs become lodged at the tip of the penis and may be removed by gently massaging the penis.

(2) Most cats require **urethral catheterization.** The plug is pushed into the bladder with pulses of saline. In most cats, the catheter is not left in place once the obstruction is cleared unless the cat is extremely ill, the obstruction was difficult to correct, the procedure was only partially successful (i.e., there is a high risk of reobstruction the next day), or detrusor atony is suspected because of bladder wall damage.

(3) In rare cases when the obstruction cannot be relieved, **repeated cystocentesis** may be required until further diagnostic tests or perineal urethrostomy can be performed.

c. Long-term management of idiopathic and struvite urolith-related FLUTD

(1) Dietary management. Magnesium intake should be limited to less than 20 mg/100 kcal. The urine pH should be maintained around 6.0, and the urine volume should be increased by placing the animal on a calculolytic diet for 4–6 weeks. This diet will usually dissolve uroliths and reduce crystalluria and should be followed with a maintenance diet (i.e., a reduced magnesium, acidifying diet) for the long-term. Less frequent feedings may also help maintain a lower urine pH.

(a) Urine acidifiers (e.g., ammonium chloride, d,l-methionine) should not be given with an acidifying diet because of the risk of overacidification, which can lead to metabolic acidosis, bone demineralization, potassium wasting, and nonstruvite urolithiasis (i.e., calcium oxalate).

(b) Urine volume can be maximized by providing plenty of fresh water, by feeding canned or moistened dry food, and by adding salt to the diet.

(2) Other measures include maintaining an ideal body weight, increasing physical activity (e.g., through playing), and encouraging frequent urination (i.e., by keeping the litter box clean).

(3) Surgery (i.e., perineal urethrostomy) is considered for urethral stricture, an obstruction that cannot be relieved by nonsurgical means, and when multiple obstructive episodes have occurred over a short period of time. The site of obstruction should be localized with a urethrogram (or other means) to ensure that a perineal urethrostomy can correct the problem. These cats will still suffer from FLUTD but are at reduced risk of obstruction. Complications include postoperative urethral stricture and an increased risk of UTI.

E. **Complications**

1. Postobstructive diuresis, which may result in dehydration or hypokalemia from fluid and potassium losses, is common following relief of the obstruction.

2. Functional urethral obstruction occurs in many cats due to urethral swelling and edema or urethral sphincter spasm.

   a. Clinical findings. Typically, the bladder remains distended, and attempts at urination produce only a thin urine stream or dribbles. Urethral catheterization reveals no physical obstruction.

   b. Treatment. Although no treatment regimen has yielded dependable results, phenoxybenzamine (an α-adrenergic receptor blocker) to reduce urethral sphincter tone, diazepam to relax the striated muscle portion of the urethral sphincter, and corticosteroids to reduce urethral edema and inflammation may be considered. Obstruction resolves in 3–5 days in most cats.

3. Reobstruction with debris or persistent urethral plugs can occur in the immediate postobstructive period.

4. Detrusor atony can result from severe distention of the bladder. The bladder should be kept small (by manual expression, intermittent catheterization, or an indwelling catheter). Cholinergic drugs (e.g., bethanechol) may be considered, but only if physical or functional urethral obstruction is not present. Decreasing urethral sphincter tone with α-adrenergic blocking agents may be beneficial.

5. UTI may be induced by urethral catheterization. The use of corticosteroids in the postobstructive period may increase risk.

F. **Prognosis.** The rate of recurrence (dysuria or hematuria) of idiopathic FLUTD is high (30%–70%). Permanent injury to the urinary tract (urethral strictures and detrusor atony) can occur. Bladder rupture occurs rarely. The mortality rate ranges from 6%–36%; animals either die from urethral obstruction or are euthanized.

XII. NEOPLASTIC DISORDERS

A. **Renal neoplasia**

1. Types. Primary renal neoplasia is rare in dogs and cats. Bilateral renal involvement occurs in over 30% of cases.

    a. Dogs
- **(1) Primary tumors.** Types found in dogs include **renal carcinoma** (69%), **transitional cell carcinoma** (9%), **renal adenoma** and **papilloma** (7%), **sarcoma** (7%), **nephroblastoma** (4%), **fibroma** (2%), and **lymphoma** (2%). In dogs, 90% of primary renal tumors are malignant.
- **(2) Metastatic tumors.** Metastatic renal neoplasia (e.g., **osteosarcoma, hemangiosarcoma, lymphoma, mast cell tumor,** and **melanoma)** is more common than primary renal tumors.

    b. Cats. The most common renal tumors in cats are (in order of decreasing frequency) **lymphoma, renal carcinoma,** and **nephroblastoma.**

2. Predisposition
    a. Age
- **(1) Dogs.** The mean age of dogs with renal neoplasia is 7–9 years. The exception is nephroblastoma, which occurs most often in dogs younger than 1 year of age.
- **(2) Cats.** The mean age of cats with renal lymphoma is 5–7 years.

    b. Sex. Renal carcinoma and transitional cell carcinoma are more prevalent in male dogs.

    c. Breed. German shepherds can develop a rare syndrome of renal cystadenocarcinoma and nodular dermatofibrosis.

3. Diagnosis is based on the exclusion of other causes of renomegaly and the detection of metastatic or paraneoplastic disease. A triad of weight loss, abdominal mass, and hematuria is indicative of renal neoplasia. Confirmation of neoplasia requires cytology or histopathology.
    a. Clinical findings
- **(1)** Nonspecific signs include weight loss, anorexia, lethargy, and hematuria (in 10%–33% of dogs). Fever, lameness (due to hypertrophic osteopathy), and vomiting may also occur.
- **(2)** An abdominal mass (possibly painful) is palpated in approximately 50% of dogs. Kidneys may be large or irregular in cats with lymphoma.
- **(3)** Signs referable to renal failure may be present.

    b. Laboratory findings
- **(1) CBC.** A nonregenerative anemia and azotemia are common. Paraneoplastic syndromes that result in polycythemia (tumor production of erythropoietin) and extreme neutrophilic leukocytosis (tumor production of colony stimulating factors) occur rarely.
- **(2) Urinalysis** may reveal hematuria (most often with hemangiosarcoma and renal pelvic tumors), proteinuria, cylinduria, and bacteriuria.

    c. Diagnostic imaging findings
- **(1) Radiographic findings.** A large abdominal mass is frequently observed on survey abdominal radiographs. Thoracic radiographs will reveal metastatic disease in approximately one-third of dogs.
- **(2) Intravenous pyelography** or **ultrasonography** will characterize renal masses.

4. Treatment and **prognosis**
    a. Renal carcinoma is highly metastatic and locally invasive. If unilateral disease is present without local involvement or distant metastasis, **nephrectomy** is the treatment of choice but has a high perioperative mortality rate. In dogs surviving longer than 21 days after surgery, the median survival is 8 months. These tumors are resistant to most chemotherapeutic drugs. Vinblastine provides the best response rates (10%–15%). There is little information on radiation therapy.

    b. Renal transitional cell carcinoma, which tends to occur in the renal pelvis, is best treated by **nephrectomy.** Postsurgical survival is 3–25 months.

    c. Nephroblastoma is best treated with **unilateral nephrectomy.** Prolonged survival has been reported in some dogs. One study reported metastatic disease in 65% of dogs at the time of diagnosis.

    d. Feline renal lymphoma is often bilateral; therefore, **combination chemotherapy** is recommended. Many cats are in renal failure at the time of diagnosis, 40% may have CNS involvement, and 50% are FeLV-positive. In one study, combination chemotherapy resulted in complete clinical remission in 60% of cats with a median survival of 169 days. Cats that are diagnosed early, are FeLV-negative, and have blood urea concentrations below 100 mg/dl (36 mmol/L) have had mean survival times of 526 days.

B. **Bladder neoplasia** is uncommon in dogs (1% of all tumors) and rare in cats. Various environmental factors (e.g., pollution, insecticides, petroleum distillates), patient-related factors (e.g., obesity, tryptophan metabolites, sex, breed), and iatrogenic factors (e.g., flea dips, cyclophosphamide) have been associated with an increased risk of bladder neoplasia.

1. **Types**
   a. **Dogs.** In dogs, tumor types include **transitional cell carcinoma** (87%), **adenocarcinoma** (6%), **squamous cell carcinoma** (2%), **undifferentiated carcinoma** (2%), **leiomyoma/sarcoma** (2%), and **adenoma** (1%).
   b. **Cats.** In cats, tumor types include **transitional cell carcinoma** (30%), **benign mesenchymal tumors** (18%), **squamous cell carcinoma** (15%), **rhabdomyosarcoma** (11%), **lymphoma** (8%), **leiomyosarcoma** (7%), **hemangiosarcoma** (7%), and **adenocarcinoma** (4%).

2. **Predisposition**
   a. **Age.** The mean age of dogs and cats with bladder tumors is 9–10 years, except for rhabdomyosarcoma, which usually occurs in large-breed dogs younger than 2 years.
   b. **Sex.** Female and neutered dogs may be at increased risk.
   c. **Breed.** Airedales, collies, beagles, Scottish terriers, and Shetland sheepdogs may be predisposed to bladder tumors.

3. **Diagnosis** is confirmed by histopathology of samples obtained by cystoscopy or laparotomy.
   a. **Clinical findings**
      (1) Most dogs will develop signs of lower urinary tract disease (i.e., dysuria, stranguria) and hematuria. Systemic illness and weight loss are less common than with renal neoplasia. However, if urinary obstruction (urethral or bilateral ureteral involvement) or advanced metastatic disease is present, anorexia, lethargy, and vomiting are common. Bone metastasis results in lameness in 5% of dogs.
      (2) A distended urinary bladder or enlarged kidneys may be palpated if the bladder or ureters are obstructed. A bladder mass may be palpable in cats and small dogs. Rectal examination may reveal sublumbar lymphadenopathy.
   b. **Laboratory findings**
      (1) **CBC.** A nonregenerative anemia (from chronic disease). Azotemia (urinary obstruction) may be detected.
      (2) **Serum biochemical profile.** Paraneoplastic syndromes that have been reported with bladder cancer include hypercalcemia, hypereosinophilia, hypertrophic osteopathy, hyperestrogenism, and cancer cachexia.
      (3) **Urinalysis.** Hematuria, pyuria, and proteinuria are common. Many dogs have concurrent UTI. Tumor cells are occasionally observed in the urine sediment. Controversy exists regarding the risk of tumor cell implantation along the needle tract when urine is collected by cystocentesis.
   c. **Diagnostic imaging findings**
      (1) **Radiographic findings.** Survey abdominal radiographs may reveal bladder distention, renomegaly (from hydronephrosis), bladder wall mineralization, and cystic calculi. Thoracic radiographs may reveal metastatic disease (10%–30% of cases).
      (2) **Contrast cystograms** and **ultrasound** can detect mucosal irregularities, masses, and bladder wall thickening. About two-thirds of transitional cell carcinomas in dogs occur in the bladder trigone area.

4. **Treatment** for transitional cell carcinoma, the most common type of bladder neoplasia, is discussed here. Treatment is similar for other types of bladder tumors.

a. **Surgery** is recommended, but because the tumor is usually in the trigone area and invades the urethra, prostate, and ureters, surgical excision is only possible in a small number of cases. The tumor has spread beyond the primary site at the time of diagnosis in 37% of dogs.

b. **Intraoperative radiation therapy** has had poor success.

c. **Chemotherapy** (with cisplatin or a combination of doxorubicin and cyclophosphamide) has achieved partial success.

5. **Prognosis.** Survival times, regardless of the treatment, range from a few months to 1 year. Metastatic disease and urinary obstruction shorten survival times considerably.

C. **Urethral neoplasia**

1. **Types**
   a. **Primary tumors.** Primary urethral neoplasia is rare in dogs and cats. The most common tumor types are **transitional cell carcinoma** and **squamous cell carcinoma.**
   b. **Secondary invasion** of the urethra from bladder or prostatic cancer is probably more common than primary disease.

2. **Predisposition.** The mean age of dogs with urethral tumors is 10 years, and there is a predilection for females and beagles.

3. **Diagnosis**
   a. **Clinical findings.** Stranguria and hematuria are common. Abdominal palpation may reveal a distended bladder. Rectal palpation of the pelvic portion of the urethra may identify a focal or diffuse urethral mass. A urinary catheter may be difficult or impossible to pass. Occasionally, distal urethral tumors in female dogs may protrude from the urethral papilla and be visualized during a vaginoscopic exam.
   b. **Laboratory findings**
      (1) **Serum biochemical profile.** Azotemia from urinary obstruction is a common finding.
      (2) **Urinalysis.** Hematuria, pyuria, or signs of UTI may be present.
      (3) **Cytology** and **histopathology.** In order to differentiate malignant urethral neoplasia from granulomatous urethritis or benign tumors, the presence of neoplasia should be confirmed by cytology or histopathology. In some animals, samples for cytology, and occasionally histopathology, can be obtained by placing a urinary catheter adjacent to the tumor and aspirating cells or tissue into the catheter.
   c. **Diagnostic imaging findings**
      (1) **Contrast urethrography** detects and characterizes urethral masses. Focal or multifocal intraluminal masses or filling defects or marked mucosal irregularity may be visualized.
      (2) **Survey radiographs** may detect metastatic disease in the sublumbar region or vertebral bodies.
      (3) **Contrast cystography** and **ultrasound** may detect bladder involvement.

4. **Treatment.** Malignant urethral tumors are usually associated with local invasion, and many are not amenable to surgical excision. Various combinations of radiotherapy and chemotherapy have yielded mixed results.

5. **Prognosis.** Metastatic disease in the thorax or abdomen is present in 20%–30% of animals at the time of diagnosis. The long-term prognosis is poor.

D. **Prostatic neoplasia** tends to occur in older (mean age: 9–10 years) intact or castrated male dogs. It is uncommon, accounting for 5% of prostatic disease in dogs.

1. **Types.** Prostatic neoplasia is usually malignant and caused by an **adenocarcinoma** or **transitional cell carcinoma.** Other tumors include **squamous cell carcinoma, leiomyosarcoma, lymphosarcoma,** and **metastatic tumors.** Metastasis to regional lymph nodes, bone, and lungs frequently occurs.

2. **Diagnosis.** The detection of prostatic enlargement, asymmetry, or nodules may suggest neoplasia, especially in a castrated male dog. Diagnosis is based on cytologic or histopathologic examination of needle aspirates or biopsy samples.
   a. **Clinical findings**
      (1) Signs of prostatic enlargement (i.e., dysuria, tenesmus), hematuria, a hemorrhagic urethral discharge, hindlimb weakness and stiffness (related to local metastasis or prostatic pain), and urinary incontinence may be seen. Rectal palpation of the prostate gland may reveal asymmetry, firm irregular nodules, enlargement, pain, or fixation to adjacent tissues.
      (2) Systemic signs of illness are common and include lethargy, depression, anorexia, fever, and weight loss. These signs may be related to the systemic effects associated with neoplasia or urinary tract obstruction (ureteral or urethral).
   b. **Laboratory findings**
      (1) **CBC.** Neutrophilic leukocytosis may be present if there is necrosis and inflammation in the prostate gland. Mild nonregenerative anemia is common.
      (2) **Serum biochemical profile.** Azotemia may occur if tumor-related urethral or bilateral ureteral obstruction has developed.
      (3) **Urinalysis** may reveal hematuria, pyuria (if there has been prostatic necrosis and inflammation), signs of UTI, or neoplastic cells in the urinary sediment.
   c. **Diagnostic imaging findings**
      (1) **Radiographic findings** usually include asymmetric prostatomegaly and, occasionally, multifocal or granular mineralization of the prostate. Thoracic radiographs may reveal metastatic disease. Regional metastasis may result in lumbar lymphadenopathy or areas of bony proliferation or lysis affecting the pelvic bones or the ventral aspect of the caudal lumbar vertebrae.
      (2) **Retrograde urethrography** may detect irregularities in the prostatic portion of the urethra.
      (3) **Ultrasonographic findings** usually include focal or multifocal areas of increased echogenicity, prostatic asymmetry, and an irregular glandular outline. Cystic hyperplasia and chronic bacterial prostatitis may have a similar ultrasonographic appearance.

3. **Treatment.** In general, response to therapy is poor.
   a. **Radiation therapy** is currently recommended if metastasis is not detected, but the median survival time is only 3–4 months.
   b. **Prostatectomy** does not yield impressive survival times and is frequently associated with postoperative problems such as urinary incontinence.
   c. **Chemotherapy** has not been evaluated in dogs. Castration or estrogen therapy appears to be of no benefit.

4. **Prognosis** is grave. Most dogs die or are euthanized within a few weeks to months following diagnosis.

PART II: FLUID AND ELECTROLYTE DISORDERS

I. SODIUM AND WATER

A. Physiology

1. **Compartments.** Approximately 60% of an animal's body weight is water.
   a. **Extracellular fluid (ECF)** comprises one-third of the water, which includes plasma or intravascular volume (about 5% of body weight) and interstitial fluid (e.g., lymph).
   b. **Intracellular fluid (ICF)** comprises the other two-thirds.

2. **Water movement.** Water moves freely between the ECF and ICF. Its direction and magnitude are determined by the **tonicity** (i.e., concentration of solutes that are re-

stricted to one compartment and cannot diffuse freely, such as glucose in the ECF). Water will move from a hypotonic to a hypertonic compartment.

3. Sodium and ECF and ICF

   a. Sodium concentration in the ECF (equivalent to that in plasma) is a measure of **ICF volume.** Hypernatremia reduces ICF volume (because water moves from the ICF to the ECF), and hyponatremia (in the absence of hyperglycemia) increases ICF volume.

   b. Sodium content. Total body sodium content (not concentration) is a measure of **ECF volume.** When ECF volume is high (e.g., edema, effusion), total body sodium is increased.

4. Sodium excretion

   a. Low body sodium content. The ECF volume is reduced, resulting in active sodium conservation by markedly reducing renal excretion. Sodium conservation is accomplished by a decrease in GFR, enhanced proximal and medullary tubular sodium reabsorption, and aldosterone-stimulated sodium reabsorption (and potassium excretion) in the distal tubule. Failure to excrete urine almost free of sodium when the ECF volume is decreased indicates a renal problem.

   b. High body sodium content. Following ingestion of a large sodium load, renal sodium excretion is enhanced as a result of an increased GFR, reduced proximal tubular sodium reabsorption, suppression of aldosterone release, and the action of atrial natriuretic peptide. Patients with congestive heart failure or hypoalbuminemia retain excessive sodium.

5. Water intake and **excretion.** Daily obligatory water losses in urine and feces and evaporative losses through the respiratory tract and skin are balanced primarily by a thirst reflex (increased intake) and ADH (decreased excretion).

   a. Thirst. Water loss increases the tonicity of body fluids, which stimulates the thirst center in the CNS and ADH release from the posterior pituitary.

   b. ADH acts on the collecting tubule of the kidney to increase water reabsorption, resulting in a small volume of maximally concentrated urine. The absence of ADH results in the production of a large volume of dilute urine.

B. **Hyponatremia** (defined as a sodium level below 140 mEq/L) is usually associated with hypoosmolality because sodium is a major contributor to plasma osmolality. However, hyponatremia can also be associated with normal or increased plasma osmolality.

1. Types

   a. Hyponatremia with normal plasma osmolality (pseudohyponatremia) is an artifact of measurement rather than true hyponatremia that can occur if significant hyperlipidemia or hyperproteinemia is present. It can be avoided by measuring sodium using ion-selective electrodes and direct potentiometry techniques.

   b. Hyponatremia with increased plasma osmolality (i.e., greater than 310 mOsm/kg) occurs when an impermeant solute (i.e., one largely confined to the ECF) other than sodium is present in the ECF (e.g., glucose, mannitol). Water moves down its concentration gradient from the ICF into the ECF and reduces the ECF sodium concentration.

   c. Hyponatremia with reduced plasma osmolality (i.e., less than 290 mOsm/kg) results from either primary water gain or sodium loss. This may occur with normal, increased, or decreased effective circulating volume. The volume status of a patient is best determined by physical parameters such as skin turgor, dryness of mucous membranes, capillary refill time, pulse rate, the size of the jugular veins, and the presence of edema or body cavity effusions.

     (1) Hypovolemic hyponatremia can be caused by sodium loss from the GI tract (vomiting, diarrhea), skin (burns), kidney (aldosterone deficiency, hypoadrenocorticism), and loss into a third space (peritonitis).

     (2) Normovolemic hyponatremia can be caused by psychogenic polydipsia, syndrome of inappropriate ADH release (SIADH), myxedema coma (due to hypothyroidism), and hypotonic (e.g., 5% dextrose in water) fluid infusion.

     (3) Hypervolemic hyponatremia is caused by severe liver disease (cirrhosis), congestive heart failure, nephrotic syndrome, and advanced renal failure.

2. **Clinical findings.** The rate of serum sodium reduction is more important than the magnitude.

   a. **Rapid reductions** are more likely to result in clinical signs, (e.g., lethargy, depression, vomiting, seizures, and coma), most of which are neurologic, relating to brain edema caused by water movement from the ECF to the ICF compartment.

   b. **Slow reductions** often do not produce signs directly attributable to the reduced sodium concentration because brain cells can accommodate to the change in ECF osmolality. Signs associated with the underlying disorder are usually dominant.

3. **Treatment** is focused on the underlying disorder.

   a. If acute and symptomatic hyponatremia has developed, isotonic (0.9%) saline should be given to correct volume and sodium deficits. If hyponatremia is severe (110–120 mEq/L) and associated with neurologic signs, hypertonic saline (3%) can be used to normalize sodium concentration more rapidly, but the serum sodium concentration should not be increased faster than 1 mEq/L per hour. When a concentration of 125 mEq/L is reached, isotonic saline is used to raise the sodium concentration to normal. Rapid elevation in sodium concentration may be associated with CNS damage.

   b. Access to water should be limited and drugs that may have an antidiuretic effect (e.g., desmopressin) should be withdrawn.

C. **Hypernatremia** reduces ICF volume, which adversely affects the brain. Hypernatremia is caused by salt gain or, more commonly, water loss. Thirst and the excretion of small volumes of concentrated urine is the normal response. Urine osmolality and the status of the effective circulating volume can help determine the cause.

1. **Types**

   a. **Hypernatremia** and **hypervolemia.** This combination usually indicates salt gain and can be caused by salt poisoning, hypertonic fluid administration (e.g., hypertonic saline, sodium bicarbonate), and hyperadrenocorticism.

   b. **Hypernatremia** and **normo-** or **hypovolemia**

      (1) **Low urine volume** and **high urine osmolality** indicate nonrenal water loss, which may be from:

         (a) GI losses (vomiting, diarrhea)
         (b) Third space (peritoneum) losses
         (c) Cutaneous losses (burns, high environmental temperature)
         (d) Hypodipsia (reduced thirst)

      (2) **Normal to increased urine volume** and **less than maximal urine osmolality** is indicative of renal losses through:

         (a) Osmotic diuresis (i.e., glucose, mannitol)
         (b) Drug-induced diuresis
         (c) Renal failure (acute or chronic)
         (d) Postobstructive diuresis

      (3) **Increased urine volume** and **very low urine osmolality** indicate a lack of ADH activity, which may be due to central or nephrogenic diabetes insipidus.

2. **Clinical findings** usually occur when the serum sodium concentration exceeds 170 mEq/L. Clinical signs include anorexia, vomiting, behavioral change, muscular weakness, disorientation, ataxia, seizures, coma, and death.

   a. Most signs relate to **neurologic dysfunction** resulting from water movement out of brain cells. If hypotonic fluid loss has resulted in hypernatremia, signs of **dehydration** and **volume depletion** may be observed. If primary salt gain is the cause, then volume overload (e.g., **pulmonary edema**) may be present. If central or nephrogenic diabetes insipidus is present, **polyuria** and **polydipsia** will be prominent.

   b. **Severity.** The severity of clinical signs is more a function of the rate than the magnitude of sodium elevation.

      (1) **Rapid reduction** in brain volume may rupture cerebral blood vessels.

(2) Gradual reduction enables brain cells to adapt by producing intracellular **substances** that counteract the increase in ECF osmolality, preventing water movement out of brain cells.

3. **Treatment**
   a. The underlying condition should be treated to stop water losses.
   b. The water deficit should be replaced. If severe dehydration is present, the ECF deficit should be corrected first using isotonic fluids (e.g., normal saline, lactated Ringer's). Water losses can then be replaced using hypotonic fluids (5% dextrose in water or half-strength (0.45%) saline). Sodium concentration should be corrected slowly over 48–72 hours, with the rate of reduction not exceeding 1 mEq/L per hour (to prevent brain edema).
   c. Sodium secretion should be augmented when primary salt gain has occurred. In animals with primary salt gain and volume overload, sodium excretion can be enhanced using loop diuretics (e.g., furosemide). Preexisting congestive heart failure or oliguric renal failure may complicate therapy.

II. POTASSIUM

A. Physiology

1. **Distribution**
   a. The ICF compartment contains 95% of the body's potassium, of which 60%–75% is within muscle cells.
   b. The ECF compartment contains only 5% of the body's potassium; however, changes in serum potassium concentration still reflect whole body changes in potassium content (i.e., reduced serum $[K^+]$ correlates with a body K^+ deficit).

2. **Membrane potential.** Diffusion of potassium down its concentration gradient into the ECF generates a resting cell membrane potential. The cell interior becomes negative relative to the exterior.
   a. **Hypokalemia** hyperpolarizes cell membranes (i.e., the resting membrane potential becomes more negative) and makes cells less excitable so that a larger stimulus is needed to reach threshold potential and depolarize the cell. Muscle weakness results.
   b. **Hyperkalemia** hypopolarizes the cell membrane (i.e., the resting membrane potential becomes less negative) and results in increased cell excitability so that a smaller stimulus is required to depolarize the cell. Cardiac rhythm disturbances result.

3. **Potassium balance**
   a. **External.** Ingestion of potassium, normally in excess of the daily requirement, necessitates net potassium excretion, 90% by the kidney and 10% by the colon. When renal function is severely impaired, colonic excretion increases.
   b. **Internal.** Alterations in serum potassium can result from large shifts between the ICF and ECF. Major factors that shift potassium from the ICF to the ECF (resulting in hyperkalemia) include:
      (1) Insulin deficiency
      (2) β_2-adrenergic blockade
      (3) Metabolic acidosis
         (a) Only normal anion gap (hyperchloremic) metabolic acidosis is associated with a significant potassium shift.
         (b) Increased anion gap metabolic acidosis (e.g., diabetic ketoacidosis) is not associated with a significant potassium shift.

4. **Renal potassium excretion** is predominantly controlled by aldosterone and the urine volume or flow rate (influenced by the GFR and a patent excretory pathway). The major stimuli for aldosterone release are ECF contraction (e.g., as a result of hypotension or hypovolemia) and hyperkalemia. Aldosterone is released from the

adrenal cortex and acts on the late distal tubule and cortical collecting duct to cause sodium reabsorption and potassium excretion.

B. Hypokalemia
1. **Etiology**
   a. **Decreased intake**
      (1) **Dietary deficiency** is a very rare cause.
      (2) **Administration of potassium-deficient intravenous fluids** is a very common cause of hypokalemia. These fluids dilute serum potassium levels and increase renal excretion as a result of fluid-induced diuresis.
   b. **Translocation (ECF to ICF)**
      (1) **Alkalemia** shifts potassium into cells in exchange for hydrogen ions (H^+).
      (2) **Insulin** and **glucose administration** results in potassium transport into the cell, most frequently during the treatment of diabetic ketoacidosis.
      (3) **Hypothermia, catecholamine release,** and a **syndrome of episodic weakness** in young Burmese cats have also been associated with hypokalemia as a result of translocation.
   c. **Increased loss** is the **most common cause** of hypokalemia.
      (1) **Gastrointestinal losses,** such as vomiting and diarrhea
      (2) **Renal losses** associated with CRF (especially in cats), dietary potassium restriction (in cats), renal tubular acidosis, postobstructive diuresis, dialysis, mineralocorticoid excess (e.g., hyperadrenocorticism), and drug therapy (e.g., furosemide)
2. **Clinical findings** are often not apparent until the serum potassium level is less than 3.0 mEq/L. Polyuria, polydipsia, reduced urine-concentrating ability, and muscle weakness are the most common signs.
   a. **Renal effects.** Polyuria and polydipsia result from increased thirst and renal tubular resistance to the action of ADH. Hypokalemia can produce peripheral vasoconstriction and reduce renal blood flow and GFR, resulting in azotemia. Sustained hypokalemia may result in morphologic damage to the kidney.
   b. **Muscle effects.** Muscle weakness (due to decreased cell membrane excitability) is a common clinical sign when the serum potassium level is less than 3.0 mEq/L. Vasoconstriction in muscle tissue occurs if the potassium level is less than 2.5 mEq/L and can lead to muscular ischemia, rhabdomyolysis, and elevations in serum creatine kinase. Death can result from hypokalemia-induced respiratory muscle weakness and paralysis.
      (1) In dogs, rear limb muscle weakness is common.
      (2) In cats, weakness of the cervical muscles (leading to ventroflexion of the head) and rear limb muscles is common. Forelimb hypermetria and a broad-based stance have also been observed.
   c. **Cardiac effects**
      (1) Electrocardiographic abnormalities include prolongation of the QT interval, U waves, sagging of the ST segment, increased amplitude of the T wave, and increased amplitude and duration of the QRS complex. Atrial and ventricular premature contractions can also be seen.
      (2) The toxic effects of digitalis, digitalis-induced arrhythmias, and depression of AV conduction are potentiated by hypokalemia. The effectiveness of class I antiarrhythmics (e.g., lidocaine, quinidine, procainamide) is reduced by hypokalemia.
3. **Treatment**
   a. **Parenteral supplementation** is typically combined with intravenous fluid administration, in an amount dependent on the severity of hypokalemia.
      (1) **Potassium chloride** is the most common intravenous formulation. **Potassium phosphate** is occasionally used when treating hypokalemia and hypophosphatemia associated with insulin therapy for diabetic ketoacidosis.
      (2) Because intravenous potassium is potentially cardiotoxic, it should be infused at a rate that does not exceed 0.5 mEq/kg/hour.
      (3) Parenteral therapy should be used with caution in animals that present with

marked hypokalemia and muscle weakness. Unless potassium supplementation in the intravenous fluids is high enough, dilution and increased excretion as a result of the intravenous fluid administration may decrease the serum potassium level, aggravating clinical signs.

 b. Oral supplementation is preferred as the initial treatment in most situations unless severe clinical signs necessitate intravenous treatment. The oral route is also used for long-term control. **Potassium gluconate** is used most often, but **potassium citrate** can also be used for oral supplementation. Dosage should be individualized.

C. Hyperkalemia

1. Etiology

 a. Decreased renal excretion. Chronic or moderate to marked elevations in serum potassium are almost always caused by decreased renal excretion, most commonly as a result of **urethral obstruction, acute oliguric renal failure, rupture of the urinary tract,** or **hypoadrenocorticism.**

 b. Excessive intake is a rare cause of hyperkalemia and is only important if potassium excretion is compromised.

 c. Translocation (ICF to ECF)

  (1) Normal anion gap metabolic acidosis. Potassium is exchanged with hydrogen ions as they move to the intracellular compartment to be buffered. This exchange does not occur with increased anion gap metabolic acidoses (e.g., lactic acidosis).

  (2) Insulin deficiency (e.g., diabetic ketoacidosis) can cause hyperkalemia due to decreased ease of intracellular movement of potassium and hypertonicity of the ECF (i.e., hyperglycemia).

  (3) Acute tumor lysis following radiation and chemotherapy in dogs with lymphoma, in which renal failure was a complicating factor, has been associated with hyperkalemia.

  (4) Reperfusion of ischemic tissue beds (e.g., relief of aortic thromboembolus) flushes out accumulated potassium, raising serum concentrations.

  (5) Administration of nonspecific β-adrenergic blocking agents (e.g., propranolol) may raise serum potassium levels, but only if additional factors such as reduced potassium excretion are present.

 d. Miscellaneous disorders (e.g., salmonellosis, ruptured duodenal ulcers, trichuriasis, and chylothorax with repeated thoracocentesis) can be associated with hyperkalemia.

 e. Drugs (e.g., ACE inhibitors, potassium-sparing diuretics, NSAIDs, heparin) can cause hyperkalemia.

 f. Pseudohyperkalemia can result from thrombocytosis or hemolysis (in Akitas).

  (1) Thrombocytosis. Platelets contain substantial amounts of potassium; and when platelet numbers are very high, potassium can seep into serum during clot formation in amounts sufficient to raise serum potassium.

  (2) Hemolysis in samples collected from Akitas may result in hyperkalemia. Akitas have higher RBC potassium concentrations than other dog breeds.

2. Clinical findings

 a. Muscle weakness occurs when serum concentrations exceed 8 mEq/L.

 b. Cardiotoxicity produces characteristic electrocardiographic findings (listed in order of increasing serum potassium levels): increased amplitude of the T wave, shortening of the QT interval, prolongation of the PR interval, widening of the QRS complex, decrease in amplitude and widening of the P wave, disappearance of the P wave, pronounced bradycardia, merging of the QRS complex and the T wave to produce a sine wave pattern, and ventricular fibrillation or asystole.

 c. Signs associated with underlying disease may also be present (e.g., vomiting with hypoadrenocorticism).

3. Treatment.
A rapid and marked increase in serum potassium necessitates prompt and aggressive therapy. Cardiotoxicity requires aggressive therapy even if serum potassium is not markedly elevated.

a. **Chronic, mild hyperkalemia** may not require immediate therapy, but its cause should be investigated.

b. **Significant hyperkalemia**

(1) Initial measures include the administration of fluids with little or no potassium (e.g., 0.9% saline, lactated Ringer's solution), withdrawal of supplements or drugs that may contribute to the hyperkalemia, and treatment of the underlying cause (e.g., urethral obstruction, ruptured bladder, hypoadrenocorticism).

(2) If hyperkalemia continues or is especially severe:

(a) **Sodium bicarbonate** administered intravenously will cause potassium to move into the ICF.

(b) **Calcium gluconate** administered intravenously will not reduce serum potassium levels, but it will counteract the cardiac toxicity. Effects last for less than 1 hour. Calcium gluconate should be administered slowly with ECG monitoring.

(c) **Glucose** or **glucose and insulin** administered intravenously will move potassium into the ICF.

(d) **Sodium polystyrene sulfonate** (administered orally or as a retention enema) is an exchange resin that will bind potassium in exchange for sodium and increase GI excretion of potassium.

(e) **Diuretics.** Administration of a loop or thiazide diuretic will help to increase urinary potassium excretion.

(f) **Peritoneal** or **hemodialysis** may be helpful.

III. CALCIUM

A. Physiology

1. **Overview.** Serum calcium concentration is maintained within a narrow range by PTH, calcitriol (1, 25 dihydroxyvitamin D_3), calcitonin, and other hormones. **Serum calcium,** or **total calcium,** is made up of an ionized fraction (50%), a complexed or chelated fraction (10%), and a protein-bound fraction (40%). Ionized calcium is biologically active and is the focus of hormonal regulation. The major target organs for these hormones are the bone, intestines, and kidneys.

a. Acute changes in the serum calcium level are made by bone, the major reservoir. Calcitriol and PTH cause osteoblasts to contract (thereby exposing bone mineral to osteoclasts) and release cytokines and growth factors, which stimulate osteoclast-mediated bone resorption.

b. Long-term regulation is controlled by the intestine and, to a lesser extent, the kidneys.

2. **Hormonal maintenance of serum calcium concentration.**

a. **PTH** is a peptide hormone secreted in response to hypocalcemia by the chief cells of the parathyroid gland. Calcitriol is important in establishing the set point for PTH secretion (e.g., calcitriol deficiency leads to excessive PTH secretion). PTH acts primarily on the kidney to increase calcium reabsorption and phosphorus excretion. It also acts on bone together with calcitriol to mobilize calcium and phosphorus.

b. **Calcitriol** is a steroid hormone and is the most biologically active of the vitamin D metabolites. Cholecalciferol (vitamin D_3) can be synthesized in the skin as a consequence of exposure to ultraviolet radiation, or it can be ingested in the diet. It is metabolized to 25 hydroxyvitamin D_3 and then to 1,25 dihydroxyvitamin D_3 (calcitriol) in the liver and kidney, respectively. Calcitriol's major action is to stimulate intestinal calcium absorption and in concert with PTH, mobilize calcium from bone. It has little effect on the kidney. Calcitriol inhibits PTH synthesis and secretion directly (at the glandular level) and indirectly (elevating blood calcium).

c. **Calcitonin** is a peptide hormone that is synthesized by C cells in the thyroid gland and secreted in response to hypercalcemia. Its main role may be to control postprandial hypercalcemia. Calcitonin's main target is bone, where it inhibits calcium mobilization. Calcitonin is considered to have a minor role in normal calcium homeostasis.

B. **Hypocalcemia**

1. **Etiology**

   a. **Hypoalbuminemia** is a common cause of mild hypocalcemia, resulting from a reduction in the protein-bound fraction of serum calcium. Ionized calcium concentrations remain normal, and no clinical signs result. Serum total calcium concentration can be adjusted to account for hypoalbuminemia according to the following formula:

   Adjusted serum total calcium (mg/dl) = serum calcium (mg/dl) − serum albumin (g/dl) + 3.5

   This formula is not valid in dogs younger than 24 weeks of age or in cats.

   b. **Renal failure.** Approximately 10% of dogs and 15% of cats with CRF are hypocalcemic. It is usually asymptomatic.

   c. **Puerperal tetany (eclampsia)** is the most common cause of symptomatic hypocalcemia and usually occurs 1–3 weeks after whelping, especially in small-breed dogs. It is thought to result from an excessive loss of calcium in milk.

   d. **Acute pancreatitis** occasionally results in mild to moderate hypocalcemia, possibly from calcium salt deposition in inflamed tissues adjacent to the pancreas.

   e. **Uncommon causes** include soft tissue trauma or rhabdomyolysis (leading to the tissue deposition of calcium), ethylene glycol intoxication, phosphate enemas, or sodium bicarbonate therapy (leading to calcium chelation), hypoparathyroidism (primary or secondary to bilateral thyroidectomy), laboratory error, severe starvation, hypovitaminosis D, and nutritional secondary hyperparathyroidism.

2. **Clinical findings** result from increased neuromuscular excitability and usually occur in dogs when the serum calcium level is less than 6.5 mg/dl (1.6 mmol/L). Rapid development of hypocalcemia is more likely to result in severe clinical signs.

   a. Signs may be intermittent or persistent and include behavioral changes (e.g., restlessness, excitation, disorientation, aggression, hypersensitivity), muscle tremors, facial rubbing, muscle cramping, pyrexia (due to muscle activity), stiff gait, seizures, and respiratory arrest.

   b. A prolapsed nictitans (cats), polyuria, polydipsia, posterior lenticular cataracts, and tachycardia can also occur.

3. **Treatment**

   a. **Asymptomatic hypocalcemia** usually does not require therapy.

   b. **Puerperal tetany** frequently requires emergency therapy.

   (1) Calcium salts (e.g., calcium gluconate) should be administered intravenously over 10–30 minutes, until severe neuromuscular signs resolve, while monitoring the ECG. Signs of toxicity include bradycardia, shortening of the QT interval, and vomiting. Behavioral signs may take another 30–60 minutes to cease.

   (2) Intravenous calcium is usually followed by diluted subcutaneous calcium gluconate until oral vitamin D (e.g., dihydrotachysterol, calcitriol) and calcium (e.g., calcium carbonate, lactate, or gluconate) supplementation can begin. The duration of oral calcium and vitamin D therapy will vary, and serum calcium should be monitored regularly. Hypercalcemia may develop when using vitamin D and calcium simultaneously.

C. **Hypercalcemia**

1. **Etiology**

   a. **Neoplasia,** especially lymphosarcoma, is the most common cause of persistent hypercalcemia. It can cause hypercalcemia in two ways.

(1) **Tumor-produced circulating (humoral) substances,** such as PTH-related polypeptide, may be seen with lymphosarcoma and anal sac apocrine gland adenocarcinoma.

(2) **Local osteolysis** from multiple myeloma, lymphosarcoma, myeloproliferative disorders, and metastatic or primary bone tumors can lead to hypercalcemia.

b. **Hypoadrenocorticism** can be associated with a mild to moderate hypercalcemia.

c. **Renal failure (acute** and **chronic).** Hypercalcemia occurs in 5%–10% of dogs and 11% of cats with CRF. The cause is unknown, but may involve increased PTH secretion.

d. **Hypervitaminosis D** can be iatrogenic, associated with the ingestion of plants containing calcitriol glycosides, the ingestion of cholecalciferol-containing rodenticides, or associated with granulomatous disease (e.g., blastomycosis).

e. **Primary hyperparathyroidism,** a rare cause, occurs most often in older dogs (age 7–13 years) and results from a functional adenoma in the parathyroid gland.

f. **Miscellaneous causes** include nonmalignant skeletal lesions (e.g., osteomyelitis, hypertrophic osteodystrophy), excessive use of intestinal phosphate binders, excessive calcium supplementation, and hypervitaminosis A.

2. **Clinical findings** vary widely among animals, despite calcium values, and are influenced by the rate of calcium elevation, underlying disease, and acid–base and electrolyte disorders (i.e., acidosis increases ionized calcium and accentuates toxic effects). Most animals show signs when the serum calcium level exceeds 15 mg/dl (3.7 mmol/L).

a. Common clinical signs include polyuria, polydipsia, anorexia, lethargy, weakness, vomiting, and, possibly, prerenal azotemia and CRF.

b. Infrequent clinical signs include constipation, cardiac arrhythmias, seizures, twitching, and death. Rarely, ARF and calcium urolithiasis occur.

3. **Treatment.** The underlying cause should be addressed. Animals with serum calcium levels greater than 16 mg/dl (4.0 mmol/L), those with clinical signs at lower serum values, and those poisoned with cholecalciferol rodenticides should be treated aggressively to help prevent renal injury and failure.

a. **General measures**

(1) **Fluid therapy,** administered either subcutaneously (with mild hypercalcemia) or intravenously (with moderate to severe hypercalcemia) using 0.9% saline, will help increase urinary excretion of calcium and correct any prerenal factors (i.e., dehydration).

(2) **Diuretics** (e.g., furosemide) increase calcium excretion.

(3) **Sodium bicarbonate** binds with calcium to decrease blood concentrations. Its use necessitates close patient monitoring (i.e., blood gas analyses).

(4) **Glucocorticoids** (e.g., prednisone, dexamethasone) are most useful when the hypercalcemia is caused by lymphosarcoma, multiple myeloma, thymoma, vitamin D toxicity, granulomatous disease, or hypoadrenocorticism. These agents reduce serum calcium by increasing urinary calcium excretion and decreasing bone resorption and intestinal calcium absorption. They are also cytotoxic to some tumor cells (i.e., lymphosarcoma). The use of glucocorticoids may interfere with diagnostic testing.

(5) **Other treatments.** Diphosphonates, calcitonin, mithramycin, sodium ethylenediamine tetraacetic acid (EDTA), and peritoneal dialysis can be considered for unresponsive hypercalcemia.

b. **Treatment for cholecalciferol rodenticide ingestion** is usually required for several weeks because of the long half-life of cholecalciferol and its metabolites.

(1) Initial therapy should include **intravenous saline, prednisone,** and **furosemide** for 1–2 weeks, followed by **prednisone, furosemide,** and a **low-calcium diet** for another month.

(2) **Oral phosphate binders** may decrease serum phosphorus concentrations and help prevent soft-tissue mineralization and organ injury.

(3) Calcitonin has been used in the acute management of affected dogs with some success, but side effects (e.g., anorexia, vomiting) and expense have limited its use.

IV. PHOSPHORUS

A. **Physiology.** Phosphorus is the major intracellular anion of the body and plays an important role in the structure (phospholipids in cell membranes, hydroxyapatite in bone),
function (nucleic acids, enzymes), and energy storage [adenosine triphosphate (ATP)] of cells and tissues.

1. **Serum phosphorus.** Most body phosphorus is in the organic form; however, serum phosphorus measurements detect only inorganic phosphorus (orthophosphoric acid, H_2PO_4). Although less than 1% of body phosphorus is in the ECF, serum phosphorus correlates with body content. Serum phosphorus is elevated postprandially and in dogs younger than 1 year of age. Hemolysis, hyperlipidemia, and hyperproteinemia can increase serum phosphorus.

2. **Intake.** Approximately 60%–70% of ingested phosphorus is absorbed in the small intestine. Calcitriol or an increase in dietary phosphorus will increase absorption.

3. **Excretion.** Phosphorus excretion occurs primarily through the kidney in proportion to amount absorbed from the intestinal tract. PTH is the main regulator of renal phosphorus excretion.

B. **Hypophosphatemia**

1. **Etiology**
   a. **Translocation (ECF to ICF)**
      (1) **Treatment of diabetic ketoacidosis** with insulin results in the intracellular movement of phosphorus. These animals have a body phosphorus deficit caused by loss of muscle mass, urinary losses, and an inability to use tissue phosphorus (due to insulin deficiency). However, serum phosphorus is usually normal before therapy. Hypophosphatemia can be severe and result in clinical signs.
      (2) **Other causes** include **infusion of a carbohydrate load** (i.e., 5% dextrose intravenously), **total parenteral nutrition, respiratory alkalosis,** and **hypothermia.**
   b. **Excess urinary loss**
      (1) **Primary hyperparathyroidism** is associated with PTH-induced inhibition of phosphorus reabsorption in the kidney, usually resulting in moderate hypophosphatemia that does not require therapy.
      (2) **Other causes** include **Fanconi's syndrome, puerperal tetany,** therapy with **carbonic anhydrase inhibitors,** and **hyperadrenocorticism.**
   c. **Reduced intestinal absorption** of phosphorus can result from therapy with **oral phosphate binders** (e.g., aluminum hydroxide), **calcitriol deficiency, dietary deficiency, vomiting,** and **malabsorption.**
   d. **Laboratory error.** Mannitol interferes with the measurement of serum phosphorus.

2. **Clinical findings** are uncommon unless severe hypophosphatemia is present. Signs may include anorexia, vomiting (due to intestinal ileus), muscle weakness and pain (rhabdomyolysis), hemolytic anemia (reduced erythrocyte ATP leads to increased fragility), thrombocytopenia, and sepsis (caused by decreased neutrophil function).

3. **Treatment** is dictated by the severity of the hypophosphatemia or the presence of clinical signs. Phosphorus requirements in hypophosphatemic animals are difficult to estimate, so a conservative approach is warranted.

a. **Parenteral phosphorous solutions** (i.e., potassium phosphate) can be used, but electrolytes should be monitored closely to prevent hypocalcemia, tetany, or soft tissue mineralization.

b. **Oral supplementation** (i.e., with potassium or sodium phosphate) is safer but can be associated with diarrhea.

C. **Hyperphosphatemia**

1. **Etiology**

a. **Translocation (ICF to ECF)**

(1) **Tumor lysis syndrome** is a rare cause of hyperphosphatemia but has been documented in dogs with lymphosarcoma treated with chemotherapy. Acute tumor cell lysis can lead to massive release of phosphate-rich intracellular material, resulting in hyperphosphatemia, hypocalcemia, hyperkalemia, and oliguric acute renal failure.

(2) **Other causes** include **massive tissue trauma, rhabdomyolysis,** and **metabolic acidosis.**

b. **Increased intake**

(1) **Phosphate-containing enemas.** Small-breed dogs and cats may develop severe hyperphosphatemia, hyperglycemia, and metabolic acidosis following the administration of phosphate-containing enemas. Lethargy, ataxia, vomiting, mucous membrane pallor, bloody diarrhea, and stupor may also be seen.

(2) **Vitamin D intoxication** (e.g., cholecalciferol rodenticides)

(3) **Overzealous parenteral phosphate administration**

c. **Decreased excretion**

(1) **Acute** or **chronic renal failure** is the most common cause of hyperphosphatemia.

(2) **Uroabdomen** and **urethral obstruction**

(3) **Hypoparathyroidism**

(4) **Hyperthyroidism** in cats (possibly via thyroxine-induced increase in renal phosphate reabsorption) has been associated with hyperphosphatemia in 20% to 50% of cases.

d. **Physiologic** hyperphosphatemia may be seen in young, growing animals.

e. **Laboratory error.** Lipemia or hyperproteinemia can lead to a misdiagnosis of hyperphosphatemia.

2. **Clinical findings** are related to the hypocalcemia and soft tissue mineralization (and organ injury) that hyperphosphatemia may induce.

3. **Treatment.** The underlying cause should be corrected, if possible.

a. **Intravenous saline administration** will increase the GFR and phosphorus excretion.

b. **Intravenous glucose administration** (with or without insulin) may temporarily shift phosphorus intracellularly and reduce serum phosphorus. This treatment is only necessary if severe hyperphosphatemia and clinical signs are present.

c. **Diet modification.** Dietary intake of phosphorus should be reduced through the use of reduced-protein diets.

d. **Oral phosphate binders** (e.g., aluminum hydroxide) can be used in addition to reduced-protein diets to further restrict phosphorus intake.

V. **ACID–BASE**

A. **Physiology.** Hydrogen ions are highly reactive, and their concentration is closely controlled through body buffer systems and respiratory and renal regulation. These systems respond to changes in pH in minutes (buffers), hours (respiratory), and days (renal).

1. **pH** and **hydrogen ion concentration $[H^+]$.** The normal blood pH is 7.4 and the normal hydrogen ion concentration is 40 nEq/L (40 nmol/L).

2. **Generation of hydrogen ions.** Hydrogen ions result from the generation of carbonic (H_2CO_3) and organic (nonvolatile) acids (e.g., β-hydroxybutyrate), and from protein metabolism (e.g., sulphuric and phosphoric acid).

3. **Buffer systems** blunt changes in the hydrogen ion concentration by binding with free hydrogen ion. The bicarbonate buffer system is the main ECF buffer; proteins and organic and inorganic phosphorus are the main ICF buffers. During metabolic acidosis, 60% of the buffering occurs in the ICF and 40% in the ECF.
   a. **Bicarbonate buffer system.** This system provides the basis for clinical acid–base monitoring. The constituents of the bicarbonate buffer system and their relationship to one another are represented as follows:

$$CO_2 + H_2O \; D \; H_2CO_3 \; D \; H^+ + HCO_3^-$$

   The reactions are catalyzed by carbonic anhydrase. The bicarbonate buffer system is related to pH by the Henderson-Hasselbalch equation:

$$pH = 6.1 + \log\left(\frac{[HCO_3^-]}{0.03 \; P_{CO_2}}\right)$$

   b. **Bone carbonate** is also a substantial buffer.

4. **Respiratory regulation** of the hydrogen ion concentration is by excretion of carbon dioxide by the lungs. The reaction equilibrium of the bicarbonate buffer system is shifted to the left, which results in a reduction in hydrogen ion concentration.

5. **Renal regulation** is responsible for long-term control of hydrogen ion concentration. The kidney responds to an increase in hydrogen ion concentration or a decrease in bicarbonate concentration by reabsorbing 100% of filtered bicarbonate (in the proximal tubule) and generating "new" bicarbonate to replace that lost in buffering hydrogen ion. New bicarbonate is produced by hydrogen ion secretion in the distal tubule. The excretion of titratable acids and ammonium facilitates this process. Carbonic anhydrase catalyzes the tubular reactions, which result in bicarbonate reabsorption and hydrogen ion secretion.

B. **Metabolic acidosis** is the most common acid–base disorder.

1. **Types.** Metabolic acidosis can be associated with an increased anion gap or a normal anion gap.
   a. **Definitions**
      (1) **Electroneutrality** must be satisfied. Therefore:
         $Na^+ + K^+ + UC = Cl^- + HCO_3^- + UA$, where
         UC = unmeasured cations and UA = unmeasured anions.
      (2) The **anion gap** equals:
         $(Na^+ + K^+) - (Cl^- + HCO_3^-)$
   b. **Differentiation of metabolic acidoses.** The anion gap helps to differentiate metabolic acidoses caused by bicarbonate loss (e.g., diarrhea) or lack of bicarbonate generation (e.g., renal tubular acidosis) from those caused by acid overproduction (usually the overproduction of organic acids, such as lactic acidosis or ketoacidosis).
      (1) **Increased anion gap metabolic acidosis.** Organic acids (e.g., lactate) and other unmeasured anions (e.g., sulfate) accumulate to cause metabolic acidosis. They also increase the anion gap because the chloride ion concentration decreases to accommodate the increase in unmeasured anions (to maintain electroneutrality).
      (2) **Normal anion gap metabolic acidosis.** When the metabolic acidosis is due to bicarbonate loss or gain of a mineral acid (e.g., ammonium chloride), there is no increase in unmeasured anions and the anion gap remains normal.

2. **Etiology**
   a. **Increased anion gap metabolic acidosis**
      (1) **Diabetic ketoacidosis** results from the accumulation of organic acids in the form of ketone bodies (i.e., acetate, acetoacetate, β-hydroxybutyrate).

      (2) Lactic acidosis is usually associated with hypoxia related to decreased tissue perfusion (e.g., shock, hypovolemia, cardiac arrest), a marked increase in tissue oxygen demand (e.g., severe exercise, seizures), or reduced arterial oxygen content. In rare instances, lactic acidosis may be associated not with hypoxia but with abnormal mitochondrial oxidative function or carbohydrate metabolism (e.g., drugs, toxins).

      (3) Renal failure results in diminished acid excretion and is typically associated with a mild to moderate metabolic acidosis until renal function is severely impaired (in the case of CRF). Moderate to severe acidosis usually accompanies acute oliguric renal failure or urethral obstruction.

      (4) Intoxication with ethylene glycol is the most common toxin associated with an increased anion gap metabolic acidosis. Initially, acidosis arises from the organic acid metabolites (glyoxylate, glycolate) of ethylene glycol. Later, acute renal failure contributes to the acidosis.

   b. Normal anion gap metabolic acidosis

      (1) GI bicarbonate loss. Diarrhea is the most common cause of GI bicarbonate loss.

      (2) Reduced renal acid secretion can result from proximal and distal renal tubular acidosis.

      (3) Hypoadrenocorticism. Aldosterone stimulates distal nephron hydrogen ion secretion; therefore, when aldosterone is decreased, hydrogen ion accumulates and leads to acidosis. The acidosis is mild to moderate.

      (4) Mineral acid administration (e.g., ammonium chloride) can lead to a normal anion gap metabolic acidosis.

3. Diagnosis

   a. Clinical findings usually reflect the underlying disease. The depth and rate of respiration may increase. Severe acidosis may result in lethargy, depression, anorexia, decreased myocardial contractility, and ventricular arrhythmias.

   b. Laboratory findings. Blood gas findings and the **expected compensatory response** are summarized in Table 43-9.

4. Treatment

   a. Initial measures. The underlying cause should be treated, and ventilation, oxygenation, and tissue perfusion should be ensured (e.g., with oxygen supplementation and intravenous fluid therapy).

   b. Bicarbonate therapy. Sodium bicarbonate ($NaHCO_3$) is the agent of choice for parenteral bicarbonate therapy.

      (1) The dose and frequency of administration of sodium bicarbonate are dictated by the severity of the acidosis, the reversibility of the underlying disorder, pulmonary function, renal function, and whether the acid is metabolizable or nonmetabolizable.

         (a) In acute acidosis, sodium bicarbonate is indicated if the blood pH is less than 7.15 or the bicarbonate concentration is less than 5 mEq/L (5 mmol/L). The dose of sodium bicarbonate is calculated with the objective of increasing the blood pH to 7.20, which will ameliorate most of the detrimental effects of acidosis and decrease the risk of adverse effects associated with sodium bicarbonate therapy.

         (b) In chronic acidosis (e.g., chronic renal failure), the blood bicarbonate concentration should be maintained at a level greater than or equal to 18 mEq/L (18 mmol/L) by administering oral sodium bicarbonate or potassium citrate.

      (2) Potential adverse effects of sodium bicarbonate therapy include:

         (a) Volume overload (due to administered sodium),

         (b) A decrease in ionized calcium (which increases the potential for tetany)

         (c) Hypokalemia

         (d) Decreased oxygen delivery to the tissues (as a result of increased oxygen affinity for hemoglobin)

TABLE 43-9. Acid–Base Disorders and Expected Compensatory Responses in Dogs

Acid–Base Disorder	Primary Defect	Effect on Blood pH	Compensatory Response	Range of Compensation
Metabolic acidosis	Loss of HCO_3^- or gain of H^+ ($\downarrow$ [HCO_3^-])	Decreased	Alveolar hyperventilation to increase CO_2 excretion ($\downarrow$ P_{CO_2})	P_{CO_2} $\downarrow$ 0.7 mm Hg for each 1.0 mEq/L $\downarrow$ in [HCO_3^-]
Metabolic alkalosis	Gain of HCO_3^- or loss or H^+ ($\uparrow$ [HCO_3^-])	Increased	Alveolar hypoventilation to decrease CO_2 excretion ($\uparrow$ P_{CO_2})	P_{CO_2} $\uparrow$ 0.7 mm Hg for each 1.0 mEq/L $\downarrow$ in [HCO_3^-]
Respiratory acidosis	Alveolar hypoventilation ($\uparrow$ P_{CO_2})	Decreased	$\uparrow$ Renal HCO_3^- reabsorption ($\uparrow$ [HCO_3^-])	Acute: [HCO_3^-] $\uparrow$ 0.15 mEq/L for each 1.0 mm Hg $\uparrow$ in P_{CO_2} Chronic: [HCO_3^-] $\uparrow$ 0.35 mEq/L for each 1.0 mm Hg $\uparrow$ in P_{CO_2}
Respiratory alkalosis	Alveolar hyperventilation ($\downarrow$ P_{CO_2})	Increased	$\downarrow$ Renal HCO_3^- reabsorption ($\downarrow$ [HCO_3^-])	Acute: [HCO_3^-] $\downarrow$ 0.25 mEq/L for each 1.0 mm Hg $\downarrow$ in P_{CO_2} Chronic: [HCO_3^-] $\downarrow$ 0.55 mEq/L for each 1.0 mm Hg $\uparrow$ in P_{CO_2}

CO_2 = carbon dioxide; H^+ = hydrogen ion; HCO_3^- = bicarbonate; P_{CO_2} = arterial carbon dioxide tension; $\uparrow$ = increase; $\downarrow$ = decrease.

    (e) Paradoxical CNS acidosis (occurring when the hyperventilation abates and carbon dioxide diffuses into the cerebrospinal fluid)
    (f) Hypercapnia
    (g) Metabolic alkalosis [due to overzealous dosing or a late development as organic acids (e.g., β-hydroxybutyrate, lactate) are metabolized to bicarbonate]

C. **Metabolic alkalosis**

    1. Types and **etiology**
       a. Chloride-responsive metabolic alkalosis is the most common type of metabolic alkalosis in dogs and cats. It is usually caused by vomiting (resulting in the loss of HCl) or overzealous diuretic therapy. The blood bicarbonate concentration is elevated due to:
          (1) ECF volume contraction, reduced GFR, and a decrease in the filtered load of bicarbonate
          (2) Chloride depletion, which encourages avid bicarbonate reabsorption in the proximal tubule
          (3) Aldosterone release (as a result of ECF volume contraction), which stimulates sodium reabsorption and potassium and hydrogen ion secretion, leading to hypokalemia and exacerbation of the alkalosis

(4) Renal ammoniagenesis, which leads to the generation of new bicarbonate and exacerbation of the alkalosis and is stimulated by hypokalemia

b. Chloride-resistant metabolic alkalosis is rare and is usually associated with hyperaldosteronism (e.g., hyperadrenocorticism).

2. Diagnosis

a. Clinical findings usually reflect the underlying disorder.

(1) Neurologic signs (e.g., disorientation, agitation, stupor) may accompany severe alkalosis.

(2) Muscle weakness may be observed with significant hypokalemia. Muscle twitching may occur if alkalosis reduces the ionized calcium concentration.

b. Laboratory findings. Blood gas findings and the **expected compensatory response** are summarized in Table 43-9.

3. Treatment. The underlying disorder and fluid and electrolyte deficits should be corrected. The administration of normal saline and additional potassium will resolve chloride-responsive metabolic alkalosis. Therapy for chloride-resistant disorders is difficult unless the underlying cause can be corrected.

D. **Respiratory acidosis** is the second most common acid–base disorder.

1. Etiology. Respiratory acidosis will accompany any disease process that decreases alveolar ventilation. Reduced ventilation results in progressive elevations in the arterial carbon dioxide tension (Pco_2), which, in turn, generates hydrogen ion. Causes of reduced ventilation include:

a. CNS disease (e.g., brain stem trauma, anesthetic or sedative overdose), which can depress respiratory centers

b. Respiratory muscle disease (e.g., myasthenia gravis, tetanus, botulism, polyradiculoneuritis, hypokalemic myopathy, polymyositis, tick paralysis)

c. Pulmonary disease (e.g., pneumonia, pulmonary thromboembolism, chronic obstructive lung disease, acute respiratory distress syndrome, diffuse metastatic disease)

d. Airway obstruction (e.g., tracheal foreign body, tumor, asthma)

e. Restrictive disease (e.g., pneumothorax, diaphragmatic hernia, pleural effusion, chest wall trauma, pulmonary fibrosis)

2. Pathogenesis. Acute hypoventilation can result in fatal hypoxemia before significant hypercapnia (i.e., an elevated Pco_2) and respiratory acidosis develop. Acute respiratory acidosis will reach a compensatory steady state in 2–5 days, after which chronic respiratory acidosis is present.

3. Diagnosis

a. Clinical findings. Signs reflect the underlying cause.

b. Laboratory findings. Blood gas findings and the **expected compensatory responses** are summarized in Table 43-9.

4. Treatment of the underlying cause (e.g., relief of airway obstruction, removal of pleural fluid) is most effective.

a. Ventilatory assistance and supplemental oxygen may be required if the condition is acute. Oxygen therapy is less useful in chronic situations because it may aggravate hypercapnia by reducing hypoxia-stimulated ventilation.

b. Intravenous saline facilitates recovery from chronic respiratory acidosis by preventing the development of metabolic alkalosis following the decrease in Pco_2. The Pco_2 should be decreased slowly in animals with chronic respiratory acidosis. Rapid reduction in Pco_2 can lead to cardiac arrhythmias, reduced cardiac output, decreased cerebral blood flow, and cerebrospinal fluid alkalosis (i.e., the rapid diffusion of carbon dioxide out of the cerebrospinal fluid).

c. Bicarbonate is not indicated in respiratory acidosis. It decreases the concentration of hydrogen ion in the CNS, which reduces the ventilatory drive and aggravates hypoxemia and hypercapnia.

E. **Respiratory alkalosis** is the least common acid–base disorder.

1. Etiology. Respiratory alkalosis results from expiration or excretion of carbon dioxide in excess of metabolic production.

    a. Hypoxemia stimulates peripheral chemoreceptors to increase ventilation. Causes of hypoxemia include right-to-left shunting [e.g., reverse patent ductus arteriosus (PDA)], congestive heart failure, severe anemia, hypotension, and pulmonary diseases causing ventilation–perfusion mismatch (e.g., pulmonary embolism).

    b. Pulmonary disease (e.g., interstitial lung disease, edema) can stimulate nocioceptors to increase ventilation in the absence of hypoxemia.

    c. Direct stimulation of medullary respiratory centers by liver disease, Gram-negative sepsis, drugs (e.g., salicylate intoxication), CNS disease, or heat stroke can result in excessive ventilation.

    d. Overzealous mechanical ventilation can lead to respiratory alkalosis.

2. Diagnosis

    a. Clinical findings. Signs of the underlying disease dominate.

        (1) Acute hypocapnia may reduce cerebral blood flow, resulting in neurologic signs.

        (2) Chronic hypocapnia rarely results in symptoms because the degree of alkalosis is mild.

    b. Laboratory findings. Blood gas findings and **expected compensatory responses** are summarized in Table 43-9.

3. Treatment should be focused on reversing the underlying abnormality.

DIRECTIONS: Each of the numbered items or incomplete statements in this section is followed by answers or by completions of the statement. Select the ONE numbered answer or completion that is BEST in each case. Please see appendix for normal reference ranges for laboratory data.

1. When does renal azotemia develop?

(1) When renal function, or the glomerular filtration rate (GFR), is less than or equal to 50% of normal
(2) When the GFR is less than or equal to 75% of normal
(3) When the GFR is less than or equal to 25% of normal
(4) When one kidney is obstructed
(5) Before the onset of polyuria and polydipsia

2. A 7-year-old neutered male cat is presented for weight loss of 2 months' duration. The cat's appetite is good, and no vomiting, diarrhea, or alteration in water intake or urination has been noted. The cat is in thin body condition with normal vital signs. A complete blood count (CBC) is normal. Serum biochemistry reveals the following: albumin, 1.4 g/dl (14 g/L); cholesterol, 426 mg/dl (11 mmol/L). Urinalysis reveals a specific gravity of 1.040 and 3 + protein; there are no abnormalities in the sediment. The urine protein:creatinine ratio ($U_{Pr}:U_{Cr}$) is 5.2. This cat has:

(1) chronic renal failure.
(2) glomerular disease.
(3) chronic tubulointerstitial disease.
(4) neoplasia.
(5) urinary tract inflammation.

3. A 2-year-old, neutered male cat is presented in a moribund state. The cat has not been well, in that the owner noted only a decreased appetite for the last day. The cat has a rectal temperature of 98.6°F (37°C), a heart rate of 90 beats/minute and a respiratory rate of 30 beats/minute. He is minimally responsive to external stimulation. A large, turgid urinary bladder is palpated. What is the tentative diagnosis and initial plan?

(1) Probable trauma. Start intravenous fluids and shock doses of corticosteroids immediately.
(2) Acute renal failure (ARF). Start on intravenous fluids and provide supplemental heat to increase body temperature.
(3) Probable toxin ingestion. Start on intravenous fluids to increase toxin excretion and provide supplemental heat.
(4) Urethral obstruction. Immediately start intravenous saline and obtain an electrocardiogram (ECG).
(5) Urethral obstruction. Catheterize the urinary bladder to relieve the obstruction.

4. An 8-year-old neutered male golden retriever is presented because of lethargy, anorexia, polyuria, and polydipsia. The dog is depressed, and marked lymphadenopathy of the prescapular and popliteal lymph nodes is detected. Serum biochemical profile abnormalities include: serum calcium, 16.5 mg/dl (4.12 mmol/L); serum creatinine, 3.4 mg/dl (300 μmol/L); serum urea, 45 mg/dl (16.1 mmol/L). Urinalysis reveals a urine specific gravity of 1.018. What is the most likely explanation for the hypercalcemia?

(1) Lymphosarcoma
(2) Chronic renal failure (CRF)
(3) Acute renal failure (ARF)
(4) Cholecalciferol rodenticide intoxication
(5) Hypoadrenocorticism

5. A 10-year-old spayed female Sheltie is presented because of lethargy, anorexia, and intermittent vomiting of 3 days' duration. The dog is thin, depressed, and 5%–6% dehydrated. Vital signs are normal. Laboratory blood analysis reveals a total white blood cell (WBC) count of $19 \times 10^3/\mu l$ (neutrophils: $15 \times 10^3/\mu l$, bands $0.1 \times 10^3/\mu l$), hematocrit of 25% (0.1% reticulocytes), a serum creatinine level of 6.7 mg/dl (592 μmol/L), a serum urea level of 125 mg/dl (44.6 mmol/L), and a serum phosphorus level of 10.2 mg/dl (3.29 mmol/L). Urinalysis reveals a specific gravity of 1.016 with an inactive sediment. What are the diagnosis and best initial treatment?

(1) Acute renal failure (ARF)— intravenous fluid therapy with lactated Ringer's solution
(2) ARF— diuretics and mannitol to increase urine volume and decrease azotemia
(3) Chronic renal failure (CRF)— reduced-protein diet and oral phosphorus binders
(4) Acute gastritis with prerenal azotemia— intravenous fluid therapy with lactated Ringer's solution
(5) CRF— intravenous fluid therapy with lactated Ringer's solution

6. A 5-year-old, spayed female Doberman pinscher is presented because of inappropriate urination. There have been wet spots on the dog's blanket after she has slept there. The dog is not on any medications. There are no abnormalities on physical examination. The dog is taken outside to urinate and does so normally. A free-flow urine sample is collected. The bladder is nonpalpable after urination. Urinalysis reveals the following: specific gravity, 1.035; pH, 5.5; negative glucose, protein, ketones, and bilirubin; red blood cells (RBCs), 0–1 per high-power field; white blood cells (WBCs), 1–2 per high-power field; trace bacteria; 2 + phosphate crystals. What is the most likely diagnosis?

(1) Urinary tract infection (UTI) causing urge incontinence
(2) Urinary incontinence due to urethral sphincter incompetence
(3) Struvite urolithiasis due to UTI
(4) Urinary incontinence due to polyuria
(5) Urinary incontinence due to partial urethral obstruction

7. A 4-year-old, neutered male cat was referred for a neurologic evaluation. The cat had been treated 3 days ago for idiopathic lower urinary tract disease and urethral obstruction. The cat had received subcutaneous lactated Ringer's solution and amoxicillin orally twice daily. The cat had not eaten for 4 days. This morning the cat was weak with his head flexed ventrally. The cat could sit sternally but could not lift his head from the flexed position. Laboratory evaluation reveals: serum potassium, 1.9 mEq/L (1.9 mmol/L); creatinine, 2.8 mg/dl (248 μmol/L); urea, 42 mg/dl (15 mmol/L); and creatine kinase, 850 IU/L (850 U/L). Urinalysis reveals: specific gravity, 1.015; pH, 6.5; protein 2 +; red blood cells (RBCs), 40–50 per high-power field; white blood cells (WBCs), 2–4 per high-power field; bacteria, negative; crystals, amorphous phosphate 3 +. The sudden change in this cat's condition is best explained by:

(1) weakness and lethargy due to renal failure.
(2) weakness and lethargy due to pyelonephritis.
(3) weakness due to muscle trauma and renal failure.
(4) weakness due to hypokalemia.
(5) drug reaction due to the amoxicillin.

8. Urine is collected by cystocentesis from a dog with dysuria and hematuria. Urinalysis reveals: specific gravity, 1.037; pH, 8.0; protein, 3 +; glucose, ketones, and bilirubin, negative; white blood cells (WBCs), 30–40 per high-power field; red blood cells (RBCs), 30–40 per high-power field; bacteria, numerous; crystals, 3 + amorphous phosphate. What is the most likely bacterial pathogen and the appropriate treatment?

(1) *Staphylococcus* species— amoxicillin
(2) *Escherichia coli* — trimethoprim/sulfa
(3) *Klebsiella* species— tetracycline
(4) *Staphylococcus* species— gentamicin
(5) *Pseudomonas* species— amoxicillin

9. A 7-month-old female Yorkshire terrier is presented for stranguria and hematuria of 1 week's duration. Findings on urinalysis (cystocentesis) are: specific gravity, 1.020; pH, 6.0; protein, 2+; glucose, ketones, and bilirubin, negative; red blood cells (RBCs), 30–40 per high-power field; white blood cells (WBCs), 10–15 per high-power field; bacteria, negative. A radiograph of the bladder reveals no abnormalities. A double-contrast cystogram reveals several small uroliths. A complete blood count (CBC) is normal. Serum biochemistry reveals: urea = 4.0 mg/dl (1.4 mmol/L), albumin, 1.8 g/dl (18 g/L). What is the most likely mineral composition of the uroliths?

(1) Struvite (magnesium ammonium phosphate)
(2) Cystine
(3) Urate
(4) Calcium oxalate
(5) Silica

10. An 11-year-old, mixed-breed, neutered male dog is presented because of weight loss and a reduced appetite. On examination, the dog is quiet and vital signs are normal. A 5″ × 4″ abdominal mass is palpated in the cranial abdomen. Laboratory abnormalities are: hematocrit, 27% (reticulocytes = 0.1%); creatinine, 2.2 mg/dl (195 μmol/L); urea, 35 mg/dl (12.5 mmol/L). Urinalysis (free-flow) reveals: specific gravity, 1.019; pH, 6.5; protein, 1+; glucose, ketones, and bilirubin, negative; red blood cells (RBCs), 20–30 per high-power field; white blood cells (WBCs), 10–15 per high-power field; bacteria, negative; crystals, negative. A radiograph identifies the abdominal mass as an enlarged left kidney. Thoracic radiographs are normal. Which one of the following assessments would be most correct?

(1) Renal neoplasia and renal azotemia (failure), most likely as a result of renal lymphosarcoma
(2) Renal amyloidosis and renal azotemia
(3) Chronic pyelonephritis and prerenal azotemia
(4) Renal neoplasia and prerenal azotemia, most likely as a result of renal carcinoma
(5) Renal neoplasia and renal azotemia (failure), most likely as a result of renal carcinoma

11. A 3-year-old, neutered male Labrador retriever is brought to the veterinarian because of lethargy and vomiting. Blood gas results are: pH = 7.22, serum bicarbonate concentration = 12 mEq/L (12 mmol/L), arterial carbon dioxide tension (Paco$_2$) = 30 mm Hg, arterial oxygen tension (Pao$_2$) = 96 mm Hg. Which acid–base disorder is present?

(1) Uncompensated metabolic acidosis
(2) Uncompensated metabolic alkalosis
(3) Compensated respiratory acidosis
(4) Compensated metabolic acidosis
(5) Uncompensated respiratory acidosis

12. A 1-year-old male Irish setter is brought to the veterinarian following the acute onset of lethargy and vomiting. The dog is very depressed and weak; he cannot stand up. Laboratory abnormalities are: potassium, 7.0 mEq/L (7.0 mmol/L); phosphorus, 13.9 mg/dl (4.49 mmol/L); creatinine, 9.6 mg/dl (849 μmol/L); urea, 140 mg/dl (50 mmol/L). Urinalysis reveals: specific gravity, 1.015; pH, 5.5; protein, trace; glucose, ketones, and bilirubin, negative; red blood cells (RBCs), 2–3 per high-power field; white blood cells (WBCs), 1–2 per high-power field; bacteria, negative; granular casts, 5 per low-power field; calcium oxalate monohydrate crystals, 3+. Blood gases reveal: pH, 7.12; bicarbonate concentration, 9 mEq/L (9 mmol/L); arterial carbon dioxide tension (Pco$_2$) = 28 mm Hg. What is the most likely diagnosis?

(1) Chronic renal failure (CRF) due to urinary tract obstruction
(2) Acute renal failure (ARF) due to calcium oxalate nephrolithiasis
(3) Urinary tract obstruction due to urethral calcium oxalate urolithiasis
(4) ARF due to ethylene glycol intoxication
(5) Hypoadrenocorticism

13. A 5-year-old spayed female dachshund is presented because of chronic small bowel diarrhea, intermittent vomiting, and weight loss. The dog is bright and alert, but thin. The complete blood count (CBC) is normal. Biochemistry reveals: serum alanine aminotransferase (sALT), 100 IU/L (100 U/L); serum alkaline phosphatase (SAP), 215 IU/L (215 U/L); albumin = 1.3 g/dl (13 g/L); calcium, 7.2 mg/dl (1.8 mmol/L). Urinalysis reveals: specific gravity, 1.017; pH, 6.5; protein, glucose, ketones, and bilirubin, negative; red blood cells (RBCs), 0–1 per high-power field, white blood cells (WBCs), 0–1 per high-power field; bacteria, negative. The hypocalcemia is most likely due to:

(1) hypoalbuminemia.
(2) acute pancreatitis.
(3) primary hypoparathyroidism.
(4) gastrointestinal (GI) malabsorption.
(5) kidney disease.

14. An 8-year-old neutered male boxer is presented for polyuria and polydipsia of 3 weeks' duration. The results of a complete blood count (CBC), serum biochemical profile, urinalysis, low-dose dexamethasone response test, and endogenous creatinine clearance evaluation are normal. The urine specific gravity has ranged from 1.004 to 1.007 on repeated measures. A water deprivation test is performed. After 4 hours and loss of 5% of body weight, the urine specific gravity is 1.008. Following antidiuretic hormone (ADH) administration, the urine specific gravity ranges from 1.007 to 1.010 for the next 3 hours. What is the reason for the polyuria and polydipsia?

(1) Hyperadrenocorticism
(2) Chronic renal failure (CRF)
(3) Psychogenic polydipsia
(4) Central diabetes insipidus
(5) Nephrogenic diabetes insipidus

15. A 3-year-old spayed female Border collie is presented because of the acute onset of vomiting and depression. The dog is quiet, with tacky mucous membranes and a prolonged capillary refill time. Her vital signs are normal, and a complete blood count (CBC) is unremarkable. Serum biochemistry reveals: sodium, 133 mEq/L (133 mmol/L); potassium, 7.0 mEq/L (7.0 mmol/L); creatinine, 2.8 mg/dl (246 μmol/L); urea, 42 mg/dl (15.4 mmol/L); osmolality, 285 mOsm/kg. Urinalysis reveals: specific gravity, 1.025; pH, 7.0; protein, glucose, ketones, and bilirubin, negative; red blood cells (RBCs), 0 per high-power field; white blood cells (WBCs), 0–1 per high-power field; bacteria, negative. What would be the next best diagnostic test?

(1) An adrenocorticotrophic hormone (ACTH) response test
(2) Endogenous creatinine clearance test
(3) Abdominal radiographs
(4) Fractional excretion of sodium
(5) Urine osmolality

16. A 4-year-old, spayed female miniature schnauzer is presented for pollakiuria and hematuria of 1 week's duration. The dog is bright and alert with no abnormal physical findings. Urinalysis (cystocentesis) reveals specific gravity, 1.028; pH, 8.0; protein, 2 + ; glucose, ketones, and bilirubin, negative; red blood cells (RBCs), too numerous to count; white blood cells (WBCs), 30–40 per high-power field; bacteria, 2 + ; crystals, amorphous phosphate. An abdominal radiograph reveals a 2″ × 1″ radiodense urolith in the bladder. What is the most likely mineral composition of the urolith?

(1) Calcium oxalate
(2) Silica
(3) Struvite
(4) Urate
(5) Cystine

17. Urethral sphincter incompetence is suspected to be the cause of incontinence in a 4-year-old spayed female German shepherd. Which one of the following drugs would be an appropriate consideration?

(1) An α-adrenergic receptor blocker
(2) Progesterone
(3) A β-adrenergic receptor blocker
(4) An α-adrenergic receptor agonist
(5) A parasympathomimetic drug

DIRECTIONS: Each of the numbered items or incomplete statements in this section is negatively phrased, as indicated by a capitalized word such as NOT, LEAST, or EXCEPT. Select the ONE numbered answer or completion that is BEST in each case.

18. Which one of the following would NOT be an appropriate choice for the treatment of chronic bacterial prostatitis in a dog?

(1) Trimethoprim/sulfonamide
(2) Amoxicillin
(3) Erythromycin
(4) Enrofloxacin
(5) Chloramphenicol

19. Which one of the following would NOT be associated with renal amyloidosis?

(1) Intermittent fevers
(2) White blood cell (WBC) casts
(3) Acute blindness
(4) Dyspnea and hypoxemia
(5) Subcutaneous edema

20. Which one of the following measures is NOT effective for reducing the serum phosphorus concentration?

(1) Aluminum hydroxide
(2) Calcium carbonate
(3) Reduced protein diet
(4) Calcitriol therapy
(5) Intravenous glucose administration

1. The answer is 3 [Part I:I A 2 b]. Azotemia occurs when renal function, as measured by the glomerular filtration rate (GFR), has been reduced to less than or equal to 25% of normal. Both kidneys have to be obstructed (urethral or bilateral ureteral obstruction) before azotemia will develop. Once renal function is decreased to less than or equal to 33% of normal, tubular concentrating ability is diminished and polyuria and polydipsia result; therefore, polyuria and polydipsia precede the development of azotemia.

2. The answer is 2 [Part I:V C 2]. Proteinuria in the absence of an active urinary sediment (i.e., hematuria or pyuria) is indicative of glomerular protein loss. A urine protein:creatinine ratio ($U_{pr}:U_{Cr}$) greater than 1.0 suggests the glomerular protein loss is significant or abnormal and indicative of glomerular disease. Hypoalbuminemia (from a variety of causes) is commonly accompanied by hypercholesterolemia. Adequate tubular concentrating capacity (as indicated by the specific gravity of 1.040) and the absence of azotemia make chronic renal failure and tubulointerstitial disease unlikely. The lack of hematuria or pyuria rules out urinary tract inflammation. The cat does not have physical or laboratory signs suggestive of neoplasia. Weight loss could be accounted for by urinary protein loss.

3. The answer is 4 [Part I: XI D 2]. The presence of a large, turgid urinary bladder suggests urethral obstruction. Complete obstruction results in severe illness within 24–72 hours. Hyperkalemia is the most life-threatening aberration and results in weakness, bradycardia (which this cat has), and cardiac rhythm disturbances. As such, hyperkalemia becomes a therapeutic priority, and an attempt should be made to reduce the hyperkalemia as soon as possible with potassium-free intravenous fluids (i.e., 0.9% saline). An electrocardiogram (ECG) should be obtained to assess cardiotoxicity and determine if other potassium-reducing measures are needed. The urethral obstruction can be addressed after these measures have been taken.

4. The answer is 1 [Part II: III C 1 a]. The most common cause of hypercalcemia is neo-plasia, especially lymphosarcoma. Although inflammatory and infectious disease may cause peripheral lymphadenopathy, the presence of marked enlargement with severe hypercalcemia is highly suggestive of lymphosarcoma. The clinical signs (polyuria, polydipsia) and azotemia can be attributed to hypercalcemia. Renal failure could result in similar clinical signs, but the lymphadenopathy and the degree of hypercalcemia are not consistent with this disorder. Cholecalciferol rodenticide toxicity and hyperadrenocorticism are not associated with lymphadenopathy. Hypercalcemia associated with hypoadrenocorticism is usually mild.

5. The answer is 5 [Part I:IV C, D]. The presence of azotemia with a urine specific gravity of less than 1.030 indicates renal azotemia (i.e., renal failure). The thin body condition and nonregenerative anemia suggest chronic renal failure (CRF), rather than acute renal failure (ARF). The dog is uremic and should be rehydrated, which will hopefully reduce the azotemia, vomiting, and lethargy. A reduced-protein diet and oral phosphorus binders would be appropriate considerations after the animal is feeling better.

6. The answer is 2 [Part I: X B 2 b]. The involuntary nature of the dog's inappropriate urination suggests incontinence. The absence of neurologic deficits, lack of bladder distention before or after urination and no dysuria or stranguria is consistent with bladder hypercontractility, reduced bladder storage, or urethral sphincter incompetence. Urethral sphincter incompetence is the most common cause of incontinence in dogs and typically occurs in young to middle-aged, large-breed, spayed female dogs. The urine red blood cells (RBCs), white blood cells (WBCs), and trace bacteria could all be considered normal for a free-flow sample. A urine specific gravity of 1.035 makes polyuria unlikely. Phosphate crystalluria is a common finding and does not indicate the presence of urolithiasis.

7. The answer is 4 [Part II:II B]. The profound hypokalemia could easily account for the muscle weakness and damage (as evidenced by the increased serum creatine kinase level) observed in this cat. Weakness of the cervical muscles results in ventroflexion of the head. Hypokalemia probably developed from decreased potassium intake (anorexia) and increased urinary losses due to postobstructive and fluid diuresis (induced by the earlier administration of lactated Ringer's solution). Hypokalemia can also result in renal vasoconstriction and the development of azotemia. Fluid therapy usually results in isosthenuric urine (specific gravity 1.007–1.015). Therefore, specific gravity cannot be used to localize the azotemia in this cat. The urine sediment abnormalities and proteinuria are consistent with the preexisting idiopathic lower urinary tract disease.

8. The answer is 1 [Part I:VII B 2, C 1]. The urine pH is very alkaline, which suggests that the bacterial pathogen is a urease-producer. Urease splits urea to ammonia, thus increasing the urine pH. The most common urease producers encountered in urinary tract infections (UTIs) are *Staphylococcus* species and *Proteus* species. Although other antibiotics are effective against staphylococcal UTI, amoxicillin is the best choice based on its effectiveness, low price, and infrequent side effects.

9. The answer is 3 [Part I:VIII E 3]. The radiolucent nature of the uroliths suggest either ammonium urate or cystine uroliths. The decreased urea and albumin level suggests impaired hepatic function. This, in conjunction with the young age and breed (portosystemic shunts are common in Yorkshire terriers), makes portosystemic shunt a strong possibility. Given this, the identity of the urolith is most likely urate. Cystine stones occur almost exclusively in males and are most prevalent in bulldogs and dachshunds. Struvite stones are radiodense and usually occur in an alkaline environment secondary to bacterial urinary tract infection (UTI) in dogs. Calcium oxalate and silica stones are radiodense and would have been visible on survey radiographs.

10. The answer is 5 [Part I: XII A 3]. This dog has a triad of clinical signs that is common with renal neoplasia; namely, weight loss, abdominal mass, and hematuria. The most common reason for marked unilateral renomegaly in a dog of this age would be neoplasia. A primary renal tumor is likely because there is no evidence of neoplastic disease elsewhere. The most common primary renal tumor in dogs is renal carcinoma. Renal amyloidosis may re-

sult in renal enlargement but not unilaterally. In addition, amyloid would be associated with more severe proteinuria. Chronic pyelonephritis is usually not associated with unilateral renal enlargement. The fact that the urine specific gravity is less than 1.030 indicates that the azotemia is renal in origin. The nonregenerative anemia is likely an anemia of chronic disease, and is not uncommon in animals with neoplasia and weight loss.

11. The answer is 4 [Part II:V B; Table 43-9]. The blood pH is acid and the bicarbonate concentration is reduced. These findings are consistent with metabolic acidosis. The metabolic acidosis is compensated. In dogs, if the normal bicarbonate concentration is 22 mEq/L (22 mmol/L) and the arterial carbon dioxide tension (P_{CO_2}) is 37 mm Hg, then the bicarbonate concentration has decreased 10 mEq/L and the P_{CO_2} has decreased 7 mm Hg. This is the expected compensatory response in metabolic acidosis.

12. The answer is 4 [Part I:III]. The Irish setter most likely has acute renal failure (ARF) due to ethylene glycol intoxication. The azotemia is renal in origin. Hyperkalemia, severe metabolic acidosis, the acute clinical course, and lack of anemia and historical polyuria and polydipsia support a diagnosis of acute rather than chronic renal failure. There are no physical findings to support urinary tract obstruction (e.g., bladder distention). Marked calcium oxalate crystalluria in the face of marked renal azotemia is highly suggestive of ethylene glycol-induced ARF. The severe metabolic acidosis is also a common feature of ethylene glycol intoxication. Acute, severe hypoadrenocorticism can mimic the clinical and laboratory abnormalities observed with acute renal failure; however, calcium oxalate crystalluria would not be observed. ARF as a result of calcium oxalate nephrolithiasis is rare.

13. The answer is 1 [Part II: III B]. Hypoalbuminemia is a common cause of mild to moderate hypocalcemia and is caused by a reduction in the protein-bound fraction of total measured calcium. Total calcium can be adjusted for hypoalbuminemia using the formula: serum calcium (mg/dl) − serum albumin (g/dl) + 3.5. Therefore, for this patient, the adjusted serum total calcium is 9.4 mg/dl, which is in the normal range: 7.2 − 1.3 + 3.5 = 9.4 mg/dl. The historical signs are not consistent with acute pancreatitis. Primary hypothyroidism is rare and not associated with chronic gastrointestinal

(GI) signs. GI malabsorption is a rare cause of hypocalcemia. The laboratory results do not support kidney disease.

14. The answer is 5 [Part I:I B 4 c (2); VI F]. The laboratory work has ruled out many common causes of polyuria and polydipsia (i.e., electrolyte disturbances, renal failure, hyperadrenocorticism). The lack of urine concentration following water deprivation rules out psychogenic polydipsia (in most cases) and is consistent with diabetes insipidus. The lack of response to antidiuretic hormone (ADH) is consistent with tubular resistance to the action of ADH; therefore, nephrogenic diabetes insipidus is the most likely diagnosis.

15. The answer is 1 [Part II:I B 1 c (1), II C 1 a]. One of the most common causes of combined hyponatremia and hyperkalemia (as evidenced by a sodium:potassium ratio of less than 25) is hypoadrenocorticism (aldosterone and cortisol deficiency). As such, an adrenocorticotropic hormone (ACTH) response test to evaluate resting and stimulated plasma cortisol concentrations would be the most specific and cost-effective diagnostic test in this situation. An endogenous creatinine clearance test [to measure the glomerular filtration rate (GFR)] or a fractional excretion of sodium (to rule out renal sodium loss) would not be worth pursuing unless the ACTH response was normal. It is difficult to localize the azotemia in this patient. On the surface, it appears renal in origin, but dogs with hypoadrenocorticism cannot maximally concentrate their urine. Therefore, a prerenal azotemia may be present in this dog. An abdominal radiograph could be justified [some gastrointestinal (GI) diseases can have these electrolyte aberrations], but it would be less specific than an ACTH response test. Evaluation of urine osmolality would not provide any diagnostically useful information at this time.

16. The answer is 3 [Part I: VIII E 1]. Urinary tract infection (UTI) with urease-producing bacteria will alkalinize the urine. The high pH favors precipitation of struvite (magnesium ammonium phosphate) crystals. Infection-induced struvite stones are the most common urolith in dogs. Therefore, the most likely identity of a radiodense urolith associated with an alkaline urine pH is struvite. All the other uroliths are associated with acidic or neutral urine. Calcium oxalate and silica uroliths are radiodense, but cystine and urate uroliths are not.

17. The answer is 4 [Part I:X C 3]. Urethral sphincter tone is increased by sympathetic nervous activity via α receptors in the smooth muscle of the sphincter and bladder neck. Therefore, an α-adrenergic receptor agonist will increase urethral sphincter tone and ameliorate incontinence associated with decreased sphincter tone or competence. An α-adrenergic receptor blocker, parasympathomimetic agent (which would stimulate detrusor muscle contraction), or β-adrenergic receptor blocker (which would decrease bladder storage) would likely aggravate the incontinence. Progesterone would have no effect.

18. The answer is 2 [Part I:IX B 2 b (2)]. Special consideration must be given to the ability of an antimicrobial to penetrate the prostate gland in a patient with chronic prostatitis. Amoxicillin is a poor choice because of its inability to penetrate the prostate gland to any great degree. The acidic nature and low lipid solubility of amoxicillin are the factors most likely responsible for this.

19. The answer is 2 [Part I:V]. White blood cell (WBC) casts are seen infrequently in dogs. They are usually associated with renal inflammation and pyelonephritis. Intermittent fevers may be associated with familial amyloidosis syndromes (e.g., in Shar pei dogs) and underlying inflammatory diseases. Acute blindness can result from retinal detachment secondary to hypertension (which is common in glomerular disease). Dyspnea and hypoxemia accompany pulmonary thromboembolism, and can occur secondary to a hypercoagulable state, which may accompany significant glomerular protein loss. Subcutaneous edema may occur if hypoalbuminemia (resulting from proteinuria) is severe.

20. The answer is 4 [Part I:IV D 3; Part II:IV C 3]. Calcitriol therapy will not decrease serum phosphorus. At a proper dose, it will not alter serum phosphorus, but at a high dose it will increase it. Aluminum hydroxide and calcium carbonate are oral phosphate binders and are commonly used to reduce serum phosphorus in patients with chronic renal failure (CRF). Reduced protein diets are always reduced in phosphorus because protein is a significant source of phosphorus. Reduced phosphorus intake will tend to reduce serum levels, especially in the context of CRF. Insulin administration will cause phosphorus to move intracellularly, thereby decreasing extracellular fluid (ECF) and serum concentrations.

Chapter 44

Endocrine Diseases

PITUITARY AND HYPOTHALAMIC DISORDERS

A. **Hypopituitarism** results in a deficiency of one or more of the pituitary hormones [e.g., adrenocorticotrophic hormone (ACTH), thyroid-stimulating hormone (TSH), growth hormone (GH), luteinizing hormone (LH), follicle-stimulating hormone (FSH)]. Without these hormones to stimulate the corresponding endocrine glands, deficiencies of other hormones (e.g., cortisol, thyroxine) result. Hypopituitarism can be congenital or acquired as a result of trauma, neoplasia, medications, irradiation, or as idiopathic disease.

1. **Pituitary dwarfism**
   a. **Etiology.** A deficiency of GH (and sometimes other pituitary hormones) in a young animal results in pituitary dwarfism. Many affected animals have a pituitary cyst.
   b. **Predisposition.** Pituitary dwarfism occurs in German shepherds and Carnelian bear dogs as an autosomal recessive disorder but has also been reported in other breeds.
   c. **Diagnosis.** A tentative diagnosis may be based on the signalment, history, and clinical signs.
      (1) **Clinical findings**
         (a) Affected animals fail to grow and mature normally. They are short, have retained deciduous teeth and delayed eruption of the permanent teeth, and often have testicular hypoplasia or anestrus.
         (b) The hair may be soft and fine (i.e., only secondary lanugo hairs with no primary guard hairs), or there may be bilaterally symmetrical truncal alopecia and thinning and scaling of the skin.
         (c) Other signs may be seen if concurrent secondary hypothyroidism, secondary hypoadrenocorticism, or hypogonadotropism are present.
      (2) **Laboratory findings**
         (a) A **complete blood count (CBC), serum biochemical profile,** and **urinalysis** will help rule out other causes of poor growth. Mild anemia, hypoalbuminemia, and azotemia may be seen.
         (b) A **skin biopsy** may just show nonspecific changes consistent with an endocrinopathy. Decreased dermal elastin may also be noted and is suggestive of hyposomatotropism.
         (c) **Secondary hypothyroidism** or **atypical hypoadrenocorticism** may also be present; an exaggerated response on an insulin response test can help support the tentative diagnosis.
         (d) A **GH stimulation test** (i.e., clonidine or xylazine stimulation test) or **measurement of insulin-like growth factor-1** can be used to establish a definitive diagnosis, but these assays are not currently commercially available.
   d. **Treatment** is with human, porcine, or bovine GH. Potential side effects include diabetes mellitus and hypersensitivity to the exogenous hormone. Concurrent hypothyroidism or hypocortisolemia should also be treated.
   e. **Prognosis.** Treatment usually results in little change in stature, but hair growth is often seen after 4–6 weeks.

2. **Adult-onset GH deficiency/GH-responsive dermatosis**
   a. **Etiology**
      (1) Adult-onset GH deficiency/GH-responsive dermatosis can result from nonfunctional pituitary neoplasia, trauma, or pituitary irradiation, or it can be idiopathic.

       (2) Decreased secretion of GH-releasing hormone (GRH), decreased GH secretion, increased somatostatin secretion, inactivation of GH, and poorly responsive peripheral tissues may cause adult-onset GH deficiency/GH-responsive dermatosis.

       (3) In Pomeranians, the GH deficiency may be secondary to aberrant adrenal sex hormone production and increased ACTH secretion.

  b. Predisposition. The disorder is hereditary in American water spaniels, chow chows, keeshonds, Lhasa Apsos, Pomeranians, poodles, and Samoyeds.

  c. Diagnosis

    (1) Clinical findings. The main clinical signs are bilaterally symmetrical alopecia (i.e., endocrine alopecia) and hyperpigmentation.

    (2) Laboratory findings. A **TSH stimulation test, ACTH stimulation test,** and **dexamethasone suppression test** can rule out other causes of endocrine alopecia. Definitive diagnosis requires evaluation of GH response to clonidine, xylazine, or GRH, but **GH assay** is not currently commercially available.

  d. Treatment is the same as for pituitary dwarfism (see I A 1 d). If abnormal adrenal sex hormone production is involved (as is the case in Pomeranians), treatment with mitotane or ketoconazole (see V C 4) may be useful.

  e. Prognosis is good, even without treatment.

3. Nonfunctional pituitary neoplasms (e.g., **craniopharyngiomas, astrocytomas,** and **metastatic lesions** from **lymphosarcoma, melanoma, mammary carcinomas,** and others)

  a. Pathogenesis. These neoplasms can cause hypopituitarism by destroying or displacing functional pituitary cells.

  b. Diagnosis. Clinical findings may be those of hormone deficiency or those that result from impingement by the tumor on the hypothalamus or brain (e.g., diabetes insipidus, obesity, anorexia or polyphagia, blindness, abnormal thermoregulation). Definitive diagnosis is based on identification of a pituitary lesion with computed tomography (CT) and possibly, concurrent identification of a pituitary hormone deficiency.

  c. Prognosis is guarded to poor with an expanding pituitary tumor.

4. Functional pituitary neoplasms

  a. Pathogenesis. Functional pituitary neoplasms may arise from the pars distalis or pars intermedia. Hypersecretion of ACTH is most common, although excessive secretion of GH also sometimes occurs.

  b. Diagnosis. Clinical findings are those of hormone excess (from the tumor cells). Concurrent deficiency from secondary hypopituitarism (e.g., polyuria and polydipsia, weight loss, sex gland atrophy, adipsia, hyper- or hyponatremia, listlessness, anorexia, pacing, dull behavior) may also be noted if the tumor expands, displacing functional pituitary tissue or compressing adjacent brain tissue. Diagnosis is made based on hormonal tests (chosen according to the clinical signs) and possibly, CT of the pituitary region.

  c. Prognosis varies with a microscopic pituitary tumor but is guarded to poor with a macroscopic or expanding pituitary tumor.

B. Diabetes insipidus

1. Etiology

  a. Central diabetes insipidus is characterized by a relative or absolute decrease in antidiuretic hormone (ADH). It may be idiopathic or congenital (primary), or may occur secondary to head trauma, inflammation, or neoplasia. The congenital form is seen in very young animals. The other forms may occur in dogs and cats of any age.

  b. Nephrogenic diabetes insipidus is characterized by renal tubular resistance to ADH. Primary nephrogenic diabetes insipidus is very rare, but nephrogenic diabetes insipidus secondary to renal failure, pyelonephritis, hypercalcemia, hyperkalemia, hyperadrenocorticism, hyperthyroidism, liver failure, pyometra, medications, and other disorders is common.

2. Diagnosis

   a. Clinical findings include polyuria with a compensatory polydipsia. Nocturia and mild weight loss may also occur. There are usually no other clinical signs, and physical examination is unremarkable. Neurologic signs may be present if a mass or head trauma is the cause of central diabetes insipidus.

   b. Laboratory findings

     (1) CBC and **serum biochemical profile.** Routine laboratory studies should be performed to rule out more common causes of secondary nephrogenic diabetes insipidus.

     (2) Urinalysis. The urine specific gravity is usually less than 1.010, and the **serum osmolality** is mildly increased with both types of diabetes insipidus.

     (3) Screening tests for hyperadrenocorticism may be useful [see V C 3 b (4)].

     (4) Modified water deprivation test. This test of an animal's ability to secrete and respond to ADH is most commonly used to differentiate central diabetes insipidus, nephrogenic diabetes insipidus, and psychogenic polydipsia. A modified water deprivation test should not be performed if the animal is dehydrated, azotemic, or has other laboratory abnormalities.

       (a) Procedure. Details of the test protocol can be found in various texts. In summary, water is withheld until the animal has lost 3%–5% of its body weight, the urine specific gravity is greater than 1.030–1.035, or the animal becomes azotemic. With the latter two results, the test is then finished. If only weight loss (due to fluid loss) has occurred, then ADH is administered and the urine specific gravity reassessed.

       (b) Interpretation of test results

         (i) Normal dogs and **cats** will slowly become dehydrated (i.e., over 40–80 hours) with an end urine osmolality greater than 1000 mOsm and an end urine specific gravity greater than 1.030. No additional increase in urine osmolality or specific gravity is seen in response to vasopressin administration.

         (ii) Animals with **complete central diabetes insipidus** will become rapidly dehydrated (i.e., over 3–5 hours) with an end urine osmolality less than 300 mOsm and an end urine specific gravity less than 1.008, but a 50%–800% increase in urine osmolality or a urine specific gravity greater than 1.012 following vasopressin administration.

         (iii) Animals with **partial central diabetes insipidus** will experience a mild increase in urine osmolality and urine specific gravity with dehydration and in response to exogenous vasopressin.

         (iv) Animals with **complete nephrogenic diabetes insipidus** will become rapidly dehydrated (i.e., over 3–5 hours) with an end urine osmolality less than 200 mOsm and an end urine specific gravity less than 1.008, with no increase in urine osmolality following vasopressin administration.

         (v) Animals with **partial nephrogenic diabetes insipidus** will have an end urine osmolality of 300–1000 mOsm and an end urine specific gravity of 1.008–1.019 with a 10%–50% increase in urine osmolality following vasopressin administration. Many of the disorders that cause polyuria and polydipsia (e.g., renal failure, pyelonephritis, hypercalcemia, hypokalemia, some medications, hepatic failure, hyperthyroidism, hyperadrenocorticism, pyometra, *Escherichia coli* infection) do so through mechanisms that result in a secondary nephrogenic diabetes insipidus. These disorders will cause water deprivation/vasopressin response test results similar to those of partial nephrogenic diabetes insipidus and can lead to an incorrect diagnosis if the animal is not evaluated for these primary disorders.

         (vi) Animals with **psychogenic polydipsia** will have normal test results. However, an animal with psychogenic polydipsia may also have a response suggestive of partial nephrogenic diabetes insipidus as a result of secondary medullary washout.

(5) **ADH trial.** Water intake is measured for 2–3 days, and then synthetic vasopressin is administered for 5–7 days while continuing to measure water consumption. If there is a greater than 50% decrease in water consumption, central diabetes insipidus or partial nephrogenic diabetes insipidus is diagnosed. Caution must be used so that a polydipsic animal does not become overhydrated.

3. **Treatment**
   a. **Diabetes insipidus.** Large amounts of water must always be available for untreated animals.
      (1) **Central diabetes insipidus** is treated with synthetic vasopressin (DDAVP) or ADH.
      (2) **Primary nephrogenic diabetes insipidus** is treated with thiazide diuretics.
   b. **Psychogenic polydipsia.** Treatment entails the gradual restriction of water to a normal amount. In some animals, long-term restriction is needed. In others, after a few weeks, unlimited water can be offered without return of the clinical signs.

4. **Prognosis.** The prognosis for animals with idiopathic or congenital central diabetes insipidus is good with treatment. Central diabetes insipidus resulting from trauma may be transient. The prognosis for primary nephrogenic diabetes insipidus or untreated central diabetes insipidus is guarded if water intake is decreased because of lack of access or illness.

C. **Syndrome of inappropriate secretion of ADH (SIADH)**

1. **Pathogenesis.** This rare disorder is characterized by nonphysiologic ADH secretion or decreased water excretion despite normal sodium excretion. The result is hyponatremia and fluid retention.

2. **Etiology.** In dogs, SIADH can be idiopathic or may occur secondary to dirofilariasis, hypoadrenocorticism, or neoplasia.

3. **Diagnosis**
   a. **Clinical findings** include weight gain, lethargy, and neurologic signs (e.g., confusion, seizures, coma).
   b. **Laboratory findings.** The diagnosis is based on finding hyponatremia and a urine osmolality that is greater than the plasma osmolality. Other causes of hyponatremia (e.g., renal disease, hypoadrenocorticism, thyroid disease, hepatic disease, heart failure) must be excluded.

4. **Treatment** requires fluid restriction. If the clinical signs are severe, administration of hypertonic saline may be useful. Any underlying disease should also be identified and treated.

D. **Adipsia** and **hypodipsia** result in marked hypernatremia and central nervous system (CNS) dehydration. Adipsia or hypodipsia may be idiopathic, or it may occur as a result of a hypothalamic lesion. These disorders are most common in young animals, and miniature schnauzers are at increased risk.

1. **Diagnosis**
   a. **Clinical findings** may include mental depression, lethargy, anorexia, disorientation, personality changes, and seizures. On physical examination, the animal is usually dehydrated and has neurologic abnormalities.
   b. **Laboratory findings** include severe hypernatremia and hyperosmolality. Hyperchloremia, hyperalbuminemia, mild azotemia, and very concentrated urine may also be seen.
   c. **Diagnostic imaging findings.** Occasionally, a hypothalamic lesion is visible on a CT scan.

2. **Treatment**
   a. The hypernatremia should be slowly corrected (i.e., over 2–3 days) using 5% dextrose or 2.5% dextrose with 0.45% saline. Rapid correction can result in cerebral edema.
   b. On a long-term basis, daily maintenance fluids should be mixed with the food daily to ensure fluid intake.

3. **Prognosis** with treatment is good if irreversible neurologic damage has not occurred prior to diagnosis or during initial treatment.

E. **Acromegaly** results from excess GH secretion and is characterized by excessive growth of bone, connective tissue, and other organs.

1. **Canine acromegaly**
   a. **Etiology.** In dogs, excessive GH secretion usually results from increased progesterone secretion during diestrus or from exogenous progestin administration.
   b. **Diagnosis.** A presumptive diagnosis can often be made on the basis of the history and the presence of diabetes mellitus.
      (1) **Clinical findings**
         (a) With a short-term increase in GH secretion, polyuria, polydipsia, and polyphagia may be the only clinical signs.
         (b) With a long-term increase in GH secretion, inspiratory stridor, excess soft tissues, and widened interdental spaces may be seen.
         (c) With diestrus or short-term progestin therapy, there are often no clinical signs or only signs of insulin-resistant diabetes mellitus [see IV A 6 b (5)].
         (d) With long-term progestin therapy, other signs of acromegaly may be seen. The diabetes may be reversible or permanent, depending on the duration, severity of GH increase, and the individual animal.
      (2) **Laboratory findings.** Hyperglycemia, increased serum alanine aminotransferase (ALT) and serum alkaline phosphatase (ALP) levels, hypercholesterolemia, and glucosuria are often seen. Definitive diagnosis requires evaluation of GH concentrations, but an assay is not currently commercially available.
   c. **Treatment**
      (1) **Excessive GH secretion.** Ovariohysterectomy or discontinuation of progestin therapy is necessary.
      (2) **Diabetes mellitus.** The diabetes mellitus must also be treated. Blood glucose concentrations should be monitored after progesterone concentrations decrease because exogenous insulin requirements will usually decrease and some animals may ultimately be able to discontinue insulin therapy.
   d. **Prognosis** is good after ovariohysterectomy or withdrawal of progestin therapy. The diabetes may be reversible in some animals.

2. **Feline acromegaly**
   a. **Etiology.** In cats, acromegaly usually results from a functional pituitary adenoma.
   b. **Predisposition.** Acromegaly is most common in middle-aged to older cats, and males are at increased risk.
   c. **Diagnosis**
      (1) **Clinical findings** may include polyuria and polydipsia, inspiratory stridor, and an increase in body size and configuration. The face may become broader and blunted with widened interdental spaces. There may be increased skin folds on the face and neck, and the abdomen may enlarge. A systolic murmur and gallop rhythm may be detected on physical examination if secondary cardiomyopathy has developed. Hepatomegaly and renomegaly may also be palpable. Acromegaly should be suspected if these clinical signs are seen in a cat with diabetes mellitus and insulin resistance.
      (2) **Laboratory findings.** Azotemia and proteinuria may be found if secondary renal failure has occurred. Hypoglycemia and glucosuria are usually also seen as a result of secondary diabetes mellitus. Definitive diagnosis requires demonstration of excess GH concentrations, but a GH assay is not currently commercially available.
      (3) **Diagnostic imaging findings.** Thoracic radiographs may reveal cardiomegaly, and abdominal radiographs may show hepatomegaly and renomegaly. A presumptive diagnosis may be made if a pituitary mass is seen on a CT scan and hyperadrenocorticism has been ruled out.

    d. Treatment. Cobalt irradiation of the pituitary mass has been tried, but is of variable efficacy and is limited in availability. More commonly, treatment is aimed at managing the diabetes mellitus, cardiomegaly, or other secondary clinical syndromes.

    e. Prognosis. The long-term prognosis is guarded because within 2–3 years, most cats die of renal failure, congestive heart failure, or progressive neurologic signs.

II. PARATHYROID DISORDERS

A. Primary hypoparathyroidism

1. **Etiology.** The cause of primary hypoparathyroidism is unknown, but immune-mediated mechanisms are suspected.

2. **Predisposition**
   a. **Dogs.** The disorder can occur in dogs of any age. There is a slight increased incidence in females and in German shepherds, Labrador retrievers, miniature schnauzers, terriers, and toy poodles.
   b. **Cats.** Primary hypoparathyroidism is rare in cats, but males are at increased risk. Iatrogenic hypoparathyroidism following thyroidectomy is seen with greater frequency.

3. **Diagnosis.** A presumptive diagnosis is often based on the history (e.g., no recent thyroid surgery or lactation), clinical signs, and appropriate laboratory findings.
   a. **Clinical findings** may include nervousness, facial rubbing, twitching, a stiff or stilted gait, lethargy, weakness, anorexia, bradycardia, and seizures. The signs may be exacerbated by excitement or exercise.
      (1) In dogs, pain, weakness, fever, cramping, and lenticular cataracts may be seen.
      (2) In cats, weakness, fever, and lenticular cataracts are most common, and the nictitating membranes may be raised.
   b. **Laboratory findings.** The presence of **hypocalcemia** and **hyperphosphatemia** on a serum biochemical profile in the absence of other abnormalities is suggestive. Serum parathyroid hormone (PTH) concentrations will be low.
   c. **Differential diagnoses for hypocalcemia** include **renal failure, hypoalbuminemia, pancreatitis, eclampsia, malabsorption, ethylene glycol toxicity,** and **phosphate enema administration.** Only hypoparathyroidism, eclampsia, ethylene glycol toxicity, and the use of phosphate enemas result in clinical signs of hypocalcemia.

4. **Treatment**
   a. **Acute therapy.** Emergency treatment is needed if tetany or other severe clinical signs are present, especially if the onset is acute.
      (1) **10% Calcium gluconate** should be administered intravenously slowly (i.e., over 10–30 minutes) while monitoring an electrocardiogram (ECG) or the heart rate. If bradycardia or premature ventricular contractions occur, the infusion should be stopped for several minutes and then continued at a slower administration rate. Other forms of intravenous calcium can also be used but are caustic if given perivascularly.
      (2) **Lowering of the body temperature** to a normal range may be necessary if hyperthermia has occurred secondary to the tetany.
   b. **Subacute therapy** is needed if the cause of the hypocalcemia is a persistent problem (e.g., hypoparathyroidism). **Diluted calcium gluconate** should be given subcutaneously every 6–8 hours to keep serum calcium slightly below the lower range of normal until oral maintenance medications become effective.
   c. **Chronic maintenance therapy**
      (1) **Vitamin D supplementation**
         (a) **Preparations**

(i) **Vitamin D$_2$ (ergocalciferol)** is the least expensive form but takes 5–14 days to become effective. Hypercalcemia resulting from overdosage requires prolonged symptomatic treatment.

(ii) **Dihydrotachysterol** is moderate in cost and becomes effective in 1–7 days with less risk of prolonged hypercalcemia.

(iii) **1,25-Dihydroxyvitamin D$_3$ (calcitriol)** becomes effective in 1–4 days with minimal risk of prolonged hypercalcemia. However, it is the most expensive form of vitamin D, and the tablet size makes correct dosing of small dogs and cats difficult.

(b) Whichever form of vitamin D is used, serum calcium must be monitored until the medication becomes effective and then periodically thereafter to ensure hypercalcemia does not occur. Subcutaneous calcium gluconate administration every 6–8 hours is continued until the serum calcium level is just below the normal range immediately prior to the time of the next scheduled calcium injection.

(c) If the hypoparathyroidism is iatrogenic and a return of parathyroid function is possible (e.g., following thyroidectomy in a cat or surgical treatment of hyperparathyroidism), an attempt can be made to slowly withdraw the vitamin D supplementation.

(2) **Oral calcium supplementation** is not usually needed if the animal is eating a balanced diet but may be used early in the course of treatment. Many forms of calcium are available, but calcium carbonate has the highest calcium concentration.

5. **Prognosis** is good with proper treatment and monitoring to prevent hypercalcemia.

B. Primary hyperparathyroidism

1. **Etiology.** Primary hyperparathyroidism usually results from parathyroid adenoma or hyperplasia, occasionally from adenocarcinoma.

2. **Predisposition**
   a. Primary hyperparathyroidism is most common in older dogs, but hereditary neonatal hyperparathyroidism also occurs as an autosomal recessive disorder in German shepherds.
   b. The disorder is rare in cats, but females may be at increased risk.

3. **Diagnosis**
   a. **Clinical findings** are those of hypercalcemia (see Chapter 43 Part II:III C 2) and are usually mild.
      (1) Anorexia, vomiting, constipation, polyuria and polydipsia, and lethargy may be seen. Pollakiuria may be seen if calcium oxalate or calcium phosphate calculi have formed. In cats, anorexia and lethargy are most common.
      (2) Physical examination is usually normal, but mild muscle weakness may be seen, and cystic calculi may be palpable. A cervical mass may be palpable in cats.
   b. **Laboratory findings.** The diagnosis is based on finding hypercalcemia, a normal or decreased serum phosphorus concentration, and an increased serum PTH concentration. A presumptive diagnosis may be based on elimination of other possible causes of hypercalcemia if PTH assay is not readily available but hypercalcemia and normophosphatemia are present.
   c. **Differential diagnoses**
      (1) **Hypercalcemia of malignancy** is the most common cause of hypercalcemia. It has been reported with lymphosarcoma (most common), multiple myeloma, apocrine gland adenocarcinoma, mammary adenocarcinoma, nasal adenocarcinoma, thyroid carcinoma, squamous cell carcinoma, and others. Direct osteolytic effects (exerted by tumor cells in the bone marrow) and humoral factors (e.g., PTH-related protein, 1,25-dihydroxycholecalciferol) may be involved. A CBC, serum biochemical profile, urinalysis, thoracic and abdominal radiographs, ultrasound, and lymph node and bone

marrow aspirates can help rule out malignancy. If these results are all normal, then PTH concentration should be evaluated or a cervical exploratory or trial chemotherapy may be considered.

    (2) Hypoadrenocorticism can cause a mild increase in serum calcium.

    (3) Renal failure can cause renal secondary hyperparathyroidism.

    (4) Vitamin D toxicosis usually results from accidental ingestion of a vitamin D rodenticide.

        (a) Clinical findings usually include weakness and anorexia and may include hematemesis and shock. The diagnosis is based on the history, the presence of severe hypercalcemia and hyperphosphatemia, and a high serum 25(OH)-cholecalciferol concentration.

        (b) The prognosis is fair to guarded because of the need for prolonged symptomatic treatment while the drug is metabolized. Treatment with oral phosphate binders, glucocorticoids, and calcitonin may also be useful.

    (5) Granulomatous disease

    (6) Lytic bone disease

  4. Treatment

    a. Acute therapy to lower the serum calcium concentration

      (1) Indications. If severe hypercalcemia is not treated, there is increased risk of renal failure and cardiac arrhythmias. Acute therapy to lower the serum calcium concentration is needed in the presence of:

        (a) Dehydration, azotemia, severe weakness, neurologic signs, or arrhythmias

        (b) A serum calcium level greater than 16 mg/dl (4 mmol/L)

        (c) A serum calcium x serum phosphorus product greater than 60–80 (mg/dl)^2 [5.7 (mmol/L)^2]

      (2) Approaches

        (a) Saline diuresis and **furosemide therapy** will increase urinary excretion of calcium and will lower serum calcium levels to below the critical zone. This treatment will not usually return serum calcium levels to normal unless hypoadrenocorticism is the underlying cause.

        (b) Glucocorticoids can be added if diuresis and furosemide treatment are insufficient. Glucocorticoids have a direct lympholytic effect and will lower serum calcium levels in animals with lymphosarcoma and some other disorders. Administration of glucocorticoids can make it difficult to identify lymphosarcoma, so they should ideally not be used until all diagnostic tests have been completed or a diagnosis has been established.

    b. Specific therapy of primary hyperparathyroidism requires removal of the hyperfunctional parathyroid gland or glands.

      (1) Dogs. If the initial serum calcium level is greater than 14 mg/dl (3.5 mmol/L), most dogs will require postoperative supplementation with vitamin D and possibly calcium for several weeks to months because of atrophy of the remaining parathyroid glands. Once the animal is stable, vitamin D therapy can be slowly withdrawn.

      (2) Cats. Few cats become clinically hypocalcemic following surgery, so they should receive supplementation only if signs of hypocalcemia are seen in association with low serum calcium concentration.

  5. Prognosis. In dogs, the prognosis is good if there is little or no secondary renal damage and postoperative hypocalcemia can be managed. In cats, the prognosis is good.

III. THYROID DISORDERS

A. **Hypothyroidism** is one of the most common endocrinopathies in dogs.

  1. Types

    a. Congenital (juvenile-onset) hypothyroidism is rare.

b. Acquired hypothyroidism

    (1) Primary. Hypothyroidism can be caused by lymphocytic thyroiditis or thyroid atrophy. Primary hypothyroidism is rare in cats.

    (2) Secondary. Hypothyroidism can occur secondary to pituitary or thyroid neoplasia (rare) or iatrogenic procedures (e.g., bilateral thyroidectomy or radioactive iodine treatment for hyperthyroidism).

2. Predisposition

  a. Congenital hypothyroidism is most common in Abyssinian cats, American shorthair cats, German shepherd mix dogs, Malamute mix dogs, and Scottish deerhounds.

  b. Primary acquired hypothyroidism is most common in middle-aged dogs. Airedale terriers, cocker spaniels, dachshunds, Doberman pinschers, golden retrievers, Great Danes, Irish setters, miniature schnauzers, and Old English sheepdogs may be at increased risk.

3. Diagnosis

  a. Acquired hypothyroidism is often diagnosed on the basis of clinical signs and the presence of low serum thyroxine (T_4) concentrations.

    (1) Clinical findings

      (a) Dogs

        (i) The most common clinical signs of hypothyroidism in dogs include bilaterally symmetrical alopecia, skin hyperpigmentation, seborrhea, a dull hair coat, and lethargy. Cold intolerance, mild weight gain, constipation, myxedema, a "tragic" facial expression, and infertility may also be seen.

        (ii) Less common or atypical clinical signs include a slow, stiff gait (myopathy), lameness, proprioceptive deficits, nystagmus or head tilt, laryngeal paralysis (peripheral neuropathy), and mental dullness, seizures, or coma (CNS dysfunction).

        (iii) Signs of concurrent endocrine disease may also be present in animals with secondary acquired hypothyroidism.

      (b) Cats. Matted hair, hair loss, and seborrhea are most common. Because most hypothyroidism in cats is iatrogenic, clinical signs are usually caught early and are mild at the time of diagnosis.

    (2) ECG findings. An ECG may show mild bradycardia and decreased P and R wave amplitude.

    (3) Laboratory findings

      (a) Hypercholesterolemia is common, and a nonregenerative anemia may be present.

      (b) Serum T_4 concentration. If the serum T_4 concentration is normal, it is unlikely that the dog is hypothyroid. If the serum T_4 concentration is not normal a TSH stimulation test, TSH assay, or therapeutic trial should be considered.

        (i) TSH stimulation test. The serum T_4 concentration is evaluated before and after administration of TSH. A hypothyroid animal will have little or no increase in serum T_4 in response to TSH. With nonthyroidal disease ("sick euthyroid syndrome"), the absolute T_4 concentrations may be somewhat low but the slope of the response to TSH similar to that of a normal animal. Disadvantages of the test are the increased cost and the limited availability of TSH.

        (ii) A serum TSH assay has recently been validated for use in dogs. The presence of increased serum TSH in conjunction with a low serum T_4 concentration should help confirm a diagnosis of hypothyroidism. If the serum T_4 concentration is normal, it is very unlikely that the dog is hypothyroid. In this case, a TSH stimulation test or therapeutic trial should be considered.

        (iii) Therapeutic trial. The clinical signs should fully resolve after 6–8 weeks of treatment with L-thyroxine (see III A 4), and the signs should recur when supplementation is discontinued. Temporary discontinuation of the supplementation is needed because some nonthyroidal dermatopathies will improve from the anabolic effects of T_4 supplementation.

(4) Differential diagnoses

(a) Nonthyroidal diseases (e.g., hyperadrenocorticism, hypoadrenocorticism, diabetes mellitus, renal failure, hepatic disease, pyoderma) and many medications [e.g., glucocorticoids, phenobarbital, nonsteroidal anti-inflammatory drugs (NSAIDs), some anesthetics] can lower serum T_4 concentrations even in a euthyroid animal.

(b) Differentiation of primary hypothyroidism and secondary hypothyroidism is possible with repeated TSH injections, a thyrotropin-releasing hormone (TRH) stimulation test, measurement of antithyroglobulin or thyroid hormone antibodies, or a thyroid biopsy. These tests are rarely done, however, because primary hypothyroidism is so much more common and the test results rarely influence treatment.

b. Congenital hypothyroidism is diagnosed based on the presence of clinical signs, decreased serum T_4 concentration, and radiographic evidence of epiphyseal dysgenesis.

(1) Clinical findings. Stunted growth (disproportionate dwarfism), mental dullness, a broad skull and short mandible, a protruding tongue, exophthalmos, alopecia, weakness, delayed dental eruption, and signs of other endocrine disorders may be seen.

(2) Laboratory findings. In addition to a decreased serum T_4 concentration, increased serum creatine kinase, hypercholesterolemia, and a nonregenerative anemia may also be seen.

4. Treatment is with **L-thyroxine.** An improvement in attitude and activity is usually seen within 1 week. The condition of the skin and haircoat usually improves within 6 weeks.

a. If a suboptimal response is seen, post-pill serum T_4 concentrations should be assessed. If low, the dose should be increased; if normal, the diagnosis should be reconsidered.

b. A dose reduction may be needed if signs of hyperthyroidism (e.g., polyuria and polydipsia, nervousness, polyphagia, weight loss, panting, tachycardia) are seen and T_4 concentrations are increased.

5. Prognosis

a. Acquired hypothyroidism. Acquired primary hypothyroidism carries an excellent prognosis if treated. Secondary or tertiary hypothyroidism carries a guarded prognosis if an enlarging or macroscopic pituitary or hypothalamic mass is the cause.

b. Congenital hypothyroidism. Animals will respond to treatment with increased growth, but treatment will not result in normal intelligence unless it is initiated very early. Even with treatment, degenerative arthritis is a common sequela.

B. **Feline hyperthyroidism** is one of the most common feline endocrinopathies.

1. Etiology. Most cats with hyperthyroidism have bilateral adenomatous hyperplasia of the thyroid glands. The cause of the hyperplasia is unknown. Adenocarcinomas are rare. Nutritional factors, environmental toxins, and immune mechanisms have all been proposed as causes of hyperthyroidism as well.

2. Predisposition. The disease is most common in middle-aged to older cats.

3. Diagnosis. The diagnosis is usually based on the presence of clinical signs and finding an increased serum T_4 concentration.

a. Clinical findings

(1) Symptoms of hyperthyroidism are usually slowly progressive and often include weight loss, polyuria and polydipsia, polyphagia, restlessness, an unkempt hair coat, and a decreased tolerance for stress. Vomiting and diarrhea may also be seen. A few cats develop "apathetic hyperthyroidism," characterized by anorexia, weakness, depression, and weight loss. Dyspnea or tachypnea may be seen, especially if secondary cardiomyopathy is present.

(2) On physical examination, cats are usually thin, may be aggressive, and may have thyroid enlargement, tachycardia, a cardiac murmur, or a gallop rhythm.

b. Laboratory findings

(1) Results of a **CBC, serum biochemical profile,** and **urinalysis** will help rule out other or concurrent disorders. A mild increase in the hematocrit, SALT, SAP, serum aspartate aminotransferase (SAST) concentration, and a stress leukogram may be seen. Azotemia may also be seen as a result of the hyperthyroidism or concurrent chronic renal disease.

(2) The **serum T_4 concentration** is usually increased. If the T_4 concentration is normal in a cat with suspected hyperthyroidism, other diseases should be ruled out and the serum T_4 level reevaluated because T_4 concentrations can sometimes drop down into the upper part of the normal range.

(3) Alternatively, a **triiodothyronine (T_3) suppression test, technetium scan,** or **TRH stimulation test** can be used to identify hyperthyroidism in cats with a normal serum T_4 concentration that are suspected of being hyperthyroid.

   (a) T_3 **suppression test.** Serum T_4 levels are evaluated before and after 2 days of oral T_3 administration. In a normal cat, T_4 concentrations will decrease, but in a hyperthyroid cat, there will be little or no decrease in the serum T_4 level. The test is very safe but does require reliable administration of the medication.

   (b) **Technetium scan.** A normal cat will have thyroid uptake of technetium equal to that of the salivary gland uptake of technetium. A hyperthyroid cat will have increased thyroid uptake. The disadvantage of the test is the need for a nuclear medicine facility to perform the scan.

   (c) **TRH stimulation test.** Serum T_4 levels are measured before and after administration of TRH. An increase in T_4 will be seen in normal cats. Hyperthyroid cats will have little or no increase in serum T_4 concentration. TRH administration may cause transient side effects (e.g., salivation, vomiting, defecation, tachypnea).

c. Diagnostic imaging findings. Increased concentrations of circulating thyroid hormones affect many organ systems.

(1) **Thoracic radiographs** may show cardiomegaly, pleural effusion, or pulmonary edema if secondary cardiomyopathy is present.

(2) **Cardiac ultrasonography** usually confirms the presence of hypertrophic cardiomyopathy, but dilated cardiomyopathy sometimes occurs (see Chapter 39 IV).

4. Treatment

a. Medical treatment. Advantages of medical treatment include lower cost, no need for special skills or facilities, minimal hospitalization, and no risk of hypothyroidism, hypoparathyroidism, or surgical and anesthetic complications. Disadvantages include the need to administer the pills for the remainder of the cat's life and the possible side effects of the medication (e.g., anorexia, vomiting, facial self-trauma, hepatic disease, thrombocytopenia, agranulocytosis). Serious or persistent side effects necessitate discontinuation of the medication.

(1) **Methimazole** is the main medical treatment for hyperthyroidism. Improvement in clinical signs is usually seen in 1–3 weeks. The medication can be used on a short-term basis to lessen the anesthetic risks during surgery or can be used for the remainder of the cat's life.

(2) **Propylthiouracil (PTU)** has a higher incidence of side effects than methimazole and is rarely used.

(3) **Calcium ipodate,** a cholecystographic contrast agent, can also be used as short-term treatment (i.e., prethyroidectomy) for hyperthyroidism in cats that cannot tolerate methimazole treatment. It will decrease serum T_3 concentrations and reverse the clinical signs of hyperthyroidism for a short time.

b. Surgical treatment. Thyroidectomy usually cures hyperthyroidism. During surgery, all functional tissue seen on a technetium scan or any visible thyroid tissue should be removed, while attempting to maintain functional parathyroid tissue.

(1) Preoperatively, medical treatment may be used to reverse some of the clinical signs of hyperthyroidism, thereby lessening the anesthetic risks. A preoperative technetium scan may also be useful to localize the hyperfunctional tissue and to rule out intrathoracic ectopic or metastatic tissue. The presence of intrathoracic tissue usually precludes surgical treatment.

    (2) Potential surgical complications include hypoparathyroidism, laryngeal paralysis, and Horner's syndrome. Transient or permanent hypothyroidism may also follow bilateral thyroidectomy, but permanent hypothyroidism is uncommon.

  c. Radioisotope treatment. Hyperfunctional thyroid tissue will take up and be destroyed by **radioactive iodine.** Normal tissue is usually relatively protected.

    (1) Advantages of radioisotope treatment include its safety and its potential capability to also destroy intrathoracic or metastatic tissue.

    (2) Disadvantages include the need for special handling facilities and prolonged hospitalization (1–4 weeks). If a larger dose is administered (e.g., with an adenocarcinoma), a longer period of hospitalization may be necessary.

  d. Secondary cardiomyopathy may also require treatment (see Chapter 39).

 5. Prognosis is good with treatment unless an adenocarcinoma is the cause of the hyperthyroidism or dilated cardiomyopathy is present.

C. **Canine thyroid tumors.** Most thyroid tumors in dogs are adenocarcinomas.

 1. Etiology. The cause is unknown.

 2. Predisposition. Thyroid neoplasia is most common in older dogs.

 3. Diagnosis. Most affected dogs are euthyroid, but a small number of dogs have hyperfunctional tumors. A serum T_4 concentration and the clinical signs will determine whether the tumor is hyperfunctional. Definitive diagnosis usually requires a surgical biopsy.

  a. Clinical findings

    (1) The most common clinical signs of thyroid neoplasia in dogs are related to the presence of a large, fixed cervical mass. Coughing, dyspnea, a hoarse bark, anorexia, regurgitation, and weight loss may be seen.

    (2) If the mass is hyperfunctional, polyuria and polydipsia, polyphagia, nervousness, weakness, and mild weight loss may also be seen.

  b. CBC, serum biochemical profile, and **urinalysis findings.** The findings of these studies are usually normal and help rule out other disorders.

  c. Cytology findings. Cytologic evaluation of a fine needle aspirate can help rule out an abscess or granuloma but will not usually provide a definitive diagnosis.

  d. Diagnostic imaging findings. Thoracic radiographs should be taken to check for pulmonary metastasis.

 4. Treatment

  a. Irradiation. If the tumor is hyperfunctional, **radioactive iodine** therapy (see III B 4 c) can be used. Prolonged hospitalization is usually required, however, and the treatment is usually palliative rather than curative.

  b. Surgery can be considered for all thyroid tumors. Unfortunately, complete excision is not usually possible because of the tumor's invasiveness and the number of critical structures in the adjacent tissue. Surgical debulking can be useful, however.

  c. Adjunct chemotherapy (e.g., with doxorubicin) or **external beam irradiation** may also be palliative.

 5. Prognosis. The long-term prognosis is usually poor because the tumor is usually advanced at the time of diagnosis.

IV. ENDOCRINE PANCREATIC DISORDERS

A. **Diabetes mellitus**

 1. Types

  a. Type I diabetes mellitus (insulin-dependent diabetes mellitus) is characterized by destruction of the beta cells and eventual complete loss of insulin secretion.

Insulin-dependent diabetes mellitus is the most common form of diabetes mellitus in dogs and is the form seen in a little over half of diabetic cats. These animals are hypoinsulinemic, show little insulin response to glucose administration, and require treatment with exogenous insulin.

    (1) In dogs, genetics, toxins, infection, insulin antagonists, immune-mediated mechanisms, pancreatitis, and chronic stress have all been speculated to be involved in development of diabetes.

    (2) In cats, islet amyloid, chronic pancreatitis, and insulin antagonists may be involved.

  b. Type II diabetes mellitus (non–insulin-dependent diabetes mellitus). Insulin resistance, beta cell dysfunction, or both, result in a relative deficiency of insulin or insulin action. Ketoacidosis is rare with this type of diabetes. Non–insulin-dependent diabetes mellitus is rare in dogs but does occur in some cats. Obesity and islet amyloid polypeptide (amylin) may be involved, especially in cats.

  c. Secondary diabetes mellitus can occur if another condition (e.g., diestrus, hyperadrenocorticism, acromegaly) causes insulin resistance. If the primary disease is treated so that the insulin resistance resolves, diabetes mellitus may not be permanent.

  d. Transient diabetes occurs in a subpopulation of cats. These cats may have subclinical diabetes that is temporarily exacerbated by concurrent disease or medication.

2. Pathogenesis

  a. Hypoinsulinemia. Inadequate insulin results in hyperglycemia and decreased utilization of glucose, amino acids, and fatty acids. Glucosuria and osmotic diuresis occur when the renal threshold for glucose [180–220 mg/dl (10–12.2 mmol/L) for dogs; 200–240 mg/dl (11–13.3 mmol/L) for cats] is exceeded. Glucose loss in the urine and decreased tissue utilization of glucose cause weight loss despite polyphagia.

  b. Diabetic ketoacidosis. Insulin deficiency, excess diabetogenic hormones, fasting, and dehydration cause excess fatty acids and ketones (i.e., acetoacetic acid, acetone, and β-hydroxybutyric acid) to accumulate, leading to ketosis and acidosis. The ketonuria worsens the osmotic diuresis and causes urinary loss of sodium and potassium. Pancreatitis, infection, renal failure, heart failure, and other disorders may initiate an episode of ketoacidosis.

  c. Nonketotic hyperosmolar diabetes mellitus is an uncommon acute complication of untreated diabetes. The signs and abnormalities of diabetes worsen but no ketosis occurs because low concentrations of insulin prevent formation of ketones.

3. Predisposition

  a. Dogs. Diabetes mellitus occurs more commonly in middle-aged to older females. Beagles, Cairn terriers, dachshunds, miniature pinschers, miniature schnauzers, poodles, and pulis are at increased risk.

  b. Cats. Diabetes is most common in middle-aged to older, neutered males.

4. Diagnosis of diabetes mellitus is based on the clinical signs and the presence of hyperglycemia and glucosuria. Other abnormalities will vary with the severity of the disease and the presence or absence of any complications.

  a. Clinical findings

    (1) Simple diabetes mellitus. Classic clinical signs of diabetes include polyuria, polydipsia, polyphagia, and weight loss. Other signs may include sudden blindness (i.e., sudden cataract formation) in dogs, or rear limb weakness and a plantigrade stance in cats. On physical examination, there may be no abnormalities, or weight loss, hepatomegaly, cataracts (in dogs), or a plantigrade stance (in cats) may be observed.

    (2) Diabetic ketoacidosis. Acute depression, weakness, dehydration, vomiting, and tachypnea or Kussmaul respiration (slow deep breaths) may be seen. An acetone odor to the breath may also be detected, as well as signs of any concurrent disease.

TABLE 44-1. Clinical Properties of Insulin Preparations in Dogs

Type of Insulin	Route of Administration	Onset of Effect	Time of Maximum Effect	Duration of Effect
Regular crystalline, semilente	IV	Immediate	$\frac{1}{2}$–2 hours	1–4 hours
	IM	10–30 min	1–4 hours	3–8 hours
	SQ	10–30 min	1–5 hours	4–10 hours
NPH (isophane)	SQ	1–3 hours	3–12 hours	8–24 hours
Lente	SQ	$\frac{1}{2}$–2 hours	3–12 hours	8–24 hours
Ultralente	SQ	2–8 hours	6–16 hours	8–24 hours

IM = intramuscular; IV = intravenous; SQ = subcutaneous.

      (3) Nonketotic hyperosmolar diabetes mellitus. Anorexia, vomiting, depression, or coma may be seen in addition to the classic signs of diabetes mellitus.
    b. Laboratory findings
      (1) Simple diabetes mellitus. Hyperglycemia and glucosuria are present. Increased SALT levels (in dogs and cats) and increased SAP levels (in dogs) may be seen if secondary hepatic lipidosis has occurred. Hypercholesterolemia and hypertriglyceridemia may also be seen.
      (2) Diabetic ketoacidosis. Hyponatremia, hypochloremia, hypokalemia, and metabolic acidosis are common, in addition to the hyperglycemia and glucosuria of simple diabetes. Ketonemia and ketonuria will be present, but it should be noted that ketone test strips will not detect β-hydroxybutyric acids.
      (3) Nonketotic hyperosmolar diabetes mellitus. Profound hyperglycemia, relative polycythemia, hyperproteinemia (dehydration), hyperosmolality, and glucosuria are seen.
      (4) Concurrent problems
        (a) Bacteriuria and leukuria are common because urinary tract infections (UTIs) are prevalent in untreated or poorly regulated diabetic patients. Proteinuria may also be seen with infection or glomerular damage.
        (b) Other changes may be seen if concurrent renal failure, pancreatitis, or other disease is present.
    c. Differentiating type I and **type II diabetes** can be difficult, even with a stimulation test (e.g., glucose or glucagon stimulation test). In the absence of definitive results:
      (1) In dogs, it should be assumed that the diabetes is insulin-dependent.
      (2) In cats, differentiation is usually based on the severity of the clinical signs and biochemical abnormalities and the response to treatment.

  5. Treatment
    a. Simple diabetes mellitus
      (1) Insulin should be given once daily initially.
        (a) Preparations. NPH, lente, or ultralente insulin can be used. Beef/pork, purified beef or pork, and recombinant human insulins are available.
          (i) In dogs, lente or NPH insulins are used most commonly (Table 44-1). Pork and human recombinant insulin preparations tend to have a quicker onset of action, a shorter duration of effect, and slightly more potency because the amino acid sequence of canine insulin is very similar to that of porcine and human insulin.
          (ii) In cats, ultralente or twice daily lente insulin is used most commonly (Table 44-2). The amino acid sequence of feline insulin is similar to that of bovine insulin.

(b) Glucose measurement

    (i) A few blood glucose concentrations should be evaluated after initiating insulin therapy to ensure that the blood glucose is not dropping too low. The animal should then be given a few days to adapt to the treatment before performing a more complete glucose curve (i.e., measurement of blood glucose every 2–3 hours for at least 10–14 hours, and ideally for 24 hours).

    (ii) In evaluating a glucose curve, it should first be determined whether or not the insulin is effective in decreasing the blood glucose. If so, then the glucose nadir should be assessed. A nadir of 100–125 mg/dl (5.6–7 mmol/L) is ideal. If the nadir is still too high, the dose should be increased and a curve reevaluated in a few days. Once the nadir is adjusted, the duration of insulin action should be assessed. If it is too short, a change to a longer-acting insulin or to more frequent administration is needed.

    (iii) Periodic glucose curves should be evaluated until treatment is optimal. Ideally, the blood glucose concentration should be 100–300 mg/dl (5.6–13 mmol/L), although this level cannot be achieved in many dogs and cats. Subsequent reevaluations are scheduled according to the animal's attitude and clinical signs at home.

(2) Diet should be used to correct obesity and minimize fluctuations in glucose. The diet should remain consistent.

    (a) A canned or dry diet high in complex carbohydrates should be fed. Semi-moist foods should be avoided because of their high concentration of simple sugars. Increased dietary fiber may also be helpful if the animal is not thin.

    (b) Feeding should be divided into multiple small meals.

    (c) If concurrent disease is present, other dietary restrictions or requirements may be more important.

(3) Ovariohysterectomy is strongly recommended for intact female patients.

(4) Exercise should be consistent.

b. Possible non–insulin-dependent diabetes mellitus in cats. Glipizide, a commonly used oral hypoglycemic medication, can be considered for treatment of healthy nonketotic cats with only mild clinical signs of diabetes mellitus. The cat should be reevaluated in 2 weeks and switched to insulin treatment if ketones have developed, or if the hyperglycemia, glucosuria, or clinical signs have worsened. Potential side effects of the drug include hypoglycemia, vomiting, increased liver enzymes, and icterus.

c. Healthy ketotic animals. Crystalline insulin should be given subcutaneously every 8 hours until ketonuria resolves. One-third of the daily caloric allotment

TABLE 44-2. Clinical Properties of Insulin Preparations in Cats

Type of Insulin	Route of Administration	Onset of Effect	Time of Maximum Effect	Duration of Effect
Regular crystalline, semilente	IV	Immediate	$\frac{1}{2}$–2 hours	1–4 hours
	IM	10–30 min	1–4 hours	3–8 hours
	SQ	10–30 min	1–5 hours	4–10 hours
NPH (isophane)	SQ	1–3 hours	2–8 hours	6–12 hours
Lente	SQ	$\frac{1}{2}$–2 hours	2–8 hours	6–14 hours
Ultralente	SQ	2–8 hours	6–16 hours	8–24 hours

IM = intramuscular; IV = intravenous; SQ = subcutaneous.

should be fed at the time of each insulin injection. When the ketones have resolved, a change can be made to a long-acting insulin.

d. Ill Ketoacidotic animals

(1) Insulin therapy

(a) Preparations. Regular crystalline insulin should be used initially because it can be administered by various routes and its shorter duration of action allows more frequent dosage adjustments if needed (see Tables 44-1 and 44-2).

(b) Regimens. With any of the following regimens, the blood glucose level should be evaluated every 1–2 hours initially and 50% dextrose added to the fluids to make a 5% solution when the blood glucose level reaches 200–250 mg/dl (11–13.9 mmol/L). The aim is to have the blood glucose level remain at 150–300 mg/dl (8.5–16.7 mmol/L).

(i) Intermittent intramuscular administration

(ii) Intramuscular administration followed by intermittent subcutaneous administration

(iii) Continuous low-dose intravenous administration

(c) Duration. Crystalline insulin therapy must be continued until the ketones are gone, the animal is clinically well, and the animal is drinking and eating. Once the ketoacidosis has resolved, longer acting insulin therapy can be initiated.

(2) Supportive measures include the correction of **fluid, electrolyte,** and **acid–base imbalances.**

(a) Intravenous 0.9% saline is commonly used because serum sodium and chloride concentrations are often decreased as a result of anorexia, vomiting, and diarrhea. Saline should not be used if serum electrolyte concentrations dictate otherwise or if the serum osmolality is greater than 350 mOsm/L. Any fluid deficit should be corrected over 24–48 hours unless shock necessitates more rapid fluid administration.

(b) Intravenous potassium supplementation helps replace total body potassium lost as a result of anorexia, vomiting, insulin treatment, urinary loss, dilution, and treatment of acidosis. The amount should be based on serum potassium concentrations.

(c) Sodium bicarbonate should be given if the serum bicarbonate or the venous total carbon dioxide is less than 12 mEq/L. If the acidosis is milder, other components of the patient's treatment will correct the imbalance without bicarbonate administration. One-half of the calculated deficit should be administered over 6 hours and then the acid–base status reassessed.

(d) Parenteral phosphorus supplementation is recommended if the serum phosphorus is less than 1.5 mg/dl (0.5 mmol/L), especially if clinical signs of hypophosphatemia (e.g., hemolysis, weakness, ataxia, seizures) are present.

(e) Monitoring of fluid status is based on urine output, central venous pressure, body weight (an anorexic animal will lose 0.5–1.0% BW/day), and thoracic auscultation.

6. Complications associated with diabetes and the treatment of diabetes

a. Hypoglycemia can occur from insulin overdosage. Lethargy, weakness, ataxia, and seizures may be seen. Emergency treatment for hypoglycemia is discussed in IV B 5 a; after resolving the acute problem, the insulin dosage should be decreased.

b. Recurrence of clinical signs. Causes include:

(1) Use of inactive insulin. Little or no decrease in blood glucose is seen on a blood glucose curve, but a response is seen when new insulin is administered. Treatment requires use of active insulin.

(2) Improper administration of insulin. Little or no decrease in blood glucose is seen on a blood glucose curve when the owner administers the insulin, but a response is seen when the veterinarian administers the insulin. Treatment requires further instruction of the owner regarding insulin administration.

(3) Rapid metabolism of insulin. A response to insulin is seen on the blood glucose curve, but the duration of action of the insulin is less than 18 hours. Treatment requires a change to a longer-acting insulin or to more frequent insulin administration.

(4) Insulin-induced hyperglycemia. Overdosage initially causes hypoglycemia. In response to the low blood glucose concentrations, glucose counterregulatory mechanisms become active but cause hyperglycemia rather than just a return to normoglycemia. Treatment requires a marked decrease in the insulin dosage and reregulation of the diabetes.

(5) Disorders causing insulin resistance. With insulin resistance, a normal amount of insulin does not cause a normal blood glucose response. Despite a relatively high dose of insulin (i.e., greater than 1.5–2 U/kg in dogs or 6 U/cat in cats), on a blood glucose curve most, if not all, of the blood glucose concentrations remain greater than 300 mg/dl (16.7 mmol/L). Use of inactive insulin or improper insulin administration should be ruled out before insulin resistance is considered. Potential causes of insulin resistance are:

(a) Diestrus or pregnancy. Increased progesterone concentrations cause an increase in GH, which in turn causes insulin resistance. The diagnosis is based on the history and a serum progesterone concentration. Treatment is by ovariohysterectomy.

(b) Hyperadrenocorticism is the most common cause of insulin resistance in dogs. The increased serum cortisol concentrations cause the insulin resistance. The diagnosis and treatment of hyperadrenocorticism are discussed in V C.

(c) Medications. Exogenous progestins and glucocorticoids are the most common iatrogenic causes of insulin resistance. Treatment requires discontinuation of the medication if possible.

(d) Infection can cause insulin resistance, possibly through increased glucagon concentrations; however, the insulin resistance is usually not severe enough to necessitate the high insulin doses recommended above. Treatment is with antibiotics.

(e) Acromegaly. In cats, increased GH concentrations cause insulin resistance.

(f) Hyperthyroidism. In cats, insulin resistance caused by hyperthyroidism is usually mild and often not identified clinically.

(g) Poor insulin absorption from subcutaneous tissues occurs in approximately 20% of cats being treated with ultralente insulin; the condition is very rare in dogs. Poor absorption should be suspected if the response to the subcutaneous long-acting insulin is little to none but the response to intravenous regular (crystalline) insulin is normal. A change to another form of insulin may be helpful.

(h) Insulin antibodies. Although dogs and cats may develop some antibodies to the exogenous insulin, the amount of antibody is rarely enough to cause significant insulin resistance. The diagnosis may be suspected after having ruled out other causes of insulin resistance. A change in the species of origin of the insulin to one more similar to the animal's own (e.g., a change to human insulin in dogs or a change to pure beef insulin in cats) may be helpful.

c. Chronic complications can occur when diabetes goes untreated or when the diabetes is poorly controlled.

(1) Cataracts are the most common chronic complication of diabetes mellitus in dogs, but they are rare in cats. In hyperglycemic dogs, sorbitol and fructose form and are trapped in the lens. The lens becomes hyperosmolar and water is drawn in, disrupting the structure of the lens so that it becomes opaque. The resulting cataracts are irreversible.

(2) Diabetic neuropathy is uncommon but can result in a plantigrade stance (i.e., "dropped hocks") in cats, proprioceptive deficits, hyporeflexia, muscle atrophy, and weakness. The signs may resolve if the diabetes is promptly treated or brought under better control.

(3) **Diabetic nephropathy** is rare, but can cause severe proteinuria and renal failure.

(4) **Diabetic retinopathy** is also rare and can result in blindness.

B. **Insulinoma (beta cell tumor)**

1. **Etiology.** The cause of the neoplastic transformation is unknown.

2. **Pathogenesis**
   a. Like normal beta cells, the neoplastic beta cells secrete proinsulin and insulin. However, the neoplastic beta cells secrete these substances, often excessively, in response to stimuli independent of glucose concentrations. The effect of the hyperinsulinemia is hypoglycemia.
   b. The tumors are usually malignant.

3. **Predisposition**
   a. Insulinomas are most common in middle-aged to older dogs. There may be an increased incidence in boxers, fox terriers, German shepherds, Irish setters, and standard poodles.
   b. Insulinomas are rare in cats.

4. **Diagnosis**
   a. **Clinical findings**
      (1) **Symptoms** are primarily those of hypoglycemia (i.e., seizures, weakness, collapse, ataxia, muscle tremors, lethargy, and odd behavior.) The symptoms are usually episodic and may be exacerbated by fasting, eating, excitement, or exercise. If the problem is chronic, clinical signs may be minimal despite biochemical hypoglycemia.
      (2) **Physical examination findings** are usually unremarkable except for possible mild weight gain. Decreased proprioception, hyporeflexia, and mild muscle atrophy consistent with a peripheral neuropathy may be seen but are uncommon.
   b. **Diagnostic imaging findings.** Thoracic and abdominal radiographs should be evaluated for evidence of other disease or for metastatic lesions. Abdominal ultrasound may reveal a pancreatic mass, but often the mass is too small to be detected. Hepatic metastasis may be visible.
   c. **Laboratory findings**
      (1) The diagnosis is based on the presence of normal or increased insulin levels in the presence of hypoglycemia. If history, signalment, and physical examination suggest insulinoma but the animal is normoglycemic, fasting blood glucose levels should be evaluated. Insulinomas will usually result in hypoglycemia after less than a 12-hour fast.
      (2) A CBC, serum biochemical profile, and urinalysis should be performed to help rule out other causes of hypoglycemia.

   d. **Differential diagnoses for hypoglycemia**
      (1) **Idiopathic "puppy hypoglycemia"** occurs most commonly in young toy and miniature breed dogs. The disorder resolves with maturity. In the interim, the signs can be prevented by frequent feedings.
      (2) **Hepatic dysfunction.** In young dogs, a portosystemic shunt should be suspected. In older dogs, cirrhosis or chronic hepatitis should be suspected.
      (3) **Sepsis.** The septic animal will be very ill and will usually demonstrate leukocytosis with a shift toward immaturity. Hypoglycemia can result from increased consumption of glucose and altered hepatic metabolism.
      (4) **Hypoadrenocorticism** is discussed in V A.
      (5) **Other neoplasms,** especially hepatic tumors, may cause hypoglycemia through consumption of glucose, secretion of insulin-like substances, and other mechanisms.

5. **Treatment**
   a. **Acute glucose replenishment.** Owners can be instructed to rub sugar syrup on the buccal mucosa. Hospitalized animals can be administered dextrose intravenously. A small meal should be fed as soon as the animal is responsive. Excessive glucose administration should be avoided because it can stimulate additional insulin secretion and a rebound hypoglycemia.
   b. **Surgery** is usually the first definitive treatment option for insulinoma. Debulking or complete excision may be possible; however, metastasis is often present at the time of surgery.
      (1) **Preoperative care.** Small, frequent meals should be fed, and glucocorticoid treatment can be considered. Intravenous dextrose administration will usually be needed during preoperative fasting, intraoperatively, and for the first 24–48 hours postoperatively.
      (2) **Postoperative care.** The animal should be monitored for hypoglycemia or hyperglycemia and for signs of pancreatitis. Because of the risk of pancreatitis following manipulation of the pancreas, oral food and water should be withheld initially and hydration maintained with intravenous fluids.
         (a) If hyperglycemia and glucosuria occur and persist, insulin therapy may be needed.
         (b) If hypoglycemia persists or recurs, metastatic disease is likely present and medical therapy (see IV B 5 c) should be instituted.
   c. **Chronic medical treatment** is aimed at decreasing the frequency and severity of the clinical signs. It is used if surgery is not an option or if the signs recur following surgery. Medical treatment is added in a stepwise fashion as needed.
      (1) **Frequent meals** of a moderate protein, moderate fat, complex carbohydrate diet should be fed. A mix of canned food and dry kibble is optimal. Soft moist foods should be avoided because they contain more simple sugars.
      (2) **Exercise** should be restricted to short walks on a leash.
      (3) **Glucocorticoids** will help antagonize the effects of insulin and stimulate hepatic glycogenolysis.
      (4) **Diazoxide,** a benzothiadiazide diuretic, can be used to decrease tissue uptake of glucose, inhibit insulin secretion, stimulate hepatic glucose output, and increase sensitivity to epinephrine. The most common side effects are vomiting and diarrhea.
      (5) **Octreotide,** a somatostatin analog, has been used experimentally to try to inhibit insulin secretion.
      (6) **Streptozocin** and **alloxan** selectively destroy beta cells, but they are rarely used because they can also cause acute renal failure and other serious problems.

V. ADRENAL DISORDERS

A. Canine hypoadrenocorticism (Addison's disease)

1. **Types**
   a. **Primary hypoadrenocorticism** is often an idiopathic disorder that results in atrophy and fibrosis of the adrenal glands. Immune-mediated destruction may play a role earlier in the course of the disorder. Other potential but less common causes include trauma, infarction, infection, metastatic neoplasia, and amyloidosis. All layers of the adrenal cortex are affected, so glucocorticoid, mineralocorticoid, and adrenal sex hormone secretion are usually deficient. However, early in the course of the disorder just hypocortisolemia may be seen.
   b. **Secondary hypoadrenocorticism** occurs as a result of ACTH deficiency with subsequent cortisol deficiency.
      (1) **Pituitary** or **hypothalamic disease** (e.g., neoplasia, trauma, inflammation, congenital abnormalities) or **abrupt discontinuation of exogenous glucocor-**

ticoid administration can cause decreased ACTH secretion and subsequent hypocortisolemia. Mineralocorticoid concentrations are usually normal.

    (2) Iatrogenic hypoadrenocorticism

        (a) Permanent hypoadrenocorticism can occur with mitotane treatment of hyperadrenocorticism.

        (b) Temporary hypocortisolemia can result from ketoconazole treatment.

  c. Atypical hypoadrenocorticism results in hypocortisolemia only. This can occur early in the course of primary hypoadrenocorticism or as a result of secondary hypoadrenocorticism.

2. Predisposition. Hypoadrenocorticism is uncommon in dogs. Young to middle-aged female dogs have the highest incidence. Primary hypoadrenocorticism is familial in a group of standard poodles and may be familial in Labrador retrievers and Portuguese water spaniels.

3. Diagnosis

  a. Primary hypoadrenocorticism. Definitive diagnosis requires an ACTH stimulation test, but results of a minimum database, ECG, and possibly radiographs can lend support to the diagnosis, identify concurrent problems, and suggest a diagnosis of hypoadrenocorticism when only a few clinical signs are present.

    (1) Clinical findings. Primary hypoadrenocorticism should always be suspected in a shocky, dehydrated, or hypotensive dog that is bradycardic.

        (a) Symptoms in dogs may include anorexia, vomiting, diarrhea, polyuria and polydipsia, lethargy, weakness, and weight loss. The symptoms may be acute, or there may be a history of waxing and waning symptoms or a previous response to symptomatic treatment (e.g., parenteral fluid administration).

        (b) Physical examination findings. Dehydration, lethargy, weakness, bradycardia, and weak pulses may be found. Shock may occur in severe cases.

    (2) Laboratory findings

        (a) CBC. A CBC may show a mild normocytic, normochromic anemia with no stress leukogram despite the apparent stress of the illness.

        (b) Serum biochemical profile

            (i) Hyperkalemia, hyponatremia, and hypochloremia are usually present, and the sodium:potassium ratio is usually less than 27:1.

            (ii) Prerenal azotemia and hyperphosphatemia are common responses to dehydration.

            (iii) Less common abnormalities include acidosis, mild hypercalcemia, mild hypoglycemia, and mild hypoalbuminemia.

        (c) Urinalysis. Although the azotemia found in many dogs with hypoadrenocorticism may result from dehydration, the urine may be isosthenuric in some affected dogs because the chronic sodium wasting of hypoadrenocorticism can cause medullary washout and an inability to concentrate urine. With replacement of total body sodium, urine concentrating ability returns.

        (d) ACTH stimulation test. A blood sample is obtained for cortisol measurement before and 1–2 hours after administration of exogenous ACTH. Dogs with hypoadrenocorticism will have basal cortisol concentrations below or near the lower end of the normal laboratory reference range and will have little or no increase in blood cortisol in response to exogenous ACTH.

    (3) ECG findings. An ECG should be evaluated if bradycardia or hyperkalemia is identified (see Chapter 43: Part II:II C 2 b). A normal ECG does not rule out hyperkalemia.

    (4) Diagnostic imaging findings. Abdominal radiographs are usually unremarkable. Thoracic radiographs may show microcardia due to severe hypovolemia.

  b. Atypical and **secondary hypoadrenocorticism**

    (1) Clinical signs. Anorexia, vomiting, diarrhea, and lethargy are the most common symptoms. Iatrogenic hypoadrenocorticism may result in signs of primary or atypical hypoadrenocorticism, depending on the cause.

(2) Laboratory findings. The CBC, serum biochemical profile, and urinalysis findings are usually normal in animals with atypical hypoadrenocorticism. An ACTH stimulation test is the only way to establish the diagnosis. Endogenous ACTH concentration evaluation will allow differentiation of early primary hypoadrenocorticism and secondary hypoadrenocorticism:

(a) Serum ACTH concentrations will be high in animals with primary hypoadrenocorticism.

(b) Serum ACTH concentrations will be low in animals with secondary hypoadrenocorticism.

(3) Diagnostic imaging findings. Radiographic findings are usually normal in animals with atypical hypoadrenocorticism.

4. Treatment

a. Primary hypoadrenocorticism

(1) Acute therapy

(a) Normal (0.9%) saline should be administered intravenously to correct dehydration and hypovolemia and to maintain hydration. The dehydration should be corrected over 24 hours, unless shock necessitates more rapid fluid administration initially. Intravenous fluid therapy will lower serum potassium by dilution and by increasing urinary excretion of potassium ions.

(b) Calcium gluconate, sodium bicarbonate, dextrose, or **dextrose and crystalline insulin** can be administered to treat hyperkalemia and its cardiac effects.

(i) Calcium gluconate will not lower the serum potassium concentration but can decrease potassium's deleterious cardiac effects.

(ii) Sodium bicarbonate, dextrose, and dextrose and crystalline insulin will decrease the serum potassium concentration by driving potassium ions into the cells.

(c) Dextrose in the intravenous fluids will correct hypoglycemia.

(d) Sodium bicarbonate will correct severe acidosis (i.e., a serum bicarbonate level less than 12 mmol/L).

(e) Glucocorticoids

(i) Parenteral dexamethasone can be administered once the ACTH stimulation test has been started. Dexamethasone will not be detected by cortisol assays and therefore will not disrupt the test.

(ii) Other glucocorticoids should be avoided, if possible, until the final sample has been obtained for the stimulation test. At that time, **prednisone sodium succinate, hydrocortisone hemisuccinate,** or **hydrocortisone phosphate** can be given if dexamethasone was not previously administered. Hydrocortisone hemisuccinate and hydrocortisone phosphate have some mineralocorticoid activity in addition to their predominant glucocorticoid activity.

(f) Parenteral mineralocorticoid preparations for acute administration are not available.

(g) Monitoring. Serum electrolytes, blood urea nitrogen (BUN) and serum creatinine levels, hydration status, and urine output should be closely monitored until normal. With treatment, azotemia will often resolve or markedly improve by the following day in dogs with hypoadrenocorticism.

(2) Chronic maintenance therapy. Maintenance therapy is initiated once the animal is stable and the diagnosis has been confirmed. Therapy must be maintained for the remainder of the dog's life.

(a) Mineralocorticoids

(i) Fludrocorticosterone is the most commonly used mineralocorticoid and is the only oral preparation. It also has sufficient glucocorticoid activity to meet the daily needs of many dogs. Additional glucocorticoid supplementation may be needed during times of stress, however.

    (ii) Desoxycorticosterone pivalate (DOCP) can be given as a monthly injection and has no glucocorticoid activity.

  (b) Glucocorticoids

    (i) Oral prednisone is the most commonly used chronic glucocorticoid supplement. It may be used to supplement fludrocorticosterone treatment during times of stress or it may be administered daily in conjunction with DOCP treatment.

    (ii) A long-acting injectable glucocorticoid can also be used in conjunction with DOCP treatment.

  (c) Oral salt supplementation may be helpful if the serum potassium concentration is controlled by the mineralocorticoid preparation but the serum sodium concentration remains low.

  (d) Monitoring. Serum electrolyte concentrations should be evaluated 1–2 times weekly for the first 1–2 weeks, then once every 3–4 months for 1 year, and then 1–2 times yearly thereafter.

  b. Atypical hypoadrenocorticism. Glucocorticoid treatment [see V A 4 a (1) (e)] alone is sufficient. Serum electrolyte levels should be evaluated monthly for several months if early primary hypoadrenocorticism was not definitively ruled out based on an endogenous ACTH concentration evaluation. Monitoring will detect electrolyte changes caused by mineralocorticoid deficiency (which will ultimately develop if primary hypoadrenocorticism is present) before they cause life-threatening problems.

5. Prognosis. With primary hypoadrenocorticism, the prognosis is good if the dog survives the acute crisis. With secondary hypoadrenocorticism, the prognosis varies with the underlying disorder.

B. **Feline hypoadrenocorticism.** Hypoadrenocorticism is rare in cats, and no age or sex predilection has been identified. The clinical signs, diagnosis, treatment, and prognosis are similar to those of dogs with primary hypoadrenocorticism with the following exceptions:

1. Diarrhea and bradycardia are rare.

2. Post-ACTH cortisol samples should be obtained 30 minutes to 1 hour following ACTH administration (versus 1–2 hours in dogs).

3. Response to acute therapy is slower.

C. **Canine hyperadrenocorticism**

1. Etiology

  a. Pituitary-dependent hyperadrenocorticism (PDH). With PDH, pituitary corticotrophs in the pars distalis (common) or pars intermedia (less common) secrete excess ACTH. Corticotroph microadenomas are most common; macroadenomas and adenocarcinomas are less common. The secretion of excess ACTH by the corticotrophs stimulates excess cortisol secretion. Normal feedback inhibition of ACTH production is lost so that both ACTH and cortisol concentrations remain high. The hypercortisolemia can cause feedback inhibition of other pituitary hormones (e.g., TSH, GH, LH, FSH), so clinical signs of other hormone deficiencies may also be seen.

  b. Adrenal tumors may be malignant or benign. The cells autonomously secrete excess cortisol. Pituitary ACTH secretion decreases as a result of normal feedback inhibition. The contralateral adrenal gland usually atrophies because there is little or no stimulation by ACTH.

  c. Bilateral adrenal hyperplasia is rare and may be a variation of PDH.

  d. Iatrogenic hyperadrenocorticism can occur with prolonged or high-dose glucocorticoid treatment.

2. Predisposition

    a. PDH is most common in middle-aged to older smaller breed dogs (i.e., those weighing less than 20 kg). Beagles, Boston terriers, boxers, dachshunds, German shepherds, poodles, and terriers may be at increased risk.

    b. Adrenal tumors are more common in middle-aged to older larger breed dogs. Dachshunds, German shepherds, Labrador retrievers, poodles, and terriers may be at increased risk.

3. Diagnosis. Definitive diagnosis of hyperadrenocorticism requires one or more screening tests; however, results of a minimum data base and radiographs may also provide diagnostic support, identify concurrent problems, or suggest a possible diagnosis of hyperadrenocorticism when there are few clinical signs.

    a. Clinical findings. The clinical signs are usually insidious in onset, and signs have often been present for weeks to months prior to presentation. A dog with hyperadrenocorticism may have any or all of the following symptoms:

        (1) Polyuria and **polydipsia** are common because cortisol can increase the glomerular filtration rate (GFR) and inhibit the effects of ADH on the renal tubules, and may affect ADH release.

        (2) Polyphagia is common as a direct effect of hypercortisolemia.

        (3) Abdominal enlargement or a **pot-bellied appearance** is common. Hepatomegaly, muscle weakness, and fat redistribution (e.g., increased intraabdominal fat) may contribute to this change in body conformation.

        (4) Fat redistribution may be seen as increased fat over the dorsal flank.

        (5) Alopecia and other **dermatopathies** are common. The alopecia is truncal and bilaterally symmetrical, or there may just be thinning of the truncal hair. Shaved hair is often slow to regrow, and skin hyperpigmentation or comedones may be seen. Pruritus may be noted with calcinosis cutis, secondary pyoderma, seborrhea, or demodicosis.

        (6) Lethargy and **weakness** may result from the effects of ACTH and cortisol on neuromuscular activity.

        (7) Panting may be seen, although the cause is not known. Muscle weakness, hepatomegaly, and increased intrathoracic fat may play a role.

        (8) Infertility, myotonia or **pseudomyotonia,** and **thromboembolism** may occur but are uncommon. Testicular atrophy or clitoral hypertrophy may also be seen.

        (9) Bruising after simple venipuncture is also common.

        (10) Neurologic abnormalities (e.g., listlessness, disorientation, pacing, ataxia, seizures) may be seen if a pituitary macroadenoma is present.

    b. Laboratory findings

        (1) CBC. A CBC often shows a mature neutrophilia, monocytosis, lymphopenia, and eosinopenia (i.e., stress leukogram) and sometimes mild polycythemia.

        (2) Serum biochemical profile. Very commonly, a moderate to marked increase in SAP, a steroid-induced isoenzyme, is seen. Other possible abnormalities include hypercholesterolemia, hypertriglyceridemia, mild hyperglycemia, a mildly increased SALT level, decreased BUN, and mild hypophosphatemia.

        (3) Urinalysis often reveals isosthenuric or dilute urine (i.e., urine with a specific gravity of less than 1.013). Evidence of UTI (i.e., leukuria, bacteriuria) is common. Glucosuria is not seen unless concurrent diabetes mellitus is present.

        (4) Screening tests for hyperadrenocorticism should always be interpreted in light of the history, clinical signs, and results of prior tests.

            (a) ACTH stimulation test. An exaggerated response to ACTH is suggestive of hyperadrenocorticism. Approximately 80%–85% of dogs with PDH and 60%–80% of dogs with an adrenal tumor will show such a response. Normal results on an ACTH stimulation test do not completely rule out hyperadrenocorticism.

(i) Post-ACTH cortisol concentrations only slightly above the laboratory reference range should be interpreted with caution because stress, especially chronic stress, and some medications (e.g., anticonvulsants) can also cause cortisol elevations.

(ii) A pre-ACTH cortisol concentration near the lower end of the normal reference range and little or no response to exogenous ACTH administration in a dog with clinical signs of hyperadrenocorticism is consistent with iatrogenic hyperadrenocorticism. This test is the only screening test that will identify iatrogenic hyperadrenocorticism.

(b) **Low-dose dexamethasone suppression test.** Blood samples are taken for serum cortisol measurement prior to and 4 and 8 hours following the intravenous administration of 0.01–0.015 mg/kg of dexamethasone.

(i) Insufficient suppression of serum cortisol at the 8-hour sampling time is indicative of hyperadrenocorticism for nearly 100% of dogs with adrenal tumors and 90%–95% of dogs with PDH.

(ii) Serum cortisol levels only slightly above the laboratory reference range for the 8-hour sampling time should be interpreted with caution because stress can affect the results.

(iii) Serum cortisol suppression at the 4-hour, but not the 8-hour, sampling time suggests that PDH, not an adrenal tumor, is the cause of the hyperadrenocorticism.

(c) **Urine cortisol:creatinine ratio.** Cortisol and creatinine concentrations in a morning urine sample are measured.

(i) If the ratio is normal, hyperadrenocorticism is unlikely.

(ii) If the ratio is increased, hyperadrenocorticism or another disorder may be present.

(d) **Steroid-induced SAP isoenzyme concentration**

(i) If the isoenzyme concentration is normal, then hyperadrenocorticism is unlikely.

(ii) If the isoenzyme concentration is increased, both hyperadrenocorticism and other disorders must be considered.

(5) **Hepatic biopsy.** Although not recommended as a first-line screening test, because of the increased hepatic enzymes and hepatomegaly in many dogs with hyperadrenocorticism, a hepatic biopsy may be considered in dogs with few other signs of hyperadrenocorticism or in dogs with conflicting results on other tests. Histologic evidence of steroid hepatopathy includes centrilobular vacuolization, glycogen accumulation, and focal centrilobular necrosis.

c. **Diagnostic imaging findings.** Abdominal and thoracic radiographs often show hepatomegaly and a large urinary bladder. Decreased bone density and ectopic calcification of the kidneys, skin, or tracheal rings are less common. A mineralized mass is sometimes visible if an adrenal tumor is present. Pulmonary metastasis of an adrenal tumor is rare.

d. **Differentiating tests.** Once a diagnosis of hyperadrenocorticism has been established, it is necessary to determine whether the hyperadrenocorticism is caused by PDH or an adrenal tumor. Unless results of the low-dose dexamethasone suppression test provided this differentiation, one or more of the following tests is usually needed.

(1) **High-dose dexamethasone suppression test.** A blood sample is obtained for cortisol measurement prior to and 4 and 8 hours following the intravenous administration of 0.1–1.0 mg/kg of dexamethasone.

(a) Suppression of one or both post-dexamethasone cortisol sample concentrations to less than 50% of the baseline value occurs in most dogs (i.e., 75%–85%) with PDH.

(b) Little or no suppression is indicative of either an adrenal tumor or PDH.

(2) Endogenous ACTH concentration. A blood sample is obtained in the morning following a night's acclimatization in the hospital. Special sample handling is required. In a dog with documented hyperadrenocorticism:

(a) A low ACTH concentration is consistent with an adrenal tumor.

(b) A high ACTH concentration is consistent with PDH.

(c) An intermediate ACTH concentration does not provide differentiation.

(3) Diagnostic imaging studies

(a) Abdominal radiographs may reveal an adrenal tumor.

(b) Abdominal ultrasonography

(i) If both adrenal glands are visible and approximately equal in size, PDH is suggested.

(ii) If one adrenal gland is enlarged and the contralateral adrenal gland is small, an adrenal tumor is likely.

(iii) Ultrasound may also identify hepatic metastatic lesions if a malignant adrenal tumor is present.

(c) CT can also be used to identify bilateral adrenal gland enlargement (suggestive of PDH) or unilateral enlargement (suggestive of an adrenal tumor). However, CT is more expensive and more limited in availability than ultrasonography. If a pituitary macrotumor is suspected, CT or magnetic resonance imaging (MRI) can be used to confirm the diagnosis.

(4) Less commonly used tests include the **corticotropin-releasing hormone (CRH) stimulation test,** which shows little or no increase in blood cortisol or ACTH if an adrenal tumor is present, and the **metyrapone test,** which shows decreases in both cortisol and 11-deoxycortisol if an adrenal tumor is present.

4. Treatment

a. PDH

(1) Mitotane selectively damages the zona fasciculata and zona reticularis of the adrenal glands.

(a) Induction therapy. It is initially given once or twice daily until polydipsia or polyphagia resolves.

(i) If anorexia, vomiting, diarrhea, or listlessness is noted, induction therapy should be stopped.

(ii) If no clinical change is seen after 8–10 days of therapy, an ACTH stimulation test should be performed to monitor the efficacy of therapy.

(iii) If the disorder is not well controlled, another 7–10 days of induction therapy should be given and the dog retested.

(iv) If the mitotane fails to control the PDH despite 2–3 weeks of induction therapy, then the dosage or diagnosis should be reassessed.

(b) Maintenance therapy. Mitotane is given every 7–14 days when the resting cortisol concentration is in the lower half of the reference range and little or no increase is seen in response to exogenous ACTH.

(i) The animal should be reassessed using an ACTH stimulation test at 1 and 3 months and 1–2 times yearly thereafter.

(ii) Treatment is required for the remainder of the dog's life, and it is not unusual for signs to recur periodically, necessitating reinduction. Some dogs may also require short-term, low-dose prednisone supplementation during periods of stress.

(c) Adverse effects

(i) Mitotane overdosage produces signs of glucocorticoid deficiency (i.e., anorexia, vomiting, diarrhea, lethargy). Other disorders should be ruled out, hypocortisolemia should be documented using an ACTH stimulation test, mitotane therapy should be temporarily discontinued, and prednisone supplementation should be initiated. This complication of therapy is usually only temporary.

(ii) Although mitotane theoretically does not affect the zona glomeru-losa, occasionally mitotane overdosage will cause full and permanent hypoadrenocorticism.

(2) **Ketoconazole** is an antifungal agent that also blocks cortisol production. Treatment efficacy is based on resolution of the clinical signs and results of ACTH stimulation testing.

(a) Advantages include its more rapid induction of hypocortisolemia and fewer complications.

(b) Disadvantages include cost, the once or twice daily dosing for the remainder of the dog's life, and the lack of response seen in some dogs.

(3) **l-Deprenyl** is a monoamine oxidase-B inhibitor that increases CNS dopamine concentrations and thereby may decrease ACTH (and consequently, cortisol) concentrations in some dogs with PDH.

(4) **Surgery**

(a) **Hypophysectomy** is not commonly performed because of the required surgical expertise.

(b) **Bilateral adrenalectomy** is not cost-effective because it necessitates life-long treatment for hypoadrenocorticism.

b. **Pituitary macrotumors** are treated with **cobalt irradiation** or **linear accelerator photon irradiation.**

c. **Adrenal tumor**

(1) **Adrenalectomy** is often the treatment of choice for a dog with an adrenal tumor because it is curative if the tumor is benign (or malignant without metastasis).

(a) Preoperative treatment with ketoconazole or mitotane can be given for a few weeks prior to surgery to lessen severe clinical signs.

(b) During surgery the animal should be supported with intravenous fluids and glucocorticoids, and mineralocorticoid supplementation should be added following surgery if hyperkalemia is seen. Temporary hormonal supplementation is often needed because the remaining adrenal gland has often atrophied.

(c) Surgery should not be performed if radiographs or ultrasonography indicate the mass is inoperable or if the animal is debilitated.

(2) **Mitotane** can be used to treat an adrenal tumor if it is inoperable, metastasis is present, the animal is debilitated, or the owner declines permission for surgery. The treatment protocol is similar to that for PDH, but dogs with an adrenal tumor often require longer induction therapy and higher dosages, and fewer respond to the drug. A high percentage of treated dogs will also show some side effects because of either direct drug toxicity or hypocortisolemia.

(3) **Ketoconazole** can also be used to control the clinical signs of hyperadrenocorticism in a dog with an adrenal tumor, but it will have no effect on the tumor or its growth. Treatment is as discussed for PDH. Ketoconazole is useful as a short-term therapy to improve the preoperative condition of the dog.

5. **Complications.** Potential complications of untreated or poorly controlled hyperadrenocorticism include infection, pancreatitis, thromboembolism, congestive heart failure, hypertension, or ketoacidosis if concurrent diabetes mellitus is present.

6. **Prognosis**

a. **PDH** has a fair prognosis if treated and there is no pituitary macrotumor or other serious complications.

b. **Pituitary macrotumors.** The prognosis is guarded, with approximately only one-third of the treated animals showing complete resolution of clinical signs. The prognosis is worse for larger tumors.

c. **Adrenal tumors** initially carry a guarded prognosis, but the prognosis improves to good if the tumor is benign and the dog survives the first postoperative month.

D. **Feline hyperadrenocorticism**

1. **Etiology.** The causes of feline hyperadrenocorticism are similar to those in dogs, but the disorder is much less common in cats.

2. Predisposition. Female, middle-aged to older cats are most commonly affected.

3. Diagnosis

    a. Clinical findings

        (1) Polyuria and polydipsia are the most common signs.

        (2) Most cats with hyperadrenocorticism also have diabetes mellitus as a result of cortisol-induced insulin resistance.

        (3) Hepatomegaly does not usually occur if only hyperadrenocorticism is present, but may be seen with concurrent poorly controlled diabetes mellitus.

        (4) Fragile skin, a pot-bellied appearance, unkempt hair, and muscle wasting may be seen.

    b. Laboratory findings

        (1) CBC, serum biochemical profile, and **urinalysis** are usually normal if just hyperadrenocorticism is present. However, if concurrent diabetes mellitus is present, hyperglycemia, hypercholesterolemia, a mild increase in SALT concentration, and glucosuria are common. Often, finding insulin resistance in a diabetic cat is what prompts investigation of possible hyperadrenocorticism. Corticosteroids do not induce SAP in the cat.

        (2) Screening tests

            (a) ACTH stimulation test. An ACTH stimulation test in the cat is performed and interpreted in the same manner as that discussed for the dog, except that the post-ACTH sample should be obtained at 30 minutes and 1 hour, or 1 and 2 hours in the cat. This test will identify approximately 60% of affected cats.

            (b) Low-dose dexamethasone suppression test. This test is also performed and interpreted in the same manner as that discussed for the dog, except that a higher dose of dexamethasone (i.e., 0.1 mg/kg intravenously) is sometimes recommended. This test will identify approximately 90%–95% of affected cats.

        (3) Differentiating tests. Once a diagnosis of hyperadrenocorticism has been established, PDH should be differentiated from an adrenal tumor. Unless results from the dexamethasone suppression test provide this differentiation, one or more of the following tests is usually needed.

            (a) High-dose dexamethasone suppression test. This test is performed and interpreted in the same manner as that discussed for the dog except that a higher dose of dexamethasone (i.e., 1.0 mg/kg intravenously) is usually recommended.

            (b) Other differentiating tests include an **endogenous ACTH concentration** and **abdominal ultrasonography.**

4. Treatment. Unilateral or **bilateral adrenalectomy** is recommended because cats tend to respond poorly or not at all to medical therapy.

    a. Medical treatment with mitotane, ketoconazole, or metyrapone can be tried preoperatively in an attempt to reverse some of the clinical signs and make the cat a better surgical candidate.

    b. Intraoperative and postoperative management is as discussed for the dog.

    c. Postoperative complications may include sepsis, wound dehiscence, hypoadrenocorticism, pancreatitis, and thromboembolism.

5. Prognosis is guarded because of the relatively high incidence of postoperative complications.

E. **Pheochromocytomas** are catecholamine-producing tumors composed of adrenal medullary cells. They are rare in dogs, and are usually found only as an incidental finding at necropsy. They have not been reported in cats.

1. Diagnosis. A noninvasive antemortem diagnosis is very difficult. Intermittent clinical signs, intermittent hypertension, and radiographic or ultrasonographic evidence of an adrenal tumor may suggest a possible pheochromocytoma.

    a. Clinical findings may include intermittent anorexia, weight loss, vomiting, weakness, and panting, or no clinical signs may be seen. Physical examination is usually unremarkable.

b. **Surgical exploratory** and **tumor excision** or **biopsy** is usually needed because measurement of urinary catecholamines or serum catecholamine response to stimuli is costly, difficult, and of limited availability.

2. **Treatment** and **prognosis.** Treatment requires surgical excision of the tumor. The prognosis varies with the location of the tumor and the extent of the disease at the time of diagnosis.

VI. GASTROINTESTINAL HORMONAL DISORDERS

A. **Gastrinomas** are gastrin-producing tumors that occur in the non-beta cell pancreas or the duodenum. The incidence is highest in middle-aged to older female dogs, but the disorder is rare overall.

1. **Pathogenesis.** The excess gastrin stimulates gastric acid secretion (and subsequent ulcer formation), gastric mucosal hyperplasia and hypertrophy, and calcitonin secretion. Early metastasis to the liver and local lymph nodes is common.

2. **Diagnosis**
   a. **Clinical findings** are primarily those of gastric hyperacidity (i.e., anorexia, vomiting, hematemesis, diarrhea, melena, weight loss). The mucous membranes may be pale if significant gastrointestinal hemorrhage has occurred. Septic shock may be seen if an ulcer has perforated.
   b. **Laboratory findings**
      (1) Nonspecific findings on preliminary tests may include leukocytosis, anemia, hypoproteinemia, hypochloremia, hypokalemia, metabolic alkalosis, gastric mucosal thickening on contrast radiographs, and endoscopic visualization of antral and duodenal ulcers.
      (2) Diagnosis is based on finding marked hypergastrinemia and concurrent gastric hyperacidity. Stimulation tests can be used if resting values are equivocal.

3. **Treatment.** Surgical excision of the tumor is required, but metastasis is often present at the time of diagnosis. Deep ulcers can be excised at the time of surgery. Symptomatic medical therapy may include histamine-2 (H$_2$)-antagonists, sucralfate, omeprazole, or a somatostatin analog.

4. **Prognosis.** The prognosis is often poor because of the high rate of early metastasis.

B. **Glucagonomas, polypeptidomas,** and **intestinal carcinoid tumors** are very rare in dogs, and only intestinal carcinoid tumors have been reported in cats.

VII. HYPERLIPIDEMIA

A. **Canine hyperlipidemia. Hypertriglyceridemia** can occur as a primary disorder or secondary to other disorders and poses a risk to the animal because increased triglycerides can trigger an episode of pancreatitis. **Hypercholesterolemia** usually occurs secondary to another disorder and does not pose a risk to the animal.

1. **Predisposition**
   a. **Primary idiopathic hyperlipidemia** occurs in miniature schnauzers and may occur in other breeds. It is characterized primarily by fasting hyperchylomicronemia.
   b. **Secondary hyperlipidemia** can occur in dogs with hypothyroidism, diabetes mellitus, hyperadrenocorticism, and protein-losing nephropathy (PLN).

2. **Diagnosis**
  a. **Primary hyperlipidemia.** The diagnosis is based on the breed, documentation of fasting lipemia, marked hypertriglyceridemia, and a positive chylomicron test in addition to exclusion of causes of secondary hyperlipidemia. Episodic vomiting and diarrhea, abdominal pain, and inappetence ("pseudopancreatitis") are the most common clinical findings. Seizures can also occur.
  b. **Secondary hyperlipidemia.** There are usually no signs related to the hyperlipidemia, but clinical signs of the primary disorder are usually present. The diagnostic approach should be aimed at discerning the possible underlying disorders (e.g., hypothyroidism, diabetes mellitus, hyperadrenocorticism, PLN).

3. **Treatment**
  a. **Primary hyperlipidemia.** A low-fat, high-fiber diet should be fed. Medication to lower serum lipid concentrations is rarely needed.
  b. **Secondary hyperlipidemia.** The underlying disorder should be treated.

4. **Prognosis.** Primary hyperlipidemia carries a good prognosis if treated. Secondary hyperlipidemia carries a variable prognosis, depending on the underlying disorder.

B. **Feline hyperlipidemia** is uncommon.

1. **Types**
  a. **Primary hyperchylomicronemia** has been reported as an autosomal recessive disorder. Affected cats may develop xanthomas and lipemia retinalis and will have fasting chylomicronemia.
  b. **Secondary hyperlipidemia** can occur with diabetes mellitus, PLN, and some medications; clinical signs are usually just those of the primary disorder.

2. **Diagnosis, treatment,** and **prognosis** are similar to those of hyperlipidemia in dogs. **Gemfibrozil** has been used in some cats with primary hyperchylomicronemia that did not respond to dietary therapy alone.

Directions: Each of the numbered items or incomplete statements in this section is followed by answers or by completions of the statement. Select the ONE numbered answer or completion that is BEST in each case.

1. What is the most likely diagnosis for a 7-year-old, overweight, spayed female poodle with weight loss, polyuria and polydipsia, and polyphagia?

(1) Diabetes insipidus
(2) Hyperparathyroidism
(3) Hyperadrenocorticism
(4) Insulinoma
(5) Diabetes mellitus

2. The most likely diagnosis for a dog with polyuria and polydipsia, a urine specific gravity of 1.002, and a normal biochemical profile is:

(1) chronic renal failure.
(2) primary hypoadrenocorticism.
(3) diabetes mellitus.
(4) central diabetes insipidus.
(5) hyperadrenocorticism.

3. The treatment of choice for long-term medical treatment of hyperthyroidism in cats is:

(1) propylthiouracil (PTU).
(2) calcium ipodate.
(3) β antagonists.
(4) diltiazem.
(5) methimazole.

4. Hypercalcemia, normophosphatemia, and a low serum parathyroid hormone (PTH) concentration are most consistent with:

(1) primary hyperparathyroidism.
(2) hypercalcemia of malignancy.
(3) vitamin D toxicosis.
(4) renal failure.

5. When evaluating a blood glucose curve on a diabetic dog, the desired peak and nadir blood glucose are:

(1) peak 125 mg/dl (6.7 mmol/L); nadir 70 mg/dl (4.0 mmol/L)
(2) peak 200 mg/dl (11 mmol/L); nadir 70 mg/dl (4.0 mmol/L)
(3) peak 300 mg/dl (16.7 mmol/L); nadir 100 mg/dl (5.6 mmol/L)
(4) peak 300 mg/dl (16.7 mmol/L); nadir 70 mg/dl (4.0 mmol/L)
(5) peak 230 mg/dl (13 mmol/L); nadir 100 mg/dl (5.6 mmol/L)

6. In hypoadrenocorticism, the sodium:potassium ratio is usually:

(1) greater than 40:1.
(2) greater than 32:1.
(3) less than 27:1.
(4) less than 15:1.

7. The most likely diagnosis in a 12-year-old dog with hypoglycemic episodes and a normal physical examination is:

(1) hypoadrenocorticism.
(2) sepsis.
(3) insulinoma.
(4) portosystemic shunt.
(5) diabetes mellitus.

8. The most likely diagnosis for an 8-year-old neutered male golden retriever with nonpruritic, bilaterally symmetrical truncal alopecia, mild weight gain, and marked hypercholesterolemia is:

(1) hypothyroidism.
(2) growth hormone (GH)–responsive dermatosis.
(3) hyperadrenocorticism.
(4) atopy.
(5) hyperestrogenism.

9. The test of choice for diagnosis of hyperthyroidism in cats is:

(1) a thyroid-stimulating hormone (TSH) stimulation test.
(2) basal serum thyroxine (T_4) concentration.
(3) basal serum triiodothyronine (T_3) concentration.
(4) a T_3 suppression test.
(5) a technetium scan.

10. The test of choice for diagnosis of iatrogenic hyperadrenocorticism is the:

(1) low-dose dexamethasone suppression test.
(2) adrenocorticotropic hormone (ACTH) stimulation test.
(3) high-dose dexamethasone suppression test.
(4) urinary cortisol:creatinine ratio.
(5) steroid-induced serum alkaline phosphatase (SAP) isoenzyme concentration.

DIRECTIONS: Each of the numbered items or incomplete statements in this section is negatively phrased, as indicated by a capitalized word such as NOT, LEAST, or EXCEPT. Select the ONE numbered answer or completion that is BEST in each case.

---

11. All of the following disorders can cause hypocalcemia EXCEPT

(1) hypoalbuminemia.
(2) hyperadrenocorticism.
(3) phosphate enema administration.
(4) eclampsia.
(5) pancreatitis.

12. All of the following are causes of clinical insulin resistance in dogs EXCEPT

(1) hyperadrenocorticism.
(2) diestrus.
(3) infection.
(4) exogenous progestin administration.
(5) hyperthyroidism.

1. The answer is 5 [IV A a a (1)]. Weight loss, polyphagia, and polyuria and polydipsia are classic signs of diabetes mellitus in dogs. With diabetes insipidus, notable weight loss is uncommon and the appetite is normal rather than increased. Weight loss is also rare with hyperadrenocorticism, although muscle atrophy may occur. With hyperparathyroidism, polyuria and polydipsia are common, but the appetite is usually normal or decreased. Mild weight gain is more typical in a dog with an insulinoma.

2. The answer is 4 [I B]. Dogs with central diabetes insipidus will usually have marked polyuria and polydipsia, hyposthenuria, and a normal serum biochemical profile. With chronic renal failure, azotemia, hyperphosphatemia, and isosthenuria are usually found. Hyponatremia and hyperkalemia are typical of primary hypoadrenocorticism. Hyperglycemia and glucosuria are always seen with diabetes mellitus. With hyperadrenocorticism, serum alkaline phosphatase (SAP) concentrations are usually increased and the urine is usually isosthenuric, although hyposthenuria is occasionally seen.

3. The answer is 5 [III B 4 a (1)]. Methimazole is the treatment of choice for long-term medical management of feline hyperthyroidism. Propylthiouracil (PTU) is also effective but has a higher incidence of side effects. Calcium ipodate will usually also control the clinical signs initially, but is thought to lose effectiveness with time. β antagonists, diltiazem, or both may be useful in management of the cardiomyopathy accompanying hyperthyroidism in some cats, but these medications will not control the other clinical signs of hyperthyroidism.

4. The answer is 2 [II B 3 c (1)]. Hypercalcemia, normophosphatemia, and a low serum parathyroid hormone (PTH) concentration are often found with hypercalcemia of malignancy. Hypercalcemia and normophosphatemia can also be seen with primary hyperparathyroidism, but serum PTH concentrations are high. With hypervitaminosis D and renal failure, serum phosphorus concentrations are usually high.

5. The answer is 5 [IV A 5 a (1) (b) (ii)]. Ideally, blood glucose concentrations should be 100–230 mg/dl (5.6–13 mmol/L). A blood glucose range of 70–125 mg/dl (4.0–6.7 mmol/L) is normal in the dog but is an unrealistic goal for the diabetic dog. A nadir of 70 mg/dl (4.0 mmol/L) is slightly lower than desired because at home the dog's blood glucose may be slightly lower (without the stress of hospitalization) and hypoglycemia should be avoided. A blood glucose peak of 300 mg/dl (16.7 mmol/L) may increase the risk of cataract development.

6. The answer is 3 [V A 3 a (2) (b) (i)]. In primary hypoadrenocorticism, hyponatremia and hyperkalemia usually result in a serum sodium:potassium ratio of less than 27:1.

7. The answer is 3 [IV B 4]. Hypoglycemic episodes in an older dog with a normal physical examination are most likely due to an insulinoma. Hypoadrenocorticism is more common in young to middle-aged dogs, the hypoglycemia is often mild and asymptomatic, and other clinical signs of hypoadrenocorticism are usually present. With sepsis, the dog is often very ill and febrile. Congenital portosystemic shunts are more common in young animals, and an older animal with acquired shunts would likely have additional signs of hepatic failure. Hypoglycemia is not a characteristic of diabetes insipidus.

8. The answer is 1 [III A 3]. Nonpruritic, bilaterally symmetrical truncal alopecia, mild weight gain, and marked hypercholesterolemia in a middle-aged golden retriever is strongly suggestive of hypothyroidism. With growth hormone (GH)–responsive dermatosis, weight gain and hypercholesterolemia do not typically occur. The alopecia could be seen with hyperadrenocorticism, along with a mild to moderate increase in cholesterol and redistribution of body fat, but a marked hypercholesterolemia and a true weight gain are uncommon. Atopy is typically pruritic and would cause no change in serum cholesterol concentration. Hyperestrogenism can also cause bilaterally symmetrical truncal alopecia but would not increase serum cholesterol and would be very rare in a neutered male dog.

9. The answer is 2 [III B 3 b (2)]. Basal thyroxine (T_4) concentrations are inexpensive and will be diagnostic in most cases of feline hyperthyroidism. Basal triiodothyronine (T_3) concentrations are less useful because most of the body's T_3 is intracellular. A thyroid-stimulating hormone (TSH) stimulation test will not aid in the diagnosis and may have deleterious effects. A thyrotropin-releasing hormone (TRH) stimulation test, T_3 suppression test, or a technetium scan can be used to diagnose hyperthyroidism, but due to the increased costs and potential side effects, these tests are reserved for the small number of cases where basal serum T_4 concentrations are nondiagnostic.

10. The answer is 2 [V C 3 b (4) (a)]. An adrenocorticotropic hormone (ACTH) stimulation test is the only test that will diagnose iatrogenic hyperadrenocorticism. The low-dose dexamethasone suppression test, urinary cortisol:creatinine ratio, and steroid-induced serum alkaline phosphatase (SAP) isoenzyme concentration are other screening tests for hyperadrenocorticism, but these tests will not identify iatrogenic disease. The high-dose dexamethasone suppression test is used to differentiate pituitary-dependent hyperadrenocorticism (PDH) from an adrenal tumor, not to diagnose hyperadrenocorticism.

11. The answer is 2 [II A 3 c]. Serum calcium concentrations are usually normal with hyperadrenocorticism. Hypoalbuminemia can cause hypocalcemia by decreasing the protein-bound fraction of calcium while ionized calcium concentrations remain normal; the net effect is a decrease in total serum calcium concentrations. Phosphate enema administration to cats or small dogs can cause hyperphosphatemia and a subsequent decrease in serum calcium. Hypocalcemia is seen in eclampsia resulting from an increase in calcium utilization. With pancreatitis, saponification of peripancreatic fats can decrease serum calcium concentrations.

12. The answer is 5 [IV A 6 b (5)]. Hyperthyroidism is very rare in dogs, and even in cats, does not usually cause clinical insulin resistance. Hyperadrenocorticism, diestrus, infection, and exogenous progestin administration can all cause significant insulin resistance.

Chapter 45

Reproductive Diseases

I. FEMALE REPRODUCTIVE DISORDERS

A. Normal physiology

1. **Estrous cycle.** Characteristics of the estrous cycle in bitches and queens are given in Tables 45-1 and 45-2, respectively.

2. **Parturition**
   a. **Initiation.** Increased fetal adrenocorticotropic hormone (ACTH) concentrations increase fetal and maternal cortisol concentrations. In turn, cortisol may stimulate prostaglandin $F_2\alpha$ ($PGF_2\alpha$) release, leading to luteolysis and a drop in progesterone concentrations. At the same time, the altered estrogen:progesterone ratio works with $PGF_2\alpha$ to dilate the cervix, cause uterine contractions, and cause the placenta to separate.
      (1) **Bitches.** The rectal temperature decreases to 37°C (99°F) or less 12–24 hours prepartum.
      (2) **Queens.** The temperature decreases within 12 hours of parturition, but this finding is less consistent than in bitches.
   b. **Stage 1.** During this stage, the cervix dilates and uterine contractions begin. There may be no clinical signs during stage 1.
      (1) **Bitches.** The bitch may be restless and anorexic. Stage 1 lasts 6–12 hours in dogs.
      (2) **Queens.** The queen may be restless, vocal, and tachypneic. Stage 1 lasts 2–24 hours in cats.
   c. **Stage 2.** Birth occurs during this stage. The mother should remove the amniotic sac and sever the umbilical cord following each delivery.
      (1) **Bitches.** The first pup is usually born within 1–2 hours of the start of strong uterine contractions with subsequent pups delivered every 15–60 minutes. Rest periods (i.e., periods without contractions) lasting up to 4 hours may also occur between births.
      (2) **Queens.** The first kitten is usually born within 1 hour with subsequent kittens delivered every 10–60 minutes. A rest period of 12–24 hours may also occur.
   d. **Stage 3.** The placenta is delivered during this stage, usually within 15 minutes of each birth.

3. **Postpartum period.** It is not uncommon for the bitch or queen to be anorexic for a short time postpartum and to have a temperature as high as 40°C (104°F) for several days. **Lochia,** a green to brick red vaginal discharge with no odor, is also normal and should decrease over several weeks.

B. Clinical evaluation

1. **Clinical signs**
   a. **Estrous cycle abnormalities** are most common.
   b. **Apparent infertility** is not a specific disorder but is a sign of reproductive dysfunction such as estrous cycle abnormalities, fetal death or abortion, uterine disease, breeding mismanagement, or aging. Diagnostic workup should include a thorough history of the female (management, breeding, and pregnancy) and breeding history of the male, evaluation of the estrous cycle, and a thorough physical examination.
   c. **Vulvar discharge**
      (1) **Normal (physiologic) causes** include discharge during proestrus and postpartum lochia.

TABLE 45-1. Characteristics of the Estrous Cycle in the Bitch

Stage	Usual Duration	Clinical Signs and Behavior	Hormonal Patterns	Vaginal Cytology Findings	Vaginoscopic Findings
Proestrus	6–11 days	Blood-tinged vulvar discharge and mild vulvar enlargement, attracts male dogs but will not allow mating	Serum estrogen increases	Early proestrus: noncornified (i.e., parabasal) and intermediate cells Mid to late proestrus: decreasing numbers of neutrophils and erythrocytes, increasing numbers of cornified (i.e., superficial) cells	Smooth, edematous mucosal folds; wrinkles on folds during preovulatory LH peak
Estrus	5–9 days	Receptive to male dogs; flaccid, edematous vulva	Serum estrogen decreases and serum progesterone begins to increase approximately 2 days prior to ovulation at the time of an LH surge	Mainly sheets of nucleated and anuclear cornified epithelial cells	Low, angular mucosal folds and wrinkles
Diestrus	60 days if the bitch is pregnant; 60–100 days if she is not	Does not attract males or allow mating	Serum progesterone increases until late diestrus, then decreases; serum prolactin increases as progesterone decreases	Noncornified epithelial cells	Low, flat folds with pale and hyperemic patches
Anestrus	4.5 months	. . .	Serum FSH increases and there are intermittent increases in serum LH	Noncornified epithelial cells	Thin, flat mucosa

FSH = follicle-stimulating hormone; LH = luteinizing hormone.

      (2) Abnormal (pathologic) causes include trauma, vaginal foreign body, vaginitis or vaginal narrowing, metritis, pyometra, and urinary incontinence.

    d. Masses. A mass or masses may be seen with inflammation, granuloma, or neoplasia.

    e. Systemic signs

      (1) Fever, depression, and anorexia may be seen with metritis, pyometra, or severe mastitis.

      (2) Other systemic signs may be seen with other infectious diseases, neoplasia, and some hormonal disorders.

2. Physical examination

    a. Digital vaginal examinations in larger bitches can be useful in identifying vaginal masses or strictures.

    b. Vaginoscopy can be used for estrous cycle staging in bitches (see Table 45-1), as well as for disease diagnosis (e.g., the identification of vaginal masses and strictures).

3. Diagnostic studies

    a. Laboratory studies

      (1) A **complete blood count (CBC), serum biochemical profile,** and **urinalysis** can help identify inflammatory disorders (e.g., pyometra), systemic disease, or concurrent urinary tract disorders.

      (2) Serum progesterone concentrations can be used to help define stages of the estrous cycle in bitches.

TABLE 45-2. Characteristics of the Estrous Cycle in the Queen

Stage	Usual Duration	Clinical Signs and Behavior	Hormonal Patterns	Vaginal Smear Results
Proestrus	1–2 days, or may be absent	Rubbing, vocalization, rolling; attracts males but does not allow mating	Serum estrogen increases rapidly	"Clearing" of vaginal mucus (i.e., absence of basophilic strands) due to liquefaction
Estrus	3–16 days	Allows mating	Estrogen is high until ovulation; copulation causes GnRH release, which causes FSH and LH release, resulting in ovulation; progesterone increases following ovulation	Cornified epithelial cells
Interestrus*	2–19 days	Normal behavior	Estrogen decreases	Basophilic background debris
Diestrus†	35–70 days	. . .	Serum estrogen is low, progesterone increases over 2–3 weeks, progesterone decreases at end of diestrus and cat returns to estrus	Basophilic background debris
Anestrus	90 days in the fall and winter	Normal behavior	Serum estrogen and progestrone are low	Thick vaginal mucus that forms strands

GnRH = gonadotropin-releasing hormone; FSH = follicle-stimulating hormone; LH = luteinizing hormone.
* If no mating, improper mating, or insufficient LH increase.
† If ovulation but not pregnancy has occurred.

    (3) Vaginal cytology has applications for estrous cycle staging (see Tables 45-1 and 45-2), as well as disease diagnosis (e.g., an increase in normal and degenerate neutrophils and intracellular bacteria may be seen with metritis, pyometra, and vaginitis).

    (4) Anterior vaginal cultures are of little use unless clinical signs of infection are present. Even then, the many normal flora of the vagina may affect interpretation.

    (5) Serologic testing can be useful for identifying *Brucella canis,* canine herpesvirus, and other infectious agents in bitches.

  b. Diagnostic imaging

    (1) Radiography. Radiographs may reveal abdominal masses (e.g., neoplasia), lymph node enlargement caused by metastasis or inflammation, or uterine enlargement caused by pregnancy, metritis, pyometra, or uterine neoplasia. Because fetal skeletal mineralization is not visible until after approximately 45 days of gestation, radiographs will not always allow differentiation of pregnancy from pathologic conditions.

    (2) Ultrasonography is useful in identifying uterine or ovarian disease or pregnancy.

      (a) Bitches. Gestational sacs can be seen by approximately 16–20 days' gestation. Fetal movement can be seen by approximately 25–30 days.

      (b) Queens. Gestational sacs can be seen by 11–14 days' gestation. Fetal movement can be seen by day 30.

  c. Other diagnostic approaches

    (1) Exploratory laparotomy with uterine biopsy can be useful in some cases of infertility if less invasive tests have not yielded a diagnosis.

    (2) Karyotyping may be considered in a young infertile animal with a suspected disorder of sexual differentiation.

C. **Specific disorders**

  1. Disorders of the estrous cycle. Because typical behavioral signs may not always accompany the stages of the estrous cycle, serial vaginal cytologic examinations, serum progesterone concentrations, and, in some cases, vaginoscopy should be used to evaluate the cycle.

a. **Delayed puberty** should be considered only in an animal older than 2 years that has not had an estrous cycle.

b. **Silent heat (estrus)** can cause an apparent failure to cycle. Silent heats can be identified through the evaluation of weekly vaginal cytologies. Housing the female near a male can induce signs of estrus.

c. **Split heats** appear to be an estrus followed by a second estrus 2–10 weeks later. Splits heats often are recurrent proestrus without progression to estrus. During a split heat, the female attracts males but will not allow mating. This disorder is most common in young animals and will usually resolve without treatment.

d. **Prolonged proestrus or estrus in bitches**

   (1) **Etiology.** Prolonged proestrus or estrus is thought to occur as a result of increased serum estrogen concentrations and possibly a mild increase in progesterone concentrations. Prolonged estrus can occur with exogenous estrogen administration, an ovarian cyst (most common in animals younger than 3 years of age), or an estrogen-secreting neoplasm (rare even in older animals).

   (2) **Diagnosis.** Prolonged proestrus or estrus must be differentiated from split heats.

      (a) **Clinical findings** include prolonged vaginal bleeding and the attraction of males.

      (b) **Laboratory findings.** Diagnosis is based on finding many cornified cells for more than 21–28 days on vaginal cytology and an elevated serum estrogen concentration.

      (c) **Diagnostic imaging findings.** Ultrasonography of the ovaries may reveal a cyst or neoplasm.

   (3) **Treatment.** If the animal is not to be used for breeding, ovariohysterectomy is recommended. Other treatment options include surgical removal of an ovarian cyst, administration of gonadotropin-releasing hormone (GnRH) or human chorionic gonadotropin (hCG) to induce ovulation, or treatment with mibolerone and breeding during the following estrus.

e. **Persistent estrus in queens**

   (1) **Seasonal persistent estrus** in queens may last up to 45 days, with multiple waves of follicles, each lasting 7–10 days. Usually, no treatment is needed and a normal estrus follows.

   (2) **Persistent estrus during seasonal anestrus**

      (a) In a younger queen (i.e., younger than 5 years), persistent estrus is usually the result of cystic follicular degeneration. Weight loss and a rough hair coat are often present. Treatment with GnRH or hCG can be tried, but because the problem tends to recur and repeated hormonal treatment increases the risk of cystic endometrial hyperplasia, removal of the cystic ovary or ovariohysterectomy is usually the best option.

      (b) In an older queen, a granulosa cell tumor should be considered, especially if persistent estrus during seasonal anestrus occurs in conjunction with signs of hyperestrogenism (e.g., bilaterally symmetrical truncal alopecia, low blood cell counts due to bone marrow suppression).

f. **Ovulatory failure in queens.** Ovulatory failure can result from inadequate mating or the presence of immature or aged follicles at the time of mating. Administration of GnRH when mature follicles are present, as determined by vaginal cytology, may induce ovulation.

g. **Estrus in spayed cats**

   (1) **Etiology.** Estrus can result from an ovarian remnant or idiopathic adrenal production of sex hormones.

   (2) **Diagnosis**

      (a) **Vaginal cytology.** True estrus should be documented by demonstration of cornified epithelial cells on vaginal cytology.

      (b) **Serum progesterone level.** If an ovarian remnant is present, administration of GnRH or hCG will produce an increase in progesterone.

(3) **Treatment**
(a) In the case of ovarian remnants, exploratory laparotomy is required to find and remove residual tissue.
(b) Adrenal sex hormone production can be suppressed by short-term glucocorticoid treatment.

h. Prolonged interestrus (failure to cycle) is anestrus lasting longer than 10–16 months.
(1) **Etiology.** Prolonged interestrus can be caused by nonfunctional ovarian cysts, premature ovarian failure, hypothyroidism, hyperadrenocorticism, and inadequate light (in queens).
(2) **Differential diagnoses** include silent heat and prolonged diestrus (i.e., increased serum progesterone levels for longer than 10–12 weeks).
(a) Silent heat should be ruled out by serial vaginal cytology samples.
(b) Prolonged diestrus should be ruled out by serial progesterone concentrations.
(3) **Treatment.** Hypothyroidism or hyperadrenocorticism should be treated appropriately. If thyroid and adrenal function are normal, induction of estrus can be attempted.

i. Shortened interestrus cycles (i.e., lasting less than 4–5 months) **in bitches.** Infertility results because the uterus does not have time to return to normal before the next estrus and implantation is disrupted.
(1) **Diagnosis** is based on serial vaginal cytology samples and serum progesterone concentrations.
(2) **Treatment**
(a) Animals younger than 3 years of age usually do not require treatment.
(b) Older animals can be treated with mibolerone for several months and then bred at the next estrus. Potential side effects of mibolerone include masculinization, vaginal discharge, and clitoral hypertrophy.

j. Primary luteal failure results in a premature decrease in serum progesterone concentrations and early abortion. Diagnosis is based on serum progesterone concentrations during a subsequent pregnancy. Treatment with progesterone can be attempted.

k. Pseudopregnancy (pseudocyesis)
(1) **Etiology.** Pseudopregnancy can result from decreasing progesterone concentrations and increasing prolactin concentrations during diestrus.
(2) **Diagnosis** is based on the clinical signs and use of abdominal ultrasonography to rule out true pregnancy. The clinical findings are those of pregnancy and may include weight gain, mammary development and lactation, restlessness, nesting, mothering of inanimate objects, and inappetence 6–12 weeks following estrus.
(3) **Treatment.** Pseudopregnancy usually requires no treatment because it resolves itself. Cessation of lactation may require restriction of nursing and other physical stimulation of the mammary glands, overnight water deprivation, furosemide, or possibly bromocriptine.

2. **Disorders of gestation (fetal death and abortion).** Early fetal death will result in fetal resorption and apparent infertility; fetal death during the second half of gestation will result in mummification or abortion, and late fetal death will result in stillbirths.
a. Etiology. Causes of gestational disorders include:
(1) **Infection**
(a) **Brucellosis** (see Chapter 49 I E) most commonly results in abortion of partially autolyzed fetuses in late gestation.
(b) **Toxoplasmosis** (see Chapter 49 III L) is a rare cause of abortion in dogs and cats.
(c) **Canine herpesvirus infection** (see Chapter 49 V G) can cause fetal death or abortion in bitches, although neonatal death is more common.
(d) **Feline herpesvirus infection** (see Chapter 49 V G) is common; the virus may be shed during times of stress. Feline herpesvirus infection most commonly causes abortion in midgestation.

(e) **Feline rhinotracheitis virus (FRV) infection** (see Chapter 40 I C 1) may cause fetal death and abortion.

(f) **Feline leukemia virus (FeLV) infection** (see Chapter 49 V D) is another common cause of fetal death, abortion, and infertility.

(g) **Panleukopenia** (see Chapter 41 IV B 3 e) can result in infertility or fetal resorption, mummification or abortion, or central nervous system (CNS) lesions or early death in kittens, depending on when infection occurs.

(h) **Feline infectious peritonitis (FIP;** see Chapter 49 V F) and **feline immunodeficiency virus (FIV) infection** (see Chapter 49 V C) have both been implicated in reproductive failure in queens, but the association has not been proven.

(i) *Mycoplasma* and *Ureaplasma* infection may be a cause of early fetal death, abortion, stillbirth, or neonatal illness. A presumptive diagnosis is made if a pure culture is grown from an anterior vaginal swab. Chloramphenicol or tetracycline may be administered if the bitch is not pregnant or nursing.

(2) **Endometritis** or **pyometra** during pregnancy can cause apparent infertility, fetal death, abortion, or stillbirths. Diagnosis and treatment are discussed in I C 7 b.

(3) **Fetal abnormalities,** both genetic and organ defects, can result in fetal death.

(4) **Iatrogenic causes** of fetal death and abortion include administration of glucocorticoids or other hormones, prostaglandins, some antibiotics (e.g., griseofulvin, fluoroquinolones), and many other medications and toxins.

(5) **Primary luteal failure** (see I C 1 j) results in early abortion.

(6) **Ectopic pregnancy** has been reported in queens, usually as a result of uterine rupture during prior pregnancy or trauma. There are often no clinical signs. Diagnosis may be suggested by radiographs and ultrasonography and confirmed at surgery.

(7) **Gestational diabetes mellitus** often results in abortion. If abortion does not occur, the fetuses are often large and necessitate a cesarean section. Because of the difficulty in controlling diabetes mellitus during pregnancy and because of the risks to the fetuses, an ovariohysterectomy is usually the best treatment option.

(8) **Uterine torsion** and **uterine prolapse** are rare causes of late fetal death.

b. **Diagnosis**

(1) Abortion or stillbirth may be observed. If early fetal death is suspected, monitoring of pregnancy via serum progesterone concentrations and ultrasonography is needed.

(2) The underlying disorder may be identified via history, physical examination, and laboratory studies (e.g., CBC, serum biochemical profile, urinalysis, vaginal cytology, *Brucella* titer). Other useful tests may include an anterior vaginal culture, abdominal radiographs and ultrasonography, other serologic tests, or postmortem evaluation of an aborted or stillborn fetus.

c. **Treatment** depends on the underlying disorder.

3. **Disorders of parturition**

a. **Dystocia** is difficulty in delivery of the fetuses.

(1) **Etiology.** Causes include:

(a) **Lack of initiation of parturition**

(b) **Abnormal progression through the stages of parturition**

(c) **Maternal problems**

(i) Narrowing of the pelvic canal, vagina, or vulva

(ii) Primary uterine inertia (i.e., uterine fatigue despite normal fetal and maternal size)

(iii) Secondary uterine inertia (i.e., uterine fatigue secondary to another cause of dystocia)

(d) **Fetal problems** (e.g., too large, congenital defects, brachycephalic breeds, malpositioning)

(2) **Diagnosis.** The diagnosis is usually based on the history, physical examina-

tion and digital vaginal examination findings, radiographic findings, and, possibly, ultrasonographic findings.

    (a) Clinical findings. Dystocia should be suspected with any of the following:

        (i) No labor within 36 hours of a drop in temperature of the bitch

        (ii) No delivery within 1 hour of initiation of stage 2 of parturition

        (iii) More than 30–60 minutes between births despite active contractions

        (iv) Prolonged rest period

        (v) Signs of illness in the bitch or queen

        (vi) Lack of stage 2 activity but the presence of a green discharge (seen with placental separation and concurrent primary uterine inertia)

    (b) Laboratory findings. If secondary uterine inertia is suspected, serum calcium and glucose concentrations should also be evaluated to rule out fatigue due to hypoglycemia or hypocalcemia.

  (3) Treatment

    (a) If the puppy or kitten is in an abnormal position, manual assistance may be helpful.

    (b) If the bitch is at least 57 days from her last breeding and primary uterine inertia and placental separation have occurred, a prompt cesarean section should be considered.

    (c) If secondary uterine inertia or primary uterine inertia without placental separation has occurred, there is no obstruction, and serum calcium and glucose concentrations are normal, oxytocin can be given. If no response is seen within 30 minutes, calcium gluconate should be administered before repeating the oxytocin injection. If there is still no response after 45 minutes, intravenous glucose and a third oxytocin injection can be given. A cesarean section is needed if there is still no response.

    (d) If the puppies or kittens are oversized or if the birth canal is too narrow, surgery is needed.

b. Uterine prolapse is a rare disorder but can occur secondary to dystocia, abortion, or metritis. The uterus should be cleaned and replaced as soon as possible. Ovariohysterectomy should be considered if the animal is not to be used for breeding or if there is damage to the uterus.

c. Uterine torsion is also rare but can occur late in gestation. Clinical findings may include those of dystocia or shock in association with severe abdominal pain. Treatment requires immediate ovariohysterectomy.

4. Postpartum disorders

  a. Behavioral abnormalities

    (1) Failure to groom. If the mother fails to groom the young, they should be rubbed with a soft, moist cloth.

    (2) Inadequate milk letdown. Stress can result in inadequate milk letdown and can be alleviated with acepromazine.

    (3) Excessive protective behavior by the bitch or queen may respond to treatment with diazepam.

  b. Eclampsia (puerperal tetany) occurs most commonly during early lactation and in small dogs with large litters. It is uncommon in cats.

    (1) Etiology. Heavy lactation, inappropriate perinatal nutrition, or lack of calcium supplementation can contribute to the drop in serum calcium concentrations that characterizes eclampsia, but the disorder can also occur independent of these factors.

    (2) Clinical findings are those of hypocalcemia (i.e., restlessness, irritability, salivation, facial pruritus, ataxia, muscle twitching, seizures). Secondary hypoglycemia sometimes occurs with eclampsia. The patient's temperature may also be elevated.

    (3) Diagnosis. The diagnosis is based on the history, clinical signs, and documentation of hypocalcemia.

    (4) Treatment should not be withheld while awaiting a serum calcium determination because even if the presumptive diagnosis is incorrect, one dose of calcium will not harm the animal.

(a) **Acute treatment** includes slow intravenous administration of calcium gluconate, administration of diazepam if needed, and correction of concurrent hypoglycemia and hyperthermia if present.

(b) **Subacute treatment,** if needed, entails the subcutaneous administration of diluted calcium gluconate three times daily. The level of nutrition should be improved, lactation demands decreased when possible (e.g., via early weaning), and oral supplementation with calcium initiated.

(5) **Prognosis** is very good with treatment.

c. **Subinvolution of placental sites.** With this disorder, the placental sites are not sloughed at the usual time and the endometrium is slow to return to its pregestational condition. Subinvolution of placental sites occurs most commonly in young dogs.

(1) **Etiology.** The cause is unknown.

(2) **Diagnosis**

(a) **Clinical findings** include a serosanguinous to hemorrhagic discharge that persists for more than 6–12 weeks postpartum in the bitch or more than 3 weeks postpartum in the queen.

(b) **Laboratory findings.** Vaginal cytology will reveal erythrocytes, normal leukocytes, and noncornified cells. Tests of hemostasis may be appropriate to rule out a systemic cause for the hemorrhage.

(c) **Other findings.** Vaginoscopy and abdominal ultrasonography are unremarkable.

(3) **Treatment** is usually not needed, but if hemorrhage is excessive, ovariohysterectomy can be considered.

d. **Metritis** is severe inflammation and bacterial infection of the postpartum uterus.

(1) **Etiology.** *Escherichia coli* is the most common pathogen involved, but previous uterine trauma (e.g., dystocia, mechanical assistance during parturition) may also play a role.

(2) **Diagnosis.** The history and clinical signs usually provide a tentative diagnosis.

(a) **Clinical findings** may include fever, dehydration, anorexia, foul-smelling brownish vaginal discharge, lethargy, and poor mothering and nursing during the early postpartum period. Uterine enlargement may be found. Shock can also occur if the disorder is not promptly diagnosed and treated.

(b) **Laboratory findings**

(i) **CBC.** A CBC will usually show a leukocytosis characterized by a neutrophilia and a shift toward immaturity.

(ii) **Serum biochemical profile.** Biochemical abnormalities may be present if septicemia has developed.

(iii) **Urinalysis.** The urine is often isosthenuric and evidence of a urinary tract infection (UTI) may be present.

(iv) **Vaginal cytology** may show red blood cells (RBCs), white blood cells (WBCs), and bacteria.

(v) **Vaginal culture.** A cranial vaginal culture will not help with diagnosis but can help identify the bacteria involved and optimal antibiotic therapy.

(c) **Diagnostic imaging findings. Abdominal ultrasonography** can help rule out pyometra or a retained fetus.

(3) **Treatment.** The young should be hand-fed until the mother's condition improves.

(a) **Acute treatment** entails intravenous fluid therapy, correction of electrolyte abnormalities, and initiation of antibiotic therapy (e.g., ampicillin, trimethoprim/sulfa). More aggressive antibiotic therapy (e.g., cephalosporin and amikacin) may be needed if the animal is septic.

(b) **Subacute treatment**

(i) If the animal is not to be used for breeding, an ovariohysterectomy should follow as soon as the animal is stable enough to undergo anesthesia.

(ii) If the animal is a breeding animal, medical treatment with $PGF_2\alpha$ can be tried, but there is some risk of uterine rupture, chronic infection, and infertility. Ovariohysterectomy may still be needed if the animal does not respond to medical therapy.

   (4) Prognosis. The prognosis is guarded to good with prompt surgical treatment and guarded to fair with medical treatment.

5. **Disorders of the mammary glands**
   a. **Agalactia** is the failure to produce or let down milk. Primary agalactia is rare. Secondary agalactia may result from stress, malnutrition, debilitation, or infection. Treatment should be aimed at the primary problem while providing nutritional supplementation for the puppies or kittens.
   b. **Galactostasis** is edema and swelling of the mammary glands.
      (1) Etiology. Galactostasis can occur as a result of teat abnormalities, inadequate nursing of all teats by the neonates, loss of a litter, or pseudopregnancy.
      (2) Diagnosis is based on clinical findings, which include swollen, painful mammary glands.
      (3) Treatment requires resolution of the primary problem, application of cool compresses (to help minimize edema and swelling), and gentle stripping of the milk. If the problem is severe, treatment may be needed to stop further milk production [see I C 1 k (3)]. Without treatment, there is an increased risk of mastitis.
   c. **Mastitis** is acute or chronic bacterial infection of one or more of the mammary glands.
      (1) Etiology. *Staphylococcus, Streptococcus* , and coliforms are the most common bacteria involved.
      (2) Diagnosis is based on history, physical examination, and cytology and culture of the milk. **Clinical findings** may include discomfort during nursing, galactostasis, discolored milk, and hyperemia and swelling of the affected glands. Anorexia, lethargy, fever, abscessation, and shock may occur with increasing severity.
      (3) Treatment
         (a) Mild to moderate mastitis may be treated with antibiotics (e.g., ampicillin, cephalexin, amoxicillin-clavulanic acid), warm packing of the affected glands, and gentle stripping of the milk. Puppies and kittens can continue to nurse unaffected glands.
         (b) Severe disease requires intravenous fluids, intensive nursing care, and possibly surgical drainage of affected glands.
   d. **Fibroadenomatous mammary hyperplasia** can occur in queens following pregnancy, pseudopregnancy, or within 1 year of ovariohysterectomy. The mammary glands are greatly enlarged and may be ulcerated, but the enlargement has well-defined borders. Fever, anorexia, and depression may also be seen. Treatment requires discontinuation or prevention of nursing and topical treatment of the mammary glands, possibly further medical treatment to stop milk production, or possibly surgery.
   e. **Mammary neoplasia**
      (1) Canine. Approximately 50% of all canine mammary tumors are fibroadenomas; a slightly lower percentage are adenocarcinomas. Some adenocarcinomas are inflammatory and tend to aggressively invade and spread.
         (a) Etiology. The etiology is not known, but because ovariohysterectomy before the first estrus dramatically decreases the risk for this neoplasm, a hormonal influence is suspected.
         (b) Predisposition. Mammary tumors are most common in older female dogs. Boston terriers, Brittany spaniels, Cocker spaniels, English setters, English spaniels, fox terriers, pointers, and poodles may be at increased risk, whereas boxers and Chihuahuas are at lower risk overall.
         (c) Diagnosis
            (i) Clinical findings include one or more mammary masses. With inflammatory carcinoma, the affected glands are often also swollen, warm, and possibly painful.
            (ii) Biopsy and **histopathology findings** form the basis for diagnosis.

        (iii) Diagnostic imaging findings. Radiographs may be helpful in determining the presence of metastasis.

    (d) Treatment is surgery, doxorubicin chemotherapy, or both.

  (2) Feline. Most feline mammary tumors are adenocarcinomas, and early metastasis is common.

    (a) Etiology. There appears to be less hormonal influence on mammary neoplasia in the cat than in the dog because early ovariohysterectomy is less protective.

    (b) Diagnosis. The diagnostic approach is the same as that for canine mammary tumors. **Clinical findings** include one or more mammary masses with possible ulceration of the overlying skin.

    (c) Treatment is the same as that for canine mammary tumors.

6. Disorders of the vagina and vulva

  a. Vaginitis is inflammation (and possible infection) of the vagina.

    (1) Etiology

      (a) Puppy vaginitis occurs in prepubertal bitches and resolves after the first estrus. The small size of the prepubertal vulva may play a role.

      (b) Adult vaginitis usually occurs secondary to vaginal stricture, an abnormal slope to the vaginal floor, neoplasia, foreign body, trauma, or a granuloma of the uterine stump.

      (c) Bacterial vaginitis usually occurs secondary to other urogenital abnormalities.

      (d) Primary vaginitis can be caused by canine herpesvirus.

    (2) Diagnosis

      (a) Physical examination findings. Digital vaginal examination and vaginoscopy of the adult dog may rule out contributing anatomic problems. Hyperemia, ulcers, exudate, and possible vesicles may be seen even in the absence of anatomic abnormalities.

      (b) Clinical findings. Vaginal discharge, licking of the vulva and perineal region, and attraction of males may be noted.

      (c) Laboratory findings

        (i) Vaginal cytology will reveal numerous normal and degenerate neutrophils and possibly bacteria. Lymphocytes and macrophages may also be seen if the problem is of long duration.

        (ii) Anterior vaginal culture may be useful if it results in the growth of primarily one type of bacteria.

    (3) Treatment

      (a) Puppy vaginitis usually does not require treatment.

      (b) Mild adult vaginitis is treated with antiseptic douches.

      (c) More severe vaginitis or nonresponsive cases may also be treated with antibiotic douches and systemic antibiotics. Underlying problems should be corrected if possible.

    (4) Prognosis is good with treatment unless an uncorrectable primary abnormality is found.

  b. Clitoral hypertrophy can occur with congenital disorders of sexual differentiation and hyperadrenocorticism. Anabolic steroid treatment of the dam may also result in clitoral hypertrophy. Clinical findings are those of vaginitis plus an enlarged clitoris. With congenital disorders, surgical amputation of the clitoris may be needed. With hormonal excess, the clitoral enlargement will usually regress when the condition is treated.

  c. Persistent hymen. A persistent band of tissue results in narrowing of the vaginal canal. Clinical findings may include difficulty in mating, signs of chronic vaginitis, or urinary incontinence as a result of urine pooling cranial to the band of tissue.

    (1) Diagnosis is based on digital vaginal examination and vaginoscopy. A contrast vaginogram may be useful if the vaginal narrowing precludes vaginoscopy.

(2) Treatment requires surgical removal of the constricting tissue. There is some risk that a stricture may recur.

d. Vaginal diverticulum, vaginal stenosis, vaginal septae, and **vulvar bands** are occasionally seen. Clinical findings are primarily those of vaginitis. Most abnormalities require surgical removal or reconstruction.

e. Vaginal fold prolapse/vaginal hyperplasia. Vaginal fold prolapse is edema and fibroplasia of the ventral vaginal fold with protrusion of the fold through the vulva. This disorder, which is most common during proestrus and estrus because of estrogen's effects on the vaginal mucosa, occurs most commonly in young large-breed dogs.

(1) Diagnosis. Clinical findings may include a vulvar "mass," excessive licking of the perineum, dysuria, perineal enlargement, and resistance to mating. The stage of the estrous cycle, results of vaginal cytology, and possibly a biopsy can help differentiate the mass of vaginal fold prolapse/vaginal hyperplasia from that of neoplasia.

(2) Treatment

(a) The problem usually resolves as the estrous cycle proceeds but may recur during subsequent cycles. The exposed vaginal mucosa should be kept clean and moist in the interim.

(b) Surgical excision is usually only considered if the exposed tissue is necrotic or the enlargement has compromised the urinary tract or vascular supply to the tissues. The problem may recur.

(c) Ovariohysterectomy is needed for permanent resolution of the problem.

f. Vaginal and **vulvar neoplasms** are uncommon; most are benign. Clinical findings may include a vaginal mass, vulvar discharge or hemorrhage, excessive licking of the perineum, tenesmus, dysuria, and perineal swelling.

(1) Types

(a) Leiomyomas are the most common type of benign tumor.

(b) Leiomyosarcomas and **squamous cell carcinomas** are the most common malignant tumors.

(2) Diagnosis is made by digital vaginal examination or vaginoscopy and subsequent biopsy.

(3) Treatment requires surgical excision and possibly adjunct radiation therapy.

g. Transmissible venereal tumors (TVTs) are spread by direct sexual or social contact and occur only in dogs, most often young, unneutered, and free-roaming.

(1) Diagnosis is based on cytology or histopathology. The tumors are usually small, raised red-pink nodules that later become proliferative and friable. Metastasis is uncommon but possible.

(2) Treatment. Some TVTs will resolve without treatment. Most TVTs are treated with surgical excision, vincristine chemotherapy, or radiation therapy.

7. Disorders of the uterus and ovaries

a. Cystic endometrial hyperplasia is characterized by hypertrophy and hyperplasia of the endometrial glands with resultant fluid accumulation in the glands and the uterine lumen. Cystic endometrial hyperplasia increases the risk of secondary uterine infection because the secretions provide a good medium for bacterial growth, and leukocyte response is diminished in patients with cystic endometrial hyperplasia.

(1) Etiology. The cause is unknown, but the uterine changes are thought to be an excessive response to repeated progesterone stimulation. The disorder is more common in older bitches and queens.

(2) Diagnosis. There are often no clinical signs other than infertility. The diagnosis is based on uterine biopsy results.

(3) Treatment. There is none. Ovariohysterectomy should be considered because animals with cystic endometrial hyperplasia are at increased risk for pyometra. The prognosis for the return of fertility is very poor.

b. Pyometra is bacterial infection of the uterus. The disorder is most common in middle-aged unspayed females, and is more common in bitches than in queens.

(1) Etiology

     (a) Pyometra usually occurs secondary to cystic endometrial hyperplasia. Recent (i.e., within the last 2 months) estrus or use of exogenous progestins increases the risk of pyometra, possibly by contributing to the initial development of cystic endometrial hyperplasia. Recent exogenous estrogen administration can also increase the risk of pyometra, possibly by potentiating progesterone's uterine effects.

     (b) Causative organisms include *E. coli* (most common), *Staphylococcus*, *Streptococcus*, and Gram-negative organisms.

(2) Diagnosis

     (a) Clinical findings are usually observed 1–2 months following estrus and may include lethargy, anorexia, weight loss, vomiting, polyuria and polydipsia, and a vulvar discharge (open-cervix pyometra). In some affected animals, vulvar discharge is absent (closed-cervix pyometra). Depression, dehydration, abdominal distention, and possibly uterine enlargement may be found. Septicemia and shock can also occur, especially with closed-cervix pyometra.

     (b) Laboratory findings

         (i) CBC. A CBC may show a leukocytosis characterized by a neutrophilia with a shift toward immaturity, monocytosis, and a nonregenerative anemia.

         (ii) Serum biochemical profile. In bitches, increased serum alkaline phosphatase (SAP), hyperproteinemia, and prerenal azotemia may be seen. In queens, increased serum alanine aminotransferase (SALT), hyperproteinemia, azotemia, and hypokalemia may be seen.

         (iii) Urinalysis commonly reveals isosthenuria and occasionally proteinuria.

         (iv) Vaginal cytology will help differentiate pyometra, characterized by degenerate neutrophils and bacteria, from a mucometra (i.e., an accumulation of sterile uterine fluid that may predispose to pyometra).

     (c) Diagnostic imaging findings

         (i) Radiography. Radiographs will often show a fluid-dense tubular structure in the caudal abdomen (i.e., uterine enlargement), but the uterus may not be as visible with an open-cervix pyometra.

         (ii) Ultrasonography should be considered to differentiate pyometra from pregnancy and to aid in the diagnosis of open-cervix pyometra.

(3) Treatment

     (a) Immediate supportive care

         (i) Intravenous fluids should be administered to correct dehydration and to meet maintenance fluid requirements.

         (ii) Antibiotic therapy effective against *E. coli* should be initiated. Trimethoprim/sulfa, amoxicillin, or cephalosporin is a good choice if the animal is not septic. If sepsis has occurred, more aggressive antibiotic treatment (e.g., with cephalosporin and amikacin) should be considered.

     (b) Definitive treatment requires removal of the infected uterus (i.e., ovariohysterectomy) or evacuation of the uterine contents (i.e., medical therapy).

         (i) Ovariohysterectomy is the treatment of choice. The procedure should be performed as soon as possible after initiation of supportive care.

         (ii) Medical abortion with **PGF$_2\alpha$** can be considered if the animal is a breeding animal, is not systemically ill, and has no concurrent medical problems. It should not be used if the animal is septic or has peritonitis or airway disease. Medical treatment is less successful and carries greater risks if the animal has a closed-cervix pyometra. PGF$_2\alpha$ is not approved for use in small animals, and potential side effects of prostaglandin treatment include salivation, panting, vomiting, diarrhea, urination, mydriasis, and treatment failure. If treatment is successful, the animal should be bred during the next estrus to prevent recurrence of pyometra.

(c) Endometritis or pyometra in pregnancy

(i) If the bitch or queen is healthy and there are live fetuses, the animal should be treated with antibiotics and monitored closely.

(ii) If the fetuses are dead, antibiotic treatment and medical abortion can be considered.

(iii) Ovariohysterectomy should be performed if the animal is not needed for future breeding or is ill or poorly responsive to medical treatment.

(4) Prognosis

(a) With surgical treatment, the prognosis is good if sepsis or peritonitis has not occurred.

(b) With medical treatment, the prognosis is fair to good with open-cervix pyometra but poor with closed-cervix pyometra. Recurrence is a risk with medical treatment.

c. Uterine tumors are rare in dogs and cats, possibly because so many animals are now spayed. When seen, they occur more commonly in older animals.

(1) Types. Leiomyomas are most common. Leiomyosarcomas are the most common uterine malignancy in the dog; adenocarcinomas are most common in the cat.

(2) Diagnosis is based on biopsy and histopathology results. There are usually no clinical signs of disease, although vaginal discharge, abdominal distention, or signs of pyometra may be present.

(3) Treatment. In dogs, ovariohysterectomy is often curative, but in cats with adenocarcinoma, metastasis is often present at the time of diagnosis.

d. Ovarian neoplasia is more common in older animals but is rare in the dog and cat overall, possibly because so many animals are now spayed.

(1) Types

(a) In dogs, adenocarcinomas and adenomas, granulosa cell tumors, and dysgerminomas/teratomas are the most common ovarian tumors. Metastasis can occur.

(b) In cats, granulosa cell tumors, dysgerminomas, and interstitial cell tumors are most common. Metastasis is more common with the former two types.

(2) Diagnosis is based on biopsy and histopathology results. There are often no clinical signs. The tumor may be detected as an incidental finding during abdominal palpation. Ultimately, estrous cycle abnormalities, abdominal distention, ascites, signs of sex hormone excess (e.g., alopecia, gynecomastia), or signs of bone marrow suppression (e.g, pale mucous membranes, petechiation) may be seen.

(3) Treatment is surgical excision.

8. Contraception and pregnancy termination

a. Contraception

(1) Ovariohysterectomy is the optimal way to prevent pregnancy. If performed before the first estrus, it has the added advantage in the bitch of decreasing the risk of mammary tumors.

(2) Suppression of estrus. Estrus can be suppressed through the use of megestrol acetate or mibolerone. Neither drug is approved for use in queens in the United States, and both drugs have significant potential side effects.

(a) Megestrol acetate is a progestin that suppresses gonadotropin secretion. It can be given in early proestrus to prevent estrus or during anestrus to prevent proestrus. Potential side effects include a change in behavior, cyclic endometrial hyperplasia, pyometra, mammary development, lactation, diabetes mellitus, acromegaly, and increased risk of mammary neoplasia.

(b) Mibolerone is an androgen that also suppresses gonadotropin secretion. It can be given during anestrus to prevent proestrus and estrus. Potential side effects include masculinization, vaginal discharge, clitoral enlargement, and possibly hepatic dysfunction. It should not be used in the queen.

(3) **Estradiol cypionate** has been used after accidental breeding (mismating) to prevent pregnancy, but carrying and delivering the litter is safer than receiving the drug. Potential side effects include pyometra and irreversible bone marrow suppression. This drug is not approved for use in dogs or cats, is not always effective, and is not recommended.

b. **Pregnancy termination (abortion).** $PGF_2\alpha$ has been used to induce luteolysis and uterine contractions after day 30–35 of pregnancy, but it is not approved for use in the dog or cat. Potential side effects include transient salivation, panting, vomiting, defecation, and urination.

II. MALE REPRODUCTIVE DISORDERS

A. Clinical evaluation

1. **Clinical signs**
   a. **Hematuria** may be seen.
   b. **Testicular pain** is most common with testicular infection, inflammation, or torsion.
   c. **Scrotal swelling** or **enlargement** may be seen with edema, infection, inflammation, neoplasia, a scrotal hernia, or testicular or epididymal enlargement.
   d. **Preputial discharge** may be seen with preputial, penile, prostatic, or urinary tract disease.
   e. **Apparent infertility** can occur with semen abnormalities, cryptorchidism, lack of libido, or breeding mismanagement. Diagnosis begins with a thorough history (including breeding management, family breeding history, and breeding histories of both the male and female), a thorough physical examination, and semen evaluation.
   f. **Masses** may be a tumor, granuloma, spermatocele, or varicocele.

2. **Diagnostic studies**
   a. **Semen evaluation.** The ejaculate can be divided into three fractions: first (pre-sperm) fraction, second (sperm-rich) fraction, and third (prostatic fluid). Semen volume, sperm numbers, sperm motility, sperm morphology, leukocyte count, sperm agglutination, and third-fraction cytology and pH should be assessed. Determination of seminal alkaline phosphatase, an indicator of epididymal fluid, may also be useful if azoospermia is found.
      (1) **Normal sperm with abnormal seminal fluid** may be seen with infection and immune-mediated disorders.
      (2) **Teratozoospermia.** More than 50% of the sperm are abnormal. Because some insults are transient, if teratozoospermia is found, the animal should be rested for 2 months and then reevaluated.
         (a) Primary abnormalities can occur with inherited defects in spermatogenesis, increased scrotal temperature, testicular disease, toxins, medications, or hormonal disease.
         (b) Secondary abnormalities are more common with epididymal disease or improper semen handling.
      (3) **Asthenozoospermia** is the presence of more than 75% hypomotile or immotile sperm. It can occur as a result of primary abnormalities, collection problems, accessory gland disease, or early in the course of infection, inflammation, fever, or drug administration. If the semen was collected properly, the animal should be evaluated for infection or inflammatory disease.
      (4) **Oligospermia** is a decrease in the number of sperm. Hormonal disorders, infection, environmental factors, aging and incomplete ejaculation can decrease sperm numbers.

(5) Azoospermia is the absence of sperm. This is uncommon but can occur with severe testicular disease or bilateral obstruction of the vas deferens. Infection, immune-mediated disorders, and abnormalities of sexual differentiation should be investigated.

(6) Aspermia is the absence of ejaculate. This may occur with retrograde ejaculation and in response to some medications.

b. Semen culture may be useful if orchitis, prostatitis, or other infection is suspected.

c. Radiographs and **ultrasonography** may help identify prostatic, urinary tract and testicular disease; metastatic disease (e.g., intra-abdominal lymphadenopathy); and discospondylitis caused by *B. canis*. Ultrasonography may also help identify a mass, abscess, scrotal hernia, or testicular torsion not identified by palpation.

d. Serologic tests for *B. canis* should be performed on all breeding dogs, even in the absence of clinical signs.

e. Hormonal tests

(1) Tests for hypothyroidism, hypoadrenocorticism, or **hyperadrenocorticism** may be useful in dogs with other clinical signs of these disorders.

(2) GnRH challenge can be used to assess the hypothalamic-pituitary-gonadal axis. For this test, testosterone and luteinizing hormone (LH) response to GnRH are measured.

(a) If testosterone concentrations are abnormal but LH concentrations are normal, testicular dysfunction is present.

(b) If both testosterone and LH concentrations are abnormal, then hypothalamic or pituitary dysfunction is present.

f. Epididymal aspiration may be performed if a mass is present. The procedure may cause an infection to spread or sperm to extravasate, and subsequent granulomas may form.

g. Testicular aspiration may be useful, especially if a mass is palpable.

h. Testicular biopsy is usually only performed when other less invasive tests have failed to yield a diagnosis and azoospermia or severe chronic oligozoospermia is present. Semen quality will decline for 2 months after a single testicular insult and will take at least 6 months to improve.

B. Specific disorders

1. Scrotal disorders

a. Scrotal dermatitis can result from abrasion, chemical irritation, insect bites, or repeated licking.

b. Scrotal hernia is herniation of abdominal contents through the inguinal ring into the scrotum. Clinical findings may include pain and scrotal enlargement. Diagnosis is based on palpation and radiographs or ultrasonography. Treatment usually requires surgery.

c. Scrotal neoplasia. Mast cell tumors and melanomas are the most common scrotal neoplasms (see Chapter 50 II A 4, Q 3 i).

2. Preputial and penile disorders

a. Persistent penile frenulum is a congenital abnormality in which a small band of connective tissue connects the tip of the penis and the prepuce or ventral penis, thereby deviating the tip of the penis. Clinical findings may include licking of the penis and preputial area or urination at an unusual angle. Diagnosis is based on physical examination. Severing the frenulum resolves the problem.

b. Penile hypoplasia is an uncommon congenital abnormality that is sometimes a result of an abnormality of sexual differentiation.

c. Balanoposthitis is inflammation of the preputial and penile mucosa. It is usually the result of a mild bacterial infection and does not require treatment; however, the prepuce and penis should also be examined for evidence of trauma, foreign body, or other abnormalities. If the discharge is copious, systemic antibiotic therapy and topical antibiotic or antiseptic douches may be indicated.

d. Phimosis is a narrowing of the preputial opening such that the penis cannot be extruded. The narrowing may be congenital or can result from inflammation, fibrosis, or a mass. Clinical findings may include discomfort, prepucial swelling, urine dribbling from the prepuce, and purulent preputial discharge. The diagnosis is based on physical examination. Treatment is surgery.

    e. Paraphimosis occurs if something (e.g., hair, foreign body) causes constriction of the penis such that venous outflow is obstructed, penile engorgement persists, and the penis cannot be returned to the prepuce. Without treatment, penile trauma or necrosis can result. Treatment involves removal of the constriction from the sedated animal, application of cool soaks to help relieve the engorgement, and returning the penis to the prepuce. If severe penile damage has occurred, amputation may be needed. Surgical enlargement of the prepucial orifice may also be needed.

    f. Penile neoplasms. TVTs are the most common penile neoplasm in dogs; all others are rare. Clinical findings may include the presence of the mass and a hemorrhagic preputial discharge. Diagnosis is by biopsy. Treatment of TVTs is discussed in I C 6 g.

3. Testicular disorders

    a. Testicular hypoplasia can occur as an isolated congenital abnormality or as part of an abnormality of sexual differentiation. Diagnosis is based on testicular biopsy results from the mature animal.

    b. Orchitis/epididymitis is inflammation or infection of one or both testicles or the epididymis.

      (1) Etiology

        (a) Infectious causes most commonly are bacterial, and *B. canis* infection should always be considered. Fungal and rickettsial infection and infection with canine distemper virus (CDV) are less common infectious causes.

        (b) Noninfectious causes are immune-mediated and can occur secondary to infection, inflammation, or trauma. Orchitis/epididymitis may also be idiopathic.

      (2) Diagnosis

        (a) Clinical findings. With acute disease, the testicle is often warm and the scrotum swollen. The dog may be febrile and reluctant to walk because of testicular pain. With chronic disease, the signs are fewer and milder.

        (b) Laboratory findings

          (i) Serologic testing for brucellosis should always be done. Testing for fungal, rickettsial or viral disease is indicated if other appropriate clinical signs are present.

          (ii) Semen culture may identify a bacterial agent.

        (c) Biopsy findings. Testicular biopsy may be necessary to evaluate the possibility of immune-mediated orchitis.

      (3) Treatment

        (a) Infectious causes should be treated. Antibiotic therapy can be used, but it may also affect semen quality. If only unilateral infection is present, cool compresses, unilateral castration, and concurrent antibiotic therapy may be most effective. If *Brucella* infection is found, the dog should not be used for breeding.

        (b) Immune-mediated orchitis/epididymitis is treated with glucocorticoids, but this treatment will decrease fertility.

      (4) Prognosis. Regardless of the cause, with bilateral disease the prognosis for return to fertility is poor.

    c. Spermatoceles and **sperm granulomas.** Spermatoceles are dilated segments of the spermatic duct. Sperm granulomas result from a secondary immune-mediated reaction to sperm that have leaked into the testicular tissue. Clinical findings may include a mass in the testes or epididymis or infertility. Diagnosis is based on biopsy and a negative culture. There is no specific treatment for either disorder.

    d. Varicoceles are dilated or thrombosed segments of the spermatic vein. The enlarged vessel may be palpable, and the affected testicle is often warm and painful. There is no specific treatment.

    e. Testicular degeneration can occur secondary to any testicular insult or it can be idiopathic. Clinical findings are mainly infertility and small, soft testicles. Diagnosis is based on semen evaluation and testicular biopsy results. There is no treatment.

f. **Testicular neoplasia** is more common in older dogs and is rare in cats. Cryptorchid animals are at increased risk, especially for the development of Sertoli cell tumors and seminomas.

  (1) **Etiology.** The etiology is unknown.

  (2) **Pathology.** The tumors are more likely to be malignant if they are intraabdominal.

   (a) Interstitial cell tumors do not metastasize.

   (b) Seminomas rarely metastasize.

   (c) Sertoli cell tumors do not commonly metastasize.

  (3) **Diagnosis** is based on biopsy and histopathology results.

   (a) **Clinical findings.** The most common clinical sign is nonpainful enlargement of one of the testicles. A palpable abdominal mass is less common. In addition, some dogs with Sertoli cell tumors will have "feminization syndrome" (i.e., bilaterally symmetrical truncal alopecia, gynecomastia, and attraction of male dogs), prostatic changes (e.g., squamous metaplasia, cysts, or hyperplasia), or perianal tumors.

   (b) **Diagnostic imaging findings.** Radiographs and ultrasonograms may reveal metastatic disease and help localize the mass in a cryptorchid animal.

   (c) **Laboratory findings.** Decreased cell counts may be seen on a CBC if a Sertoli cell tumor is secreting estrogen and has caused bone marrow suppression.

  (4) **Treatment** is castration if the tumor is localized. Radiation therapy or chemotherapy may be useful if metastasis has occurred. Bone marrow suppression caused by a Sertoli cell tumor may be irreversible.

  (5) **Prognosis** is good for most testicular tumors if castration is performed and there is no metastasis or bone marrow suppression.

 g. **Testicular torsion** is rare. Animals with a neoplastic intra-abdominal testis are at increased risk. Clinical signs include severe pain, testicular swelling, and shock, and the diagnosis is usually confirmed by ultrasonography. Immediate surgery is essential.

4. Prostatic disorders are discussed in Chapter 43 Part I:IX.

5. Hormonal disorders. Abnormal hypothalamic-pituitary-gonadal function can be congenital or acquired (most commonly resulting from neoplasia or medication). Clinical findings may include infertility and decreased libido. Diagnosis is based on a GnRH challenge test. Treatment with pulsatile administration of LH and follicle-stimulating hormone (FSH) or administration of GnRH (if deficient) can be tried. The prognosis for return to fertility is poor despite treatment.

III. CONGENITAL REPRODUCTIVE DISORDERS are most common in purebred dogs.

A. Definitions

1. Recessive-gene defects appear only in the offspring that are homozygous for the mutant genes. Because the defective offspring are unable to reproduce, the defects often skip a generation.

2. Dominant-gene defects do not skip generations. Animals with the defect can produce both normal and defective animals.

3. Incomplete dominance occurs when two severely affected animals are mated and 25% of their offspring are normal, 50% are slightly defective, and 25% are severely defective.

4. **Overdominance** occurs when two superior animals are mated and 25% of the off-spring are normal, 50% of the offspring are superior, and 25% are defective.

5. **Aneuploidy.** Aneuploid animals have an abnormal number of chromosomes. **Trisomy** is an increase in the normal number of chromosomes; **monosomy** is a decrease in the normal number of chromosomes.

B. **Diagnosis** of congenital reproductive disorders is usually based on physical examination, exploratory laparotomy, biopsy, and possibly karyotyping.

C. **Specific disorders**

1. **Defects resulting from abnormal chromosome numbers**
   a. **XXY syndrome (Klinefelter's syndrome)** is an XXY trisomy that results in sterility and hypoplasia of the testicles and tubular and accessory sex organs. In cats, this most commonly occurs in tricolor (calico) male cats.
   b. **XO syndrome (Turner's syndrome).** These animals appear to be female, but are short and have infantile genitalia. This disorder may be suspected in a "female" that has not exhibited estrus by 24 months of age. In cats, XO syndrome should be suspected if an orange female kitten or a female kitten that has no orange coloration results from the mating of an orange and a nonorange cat.
   c. **XXX trisomy.** Affected animals will usually be infertile and show abnormal estrous cycles.
   d. **True hermaphrodites** have both ovarian and testicular tissue as either ovotestes or one of each. Most have an XX chromosome pair, but occasionally other combinations (e.g., XX/XY, XX/XXY) are seen. Animals with XX/XY chromosomes usually have testicular-like tissue. Male tortoiseshell cats with XY/XY chromosomes may have normal fertility.

2. **Disorders of gonadal sex**
   a. **XX sex reversal** denotes an individual with an XX chromosome pair and testicular tissue.
   b. **XX true hermaphrodites** are discussed in III C 1 d.
   c. **XX male syndrome** denotes an individual with an XX chromosome pair and a complete uterus but undescended bilateral testes.

3. **Disorders of phenotypic sex.** With disorders of phenotypic sex, the chromosomes and gonads match but the genitalia are ambiguous.
   a. **Premature gonadal failure** should be considered if estrus is not seen by 24 months of age.
   b. **Congenital defects of the vagina and vulva** are discussed in I C 6.
   c. **Female pseudohermaphrodites** have XX chromosomes and ovaries, but the internal and external genitalia are masculinized (e.g., clitoral hypertrophy). The condition may result from endogenous androgens or progesterone administration during gestation or chronic androgen administration. The affected animal may attract males or develop cyclic endometrial hyperplasia, pyometra, or vaginal pooling of urine. Ovariohysterectomy is the recommended treatment.
   d. **Male pseudohermaphrodites** have XY chromosomes and testes, but the genitalia are feminized.
   e. **Hypospadias** is usually characterized by a urinary orifice ventral and proximal to the usual site in male animals. Surgery to reposition the urethral orifice may be needed. Affected animals are also often cryptorchid and may have concurrent penile hypoplasia.
   f. **Cryptorchidism,** failure of testicular descent, is one of the most common disorders of phenotypic sex. It is thought to be a sex-linked autosomal recessive disorder and is more common in boxers, English bulldogs, Chihuahuas, miniature dachshunds, Maltese, Pekingese, Pomeranians, toy and miniature poodles, miniature schnauzers, and Shetland sheepdogs.

(1) Diagnosis. Cryptorchidism is suspected if the testes are not present in the scrotum by 8 weeks of age. The diagnosis is confirmed if the testes have failed to descend by 4–6 months of age.

(2) Treatment usually requires castration. Hormonal treatment to try to induce testicular descent is controversial.

(3) Complications. Animals with undescended testicles are at an increased risk for the development of Sertoli cell tumors.

DIRECTIONS: Each of the numbered items or incomplete statements in this section is followed by answers or by completions of the statement. Select the ONE numbered answer or completion that is BEST in each case.

1. Which hormone causes vaginal fold prolapse/vaginal hyperplasia?

(1) Follicle-stimulating hormone (FSH)
(2) Progesterone
(3) Prolactin
(4) Gonadotropic-releasing hormone (GnRH)
(5) Estrogen

2. A hemorrhagic vulvar discharge may be normal in the bitch during:

(1) anestrus.
(2) diestrus.
(3) estrus.
(4) proestrus.
(5) diestrus and proestrus.

3. The appearance of primarily cornified epithelial cells on a vaginal smear is characteristic of which stage of the estrous cycle?

(1) Estrus
(2) Diestrus
(3) Anestrus
(4) Metestrus

4. Which of the following is a cause for concern?

(1) A brick-red vaginal discharge in a postpartum bitch
(2) A green vaginal discharge in a pregnant bitch
(3) A serohemorrhagic vaginal discharge in a nonpregnant bitch
(4) A slight mucoid vaginal discharge in a 12-week old female puppy

5. The most common pathogen involved in metritis is:

(1) *Staphylococcus aureus.*
(2) *Proteus.*
(3) *Escherichia coli.*
(4) *Candida.*
(5) anaerobes.

6. The most likely diagnosis in a 10-year-old male dog with a testicular mass, thin truncal hair, and mild gynecomastia is:

(1) seminoma.
(2) adenocarcinoma.
(3) interstitial cell tumor.
(4) Sertoli cell tumor.
(5) leiomyosarcoma.

1. The answer is 5 [I C 6 e]. Increased estrogen concentrations during proestrus and estrus cause the thickening and folding of the vaginal wall. When the thickening is excessive, then prolapse of one or more folds can occur. When serum estrogen concentrations ebb, the problem resolves.

2. The answer is 4 [Table 45-1]. During proestrus, a hemorrhagic vulvar discharge may be seen. In some bitches, this discharge may also continue into estrus. A hemorrhagic discharge during another stage of the estrous cycle should raise concern about possible pathology.

3. The answer is 1 [Table 45-1]. Primarily cornified epithelial cells are seen on a vaginal smear during late proestrus and estrus in the bitch. During diestrus, anestrus, and metestrus, mainly noncornified (i.e., parabasal cells) are seen.

4. The answer is 2 [I C 3 a (2) (a) (vi)]. A green vaginal discharge in a pregnant bitch is an indication of placental separation and is a cause for concern unless accompanied by stage 2 labor. A brick red discharge (i.e., lochia) is normal for several weeks following whelping. A serohemorrhagic discharge in a nonpregnant bitch is most likely an indication of proestrus. A mild mucoid vaginal discharge in a 12-week old female puppy is most likely caused by vaginitis and will often resolve without treatment. Cytology of the discharge and possible vaginal cytology should be assessed in the latter three cases to help rule out other disorders.

5. The answer is 3 [I C 4 d (1)]. Although many types of bacteria can cause metritis, *Escherichia coli* is the most common cause. Uterine trauma associated with parturition may also play a role in the development of metritis.

6. The answer is 4 [II B 3 f (3) (a)]. Seminomas, interstitial cell tumors, and Sertoli cell tumors are the most common testicular tumors in the dog. Of these, Sertoli cell tumors also often produce estrogen, which can cause bilaterally symmetrical truncal alopecia, gynecomastia, attraction of male dogs, and bone marrow suppression. A biopsy is required for definitive diagnosis.

Chapter 46

Joint Diseases

I. CLINICAL FINDINGS

A. **History.** Most animals have a history of lameness or gait abnormality. Lethargy and a decreased appetite may accompany immune-mediated or infectious disorders.

B. **Physical examination.** Crepitus, pain, altered range of motion, or, less commonly, joint swelling or effusion, may be noted in one or several joints. Multiple joint involvement (i.e., polyarthritis), may result in a stilted gait, reluctance to walk or stand, or pain when touched or moved. Fever may accompany infectious joint disease. The lack of physical abnormalities does not rule out significant joint disease. The clinical signs associated with arthritis can mimic neurologic or muscular disease.

II. DIAGNOSTIC APPROACHES AND TECHNIQUES

A. **Radiography.** Radiographic evaluation is necessary to differentiate erosive from nonerosive joint disease. Negative radiographic findings do not rule out joint disease. In general, nonbacterial infectious causes (i.e., borreliosis or Lyme disease, rickettsial infection, viral infection) and immune-mediated conditions are associated with mild or no radiographic lesions.

1. The joints to be radiographed should be determined by physical examination findings.
   a. Distal joints (i.e., the carpi, hocks) should be examined when immune-mediated polyarthritis is suspected.
   b. Radiographs of the thorax or vertebral column may reveal occult neoplasia or infectious disease (e.g., discospondylitis), which may be related to an immune-mediated polyarthritis.

2. Radiographic **findings** can include joint space narrowing, osteophyte formation, erosion or destruction of subchondral bone, and, in severe cases, joint subluxation, luxation, or ankylosis.

B. **Laboratory studies.** A complete blood count (CBC), serum biochemical profile, urinalysis, urine culture, synovial fluid analysis and culture, and serologic or immunologic tests (e.g., Lyme titer, rheumatoid factor) may aid in the diagnosis of inflammatory conditions (infectious or noninfectious).

1. **Hematologic, serum biochemical** and **urinalysis findings** vary, depending on the causative or associated diseases. Findings can include leukocytosis, anemia, thrombocytopenia, hypoproteinemia, proteinuria, and urinary tract infection. However, the absence of findings indicative of inflammation does not rule out inflammatory polyarthritis.

2. **Synovial fluid analysis** (Table 46-1) is inexpensive and noninvasive. It is the principal test for differentiating inflammatory and noninflammatory joint disease.
   a. In general, septic arthritis affects the larger proximal joints, while immune-mediated polyarthritis affects the distal joints (i.e., carpi, hocks). When polyarthritis is suspected, multiple joints should be aspirated.
   b. Synovial fluid should be evaluated for color, turbidity, and viscosity. Smears are examined for cell count (which may be estimated), predominant cell types, and infectious agents (i.e., bacteria, fungi). Although most bacteria induce degenerate

TABLE 46-1. Synovial Fluid Findings in Normal and Diseased Joints

Condition	Synovial Fluid Findings			
	Appearance	Viscosity	Cell Count	Cell Types
Normal joint	Clear	Normal*	Low (200–300 cells/μl)	Mononuclear cells predominate, nondegenerate neutrophils < 10%
Degenerative joint disease (DJD)	Clear to slightly turbid	Normal	Low (1000–5000 cells/μl)	Mononuclear cells predominate, nondegenerate neutrophils 0–12%
Trauma	Blood-tinged	Reduced	Variable	Erythrocytes predominate, nondegenerate neutrophils < 25%
Septic arthritis	Yellow to sanguineous, turbid to purulent	Reduced	High (40,000–280,000 cells/μl)	Degenerate neutrophils predominate, ± visible intra- or extracellular bacteria
Immune-mediated (erosive or nonerosive) polyarthritis	Yellow to sanguineous, mild to moderate turbidity	Reduced	Moderate to high (4000–370,000 cells/μl)	Nondegenerate neutrophils predominate, no visible bacteria

* Normal viscosity is present if a 1- to 2-inch continuous strand forms when a drop of joint fluid is placed on the thumb and touched by the forefinger.

or toxic changes in the neutrophils and may be visible within the sample, some infectious agents (e.g., *Mycoplasma*) may not.

3. **Synovial fluid culture,** aerobic and anaerobic, should be performed when septic arthritis is suspected or when neutrophilic inflammation is detected in the synovial fluid.
    a. Bacterial culture is positive in only approximately 50% of patients with septic arthritis.
    b. Special culture techniques are required for *Mycoplasma* species.

4. **Mucin clot test.** The mucin clot test is the most objective method of assessing joint fluid viscosity. Inflammatory disease reduces viscosity; however, this information does not help differentiate most joint diseases.

5. **Serologic** and **immunologic tests**
    a. **Enzyme-linked immunosorbent assay (ELISA)** measures antibodies against *Borrelia burgdorferi,* the organism that causes **borreliosis (Lyme disease).**
        (1) A positive titer does not necessarily indicate active disease. Many clinically unaffected dogs in areas endemic with Lyme disease and all dogs vaccinated with the Lyme bacterin will have positive titers.
        (2) A false-negative ELISA result is rare because dogs reliably generate an antibody response following infection.
        (3) In equivocal situations, a rising antibody titer over several weeks or a declining titer following treatment can be used to support a diagnosis of Lyme disease.
    b. **Rose-Waaler** and **latex agglutination tests** detect **rheumatoid factor** in serum. In dogs, rheumatoid factor is considered to be an immunoglobulin M (IgM) antibody directed at altered host IgG antibody.
        (1) Rheumatoid factor is reported to be positive in only 20%–70% of dogs with rheumatoid arthritis.
        (2) A positive result is associated with rheumatoid arthritis but can also be detected in dogs with various inflammatory diseases and in some normal dogs. Because of the many false-positive and false-negative results, a positive rheumatoid titer should be only one of several criteria in the diagnosis of rheumatoid arthritis.

c. **Other serologic tests**
   (1) **Antinuclear antibody (ANA) test.** An ANA test, along with a lupus erythematosus (LE) cell preparation and skin biopsy examination, will allow detection of systemic lupus erythematosus (SLE), which is often associated with an immune-mediated polyarthritis (see Chapter 48 V B 4 d).
   (2) **Rocky Mountain spotted fever antibody titers** are indicated in areas where the disease is endemic or when there is a history of travel to these areas. A fourfold increase in antibody titer between acute and convalescent samples will be noted. A single Rocky Mountain spotted fever antibody titer is difficult to interpret because many normal dogs will have significant Rocky Mountain spotted fever antibody titers (especially in the summer) produced by cross-reacting antibodies to nonpathogenic rickettsiae.
   (3) **Immunofluorescent antibody (IFA) test.** An IFA test can be used to detect antibodies to *Ehrlichia canis*. The IFA may not be positive in the acute phase of the disease, but in the chronic phase, it is reliably positive and remains so unless the dog is treated.

C. **Synovial membrane biopsy** may be indicated when laboratory testing or synovial fluid analysis has not provided a diagnosis (e.g., as may be the case with neoplasia or lymphocytic–plasmacytic synovitis). Samples can be submitted for culture as well as histopathologic examination.

III. **DISEASES.** Joint disease can be classified as noninflammatory or inflammatory (Table 46-2). Inflammatory causes can be further classified as infectious or noninfectious.

A. **Noninflammatory joint diseases**

1. **Degenerative joint disease (DJD, osteoarthritis),** a chronic condition characterized by progressive deterioration of the articular cartilage, is commonly seen in dogs, and to a lesser extent, in cats.
   a. **Pathogenesis.** DJD can result in osteophyte formation, remodeling of periarticular and subchondral bone, synovial effusion, and periarticular fibrosis.
   b. **Etiology.** Articular cartilage deterioration may be initiated by abnormal mechanical stresses on the joint (e.g., poor conformation, ligamentous damage) resulting in joint instability, or a fundamental defect in the ability of the articular cartilage to withstand normal stresses.
   c. **Clinical findings**
      (1) With early and mild disease, stiffness is often the main sign and may disappear after minor exercise. Dogs may show signs only after overexertion or prolonged exercise. Damp or cold weather may exacerbate signs.
      (2) As DJD worsens, the stiffness becomes persistent and overt lameness may occur in one or more limbs. If DJD is secondary to a previous joint injury, signs of lameness appear earlier and will be dominant in the affected limb. Affected joints may have swelling, reduced range of motion, pain on extension or flexion, crepitus, or instability (if ligamentous injury is the cause). Some animals with severe disease become irritable and inappetent.
   d. **Diagnosis** is usually based on clinical and radiographic findings.
      (1) **Radiographic findings** can include effusion and periarticular soft tissue swelling, osteophyte formation, subchondral bone sclerosis, attrition or wearing of subchondral bone, bone remodeling, reduction in the joint space, subluxation, intra- and periarticular soft tissue mineralization, and subchondral cyst formation.
      (2) **Synovial fluid analysis.** Although low-grade synovitis can occur, significant inflammatory changes are absent on joint fluid analysis (see Table 46-1).
   e. **Treatment**
      (1) **Weight control** and **exercise**
         (a) **Weight loss** (in obese animals) will reduce the stress on joints.

TABLE 46-2. Classification of Joint Disease in Dogs and Cats

Noninflammatory joint disease
  Degenerative joint disease (DJD)
  Traumatic joint disease
  Neoplastic joint disease
Inflammatory joint diseases
  Infectious
    Septic or bacterial arthritis
    Borreliosis (Lyme disease)
    Mycoplasma polyarthritis
    Rickettsial polyarthritis (dogs)
    Fungal arthritis
    Calicivirus arthritis (cats)
    Bacterial L-form arthritis (cats)
  Noninfectious
    Nonerosive arthritis
      Idiopathic immune-mediated polyarthritis
      Systemic lupus erythematosus (SLE) polyarthritis
      Immune-mediated arthritis secondary to chronic inflammatory disease
      Immune-mediated arthritis secondary to drug administration
      Lymphocytic–plasmacytic synovitis
    Erosive arthritis
      Rheumatoid arthritis
      Polyarthritis of greyhounds
      Feline chronic progessive polyarthritis—erosive form
    Periosteal proliferative arthritis
      Feline chronic progressive polyarthritis—nonerosive form

Reprinted with permission from Nelson RC, Couto GC (eds): *Essentials of Small Animal Internal Medicine.* St. Louis, Mosby Year Book, 1992, p 813.

(b) **Exercise** will aid in weight control and help maintain muscle and ligament tone. Exercise should be low-impact (e.g., leash walking, swimming) and moderate, to a degree the animal can tolerate without resulting in lameness or stiffness. Strict rest may be indicated in the short-term management of severely affected animals.

(2) **Drug therapy** may be used for short-term relief from an acute episode or on a long-term basis in severely affected animals.

  (a) **Nonsteroidal anti-inflammatory drugs (NSAIDs),** such as **enteric-coated** or **buffered aspirin, phenylbutazone, meclofenamic acid,** and **ketoprofen,** are commonly used.

    (i) **Adverse effects** usually result from **gastric** or **intestinal ulceration.** Coadministration of misoprostol (a prostaglandin E analogue) may reduce the ulcerogenic potential of aspirin, and perhaps other NSAIDs as well. **Blood dyscrasias** (i.e., thrombocytopenia, agranulocytosis) may occur with phenylbutazone therapy.

    (ii) Although aspirin can be used at a very low dose in cats, its effectiveness is questionable.

  (b) **Corticosteroids** (e.g., prednisone) are generally reserved for severely affected animals that fail to respond to other therapies. Before prescribing corticosteroids, the veterinarian should ensure that the benefits to the animal outweigh the long-term consequences of systemic side effects and the deleterious effect on articular cartilage. Corticosteroids are usually administered orally but can be used intraarticularly if a single joint is affected.

  (c) **Chondroprotective substances** (e.g., **polysulfated glycosaminoglycan, hyaluronic acid**) protect the articular cartilage from progressive degradation, but results are variable. Polysulfated glycosaminoglycan administration may be associated with an increased bleeding tendency.

    (3) Surgery

        (a) Surgery to correct abnormal joint stresses (e.g., ruptured cruciate ligament, fragmented coronoid process) may reduce discomfort and prevent further joint deterioration but will not reverse existing degenerative changes.

        (b) Joint arthrodesis, excision, or replacement (e.g., total hip replacement) are reserved for those patients with severe, debilitating, nonresponsive DJD.

2. Traumatic joint diseases (traumatic arthritis) may include mild synovitis (resulting from a mild sprain), ligamentous injury, damage to the articular cartilage, intra-articular fractures, and post-traumatic osteoarthritis. Treatment is dictated by the injury and may entail exercise restriction, support bandaging, anti-inflammatory drug therapy, or surgical intervention.

3. Neoplastic joint diseases. Tumors involving the joints are rare in dogs and cats.

    a. Synovial sarcoma is the most common tumor of the joints and is most often seen in male large-breed dogs. The stifle or elbow joint is most often affected. Synovial sarcomas are locally invasive and can metastasize to the regional lymph nodes or lungs.

    b. Other tumors that may involve the joints include **synoviomas, lipomas, liposarcomas, osteosarcomas,** and **fibrosarcomas.**

B. | **Inflammatory infectious joint diseases**

1. Lyme disease (borreliosis)

    a. Transmission. *B. burgdorferi* is transmitted by ticks of the *Ixodes* genus [predominantly *Ixodes scapularis* (formerly *I. dammini*) in the eastern and north central United States, *I. pacificus* in Oregon and California, and *I. ricinus* in Europe]. Feeding by adult ticks and, to a lesser extent, nymphs is responsible for transmission.

        (1) Ticks must feed for longer than 12–24 hours to transmit *B. burgdorferi*.

        (2) Transmission from dogs to humans (either directly or by transporting infected ticks) or dog to dog (via urine or other body secretions) appears to be very unlikely.

    b. Clinical findings may be episodic and often do not appear until 2–5 months after infection.

        (1) Symptomatic disease occurs most commonly in humans and dogs. A sudden onset of lameness with one or more swollen, painful joints is the most common presentation and may be accompanied by depression, lethargy, inappetence, and occasionally fever. A cutaneous rash, a common finding in humans, is very rare in dogs.

        (2) Seropositive dogs are common in endemic areas, but only a small percentage develop clinical disease. Rarely, other diseases (e.g., glomerulonephritis, complete heart block, seizures, aggression, behavioral abnormalities) have been documented in seropositive dogs.

    c. Laboratory findings

        (1) A **CBC, serum biochemical profile, urinalysis, ANA titer,** and **rheumatoid factor** are typically normal or negative. **Creatine kinase** is occasionally slightly elevated.

        (2) Synovial fluid analysis reveals an elevated cell count, predominantly neutrophils. Macrophages, monocytes, and synovial lining cells may also be seen.

        (3) Serologic tests. ELISA (see II B 5 a) will detect antibodies to *B. burgdorferi* after 4–6 weeks of infection.

    d. Diagnosis is based on a history of tick exposure in an endemic area, compatible clinical signs, positive serology, and a prompt response to antibiotic therapy.

    e. Treatment with **doxycycline** or **amoxicillin** is instituted for 3–4 weeks and usually resolves clinical signs within 24–48 hours. Antibiotic therapy may not eliminate the organism from the body. Corticosteroid administration should be avoided because it will mask clinical signs and response to antibiotic therapy.

    f. Prognosis is very good. Relapses or reinfections can occur but are responsive to antibiotic therapy. Chronic debilitating disease is very rare in dogs.

    g. Prevention

       (1) Tick control. Removal of ticks before they become engorged, daily grooming, and use of tick collars or dips is effective for preventing infection.

       (2) Vaccination. The efficacy and potential side effects of a bacterin containing killed *B. burgdorferi* is controversial.

2. Septic arthritis is more common in dogs than in cats, and large-breed male dogs are overrepresented.

    a. Etiology. Septic arthritis results from inoculation of bacteria into the joint, either directly (e.g., following a penetrating wound) or hematogenously (e.g., following bacterial endocarditis or discospondylitis).

       (1) Cats. Septic arthritis occurs most often in kittens as a result of omphalophlebitis. *Pasteurella* species is the most common isolate.

       (2) Dogs. *Staphylococcus* species, *Streptococcus* species, and coliforms are the most common isolates.

    b. Clinical findings

       (1) The carpus, hock, and stifle are the most commonly involved joints. Lameness involves one or a few joints and varies from mild to severe. Affected joints are often hot, painful, and swollen, and may be accompanied by erythema and discoloration of the overlying skin and by crepitus and regional lymphadenopathy. Edema of the affected limb may occur.

       (2) Fever, lethargy, and inappetence may also be present.

    c. Radiographic findings

       (1) Initially, soft tissue swelling around the joint and distention of the fluid-filled joint capsule are observed.

       (2) With time, radiographs may reveal a marked periosteal reaction and mineralization of the periarticular soft tissues, reduced joint space (due to loss of articular cartilage), and subchondral bone erosion (discrete areas or extensive).

       (3) In long-standing cases, secondary changes associated with DJD, subluxation or luxation (secondary to ligament injury/destruction), and fibrous or bony ankylosis may be observed.

    d. Laboratory findings

       (1) A **CBC** may reveal a leukocytosis.

       (2) Synovial fluid analysis (see Table 46-1). Approximately 50% of patients with septic arthritis will have a negative synovial fluid culture.

       (3) A positive **blood** or **urine culture** in a bacteremic animal can support a diagnosis of septic arthritis if synovial fluid examination is equivocal.

    e. Diagnosis is based on the observation of intra- or extracellular bacteria in synovial fluid, with or without a positive bacterial culture. Bacteremia should be suspected if the animal is a neonate or if multiple joints are affected. A thorough search for the source of the infection should be undertaken.

    f. Treatment

       (1) Antimicrobials should be selected based on culture and sensitivity testing. In general, a prolonged course (a total of 4–6 weeks, including 2 weeks beyond clinical resolution) is required using a bactericidal antibiotic.

       (2) Arthrotomy followed by joint lavage and drainage is indicated in the presence of severe arthritis, bacteria associated with rapid joint destruction (i.e., *Staphylococcus* sp, coliforms), or an immature animal with open growth plates.

       (3) Supportive therapy. Cage rest, supportive bandaging, physiotherapy, and a controlled return to **exercise** are helpful.

    g. Prognosis depends on the severity of damage and extent of other organ injury (in bacteremic animals). The prognosis in pups and kittens is usually poor. Chronic DJD is a common sequela.

3. *Mycoplasma* **polyarthritis** is rare in dogs and cats.
   a. **Etiology.** Although *Mycoplasma* species are part of the normal flora in the upper respiratory tract and urogenital tract, systemic infection can occur, especially in debilitated or immunosuppressed animals. *M. gatea* and *M. felis* have been associated with clinical disease in cats. *M. spumans* has been associated with polyarthritis is young greyhounds.
   b. **Clinical** and **laboratory findings** in *Mycoplasma* polyarthritis are almost identical to those seen with nonerosive immune-mediated polyarthritis (see III C 1). However, significant erosive changes can occur in some cases.
   c. **Diagnosis** is confirmed by a positive culture, but special culture techniques are required.
   d. **Treatment** with tetracycline, doxycycline, tylosin, erythromycin, or chloramphenicol is usually effective.

4. **Viral arthritis**
   a. **Etiology.** Calicivirus occasionally causes a transient polyarthritis in kittens.
   b. **Clinical findings** include lameness, stiffness, and joint pain. Clinical signs usually resolve in 2–4 days.
   c. **Laboratory findings.** Synovial fluid analysis reveals an elevated cell count of predominantly macrophages.
   d. **Treatment** is usually unnecessary.

5. **Bacterial L-form arthritis.** Bacterial L-forms are cell wall–deficient bacteria that can cause a rare syndrome of subcutaneous abscesses and polyarthritis in cats and possibly polyarthritis in dogs.
   a. **Transmission.** The infection may be transmitted by bite wounds.
   b. **Clinical findings.** Joints are swollen and painful and tend to fistulate and drain. Joint damage can be severe.
   c. **Treatment.** Tetracycline is the treatment of choice.

6. **Rickettsial polyarthritis** is occasionally observed in animals with Rocky Mountain spotted fever or ehrlichiosis (see Chapter 49 IV B, E).

7. **Fungal arthritis** is usually an extension of fungal osteomyelitis caused by *Blastomyces dermatitidis, Coccidioides immitis,* or *Cryptococcus neoformans.*

8. **Protozoal arthritis.** Infection with *Leishmania donovani* can result in polyarthritis (possibly as the result of an immune-mediated response).

C. **Inflammatory noninfectious joint diseases**

1. **Nonerosive arthritis**
   a. **Idiopathic immune-mediated polyarthritis** is a common cause of polyarthritis in dogs, most often in sporting and large-breed dogs between 2.5 and 4.5 years of age. It is rare in cats.
      (1) **Clinical findings** include a stilted gait, lameness, joint effusion (which may be mild or not detectable), and painful joints. The most commonly involved joints are the distal joints; the intervertebral joints are occasionally involved as well. Intermittent fever, lethargy, and anorexia may occur.
      (2) **Radiographic findings** are minimal and consist of joint and periarticular swelling.
      (3) **Laboratory findings**
         (a) A **CBC** may reveal a neutrophilic leukocytosis.
         (b) **Synovial fluid analysis** reveals an increased cell count that is dominated by nondegenerate neutrophils (see Table 46-1).
      (4) **Diagnosis** is based on ruling out other immune-mediated joint diseases and chronic inflammatory or infectious disorders.
      (5) **Treatment**
         (a) **Glucocorticoids** (e.g., prednisone) are initially given in immunosuppressive doses for 10–14 days; then the dose is halved for another 10–14 days, and then the dose is gradually reduced over 2–4 months. Reevaluation of synovial fluid is recommended after 1 month of therapy and at

monthly intervals thereafter until alternate-day prednisone therapy is effective, and then as needed. Treatment may be required for several months in some and for life in others. Glucocorticoids alone are effective in approximately 50% of dogs.

    (b) Azathioprine (for dogs only) can be added to glucocorticoid therapy if clinical signs are not controlled. Azathioprine is administered daily for 4–6 weeks; and then, if the response is satisfactory, on alternate days. A CBC should be performed regularly to check for myelosuppression.

    (c) Other immunosuppressive medications (e.g., cyclophosphamide, gold salts) may be required in refractory cases.

  (6) Prognosis. In many animals, symptoms can be controlled without undue side effects.

b. Polyarthritis associated with SLE. Polyarthritis is one of the most common features of SLE and occurs in 70%–90% of affected dogs. The joint signs and synovial fluid findings are identical to those of idiopathic immune-mediated polyarthritis except that other signs consistent with SLE (see Chapter 48 V B 4) are present.

c. Polyarthritis associated with chronic inflammatory disease. Polyarthritis can develop secondary to chronic inflammatory diseases (e.g., bacterial endocarditis, heartworm infection, systemic fungal infections, discospondylitis, neoplasia) or chronic antigenic stimulation. It is related to immune complex formation and deposition in joints. Clinical signs related to the joints and synovial fluid findings are indistinguishable from those of idiopathic immune-mediated polyarthritis except that an underlying chronic inflammatory disorder is identified.

d. Drug-induced polyarthritis has been associated with trimethoprim/sulfadiazine and penicillin administration in dogs.

e. Lymphocytic–plasmacytic synovitis is an uncommon disorder that primarily involves the stifle joints in small- to medium-breed dogs.

  (1) Clinical findings include synovitis, joint pain, and lameness, which may be acute or chronic and may occur in one or both stifle joints. Cruciate ligament rupture may occur secondary to synovitis and intraarticular inflammation. Systemic signs of illness are usually absent.

  (2) Laboratory findings

    (a) Synovial fluid analysis reveals an increased cell count, predominantly lymphocytes and plasma cells.

    (b) Synovial membrane biopsy. Histopathologic findings include lymphocytic–plasmacytic inflammation and villous hyperplasia. Definitive diagnosis often requires synovial membrane biopsy.

  (3) Treatment is similar to that for idiopathic immune-mediated polyarthritis.

f. Other nonerosive polyarthritis syndromes

  (1) A **polyarthritis–polymyositis syndrome** is recognized in spaniel breeds.

  (2) A **polyarthritis–meningitis syndrome** is recognized in several breeds of dogs (e.g., boxers, Weimeraners, German short-haired pointers, Bernese mountain dogs) and cats.

  (3) A **heritable polyarthritis** occurs in young Akitas.

2. Erosive joint arthritis

a. Rheumatoid arthritis is a rare disease characterized by erosive polyarthritis and joint destruction. Young to middle-aged, small- to medium-sized dogs are most commonly affected.

  (1) Pathogenesis. Rheumatoid factor represents anti-IgG antibody of the IgM class. The immune complexes that form are deposited in the synovium and incite a primarily lymphocytic–plasmacytic inflammatory response, which results in synovitis, villous hyperplasia, fibrin deposition, and articular cartilage and subchondral bone destruction. The inflammatory response can involve periarticular structures and can lead to the rupture of collateral ligaments. Subluxation, luxation, and ankylosis can occur in severely affected joints.

  (2) Clinical findings are similar to those of other polyarthritis conditions. The distal joints are the most severely affected.

  (3) Radiographic findings

    (a) Early in the disease, erosive changes may not be present, and rheumatoid arthritis may be difficult to distinguish from nonerosive polyarthritis. With time, periarticular osteophyte formation and swelling, subchondral bone destruction (i.e., "punched out" lesions, irregular articular surface), and joint space collapse occur.

    (b) With advanced disease, mineralization of periarticular tissue, subluxation, luxation, and ankylosis may be observed.

  (4) Laboratory findings

    (a) Blood analysis may reveal leukocytosis, mild anemia, increased serum globulin concentration, increased liver enzymes, and proteinuria.

    (b) Synovial fluid analysis. Findings resemble those of nonerosive polyarthritis (see Table 46-1).

    (c) Serologic tests to detect circulating rheumatoid factor include the Rose-Waaler test and the latex agglutination tests (see II B 5 b).

    (d) Synovial biopsy reveals proliferative synovitis associated with severe lymphocytic–plasmacytic inflammation.

  (5) Diagnosis is based on consistent radiographic and synovial fluid abnormalities, a positive rheumatoid factor test, and (in equivocal cases) histopathologic findings on synovial biopsy. Radiographs are most helpful in distinguishing rheumatoid arthritis from nonerosive forms of polyarthritis.

  (6) Treatment should be aggressive to suppress joint damage and ameliorate clinical signs.

    (a) Initially, a combination of **glucocorticoids** (e.g., prednisone) at immunosuppressive doses and **azathioprine** or **cyclophosphamide** is used, then tapered as described for idiopathic immune-mediated polyarthritis [see III C 1 a (5)]. If inflammatory changes are still present in the synovial fluid at a 1-month recheck, either **azathioprine** or **cylcophosphamide** (depending on which one was chosen initially) should be added. If inflammation is still present in the synovial fluid after 4 months of therapy, the use of **gold salts** should be considered.

    (b) Concomitant use of **NSAIDs** may help reduce persistent joint pain. **Weight control** and **reduced exercise** will also help most animals.

  (7) Prognosis. Rheumatoid arthritis is a progressive disorder. Although early diagnosis and treatment will slow the development of debilitating joint disease, most dogs have well-established pathologic changes in their joints at the time of diagnosis and will continue to deteriorate.

b. Feline chronic progressive polyarthritis is a rare disorder recognized exclusively in male cats. An ankylosing, **nonerosive,** nondeforming, proliferative periosteal arthritis occurs in young cats, and a more severe, deforming, **erosive** arthritis occurs in older cats. Many cats are infected with both **feline syncytium-forming virus (FeSFV)** and **feline leukemia virus (FeLV),** but the role of viral infection is unclear.

  (1) Clinical findings

    (a) In both forms of the disorder, an acute onset of fever, lethargy, lymphadenopathy, joint swelling, and joint pain occurs.

    (b) In untreated cats, the acute stage will resolve, followed by a chronic stage where joint damage continues and cats become debilitated and thin.

  (2) Radiographic findings

    (a) Nonerosive form. Findings include joint swelling followed by periarticular osteoporosis and then by periarticular periosteal new bone formation.

    (b) Erosive form. Radiographic findings resemble those of rheumatoid arthritis and can include the collapse of subchondral bone and joint subluxation in advanced cases.

  (3) Laboratory findings

    (a) Tests for **FeLV** and **FeSFV** may be positive, but the latter test is not readily available.

    (b) Synovial fluid analysis may reveal an increased cell count composed primarily of nondegenerate neutrophils.

(4) Diagnosis is based on characteristic signalment, clinical signs, and radiographic signs.

(5) Treatment is usually required for the remainder of the cat's life. **Prednisone** in immunosuppressive doses will slow progression and reduce the severity of clinical signs in most cats. **Additional immunosuppressive drugs** (e.g., cyclophosphamide) may aid in control.

(6) Prognosis is reasonably good for the control of clinical signs, but treatment will not completely halt progression of the disease. Cats that test positive for FeLV will eventually develop FeLV-related disease (e.g., lymphosarcoma).

c. Polyarthritis of greyhounds may be related to *M. spumans* infection and occurs in young animals (e.g., between the ages of 3 and 30 months). The arthritis is erosive and can result in severe damage to the articular surfaces, primarily of the interphalangeal and other distal joints.

STUDY QUESTIONS

DIRECTIONS: Each of the numbered items or incomplete statements in this section is followed by answers or by completions of the statement. Select the ONE numbered answer or completion that is BEST in each case.

1. An 8-year-old male Shetland sheepdog is brought to the veterinarian because of generalized stiffness and lameness in the right forelimb. When the right forelimb is examined, manipulation of the carpal joint elicits some discomfort. No crepitation or swelling of this joint is noted. Synovial fluid collected from this joint reveals a normal cell count. Mononuclear cells are the predominant cell type, but a few (3%) nondegenerate neutrophils are observed. Bacterial culture is negative. Radiographs of the right carpus reveal a mild degree of osteophyte formation. What is the most likely disease process in this joint?

(1) *Mycoplasma* arthritis
(2) Idiopathic immune-mediated polyarthritis
(3) Rheumatoid arthritis
(4) Degenerative joint disease (DJD)
(5) Lyme disease

2. An owner of a large kennel of hunting dogs in Connecticut is concerned about Lyme disease in his dogs. Which of the following methods will best help him prevent transmission of the disease?

(1) Mouse eradication on the premises
(2) Implementation of a good tick control program
(3) Intermittent prophylactic antibiotic therapy for all dogs
(4) Rigorous disinfection of the premises
(5) Isolation of seropositive dogs

3. Which one of the following viruses has been associated with polyarthritis in kittens?

(1) Feline calicivirus (FCV)
(2) Herpesvirus
(3) Panleukopenia virus
(4) Feline leukemia virus (FeLV)
(5) Feline immunodeficiency virus (FIV)

4. Rheumatoid arthritis in dogs is characterized by:

(1) erosive arthritis in only one or two distal joints (i.e., carpi, hocks).
(2) nonerosive polyarthritis in proximal joints (i.e., shoulder, hip).
(3) nonerosive polyarthritis in distal joints.
(4) erosive polyarthritis in proximal joints.
(5) erosive polyarthritis in distal joints.

5. Which one of the following antibiotics would be most effective against *Borrelia burgdorferi*?

(1) Trimethoprim/sulfonamide
(2) Gentamicin
(3) Doxycycline
(4) Lincomycin
(5) Tylosin

1. The answer is 4 [III A 1; Table 46-1]. The low cell count in the synovial fluid, composed primarily of mononuclear cells, is most consistent with degenerative joint disease (DJD). *Mycoplasma* arthritis, idiopathic immune-mediated polyarthritis, rheumatoid arthritis, and Lyme disease would all be characterized by much higher cell counts with neutrophils predominating. In addition, the radiographic changes would be more severe with rheumatoid arthritis (except very early in the disease).

2. The answer is 2 [III B 1 g]. The organism that causes Lyme disease, *Borrelia burgdorferi,* is transmitted by ticks (e.g., *Ixodes scapularis*). Ticks must feed for at least 12–24 hours before the infection can be transmitted. Therefore, good tick control (i.e., regular grooming, tick collars, insecticidal dips) can be very effective at preventing transmission. Mouse eradication on the premises may reduce tick populations on the premises, but the major exposure would be off the premises in woods and fields. The majority of dogs in an endemic area, such as Connecticut, may be seropositive with no clinical signs of disease. As a result, prophylactic antibiotic therapy or the isolation of seropositive dogs would not be useful or indicated. Similarly, because direct dog-to-dog transmission has not been documented and is unlikely to occur, disinfection of the premises would not be helpful for this infectious disease.

3. The answer is 1 [III B 4 a]. Feline calicivirus (FCV) has been associated with a transient polyarthritis in kittens. Feline leukemia virus (FeLV) infection has been documented in older cats in association with feline chronic progressive polyarthritis.

4. The answer is 5 [III C 2 a]. Rheumatoid arthritis affects multiple joints, usually distal joints, in an erosive and destructive fashion.

5. The answer is 3 [III B 1 e]. Doxycycline or other tetracyclines, in addition to amoxicillin or erythromycin, are the most commonly recommended antibiotics to treat borreliosis (Lyme disease).

Chapter 47

Neuromuscular Diseases

I. CLINICAL ASSESSMENT

A. Signalment

1. **Breed.** Neurologic disorders associated with certain breeds are summarized in Table 47-1.

2. **Age**
   a. Animals younger than 6 months are more likely to have congenital or inherited disorders or infectious disease.
   b. Older animals are more frequently affected with degenerative or neoplastic disorders.

B. History

1. **Onset and progression.** Particular attention should be given to characterizing the clinical course of the disease (Figure 47-1).
   a. **Peracute** and **acute disorders** develop quickly and reach their maximal intensity within minutes or several hours, respectively. Examples include trauma, intoxication, metabolic disorders (e.g., hypoglycemia), and vascular disorders (e.g., infarction).
   b. **Subacute disorders** develop over days or weeks. Examples include inflammatory and metabolic diseases, and some neoplastic disorders.
   c. **Chronic disorders** develop over months or years. Examples include degenerative, nutritional, metabolic, or neoplastic diseases.

2. **Potential causes.** The DAMNIT-V scheme of organizing potential differential diagnoses is often helpful. D = degenerative disease; A = anomalous (congenital) disease; M = metabolic disease; N = neoplastic or nutritional diseases; I = inflammatory, idiopathic, or immune-mediated diseases; T = traumatic disorders; and V = vascular diseases.

C. Physical examination

1. **General examination.** A complete physical examination may detect disorders that mimic or induce secondary neurologic signs. Primary nervous system signs include seizures, altered mental state (e.g. stupor, coma, behavioral changes), paresis, paralysis, proprioceptive deficits, ataxia, head tilt, circling, tremors and other abnormal movements, dysmetria, nystagmus, hyperesthesia, and analgesia.

2. **Neurologic examination.** A neurologic examination helps to localize clinical abnormalities first to the nervous system and then to a specific site within the nervous system.
   a. **Mental state** is classified as alert, depressed, stuporous, or comatose.
      (1) **Depressed, stuporous,** or **comatose** animals usually have cerebrocortical or brain stem disease (see Chapter 22).
      (2) **Behavioral abnormalities** such as aggression, fear, withdrawal, and disorientation may indicate brain disease (i.e., limbic system abnormalities) or may reflect the animal's personality and environment.
   b. **Posture**
      (1) **Head.** A persistent **head tilt** (see Chapter 25) is indicative of vestibular disease.
      (2) **Trunk.** Abnormal posture of the trunk can occur from vertebral abnormali-

TABLE 47-1. Common Neurologic Diseases and Breed Associations

Disease	Breed
Myelodysplasia (e.g., spina bifida, meningocele, myelomeningocele)	Manx cat, English bulldog, Boston terrier, Rhodesian ridgeback
Hemivertebra, incomplete segmentation	Brachycephalic dogs
Spinal dysraphism	Weimaraner
Atlantoaxial luxation	Toy breeds
Cervical spondylomyelopathy (wobbler syndrome)	Doberman pinscher, Great Dane
Lumbosacral stenosis	German shepherd
Spondylosis	Large-breed dogs
Intervertebral disk disease	Chondrodystrophic dog breeds (e.g., dachshund, Pekingese, beagle)
Degenerative myelopathy	German shepherd
Hydrocephalus	Toy breeds (e.g., Chihuahua)
Cerebellar hypoplasia	Cats*
Congenital deafness	Dalmatian, bull terrier, white-coated, blue-eyed cats
Idiopathic epilepsy	Beagle, poodle, German shepherd, Keeshond, fox terrier

* Associated with panleukopenia virus infection.

ties or an alteration in muscle tone associated with a brain or spinal cord lesion. Abnormalities include:

   (a) **Scoliosis** (lateral deviation of the spine)
   (b) **Kyphosis** (dorsal deviation of the spine, humpback)
   (c) **Lordosis** (ventral deviation of the spine, swayback)

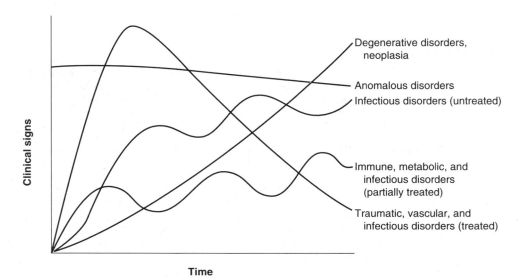

FIGURE 47-1. Graph demonstrating the onset and progression of pathologic processes within the nervous system. (Redrawn with permission from Fenner WR: Diseases of the brain. In *Textbook of Veterinary Internal Medicine,* 4th ed. Edited by Ettinger SJ and Feldman EC. Philadelphia, WB Saunders, 1995, p 581.)

(3) Limbs. Abnormal posture of the limbs results from improper positioning or from increased or decreased extensor muscle tone.

    (a) A. **wide-based stance** is commonly associated with ataxia.

    (b) Knuckling (weight placed on the dorsal surface of the paw) can be caused by decreased proprioception from an upper motor neuron (UMN) or lower motor neuron (LMN) lesion.

        (i) UMN lesions are associated with increased extensor muscle tone.

        (ii) LMN lesions are associated with decreased extensor tone (flaccid paralysis).

    (c) Decerebrate rigidity (extensor rigidity in all four limbs, with opisthotonus if the cerebellum is involved) can result from severe head trauma.

    (d) The **Schiff-Sherrington sign** (increased extensor tone in the thoracic limbs and hyperextension of the neck) results from a severe spinal cord injury caudal to C6–T2.

c. Gait

  (1) Proprioceptive deficits. Proprioception is the sense of knowing where the limbs are without visual input. It is one of the first functions to be affected in compressive spinal cord diseases (e.g., intervertebral disk prolapse). Proprioceptive deficits cause knuckling, misplacement, and dragging of a foot, which may be associated with wear on the dorsal aspect of the claws.

  (2) Paresis or **paralysis** results from damage to the voluntary motor pathways and is a feature of UMN or LMN disease.

  (3) Circling (wide, somewhat aimless circles, tight circles, or spinning) is generally not a very localizing sign, but tight circles can be associated with caudal brain stem lesions. Circling usually occurs toward the side of the lesion if the lesion is caudal to the midbrain. Twisting or circling may be apparent in animals with a head tilt.

  (4) Ataxia (lack of coordination) may be associated with abnormal cerebellar, vestibular, spinal cord, or proprioceptive function (see Chapter 21).

  (5) Dysmetria refers to movements that are too long (hypermetria) or too short (hypometria). Dysmetria is usually a sign of cerebellar (or cerebellar pathways) disease. Hypermetria is characterized by a stride described as "goose-stepping."

  (6) Abnormal movements may include tremors (see Chapter 20), myoclonus, and intention tremors (indicative of cerebellar disease).

d. Postural reactions (proprioceptive or motor) maintain an animal's upright position via intact spinal reflexes and input from the sensory and motor systems of the brain. Proprioceptive positioning and hopping are the most useful screening tests.

  (1) Proprioceptive positioning abnormalities can arise from brain, spinal cord, or peripheral nerve disease. Abnormal conscious proprioception is an early and sensitive indicator of spinal cord compression.

  (2) Hopping reaction. This reaction is slow to initiate with a conscious proprioception abnormality, has a poor follow through with motor deficits, and may be inaccurate (dysmetria) with cerebellar dysfunction.

e. Spinal reflexes are integrated in the spinal cord in very localized areas and are modified by input, or lack thereof, from the brain. Their assessment is critical in determining whether a disease process is UMN (hyperreflexic responses) or LMN (hyporeflexic or absent responses) in nature. Reflex responses are graded as normal, hyperreflexic, or hyporeflexic.

  (1) Pelvic limb

    (a) Patellar (quadriceps, knee-jerk) reflex. The stretch sensation induced in the patellar ligament is transmitted to the spinal cord and integrated in segments **L4–L6.** The motor response travels down the femoral nerve to the quadriceps muscle and results in extension of the stifle.

        (i) Hyporeflexia. Unilateral hyporeflexia usually indicates a peripheral (i.e., femoral) nerve disorder. **Bilateral hyporeflexia** indicates a spinal cord lesion in the L4–L6 region (i.e., LMN disease).

        (ii) Hyperreflexia results from the loss of inhibitory influences on the reflex from the brain and, therefore, is indicative of a spinal cord lesion cranial to spinal cord segments **L4–L6** (i.e., UMN disease). **Clonus** (repetitive muscle contraction to a single stimulus) may accompany a hyperreflexia and is associated with a chronic (i.e., weeks to months) UMN lesion.

  (b) **Withdrawal reflexes** are integrated in spinal cord segments **L6–S1**. The motor response to flex the limb travels down the sciatic nerve to flexor muscles.

    (i) **Hyporeflexia** or **areflexia.** A **unilateral** absent or reduced response usually indicates peripheral nerve disease (i.e., sciatic nerve involvement). A **bilateral** absent or reduced response indicates spinal cord disease in the L6–S1 segments.

    (ii) **Normal response.** The response will be normal as long as the peripheral (i.e., sciatic) nerves and spinal cord segments at L6–S1 are intact; therefore, severe spinal cord lesions cranial to L6 will not alter the reflex. An intact withdrawal reflex does not require any conscious perception of pain and, therefore, does not indicate normal pain sensation.

    (iii) **Hyperreflexia.** An increased withdrawal response is rare.

  (2) **Thoracic limb.** The **withdrawal reflex** can also be evaluated in the thoracic limb.

    (a) **Hyporeflexia** or **areflexia.** A **unilateral** absent or reduced withdrawal response indicates peripheral nerve disease. A **bilateral** absent or reduced response indicates a spinal cord lesion in the C6–T1 region.

    (b) **Normal response.** Normal withdrawal reflexes are seen with spinal cord lesions cranial to C6 or caudal to T1.

  (3) **Perineum.** The **perineal reflex** (contraction of the anal sphincter and a downward flexion of the tail) is integrated in spinal cord segments S1–S3. An absent or reduced response is indicative of pudendal nerve or spinal cord disease (S1–S3). The sensory and motor components of the reflex travel through the pudendal nerve, and the reflex can be used to evaluate neurologic causes of urinary or fecal incontinence.

  f. **Cranial nerves.** Signs of cranial nerve (CN) dysfunction are summarized in Table 47-2.

  g. **Sensation.** Palpation and flexion of the limbs, spinal cord, and neck detect areas of pain or increased sensitivity (hyperesthesia).

    (1) **Superficial.** In order to assess superficial sensation, just enough stimulus is applied to generate a behavioral response (e.g., the animal turns his head toward the stimulus or vocalizes, which indicates conscious pain sensation). The distribution of affected superficial sensation will help determine the nerves involved.

    (2) **Deep.** Deep pain fibers are small fibers deep within the spinal cord. Deep pain sensation assessment is only necessary if superficial sensation is absent. Absence of deep pain sensation bilaterally indicates severe spinal cord injury.

  h. **Muscle tone**

    (1) **Atrophy** of the muscles of the head, limbs, and trunk may be related to denervation. Atrophy from denervation occurs more rapidly and to a greater extent than atrophy from disuse.

    (2) **Increased muscle tone** is generally associated with UMN disease.

    (3) **Decreased muscle tone** is generally associated with LMN disease.

D. Diagnostic studies

  1. Laboratory studies

    a. **Hematology**

      (1) **Normal peripheral blood** is common in primary neurologic diseases.

      (2) An **inflammatory leukogram** may be present with infectious disorders [e.g., canine distemper virus (CDV) infection, cryptococcosis, bacterial meningitis], as well as with noninfectious disorders (e.g., nonseptic meningitis).

      (3) **Microcytosis** may be associated with a portosystemic shunt that is causing encephalopathic signs.

TABLE 47-2. Structures Innervated by Cranial Nerves and Signs of Dysfunction

Cranial Nerve	Summary of Function	Signs of Dysfunction
I Olfactory	Sensory for smell	Loss of sense of smell
II Optic	Sensory for vision and pupillary light reflexes (PLR)	Blindness, loss of PLR, mydriasis, loss of menace reflex
III Oculomotor	Motor to pupil, extraocular muscles	Loss of PLR, dilated pupil, ventrolateral strabismus
IV Trochlear	Motor to extraocular muscles (dorsal oblique)	Slight dorsomedial eye rotation
V Trigeminal	Motor to muscles of mastication, sensory to face	Atrophy of temporalis and masseter muscles; loss of jaw tone and strength; dropped jaw (if bilateral); loss of sensation to eyelid, nasal mucosa, cornea, and face; absent palpebral reflex
VI Abducens	Motor to extraocular muscles (lateral rectus) and retractor bulbi muscle	Medial strabismus, poor retraction of the globe
VII Facial	Motor to facial muscles, sensory for taste (palate, rostral tongue)	Droop of eyelid, ear, or lip, loss of ability to blink (absent palpebral reflex) or retract lip
VIII Vestibulocochlear	Cochlear branch: hearing	Deafness
	Vestibular branch: maintenance of balance and head position	Ataxia, head tilt, nystagmus
IX Glossopharyngeal	Motor to pharynx, parasympathetic innervation to salivary glands, sensory to caudal tongue and pharynx	Loss of gag reflex, dysphagia
X Vagus	Motor to pharynx and larynx, parasympathetic innervation to viscera, sensory to caudal pharynx, larynx and viscera	Loss of gag reflex, laryngeal paralysis, dysphagia
XI Accessory	Motor to trapezius, sternocephalicus, and brachiocephalicus muscles	Atrophy of innervated muscles
XII Hypoglossal	Motor to tongue	Loss of tongue strength, deviation of tongue if lesion is unilateral

b. Serum biochemical profile
   (1) Hypoglycemia, uremia, hypokalemia, hypocalcemia, diabetes mellitus, and **hypothyroidism** are metabolic disorders that may cause neuromuscular signs.
   (2) Serum liver enzymes. Serum alkaline phosphatase (ALP) and serum alanine transferase (ALT) may be elevated in the presence of liver disease that is causing hepatic encephalopathy.
   (3) Serum albumin may be decreased with hepatic encephalopathy.
   (4) Serum cholesterol may be elevated with hypothyroidism.
   (5) Serum creatine kinase or **aspartate aminotransferase (AST)** may be elevated with inflammation or damage to muscles.

TABLE 47-3. Cerebrospinal Fluid (CSF) Findings in Selected Central Nervous System (CNS) Diseases

Condition	White Blood Cell (WBC) Count*	Cytology	CSF Protein*
Steroid-responsive (aseptic) meningitis	+ + +	Nondegenerate neutrophils	+ + +
Breed-associated meningeal vasculitis	+ + +	Nondegenerate neutrophils	+ + +
Granulomatous meningoencephalitis	+ +	Lymphocytes, monocytes, occasional plasma cell and anaplastic mononuclear cells, neutrophils (usually <20% of total cells)	+ +
Pug dog meningoencephalitis	+ + +	Small lymphocytes	+ +
Bacterial meningitis	+ + +	Degenerate (toxic) neutrophils, bacteria	+ + +
Canine distemper	+	Small lymphocytes	+
Rabies	+	Small lymphocytes	+
Toxoplasmosis	+ +	Lymphocytes, macrophages, occasional neutrophils, organism may be observed	+ +
Neospora caninum infection	+ +	Lymphocytes, macrophages, occasional neutrophils, organism may be observed	+ +
Cryptococcosis	+ +	Neutrophils, monocytes, occasional eosinophils, organism (detected in 60% of samples)	+ +
Rocky Mountain spotted fever	+	Neutrophils	+
Ehrlichiosis	+ +	Lymphocytes	+
Feline infectious peritonitis (FIP)	+ + +	Lymphocytes, monocytes, neutrophils	+ + +
CNS parasite migration	+	Monocytes, neutrophils, occasional eosinophils	+
Brain or spinal cord infarct	Normal or +	Mononuclear cells, ± neutrophils	+
CNS neoplasia (except meningioma and lymphosarcoma)	Normal or +	Mononuclear cells	+
Meningioma	Normal or + +	Mononuclear cells, neutrophils	+ +
CNS lymphosarcoma	+ +	Lymphocytes, neoplastic cells	+

(continued)

TABLE 47-3. *(continued)*

Condition	White Blood Cell (WBC) Count*	Cytology	CSF Protein*
Hydrocephalus	Normal	Normal	Normal
Degenerative myelopathy	Normal	Normal	Normal or +
Intervertebral disk prolapse	Normal	Normal	Normal or +
Polyradiculoneuritis	Normal	Normal	Normal or +

Modified with permission from Nelson RW, Couto GC (eds.): *Essentials of Small Animal Internal Medicine,* St. Louis, Mosby-Year Book, 1992, p 734.
 * Relative to normal:

	WBC Count	CSF Protein Concentration
Normal	<6 cells/μl	<25 mg/dl
+	<50 cells/μl	25–50 mg/dl
+ +	50–100 cells/μl	50–100 mg/dl
+ + +	>100 cells/μl	>100 mg/dl

    c. Urinalysis can be used to support a diagnosis of renal failure (uremia).
        (1) Ammonium biurate crystals may be indicative of a portosystemic shunt.
        (2) Calcium oxalate crystalluria (marked) is indicative of ethylene glycol intoxication.
    d. Cerebrospinal fluid (CSF) analysis is indicated when less invasive tests are not diagnostic. CSF findings in disease are described in Table 47-3.
        (1) Indications include focal, multifocal, or diffuse disease in the brain or spinal cord. Analysis of CSF is most useful in inflammatory central nervous system (CNS) disorders.
        (2) Contraindications include excessive anesthetic risk, presence of a coagulopathy, or suspicion of increased intracranial pressure (most often associated with head trauma and brain tumors). Increased intracranial pressure is associated with a significant risk of brain herniation, which involves either the caudal movement of the cerebellum toward the foramen magnum or the temporal cerebral cortex under the tentorium cerebelli, resulting in compression of the medullary oblongata or midbrain, respectively (and frequently resulting in death).
    e. Serology
        (1) Canine distemper. The detection of anti-CDV antibody in CSF is definitive evidence for CDV infection. The antibody is produced locally within the CNS and does not cross the blood–brain barrier, so previous vaccination will not influence the result.
        (2) Toxoplasmosis. Serum antibodies [immunoglobulin M (IgM) or immunoglobulin G (IgG)] can be detected by an enzyme-linked immunosorbent assay (ELISA), immunofluorescent antibody (IFA) technique, and an agglutination assay. ELISA techniques have also been developed to detect antibody in CSF and aqueous humor and *Toxoplasma gondii*-specific antigens and immune complexes in serum. Active *T. gondii* infection is indicated by a serum IgM titer greater than 1:64, a fourfold or greater increase in a serum IgG titer over 2–3 weeks, *Toxoplasma*-specific antigen or immune complexes in serum, or *Toxoplasma* antibodies in aqueous humor or CSF.
        (3) Myasthenia gravis. Acetylcholine receptor antibody directed at the acetylcholine receptor in muscle tissue establishes a definitive diagnosis of acquired myasthenia gravis when present in sufficient quantity.
        (4) Other diseases. Serum antibody titers to *Rickettsia rickettsii* (which causes Rocky Mountain spotted fever) and *Ehrlichia canis* and tests to detect the capsular antigen from *Cryptococcus neoformans* are also available.

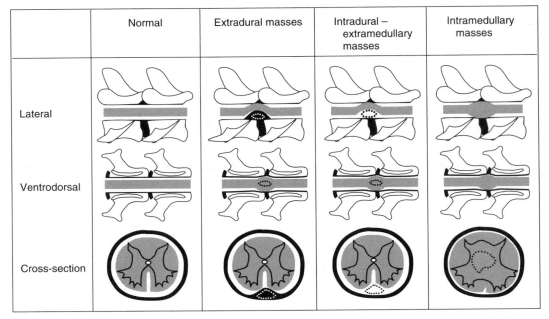

	Normal	Extradural masses	Intradural – extramedullary masses	Intramedullary masses
Lateral				
Ventrodorsal				
Cross-section				

FIGURE 47-2. Diagrammatic representation of myelographic abnormalities associated with extradural, intradural–extramedullary, and intramedullary spinal cord masses. (Redrawn with permission from Nelson RW, Couto GC (eds): *Essentials of Small Animal Internal Medicine*, St. Louis, Mosby–Year Book, 1992, p 736.)

2. **Diagnostic imaging**
    a. **Radiography**
        (1) **Survey radiographs** of the spine can detect intervertebral disk disease, discospondylitis, fractures, luxations, and some neoplasms. Intracranial masses are not usually visualized unless there is a bony reaction in the skull bones adjacent to a tumor or calcification of the mass itself. Nasal neoplasia extending across the cribriform plate may be visible.
        (2) **Contrast radiographs**
            (a) **Myelography** is used to confirm, localize, and characterize spinal cord lesions in surgical or radiotherapy candidates (Figure 47-2).
                (i) **Indications** include suspected intervertebral disk herniation, mass lesions in and around the spinal cord, and other causes of spinal cord compression.
                (ii) **Contraindications** may include the presence of CNS inflammation or seizures.
                (iii) **Complications.** The potential for seizures is greatest if contrast is placed at the cerebellomedullary cisternal site (because the contrast material is more likely to reach the brain) and if the contrast agent metrizamide is used. Newer contrast agents (e.g., iohexol) are associated with a much lower risk of seizures.
            (b) **Epidurography** (contrast injected into the lumbosacral epidural space), **transosseous vertebral sinus venography** (contrast injected into the vertebral sinuses), and **discography** (contrast injected into the nucleus pulposus of the lumbosacral disk) are used to detect lesions in the lumbosacral area because myelography does not readily image this area.
            (c) **Pneumoventriculography** (injection of air into the lateral ventricles of the cerebral hemispheres) is rarely performed. This technique may be used to document the presence of hydrocephalus.
            (d) **Angiography** (i.e., arteriography, cavernous sinus venography) is occasionally used to examine the integrity of the cerebral or cerebellar blood

supply or to detect deviations in the venous sinuses resulting from mass lesions.

b. **Ultrasonography** is of limited usefulness in neurologic disease because of interference by overlying bone. However, it can be very useful in detecting hydrocephalus if the animal has open fontanelles through which the ultrasound beam can be directed.

c. **Computed tomography (CT)** generates a detailed image of intracranial structures.

   (1) CT is one of the best techniques to detect and localize intracranial mass lesions. Contrast material is often injected intravenously to enhance the image of a mass.

   (2) Diffuse inflammatory disease may not be easily detected with a CT scan.

d. **Magnetic resonance imaging (MRI)** is used less often than CT in veterinary medicine because of its high cost. It produces a more detailed image than CT and as a result is more sensitive in detecting alterations resulting from neoplasia and inflammatory disease.

3. **Electrodiagnostic testing** is used to characterize specific neurologic deficits.

a. **Electromyography** is the passive recording of electrical activity within muscle. Normal muscle is electrically silent. The electromyogram (EMG) can help localize an LMN disorder based on the distribution of denervated muscle) or detect primary muscle disease.

   (1) **LMN disease** (from spinal cord, nerve root, or peripheral nerve disease) results in denervation of muscle, which produces prolonged electrical activity and resting spontaneous activity (fibrillation or denervation potentials).

   (2) **Muscle damage** or **inflammation** produces abnormal electrical activity.

b. **Nerve conduction velocity** is useful in assessing LMN disease. Demyelinating peripheral neuropathies and localized peripheral nerve injury will reduce or, if a peripheral nerve has been severely damaged distal to the stimulation site, eliminate conduction velocity.

c. **Electroretinography** is used to assess retinal function, often prior to cataract removal.

   (1) **Abnormal.** An abnormal electroretinogram (ERG) is produced if the retina is diseased, detached, or atrophied.

   (2) **Normal.** A normal ERG may be produced in a blind eye if the cause of the blindness is at the level of the optic nerve, optic chiasma, optic tract, or cerebral cortex.

d. **Brain stem auditory evoked response (BAER)** is a test to objectively assess bi- or unilateral loss of hearing or deafness. BAER is especially useful as a screening tool to detect congenital deafness in puppies at high-risk (e.g., Dalmatians).

   (1) **Congenital** or **acquired deafness.** The waveform is completely absent (i.e., flat line).

   (2) **Brain stem disease.** The areas in the waveform associated with brainstem centers are altered or delayed.

e. **Electroencephalography** records cerebral cortical electrical activity from many sites over the skull. Alterations in the electroencephalogram (EEG) are often nonspecific but may support a diagnosis of diffuse or focal cerebrocortical disease. CT and MRI usually provide superior information, especially if mass lesions are suspected.

4. **Biopsy procedures**

a. **Muscle biopsies** can detect inflammatory and neoplastic disorders. Histochemical staining to identify abnormalities affecting specific muscle fiber types (i.e., type I and II fibers) is helpful in identifying some disorders (e.g., Labrador retriever myopathy). Special handling techniques and a laboratory capable of performing the histochemical staining are required.

b. **Nerve biopsies** are used to confirm and characterize peripheral neuropathies. The common peroneal nerve and ulnar nerve are frequently biopsied in diffuse peripheral neuropathies.

c. Brain biopsies can be performed in select cases to identify superficial mass lesions.

II. DISORDERS OF THE BRAIN

A. Localizing signs

1. **Cerebral cortex.** Unexplained changes in learned behavior or personality, changes in mentation, seizures, cortical blindness (i.e., blindness with normal pupil size and light reflexes), circling (toward the side of the lesion), head pressing, postural or proprioceptive deficits (contralateral to the lesion) can result from cerebral cortical disease. Gait is normal or near normal.

2. **Cerebellum.** Ataxia and hypermetria with normal strength and a broad-based stance and intention tremors of the head and eye are common. The menace response may be absent ipsilateral to the lesion. Mentation is normal.

3. **Thalamus** and **hypothalamus (diencephalon).** Signs of dysfunction may include altered personality or mentation, changes in body temperature or eating, drinking or sleeping habits, diabetes insipidus, hyperadrenocorticism, acromegaly, and postural or proprioceptive deficits (contralateral to the lesion). Because of the presence of the optic chiasma in this area, hypothalamic disease may also result in bilateral visual impairment with dilated pupils and decreased pupillary light responses.

4. **Brain stem (pons, medulla oblongata).** Hemiparesis (UMN) ipsilateral to the lesion, tetraparesis, altered mental status, or an irregular respiratory pattern may result from a brain stem lesion. Most of the CNs (III to XII) are in the brain stem, and an abnormality in CN function can specifically indicate the location of the lesion.

5. **Vestibular system.** A head tilt, falling, or rolling (all toward the side of the lesion) are common with central or peripheral vestibular disease. Asymmetrical ataxia and spontaneous or positional nystagmus (fast phase away from the side of the lesion) also occur.
   a. **Peripheral vestibular disease.** Signs result from dysfunction of CN VIII outside of the skull or they may be idiopathic. Because CN VIII passes close to the inner and middle ear (as does the facial nerve, CN VII), inflammation, infection, or neoplasia in this area can result in vestibular signs. Signs that suggest peripheral disease include a horizontal or rotatory nystagmus that does not change direction with head position, absence of postural or proprioceptive deficits, concomitant facial nerve paralysis (may also occur with central disease but is more commonly associated with peripheral disease), and Horner's syndrome (miosis, ptosis, enophthalmos).
   b. **Central vestibular disease.** Signs result from a brain stem lesion and may include postural or proprioceptive deficits or paresis (ipsilateral to the lesion), vertical nystagmus, nystagmus that changes direction with the head position, or other signs of brain stem dysfunction. Both peripheral and central vestibular disease can produce horizontal and rotatory nystagmus, but vertical nystagmus only occurs with central vestibular disease.

B. Degenerative disorders

1. **Storage diseases.** Metabolic or lysosomal storage diseases are rare disorders that are inherited in an autosomal recessive fashion and tend to occur in highly inbred lines of purebred dogs and cats.
   a. **Pathogenesis.** When a lysosomal enzyme responsible for the degradation of a metabolic substance is deficient or absent, lipids (e.g., gangliosides), carbohydrates (e.g., mannoside, glycoprotein), mucopolysaccharides, or ceroid lipofuscins can accumulate within cells of the nervous system (and other organs) and lead to neurologic signs.

b. Clinical findings. Animals are usually normal at birth but fail to thrive, with progressive clinical signs usually noted within several weeks of birth. Clinical signs vary, but UMN spinal cord, cerebellar, and cerebral signs are common. Visual deficits are also frequent. Organ enlargement (e.g., hepatomegaly, splenomegaly) may occur.

c. Prognosis. Most animals die or are euthanized by 4–6 months of age.

2. Cerebellar abiotrophy. Progressive degeneration of the cerebellum has been documented and is known or suspected to be inherited in many breeds of dogs. Signs of cerebellar dysfunction are usually noted around 2 months of age and worsen over time. Some breeds develop signs later (e.g., in Gordon setters, the onset is often at 6–30 months of age). Diagnosis is by exclusion of all other causes of cerebellar dysfunction.

3. Neuroaxonal dystrophy is a progressive, inherited degenerative condition that disrupts axonal function. The signs are predominantly cerebellar and begin at a young age. Affected breeds include Rottweilers, Chihuahuas, Jack Russell terriers, and tricolor cats. The signs progress relatively more slowly in Rottweilers (over several years) than in other breeds.

4. Rottweiler leukoencephalomyelopathy is an inherited disorder that results from the progressive degeneration of white matter in the spinal cord, brain stem, and cerebellum. Clinical findings such as symmetric limb ataxia and weakness begin between 1.5–3.5 years of age and slowly progress. Diagnosis is based on the exclusion of other conditions, and there is no treatment.

C. Anomalous disorders

1. Hydrocephalus

a. Pathogenesis. Hydrocephalus results from the excessive accumulation of CSF in the ventricular system of the brain. Dilation of the lateral ventricles in the cerebral hemispheres results in compression and atrophy of cerebrocortical tissue.

(1) Congenital hydrocephalus may be due to decreased reabsorption of CSF by the arachnoid villi or by stenosis of the mesencephalic aqueduct. Pressure is normal to low. Hydrocephalus is one of the most common congenital malformations of the CNS in dogs and cats; toy and brachycepahlic breeds of dogs (e.g., Chihuahuas, Pomeranians) are predisposed.

(2) Secondary or **acquired hydrocephalus** may result from similar mechanisms but is the result of inflammation (e.g., infection, cranial trauma) or neoplasia. Secondary hydrocephalus is usually associated with increased CSF pressure.

b. Diagnosis (congenital)

(1) Clinical findings. Signs are apparent in about 50% of affected dogs by 1 year of age and include an enlarged, domed cranium with open fontanelles (may be absent in affected animals and present in unaffected animals), altered mental status (hyperexcitability to severe depression), seizures, ataxia, head tilt, circling, head pressing, dilated and fixed pupils, and visual or auditory deficits. Ventrolateral strabismus may result from encroachment on the orbit from expanding frontal bones.

(2) Radiographic findings. Survey radiographs may reveal open skull suture lines and fontanelles after the age of usual closure.

(3) Other findings. Pneumoventriculography, ultrasound examination through an open fontanelle, CT, or MRI can be used to confirm the diagnosis.

c. Treatment

(1) Medical treatment

(a) Corticosteroids increase CSF reabsorption and decrease production.

(b) Mannitol, acetazolamide, or **diuretics** may be helpful in animals that are suspected of having increased intracranial pressure.

(c) Anticonvulsants may help control seizure activity.

(2) Surgical treatment. The placement of ventriculovenous or ventriculoperitoneal shunts to establish an alternate route of drainage has been performed successfully in some animals.

    d. Prognosis
       (1) Congenital hydrocephalus may carry a fair prognosis, depending on the severity of the clinical signs and the response to treatment.
       (2) Acquired hydrocephalus can be rapidly progressive in some animals and is associated with a poorer prognosis.

2. Cerebellar hypoplasia is most common in cats but can occur in dogs.
    a. Etiology. Cerebellar hypoplasia may result from an inherited defect in development or *in utero* damage from toxins or infectious agents (e.g., panleukopenia virus in cats).
    b. Diagnosis. Signs are usually noted when animals start to ambulate and consist of typical cerebellar signs (i.e., ataxia with normal strength, hypermetria, intention tremors). Signs are not progressive. Diagnosis is made by exclusion of other causes of cerebellar disease.
    c. Prognosis. Depending on the severity of signs, some animals can make acceptable pets, particularly if kept indoors.

3. Lissencephaly is the absence of gyri and sulci in the cerebrum. It is a rare disorder apparent in neonates, most frequently Lhasa apsos, Irish setters, and wire-haired fox terriers. Signs include dementia, seizures, severe behavioral abnormalities, and blindness; definitive diagnosis is made at necropsy. There is no treatment.

4. Abnormalities in myelinogenesis can be inherited, occurring in several breeds of dogs (e.g., chow chows, Weimaraners, Dalmatians, Samoyeds). They are diffuse disorders that affect the spinal cord, brain stem, and cerebellum. Clinical signs appear in neonates and resemble those of cerebellar disease; abnormal proprioception is common. The diagnosis is confirmed by histopathology. There is no treatment, but the prognosis is generally good because the signs are nonprogressive and may improve (or disappear) over several weeks to months.

5. Scotty cramp, an inherited syndrome exclusive to Scottish terriers, is believed to be related to abnormal serotonin metabolism.
    a. Diagnosis is usually based on the characteristic breed and clinical signs.
       (1) The onset of clinical signs occurs between 6 weeks and 18 months of age.
       (2) Episodes of spasticity and alternating hyperflexion and hyperextension of the limbs, lasting 1–30 minutes, are often associated with exercise and excitement. There is no alteration in mental status before, during, or after the episodes. Administration of methysergide maleate blocks the effect of serotonin and exacerbates the signs in affected animals.
    b. Treatment
       (1) Diazepam relaxes skeletal muscle and may reduce the severity of the episodes. **Vitamin E** administration can also reduce the frequency and severity of the events. **Avoidance of stress** is beneficial.
       (2) Nonsteroidal anti-inflammatory drugs (NSAIDs) and penicillin are contraindicated because they can exacerbate the clinical signs.

D. **Metabolic disorders** that can result in neurologic signs include **hepatic encephalopathy, hypoglycemia, uremia, hypoxia** or **anoxia, hypocalcemia,** and **hyper-** or **hyponatremia.** Neurologic signs can occur as a result of processes that deprive the brain of fuel (i.e., glucose, oxygen), disorders that generate endogenous neurotoxins (e.g., hepatic failure), or from processes that alter water or electrolyte concentrations in the brain. Clinical findings include alterations in mentation and nonspecific motor abnormalities (e.g., muscle spasms, tremors, flaccidity, seizures).

E. **Neoplastic disorders.** Neoplasms of the brain are relatively common in dogs and cats and include **astrocytoma, oligodendroglioma, choroid plexus tumors, meningioma, primary lymphoma, pituitary adenoma,** and **metastatic tumors** (e.g., mammary carcinoma, hemangiosarcoma). Approximately 50% of all brain tumors are metastatic in origin.

    1. Predisposition
       a. Meningioma is the most common brain tumor in cats and is one of the most

common brain tumors in dogs. Dolichocephalic breeds have a predisposition for meningiomas.

   b. Brachycephalic dog breeds are predisposed to astrocytomas, oligodendogliomas, and pituitary adenomas.

   c. Brain tumors usually affect middle-aged to older dogs and cats.

2. Diagnosis should be based on age, neurologic signs, and imaging (especially CT or MRI) results.

   a. Clinical findings. Clinical signs tend to be focal, slowly progressive, and reflect the tumor location within the brain. Signs can include:

     (1) Seizures (cerebral tumors)

     (2) Endocrine signs (pituitary tumors)

     (3) Vestibular signs (brain stem tumors)

     (4) Intention tremors, hypermetria, vestibular signs, and ataxia (cerebellar tumors)

     (5) Rapid death from respiratory paralysis due to increased intracranial pressure and brain herniation (brain stem tumors)

   b. Laboratory findings

     (1) CSF analysis findings are useful in confirming the presence of CNS disease but will not absolutely rule in or rule out a tumor.

       (a) Typically, brain tumors are associated with an **increased protein concentration** and a **normal** or **minimally elevated cell count.**

         (i) Meningiomas and **choroid plexus tumors** are associated with an increased cell count in about 60% of cases.

         (ii) Lymphoma may increase the number of lymphocytes in the CSF.

       (b) Brain tumors are frequently associated with an increase in CSF pressure; therefore, CSF collection carries an added risk of herniation. Examination of the optic disk for papilledema may provide advanced warning of increased pressure.

     (2) Diagnostic imaging findings

       (a) Survey radiographs of the skull are often unrewarding with most brain tumors except those involving bone or causing a bony reaction adjacent to the tumor (e.g., meningioma).

       (b) CT (especially with contrast enhancement) and/or **MRI** are the diagnostic techniques of choice.

3. Treatment

   a. Supportive therapy

     (1) Corticosteroids will decrease tumor blood flow and size, edema, and inflammation in many animals.

     (2) Anticonvulsant medications may be required.

   b. Surgery (excision, decompression, or **debulking), radiation therapy,** and **chemotherapy** may be used to prolong survival. Superficial masses (especially meningiomas) can be surgically removed quite successfully in some animals, producing good long-term survival (1–2 years).

4. Prognosis. In general, the long-term prognosis is poor unless complete surgical excision is possible.

F. **Nutritional disorders. Thiamine (vitamin B$_1$)** is required for aerobic metabolism in the CNS, and its absence or deficiency results in anaerobic glycolysis, lactic acid production, and subsequent neuronal dysfunction.

1. Etiology. Dogs and cats are dependent on dietary sources of thiamine. Some cats develop thiamine deficiency if fed a diet of raw fish (e.g., salmon, tuna) because of the presence of thiaminase enzymes.

2. Diagnosis is made by history, clinical signs, and response to therapy.

   a. Clinical findings are acute in onset.

     (1) Dogs may exhibit anorexia, depression, progressive spastic paraparesis, circling, torticollis, seizures, recumbency, and death.

     (2) Cats may exhibit vestibular signs, head tremors, depression, seizures, ventroflexion of the head, dilated and poorly responsive pupils, opisthotonus and limb spasticity, coma, and death.

    b. Laboratory findings. Serum thiamine concentration is decreased.

  3. Treatment. If thiamine is given early in the clinical course, the response is often dramatic and recovery is usually complete.

G. **Inflammatory disorders**

  1. General considerations

    a. Terminology. Meningitis, myelitis, and encephalitis refer to inflammation of the meninges, spinal cord, and brain, respectively. Meningitis commonly results in cervical pain and fever whereas encephalitis is characterized by CNS dysfunction (e.g., altered mental state). Meningoencephalitis results in a combination of signs.

    b. Diagnosis. Analysis of CSF is central to identifying and characterizing the inflammatory process. The CSF may yield an etiologic agent when examined, or it can be cultured for bacteria or used for serologic testing (e.g., CDV antibody).

  2. Infectious causes

    a. Rabies. Rabies virus infection results in a rapidly progressive, fatal encephalomyelitis in dogs and cats. Rabies virus can infect any warm-blooded animal, although the susceptibility varies between species. Dogs and cats are moderately susceptible, whereas foxes, skunks, cows, and bats (among others) are highly susceptible to infection.

      (1) Transmission. In dogs and cats, the majority of infections result from a bite wound by an animal shedding virus in the saliva. The main reservoir in North America is wildlife, with skunks being perhaps the most common reservoir, but raccoons (especially in the eastern United States) and foxes (in Ontario, Canada) are also important. Dogs and cats are important vehicles for the transmission of rabies from the wildlife to human population.

      (2) Pathogenesis. Virus replicates at the site of inoculation and travels up the peripheral nerves to the CNS. The incubation period is variable (2 weeks to 6 months), but averages 3–8 weeks in dogs and 2–6 weeks in cats. Once in the CNS, the virus replicates and spreads up the spinal cord and into the brain. Virus can then travel back out of the CNS down peripheral nerves into other tissues (i.e., salivary glands). Dogs can shed rabies virus in the saliva for up to 13 days prior to the onset of clinical signs.

      (3) Diagnosis

        (a) Clinical findings. It is important to note that not all dogs or cats develop the following phases in order or at all. Rabies should be considered in any animal with rapidly progressive signs of encephalitis, sudden profound behavioral changes, or ascending paralysis.

          (i) Prodromal phase. This phase lasts 2–3 days and is characterized by restlessness and nervousness.

          (ii) Excitative ("furious") phase . This phase lasts 1–7 days and may be characterized by aggression, photophobia, pica, and biting at imaginary objects. Cats tend to develop the furious phase more consistently than dogs.

          (iii) Paralytic ("dumb") phase. This phase lasts 2–4 days. Ascending progressive LMN paralysis beginning at the site of infection and eventually resulting in tetraparesis, excessive salivation, an inability to swallow (as a result of pharyngeal paralysis), an altered bark (as a result of laryngeal paralysis), and a dropped jaw (as a result of trigeminal nerve paralysis) may be noted. Eventually, the animal goes into a coma and dies of respiratory failure.

        (b) Laboratory findings

          (i) Antemortem. There are no characteristic findings on hematology, serum biochemical analysis, or in the CSF. An antemortem diagnosis can sometimes be made by direct fluorescent antibody (DFA) staining of skin biopsies (from the whiskered area of the muzzle).

However, if the likelihood of rabies is high, clinical examination and further diagnostic testing should be performed with great caution, if at all, because of the risk of transmission to humans.

    (ii) Postmortem. A definitive diagnosis is usually made by DFA staining of brain tissue collected during necropsy.

(4) Treatment is not recommended because of the human health hazard. Dogs or cats suspected of having rabies should be quarantined or euthanized.

(5) Prognosis. Almost all animals die within 7–10 days of the onset of clinical signs; however, in experimental infections, spontaneous recovery has been noted.

(6) Prevention. Vaccination of dogs and cats at 1- or 3-year intervals (depending on the vaccine product and local regulations) is effective at preventing the development of clinical rabies and reducing the risk of transmission of rabies to people. In rare instances, vaccine-induced rabies can occur with the use of modified live-virus vaccines in dogs and cats. However, most rabies vaccines currently on the market are killed-virus products, so vaccine-induced rabies has ceased to be a major concern.

b. Canine distemper is caused by a paramyxovirus of the *Moribillivirus* genus that causes multiorgan disease, predominantly respiratory, gastrointestinal (GI), and CNS disease.

  (1) Pathogenesis and clinical findings. It is estimated that 50%–75% of dogs develop subclinical infection. If dogs are unvaccinated or develop a poor antibody and cell-mediated immune response, virus spreads to all epithelial tissues of the body and the CNS. Neurologic disease may develop following subclinical, mild, or severe clinical illness, but the likelihood of neurologic disease increases with the severity of clinical illness. Different forms of neurologic disease can result.

    (a) Meningoencephalitis in young or unvaccinated dogs usually occurs 1–3 weeks after recovery from the acute clinical illness (i.e., fever, coughing, ocular discharge, vomiting, diarrhea). Signs can include cervical pain, seizures, cerebellar or vestibular signs, paraparesis, tetraparesis, and seizures (generalized or focal). **"Chewing gum fits"** are thought to result from focal seizure activity and are considered to be a classic finding of distemper encephalitis. **Myoclonus** (rhythmic involuntary twitching of muscle groups) may occur in some dogs and is thought to be relatively specific for CDV infection.

    (b) Encephalitis in older dogs may develop in rare instances as a consequence of previous CDV infection. Two different forms have been described.

      (i) Multifocal encephalomyelitis in mature dogs, 4–8 years of age, produces pelvic limb weakness and ataxia progressing to tetraparesis. Cerebellar signs may occur, but alterations in mental status and seizures are not present. Multifocal necrosis in the lower brain stem and spinal cord may occur.

      (ii) "Old dog" encephalitis, which typically affects dogs over 6 years of age, is characterized by visual impairment and progressive mental depression, circling, and head pressing. Diffuse sclerosis involving the cerebral cortex and upper brain stem occurs in this form of the disease.

    (c) Ophthalmic disease. Chorioretinitis, optic neuritis, or **retinal detachment** may occur.

  (2) Diagnosis is based on characteristic clinical signs and laboratory findings.

    (a) CSF analysis usually reveals an increase in protein concentration and a mild increase in lymphocyte numbers.

    (b) Serology. Confirmation of CDV infection can be obtained by immunofluorescent staining of cytologic samples from conjunctival scrapings (early in infection) or respiratory epithelium (from transtracheal wash samples) or the detection of anti-CDV antibodies in CSF.

(3) Treatment

(a) Acute distemper meningoencephalitis is best treated with supportive care, nursing care, and anticonvulsant medication (if required). A single dose of dexamethasone to suppress CNS inflammation may decrease the severity of signs.

(b) Encephalomyelitis of older dogs has no reliable treatment.

(4) Prognosis. Despite therapy, acute meningoencephalitis progresses in most dogs to tetraparesis and coma, and euthanasia is usually necessary. However, some dogs do not develop progressive signs, and the neurologic deficits may be compatible with life.

(5) Prevention. Vaccination of puppies beginning at 6–8 weeks and at 3- to 4-week intervals until 16 weeks of age, followed by annual revaccination, provides good protection. Widespread vaccination of dogs against distemper has markedly reduced the prevalence of severe clinical disease in most of North America.

c. Feline infectious peritonitis (FIP) (see Chapter 49 V F). Cats less than 2 years of age or old cats are affected most often. **Two clinical forms** of the disease are recognized, an **effusive (wet) form** and a **noneffusive (dry) form.** Occasionally, a combination of forms occurs.

(1) Pathogenesis. FIP is caused by a coronavirus that induces widespread vasculitis and pyogranulomatous inflammation.

(2) Diagnosis is established based on clinical and laboratory findings.

(a) Clinical findings

(i) Neurologic signs are commonly cerebellar, but hindlimb paresis, ataxia, tetraparesis, seizures, or central vestibular signs can also occur. Signs are progressive. If neurologic signs occur, they are usually associated with the noneffusive form.

(ii) Other signs. Affected cats may also have an intermittent fever, anorexia, lethargy, and other organ abnormalities (e.g., liver disease, uveitis, chorioretinitis).

(b) Laboratory findings

(i) Hematology. An inflammatory leukogram and increased serum globulin concentration may be present.

(ii) Serology. An FIP antibody titer can be performed, but it is difficult to interpret because infection with a relatively nonpathogenic enteric coronavirus is common in cats and will produce antibodies that cross-react with this assay. An extremely high FIP titer may indicate active clinical disease.

(iii) CSF analysis usually reveals a moderate to marked increase in protein concentration and cell count. Nondegenerate neutrophils, lymphocytes, and macrophages are the predominant cell types.

(3) Treatment is supportive. Anti-inflammatory and immunosuppressive drugs may decrease the severity of clinical signs in some cases but will not halt or reverse the progression of the disease.

(4) Prognosis is poor. Almost all cats eventually die regardless of treatment.

d. Toxoplasmosis is caused by *Toxoplasma gondii.*

(1) Diagnosis is based on supportive serologic findings or demonstration of the organism in fluid or tissue samples.

(a) Clinical findings. Asymptomatic infection is common, but clinical disease can occasionally occur in dogs and cats (most often in immunocompromised or young animals). Neurologic signs are extremely variable and reflect the multifocal nature of the CNS lesions (cerebrum, cerebellum, brain stem, spinal cord, muscle). Signs reported include hyperexcitability, tremors, ataxia, paresis, depression, and seizures.

(i) Polyradiculoneuritis and myositis may occur and result in hindlimb paresis, bilateral hind limb rigidity, and tetraparesis (occasionally). This syndrome has been observed most often in dogs younger than 4 months. When myositis occurs in cats, muscle pain is common.

(ii) When neurologic disease occurs, systemic signs of illness are often absent. However, signs of involvement of other organs (e.g., pneu-

monia, hepatitis, myositis) or ocular lesions (especially chorioretinitis or optic neuritis in cats) should raise suspicion of toxoplasmosis.
  (b) Laboratory findings
 (i) Serum biochemical profile. Serum creatinine kinase and ALT levels are commonly elevated if myositis is present.
 (ii) Serology. Findings on serology may support infection [see I D 1 e (2)]. Cats should be tested for concurrent feline leukemia (FeLV) and feline immunodeficiency virus (FIV) infection.
 (iii) CSF analysis usually reveals an elevated protein concentration and cell count (monocytes, lymphocytes, occasional neutrophils). In rare instances, *T. gondii* may be observed within cells.
 (iv) Biopsy findings. Biopsy of affected muscle (or other nonneural tissue) may also detect the organism.
  (c) Electromyographic findings in animals with myositis consist of abnormal spontaneous activity (i.e., fibrillation potentials, prolonged insertional activity).
(2) Treatment entails **supportive care** and **antimicrobial therapy. Clindamycin** is used most commonly because it crosses the blood–brain barrier. Alternative drug choices include combinations of either **trimethoprim** or **pyrimethamine** with a **sulfa drug.** However, pyrimethamine frequently results in side effects in cats.
(3) Prognosis. The prognosis is guarded to poor, especially in cats with concurrent FeLV or FIV infection. The hindlimb paresis and rigidity in young dogs usually do not respond to therapy.
e. Neosporosis. *Neospora caninum* is a protozoal parasite that can cause multifocal CNS disease, polyneuritis, and polymyositis in dogs.
  (1) Diagnosis is based on compatible serologic findings or identification of the organism in tissue samples or CSF.
  (a) Clinical findings. The clinical signs are similar to that of the polyradiculoneuritis and myositis of toxoplasmosis. An ascending LMN paralysis in young dogs can occur, with the hindlimbs being most severely affected. Rigid contracture and atrophy of the hindlimb musculature can follow.
  (b) Laboratory findings
 (i) Serology should reveal a rising serum antibody titer. Antibodies to *N. caninum* can be detected in CSF.
 (ii) CSF analysis reveals a mild elevation in protein concentration and cell count (mostly monocytes and lymphocytes). Occasionally, the organism can be identified within cells in the CSF.
 (iii) Muscle biopsies occasionally reveal the organism.
  (2) Treatment. There is no known treatment for neosporosis. Antimicrobial agents used for toxoplasmosis can be considered.
f. Mycotic infections. Although many fungal organisms can involve the CNS and eyes as part of a systemic infection, only *Cryptococcus neoformans* has a predilection for the CNS.
  (1) Pathogenesis. *C. neoformans* usually gains entry to the CNS through the nose and cribriform plate in cats and hematogenously, secondary to disseminated disease, in dogs.
  (2) Diagnosis
  (a) Clinical findings. Depression, seizures, and chronic rhinitis are common clinical signs.
  (b) Laboratory findings
 (i) Serology. Cryptococcal capsular antigen may be detected in serum or CSF using a latex agglutination test.
 (ii) CSF analysis usually reveals an elevated protein concentration and cell count (mostly neutrophils), and the organism may be detected in CSF in about 60% of the cases. A fungal culture of the CSF may also detect the organism.
 (iii) Cytology. It may be possible to detect the organism in other samples, such as nasal discharge.

(3) **Treatment** may be attempted with ketoconazole, amphotericin B, flucyto-sine, fluconazole, or itraconazole, but the prognosis with cryptococcal CNS infection is poor.

g. **Rickettsial infection.** Rocky Mountain spotted fever (caused by *Rickettsia rickett-sii*) and ehrlichiosis (caused by *Ehrlichia canis*) result in meningoencephalomye-litis in about 30% of infected dogs.

(1) **Diagnosis**

(a) **Clinical findings**

(i) **Neurologic signs** are more severe (acute and progressive) with Rocky Mountain spotted fever and can include cervical pain, hyper-esthesia, changes in mental status, ataxia, vestibular signs, stupor, and seizures.

(ii) **Systemic signs** (e.g., depression, fever, lymphadenopathy, vomiting, oculonasal discharge) always accompany CNS signs.

(b) **Laboratory findings.** Both types of rickettsial infections result in an in-crease in CSF protein concentration and cell count, but neutrophils pre-dominate in Rocky Mountain spotted fever, and lymphocytes predomi-nate in ehrlichiosis.

(2) **Treatment.** Tetracycline, doxycycline (which has good CNS penetration), or chloramphenicol are acceptable antimicrobial choices. The response to treat-ment is usually rapid, but significant neurologic involvement will slow recov-ery. Some neurologic deficits may be permanent.

h. **Bacterial meningitis** is rare in dogs and cats. Encephalomyelitis is usually a fea-ture.

(1) **Pathogenesis.** Bacteria (usually *Pasteurella, Staphylococcus , Actinomyces*, or *Nocardia*) can enter the CNS by local extension (e.g., from the ears, nose, or eyes) or hematogenously (e.g., secondary to bacteremia from infections such as endocarditis or prostatitis).

(2) **Diagnosis.** Definitive diagnosis requires the observation of bacteria in the CSF or a positive CSF culture, but a presumptive diagnosis can be based on suggestive clinical and laboratory findings.

(a) **Clinical findings** can include cervical pain, nuchal (neck) rigidity, hyper-esthesia, fever, vomiting, depression, anorexia, bradycardia, seizures, pa-resis, blindness, and vestibular signs. An extraneural focus for the infec-tion may be found. Animals may be hypotensive, in shock, or develop disseminated intravascular coagulation (DIC).

(b) **Laboratory findings**

(i) **Complete blood count (CBC).** A CBC may be normal or reveal a neutrophilic leukocytosis (with or without a left shift).

(ii) **CSF analysis** may reveal an increased (often marked) CSF protein concentration and cell count (mostly neutrophils). Neutrophils may be degenerate and intra- or extracellular bacteria may be detected.

(iii) **Culture** of the CSF for bacteria may be positive, but negative cul-tures are common. Alternatively, if an extraneural focus (e.g., blood, urine) of infection is found, it can be cultured and the re-sults used to guide antimicrobial selection.

(3) **Treatment.** Bacterial meningitis is potentially life-threatening and should be treated promptly and aggressively.

(a) **Antimicrobials** should be selected on the basis of culture and sensitivity results, should be bactericidal, and should be administered intrave-nously during initial therapy. Therapy should continue for 2–4 weeks be-yond the resolution of clinical signs.

(i) **Chloramphenicol, trimethoprim/sulfadiazine,** and **metronidazole** reach therapeutic concentrations within the CNS.

(ii) **Ampicillin** and **penicillin** penetrate well only if significant inflamma-tion is present.

(iii) Some second- and third-generation cephalosporins (e.g., **moxalac-tam, cefotaxime**) also penetrate reasonably well.

(b) **Supportive care** will be required in many cases.

(c) Corticosteroid therapy (usually contraindicated in infection) is controversial. If used during the first 24 hours of antibiotic therapy, corticosteroids may ultimately reduce the degree of CNS damage and hasten recovery.

(4) Prognosis is variable. Some animals respond very well to antibiotic therapy and are effectively cured, while others respond slowly to treatment, develop relapsed infection, or have debilitating or fatal complications (e.g., DIC, severe neurologic deficits).

3. Noninfectious causes

a. Granulomatous meningoencephalitis (GME), a progressive inflammatory disease (or group of diseases) of unknown etiology that can occur in a disseminated, focal, or ocular form, may be one of the most common inflammatory diseases of the CNS in dogs. The **disseminated form** tends to involve the lower brain stem, cervical spinal cord, and meninges. The **focal form** mostly affects the cerebral cortex, cerebellopontine angle, and the cervical spinal cord. The **ocular form** primarily affects the optic nerves, resulting in optic neuritis.

(1) Predisposition. GME tends to affect small-breed dogs 1–8 years of age. Females may be affected more often. The disorder is rare in cats.

(2) Diagnosis is based on suggestive clinical and laboratory findings. Definitive diagnosis requires histopathology, but tissue samples are rarely obtained antemortem. Many infectious causes of CNS inflammation can appear similar to GME and should be ruled out.

(a) Clinical findings

(i) Disseminated disease tends to have a rapid onset (i.e., over a period of weeks). Signs can include ataxia, circling, depression, fever, cervical pain, vestibular signs, facial or trigeminal nerve paralysis, visual deficits, and seizures.

(ii) Focal disease produces signs of a localized mass lesion and will reflect the area involved (most commonly the cerebellopontine angle). Onset is slow and insidious (over months).

(iii) Ocular disease produces primarily acute unilateral or bilateral blindness due to optic neuritis.

(b) Laboratory findings. CSF analysis is most useful in the disseminated form. Changes usually include increased protein concentration and a mild to moderate increase in the cell count. About 60%–80% of the cells are lymphocytes, 10%–20% are monocytes or macrophages, and 10%–20% are neutrophils. Changes in the CSF may be minimal with focal disease.

(c) Diagnostic imaging findings. CT or MRI should identify focal disease.

(3) Treatment. Corticosteroids given initially in immunosuppressive doses reduce clinical signs but usually do not resolve them. Other **immunosuppressive drugs** (e.g., azathioprine, cyclophosphamide) may improve and prolong remission, but the disease usually continues to progress despite therapy. The prognosis is guarded to poor.

b. Pug meningoencephalitis is a breed-specific form of GME. Pug dogs 9 months to 7 years of age are most often affected.

(1) Diagnosis is based on clinical signs, laboratory findings, and breed.

(a) Clinical findings are usually acute in onset and are referable to cerebral and meningeal involvement. Seizures, circling, dementia, depression, cortical blindness, head pressing, cervical pain, and ataxia may develop. The signs progress rapidly in most dogs (e.g., over 5–7 days); death usually results from intractable seizures or coma. Some dogs have a slower progression of signs over several weeks to months.

(b) Laboratory findings. CSF analysis reveals a mixed inflammatory response.

(2) Treatment. There is no effective treatment. Clinical signs in some dogs improve transiently with corticosteroid therapy. Survival for more than 6 months after diagnosis has not been documented.

c. Steroid-responsive (aseptic) suppurative meningitis is the most common form of meningitis diagnosed in dogs. Large-breed dogs younger than 2 years are most commonly affected.

(1) **Etiology.** The cause is unknown, but aseptic suppurative meningitis is suspected to have an immune-mediated basis.

(2) **Diagnosis** is based on clinical findings, CSF analysis, and a negative CSF bacterial culture.

    (a) **Clinical findings.** Signs of fever, cervical pain, and rigidity are common and may wax and wane. Other neurologic signs are uncommon.

    (b) **Laboratory findings**

        (i) **CBC.** A neutrophilic leukocytosis may be present.

        (ii) **CSF analysis.** Typical findings include a marked increase in the protein concentration and cell count. Nondegenerate neutrophils predominate. Bacterial culture is negative. CSF may be normal very early in the course of the illness.

(3) **Treatment.** Dogs are not responsive to antimicrobial therapy. **Corticosteroids** at immunosuppressive doses result in a reliable and rapid improvement in clinical signs. Corticosteroid therapy should be tapered off over 1–2 months. Occasionally, relapses occur and may require a more prolonged (4- to 6-month) course of therapy.

(4) **Prognosis.** The prognosis is very good. Most dogs do not require long-term corticosteroid therapy and will not experience a relapse.

  d. Breed-associated meningeal vasculitis is a severe necrotizing vasculitis recognized in beagles, Bernese mountain dogs, and German short-haired pointers. Clinical signs include cervical pain and fever. CSF changes consist of an elevated protein concentration and a marked increase in neutrophils. Treatment is with corticosteroids at an immunosuppressive dose. Some Bernese mountain dogs and most German short-haired pointers achieve long-term remission after several months of corticosteroid therapy, but severely affected dogs have a guarded prognosis.

  e. Feline polioencephalomyelitis is an uncommon disorder of unknown etiology. Cats 3 months to 6 years of age are most often affected. Clinical signs associated with spinal cord dysfunction progress over 2–3 months and can include hindlimb ataxia, paresis, and hyporeflexia. Intention tremors of the head and seizures can also occur. Laboratory findings are normal. Definitive diagnosis is made at necropsy. Treatment of affected cats has not been reported, and the prognosis is poor.

H. Idiopathic disorders

  1. Idiopathic epilepsy is the most common cause of seizures in dogs in most practices. It is less common in cats. Idiopathic epilepsy represents a functional disturbance in the brain and is not associated with any identifiable macroscopic or microscopic lesions in the CNS.

    a. Predisposition. Idiopathic epilepsy is probably related to an inherited predisposition in most animals; hence, it is relatively prevalent in many breeds of purebred dogs. Breeds with a high incidence include German shepherds, poodles, keeshonds, Irish setters, Saint Bernards, Labrador retrievers, golden retrievers, colony-bred beagles, wire-haired fox terriers, and cocker spaniels.

    b. Diagnosis. Idiopathic epilepsy is a diagnosis of exclusion— other causes of epilepsy must be ruled out (see Table 24-1).

    (1) **Clinical findings.** Seizures typically begin between 9 and 36 months of age and almost always before 5 years of age. If seizures begin before 9 months or after 5 years of age, idiopathic epilepsy is unlikely. Animals are clinically normal between seizure events, and physical and neurologic examinations are normal between seizure episodes.

        (a) Small-breed dogs tend to have **isolated generalized seizures** that gradually increase in frequency over many months to years.

        (b) Large-breed dogs have a tendency to develop **cluster seizures** (several generalized seizures in rapid succession; e.g., 10 seizures over 1 or a few days). In large-breed dogs the seizure events progress at a faster rate to become more frequent and more severe than in small-breed dogs.

   (c) **Status epilepticus,** a state of almost constant seizure activity in which the animal does not regain consciousness between seizures, will occasionally develop. This is potentially life-threatening because spasm of respiratory muscles interferes with respiration.

   (2) **Laboratory findings.** No abnormalities are apparent on a CBC, serum biochemical profile, urinalysis, or CSF analysis.

   (3) **Treatment** with anticonvulsant medication usually begins when the seizure frequency is greater than one seizure every 4–6 weeks, or earlier if the seizures are especially severe or prolonged (i.e., cluster seizures).

   (a) **Phenobarbital** is the initial drug of choice. Serum phenobarbital concentrations should be monitored at regular intervals, beginning 7–10 days after initiating therapy. Phenobarbital has a long half-life and any dosage change will take 7–10 days before a new steady state plasma concentration is reached. The side effects of phenobarbital therapy include sedation, polyuria/polydipsia, polyphagia, and elevated liver enzymes.

   (b) **Potassium bromide** can be added if seizure activity cannot be controlled with phenobarbital alone or serum concentrations are exceeding the therapeutic range.

   (4) **Prognosis.** Most dogs can be adequately controlled with anticonvulsant medications and have a good quality of life, especially small-breed dogs. Seizure activity in large-breed dogs often becomes more difficult to control over time.

2. **Idiopathic tremor syndrome (white shaker dog syndrome)** is characterized by the acute onset of diffuse tremors of the entire body. The etiology is unknown.

   a. **Predisposition.** Idiopathic tremor syndrome occurs most often in young to middle-aged West Highland white terriers, Maltese, Bichons Frisé, and poodles.

   b. **Clinical findings.** Body tremors (which can be severe and debilitating in some dogs), chaotic random eye movements, and hyperthermia (secondary to the tremors) may occur.

   c. **Treatment.** Some animals require prolonged therapy. Others may have residual tremors after therapy for the rest of their lives.

   (1) **Corticosteroid therapy** is usually effective for resolving clinical signs, and dosages are gradually reduced over several months.

   (2) **Diazepam** may benefit some patients via its muscle-relaxant properties.

3. **Prognosis.** The prognosis is good. Most dogs recover completely if treated early.

I. **Traumatic disorders.** Head trauma is a common occurrence in dogs and cats. Damage to the brain occurs as a result of direct injury and the development of secondary events such as increased intracranial pressure, brain edema, and CNS hypoxia. Seizures are a common acute sequela but can also arise later in life.

1. **Diagnosis** of head trauma is not difficult, but many patients have multiple traumatic injuries, some more immediately life-threatening than CNS malfunction.

   a. **Clinical findings.** To varying degrees, trauma to the brain can:

   (1) Alter motor activity (producing hemiparesis, tetraparesis, or decorticate rigidity)

   (2) Affect brain stem reflexes

   (3) Alter pupil size, pupil responsiveness, and the oculovestibular reflex (i.e., the normal ocular nystagmus that accompanies movement of the head from side to side)

   (4) Alter mental status (rendering the animal alert, depressed, stuporous, or comatose)

   b. **Imaging findings.** A CT or MRI scan can identify a subdural hematoma if one develops.

2. **Treatment.** After basic life-support measures have been instituted, therapy for head trauma should be promptly carried out. The immediate goals of therapy are to **reduce brain edema** and **lower the intracranial pressure.**

a. **Medical therapy.** Measures to reduce brain edema and decrease the intracranial pressure include **elevating the head** (to encourage passive venous drainage), administering **supplemental oxygen** (to reduce CNS hypoxia), administering **corticosteroids** (to reduce brain edema and the intracranial pressure), and administering **diuretics** such as furosemide (to reduce the intracranial pressure). **Intubation** and **hyperventilation** [to reduce the arterial carbon dioxide tension ($Paco_2$), which in turn induces cerebral vasoconstriction and decreases the intracranial pressure] and additional diuretic therapy (e.g., with mannitol) may benefit deteriorating patients.

b. **Surgical therapy. Reduction of severe compressive skull fractures** is also indicated. Subdural hematomas may require **surgical decompression.**

c. **Supportive care** and frequent turning of recumbent patients are indicated.

3. **Prognosis** is related to the location of predominant damage in the brain and whether the neurologic signs are progressing or improving over the first 12–48 hours.

   a. **Location of the injury**
      (1) Animals with cerebral injury have a fair prognosis.
      (2) Animals with cerebellar injury have a fair to good prognosis.
      (3) Animals with brain stem injury have a poor prognosis.

   b. **Progression of signs.** Prognosis is poor when the animal has been comatose for longer than 48 hours or exhibits rapidly deteriorating mentation, dilating pupils, progressive paresis, bradycardia, and loss of the oculovestibular reflex. These signs may indicate brain herniation.

J. Toxic disorders

1. **Lead poisoning** occurs more commonly in dogs than in cats.

   a. **Etiology.** Lead poisoning usually results from the ingestion of a lead-containing material such as lead-based paints, linoleum, automobile batteries, lead fishing weights, plumbers putty, roofing felt, or the use of improperly glazed ceramic water bowls.

   b. **Diagnosis**
      (1) **Clinical findings.** Signs are primarily GI (vomiting, anorexia, diarrhea, abdominal pain) and neurologic in origin. Neurologic signs can include depression, seizures, hysteria or dementia (continuous barking or whining, snapping at imaginary objects), ataxia, blindness, and jaw champing. Megaesophagus occasionally develops as a result of a lead-induced neuropathy.
      (2) **Laboratory and radiographic findings.** A definitive diagnosis is based on elevated blood lead concentrations. Other features that may suggest lead poisoning are basophilic stippling of red blood cells (RBCs), excessive numbers of nucleated RBCs in the absence of severe anemia, and radiopaque material in the GI tract.

   c. **Treatment**
      (1) **Removal of objects. Magnesium** or **sodium sulfate cathartics** can aid in the removal of small radiopaque objects within the bowel. **Surgical** or **endoscopic removal** of lead-containing objects within the bowel may be justified in some cases, depending on size and location.
      (2) **Chelation** with **calcium ethylenediamine tetraacetic acid (EDTA)** is indicated to remove accumulated lead within the body. Calcium EDTA binds lead and enhances its excretion in the urine. It is generally administered for 5 days, stopped for 5 days, then given again for 5 days if needed. **d-Penicillamine** will also chelate lead and can be used for prolonged therapy after calcium EDTA administration or in cases where only mild exposure is suspected. Most animals respond favorably to chelation therapy within 24–36 hours.
      (3) **Symptomatic treatment. Thiamine** may help alleviate some of the clinical signs.

   d. **Prognosis.** The prognosis is fair to good.

2. **Metronidazole toxicity.** Metronidazole, a commonly used antimicrobial drug in

dogs and cats, readily crosses the blood–brain barrier and can accumulate within the CNS, resulting in toxicity. Toxic signs in dogs and cats have been associated with high doses administered for longer than 5–10 days.

   a. Diagnosis is made on a history of drug administration and signs. Neurologic signs develop acutely and can include ataxia, weakness, diminished postural reflexes, disorientation, seizures, and apparent blindness.

   b. Treatment. Withdrawal of the drug usually results in an improvement within 48 hours, and most animals make a complete recovery.

3. **Strychnine poisoning.** Strychnine is commonly used in baits for rodents and coyotes (although its use may be decreasing in some areas). Strychnine is thought to competitively inhibit the inhibitory neurotransmitter glycine, resulting in uncontrolled muscular activity.

   a. Diagnosis is made by characteristic clinical signs and a history of exposure.

   (1) Clinical findings. Clinical signs occur within 15 minutes to 2 hours after ingestion and include nervousness and apprehension followed by severe tetanic seizures (i.e., stiff extension of the legs and body). Seizure episodes may be triggered by noise, bright light, and touch. The seizures get progressively worse and death results from respiratory muscle spasm or paralysis.

   (2) Laboratory findings. Definitive diagnosis may be made by analysis of stomach contents for strychnine.

   b. Treatment consists of the induction of emesis (if seizure activity is not present), gastric lavage with activated charcoal, anticonvulsant therapy (i.e., diazepam and/or pentobarbital as needed), and intravenous fluid administration to enhance toxin excretion.

4. **Organophosphates** and **carbamate poisoning.** Chlorpyrifos, malathion, diazinon, fenthion, and ronnel are commonly used in insecticide preparations for use as animal dips and sprays or for home and garden use. These substances are cholinesterase inhibitors, which result in the accumulation of excessive amounts of acetylcholine at neuromuscular junctions throughout the body. Exposure can occur by absorption through the skin or ingestion.

   a. Diagnosis is based on a history of exposure and characteristic clinical signs.

   (1) Clinical findings. Signs of toxicity are caused by excessive cholinergic activity and usually occur within minutes to an hour.

   (a) Salivation, lacrimation, urination, and **defecation (SLUD)** are typical findings.

   (b) Diffuse muscle fasciculations, constricted pupils, dyspnea (caused by bronchoconstriction, excessive respiratory secretions, and pulmonary edema), convulsions, depression, weakness, and paralysis also occur in many animals. Death is due to respiratory paralysis and pulmonary edema.

   (2) Laboratory findings. A definitive diagnosis can be made by analyzing anticholinesterase levels in stomach contents or serum.

   b. Treatment

   (1) Toxin removal through bathing (topical exposure) or induction of emesis and gastric lavage with activated charcoal will decrease absorption.

   (2) Atropine and **pralidoxime chloride (2-PAM)** help reverse the cholinesterase inhibition and clinical signs, usually within minutes. 2-PAM should be administered within 12–24 hours of exposure.

   (3) Supplemental oxygen may be required for animals in respiratory distress.

5. **Metaldehyde poisoning.** Metaldehyde is commonly used in snail and slug bait.

   a. Diagnosis is based on a history of ingestion and compatible clinical signs. Metaldehyde poisoning may be difficult to differentiate from other toxicities.

   (1) Clinical findings

   (a) Hypersalivation, abdominal pain, tremors, hyperesthesia, nystagmus (most severe in cats), incoordination, and hyperthermia (from muscle activity) are characteristic.

   (b) Tonic–clonic seizures are common with moderate to severe intoxication but are not stimulated by noise or touch as they are with strychnine poisoning. Metabolic (lactic) acidosis can develop secondary to seizure activity.

  (c) Cholinergic signs [see II J 4 a (1)] may also be present because carbamates may also be included in commercial bait preparations.

  (d) A formaldehyde-like odor may be detected on the breath.

  (2) Laboratory findings. Definitive diagnosis requires analysis of stomach contents for metaldehyde or acetaldehyde.

b. Treatment. Measures include inducing emesis (if the animal is not seizuring), gastric lavage with activated charcoal, diazepam and/or pentobarbital to control seizures, intravenous fluid therapy to enhance urinary excretion, treatment of metabolic acidosis (if required) and supportive care.

6. Other toxicities. Other toxins that can be associated with prominent neurologic signs include organochlorine (chlorinated hydrocarbon) compounds, ethylene glycol, zinc phosphide, pyrethroids, salicylates, bromethalin, solvents, and plant toxicants.

K. Vascular disorders

1. General considerations

  a. Etiology. Vascular disorders of the CNS arise from either **hemorrhage** or **ischemia.** Most vascular injuries in the CNS result from systemic illnesses such as sepsis, hypothyroidism, coagulopathies, or head trauma.

  b. Diagnosis

  (1) Clinical findings. Vascular events are usually acute in onset and result in focal neurologic signs.

  (2) Laboratory findings

  (a) In patients with ischemic injury, CSF analysis usually reveals a mild to moderate elevation in protein and a minimal alteration in the cell count. Severe necrosis may elevate CSF leukocyte numbers.

  (b) Increased numbers of erythrocytes, erythrophagocytosis, and xanthochromia may be observed following hemorrhage.

  (3) Diagnostic imaging findings. CT or MRI may demonstrate a mass effect associated with the area of hemorrhage or infarction.

  c. Treatment includes supportive care and corticosteroids. The administration of diuretics (to help reduce brain edema) and anticonvulsant drugs (to control seizures) may be required.

  d. Prognosis. The prognosis depends on the nature of any systemic illnesses and the location and extent of the CNS injury.

2. Feline ischemic encephalopathy is a sporadic disease of unknown etiology that affects adult cats. Most cases occur in the northeastern United States in the late summer. The middle cerebral artery is most commonly affected.

  a. Diagnosis

  (1) Clinical findings. A peracute onset of neurologic signs can include severe dementia, aggression, circling (to the side of the lesion), seizures, proprioceptive deficits, and cortical blindness (on the side opposite the lesion).

  (2) Laboratory findings. Analysis of CSF is normal, but the protein concentration may be mildly elevated in some cats.

  b. Treatment is primarily supportive. Anticonvulsant therapy is indicated for seizures.

  c. Prognosis. Most cats improve dramatically within 2–7 days, and most make a complete recovery. Aggression may persist in some cats, necessitating euthanasia.

III. DISORDERS OF THE SPINAL CORD

A. Localizing signs. Signs occur simultaneously because most spinal cord diseases affect multiple spinal tracts. An abnormality occurring in isolation would make spinal cord dis-

ease unlikely. Strictly unilateral signs are rare with spinal cord disease, but asymmetric signs are common.

1. **Lesions.** Animals with spinal cord disease have reduced or absent voluntary motor activity, altered spinal reflexes (indicative of UMN or LMN abnormalities), altered muscle tone, muscle atrophy, and sensory dysfunction.

    a. **UMN involvement** is generally present when there is paresis, paralysis, or proprioceptive deficits and when spinal reflexes are normal to hyperreflexic.

    b. **LMN involvement** is present when there is paresis, paralysis, or proprioceptive deficits and when spinal reflexes are absent or hyporeflexic.

2. **Localization of lesions.** Because the spinal cord ends before the vertebral column does, spinal cord segments are shifted cranially relative to their corresponding vertebral body (Figure 47-3). Therefore, designations such as "cervical," "thoracic," and "lumbar" indicate spinal cord segments, not vertebral bodies. Localization of lesions within the spinal cord is primarily based on the occurrence of UMN or LMN signs in the fore- and hindlimbs.

    a. **C1–C5 lesions** produce UMN signs in all four limbs. (Disorders that can cause lesions in the C1–C5 area are listed in Table 47-4.)

        (1) Associated signs can include cervical pain and rigidity, tetraparesis or hemiparesis, increased muscle tone and muscle atrophy in all limbs, ataxia, and proprioceptive and postural deficits in all limbs.

        (2) Voluntary control of urination and defecation may be absent.

        (3) Perineal reflexes as well as cutaneous and deep pain sensation are usually normal.

        (4) Severe damage in this area can result in respiratory paralysis and death.

    b. **C6–T2 lesions** produce UMN signs in the hindlimbs and LMN signs in the forelimbs. (Disorders that can cause lesions in the C6–T2 region are listed in Table 47-4.)

        (1) Associated signs can include cervical pain, thoracic limb lameness, "root signature" (i.e., compression of a nerve root causes the animal to hold the forelimb off the ground), tetraparesis or hemiparesis, normal to increased muscle tone in the hindlimbs, normal to decreased muscle tone (with or without denervation atrophy) in the forelimbs, and ataxia. Postural and proprioceptive deficits may occur in all limbs or in a forelimb and the ipsilateral hindlimb. Unilateral Horner's syndrome may occur.

        (2) Voluntary control of urination and defecation may be absent.

        (3) Perineal reflexes are normal. Cutaneous and deep pain sensation may be normal, decreased, or absent in the forelimbs and hindlimbs.

    c. **T3–L3 lesions** produce UMN signs in the hindlimbs. The forelimbs are normal. (Disorders that can cause lesions in the T3–L3 region are listed in Table 47-4.)

        (1) Associated signs can include apparent back pain (with or without a focal area of hyperpathia or pain), hindlimb paresis or paralysis and increased muscle tone (with or without disuse atrophy), and ataxia in the hindlimbs. There are proprioceptive and postural deficits in one or both hind limbs.

        (2) Voluntary control of urination and defecation may be absent.

        (3) Perineal reflexes are normal. Cutaneous and deep pain sensation may be normal, reduced, or absent in the hindlimbs. Spinal reflexes, motor activity, muscle tone, proprioception, postural reactions and pain sensation are all normal in the forelimbs.

        (4) The Schiff-Sherrington sign may accompany severe injury in this area.

    d. **L4–Cd5 lesions** produce LMN signs in the hindlimbs. The forelimbs are normal. (Disorders that can cause lesions in the T3–L3 region are listed in Table 47-4.)

        (1) Associated signs can include lumbar or lumbosacral pain (with or without a focal area of pain), hindlimb lameness, difficulty sitting or rising, hindlimb paresis or paralysis and ataxia, paralysis of the tail, and normal to decreased muscle tone in the hindlimbs (with or without denervation atrophy). Proprioception and postural reactions are reduced in the hind limbs.

        (2) Urinary and fecal incontinence may occur as a consequence of flaccid paralysis of the urinary bladder and urethral and anal sphincter.

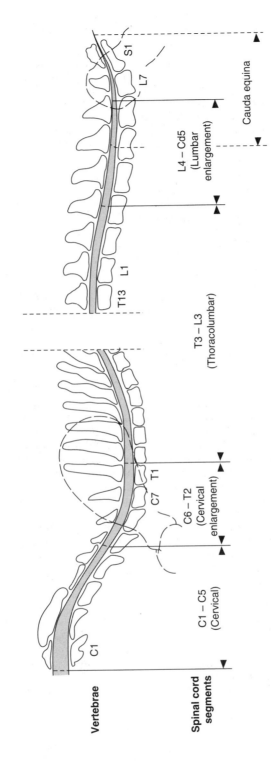

FIGURE 47-3. The anatomic relationship of the vertebrae to spinal cord segments. (Redrawn with permission from LeCouteur RA and Child G: Diseases of the spinal cord. In *Textbook of Veterinary Internal Medicine*, 4th ed. Edited by Ettinger SJ and Feldman EC. Philadelphia, WB Saunders, 1995, p 636.)

TABLE 47-4. Common Disorders Affecting Spinal Cord Regions

C1–C5	C6–T2	T3–L3	L4–Cd5
Atlantoaxial subluxation	Congenital vertebral anomalies	Congenital vertebral anomalies	Spina bifida
Congenital vertebral anomalies	Intervertebral disk disease	Intervertebral disk disease	Sacrococcygeal dysgenesis
Intervertebral disk disease	Discospondylitis	Discospondylitis	Intervertebral disk disease
Cervical spondylomyelopathy (wobbler syndrome)	Cervical spondylomyelopathy (wobbler syndrome)	Canine distemper myelitis	Lumbosacral stenosis
Steroid-responsive meningitis	Neoplasia	FIP meningitis or myelitis	Discospondylitis
Granulomatous meningoencephalitis (GME)	Trauma	Neoplasia	Protozoal myelitis (e.g., toxoplasmosis, neosporosis)
Feline infectious peritonitis (FIP) meningitis or myelitis	Fibrocartilaginous embolism	Trauma	Neoplasia
Discospondylitis		Fibrocartilaginous embolism	Trauma
Canine distemper myelitis			Fibrocartilaginous embolism
Neoplasia			
Trauma			
Fibrocartilaginous embolism			

    (3) Perineal reflexes may be normal, reduced, or absent. Cutaneous and deep pain sensation may be normal, reduced, or absent in the hindlimbs (with or without perineum and tail involvement).

    (4) The Schiff-Sherrington sign may occur with severe injuries in this area.

B. Degenerative disorders

    1. Intervertebral disk disease is one of the most common diseases affecting the spinal cord in dogs. It is rare in cats.

        a. Types. Degeneration of intervertebral disks can result in extrusion or protrusion of disk material into the spinal canal and cause compression of the spinal cord or nerve roots.

        (1) Acute (type I) disk herniation is caused by the extrusion of degenerated disk material into the spinal canal (chondroid degeneration). Injury to the spinal cord, and therefore the clinical signs, is typically more severe with type I disk herniations than with type II herniations because the velocity and force directed at the spinal cord are greater.

        (a) Chondrodystrophoid dogs (e.g., dachshunds, beagles, Lhasa apsos), poodles, and cocker spaniels over 3 years of age are most often affected.

        (b) Disk extrusion can occur at any level of the spinal cord, although 65% of herniations occur between T11 and L3.

        (2) Chronic (type II) disk herniation is associated with disk degeneration (fibroid degeneration), protrusion, and spinal cord compression.

        (a) Older, large-breed, nonchondrodystrophoid dogs are most often affected, although type II herniation can occur in any breed.

        (b) Chronic herniation is more common in the thoracolumbar region than in the cervical region. When the cervical region is affected, the caudal disks (C4, C5) are more frequently affected. Cervical disk protrusion may accompany cervical spondylomyelopathy.

b. Diagnosis is based on characteristic age, breed, neurologic signs, and radiographic findings.

(1) Clinical findings

(a) Acute (type I) disk herniation. Signs typically develop over minutes to hours, although they may be intermittent over several months or progress slowly over several days.

(i) Thoracolumbar region. Herniation can cause varying signs, from back pain with no neurologic deficits to paralysis. In its most severe form, signs resemble those of complete spinal cord transection with the loss of deep pain sensation. Pain is a consistent and prominent feature in most dogs. An arched back is a manifestation of spinal pain (also of abdominal pain), and a localized area of hyperpathia over the affected disk may be detected. UMN and LMN signs may occur and depend on the site of damage. Signs may be asymmetric.

(ii) Cervical region. Herniation in the cervical region is associated with less severe signs than herniation in the thoracolumbar region; the larger vertebral canal in the cervical region may be responsible for the less severe signs (i.e., there is less spinal cord damage and compression). Cervical pain is the most common sign, and marked neurologic deficits are uncommon. Some dogs develop forelimb lameness and a "root signature."

(b) Chronic (type II) disk herniation. Onset is chronic (over several weeks to months) and is usually associated with slowly progressive signs, although acute signs may occur. Spinal cord compression may result in ataxia, proprioceptive deficits, and paresis of the hindlimbs or all limbs. Pain can be present but is less prominent than with acute herniations.

(2) Laboratory findings. CSF analysis is usually normal, but a mild elevation in protein may occur.

(3) Diagnostic imaging findings

(a) Acute (type I) disk herniation

(i) Signs can include a narrowed or wedge-shaped disk space, a small or cloudy intervertebral foramen (from extruded disk material), narrowed facetal joints, and calcified material within the spinal canal. Calcified disks indicate disk degeneration but not necessarily herniation (unless the disk is obviously displaced).

(ii) A myelogram is often required to specifically localize the area of spinal cord compression prior to surgery. Disk herniation appears as an extradural compressive lesion.

(b) Chronic (type II) disk herniation. Signs can include disk space narrowing, sclerosis of vertebral endplates, and osteophyte formation. Calcification of disks is rare. Radiographic changes are usually evident in many disk spaces, so a myelogram is usually required to localize the site of cord compression and to rule out other causes of compression (e.g., neoplasia).

(4) Differential diagnoses

(a) Acute (type I) disk herniation. Common differential diagnoses include fibrocartilaginous embolism and trauma.

(b) Chronic (type II) disk herniation. Common differential diagnoses include neoplasia, degenerative myelopathy, and cervical spondylomyelopathy.

c. Treatment

(1) Acute (type I) disk herniation. Treatment can be primarily medical or surgical, depending on the severity of clinical signs.

(a) Cervical or thoracolumbar pain with no neurologic deficits

(i) Strict exercise restriction with only short leash walks outside is indicated for a minimum of 2 weeks.

(ii) If pain is severe, corticosteroids can be considered, but if used, strict cage rest for 5–7 days is recommended, followed by stringent exercise restriction at home for several more weeks. Anti-inflammatory or analgesic drugs are generally avoided because if mobility does not cause the animal pain, the animal may be too active, exacerbating the injury.

(b) Pain and mild neurologic deficits

(i) **Strict exercise restriction** and **corticosteroid therapy** (e.g., dexamethasone for 3 days) to decrease spinal cord swelling and edema are indicated.

(ii) **Surgery** is indicated if neurologic signs do not resolve or progress in 5–7 days.

(c) Severe neurologic deficits

(i) Immediate **corticosteroid therapy** (e.g., dexamethasone intravenously) and **surgical decompression** (e.g., dorsal laminectomy) are indicated. Corticosteroid therapy is continued for 2–3 days after surgery, then discontinued.

(ii) Postoperative care of paraplegic patients involves good nursing care, soft bedding, passive physiotherapy, supervised exercise (e.g., towel walking, swimming) and frequent emptying of the urinary bladder.

(d) Recurrent pain. Patients with recurrent pain and evidence of disk degeneration on radiographs are considered candidates for **prophylactic fenestration** (i.e., removal of disk material through a ventral approach to the intervertebral space). Prophylactic fenestration may prevent additional disk herniation in high-risk spinal regions (i.e., C2–3 to C6–7 and T11–12 to L3–4) and may be more beneficial in animals with cervical disk disease.

(2) Chronic (type II) disk herniation

(a) Corticosteroids may produce improvement but will not usually resolve the neurologic deficits. Acupuncture may aid in pain management; however, it should not replace or delay surgical procedures.

(b) Surgery is usually indicated to stabilize the neurologic status. Even with surgery, neurologic function rarely normalizes, and improvement may take months. Following surgery in some animals, neurologic signs may temporarily or permanently worsen.

(i) A dorsal laminectomy or hemilaminectomy is performed in the thoracolumbar region.

(ii) Ventral decompressive procedures are used most often in the cervical region.

(iii) Fenestration may also be performed.

d. Prognosis

(1) Acute (type I) disk herniation. Severe neurologic signs, rapid onset of signs, and a delay in surgical decompression all adversely affect the outcome. In general, the length of time from the onset of clinical signs to surgical decompression is directly proportional to prognosis (i.e., as more time passes, the prognosis worsens).

(a) The prognosis is fair to very good in dogs that retain deep pain sensation following decompressive procedures.

(b) The prognosis is poor if deep pain sensation has been absent for less than 48 hours. Up to 50% (depending on the promptness of surgical decompression) of these dogs regain the ability to walk, but retain significant neurologic deficits. If deep pain sensation has been absent for longer than 48 hours, the dog (>95% of cases) will be permanently paralyzed.

(c) The prognosis is also poor in dogs that show no improvement in neurologic signs within 3 weeks of decompressive surgery.

(2) Chronic (type II) disk herniation. The prognosis for a return to normal neurologic function is guarded, although if signs can be stabilized or improved, then a reasonably good quality of life may be possible.

2. Cervical spondylomyelopathy, also known as **wobbler syndrome, cervical vertebral instability, cervical vertebral malformation or malarticulation, cervical spondylopa-**

thy, and **cervical vertebral stenosis,** is a disease of large-breed dogs, most notably Great Danes younger than 2 years and Doberman pinschers between the ages of 3 and 9 years.

a. **Pathogenesis.** Chronic compression of the cervical spinal cord results in ataxia and tetraparesis. Spinal cord compression may occur ventrally from a hypertrophied ligamentum flavum, dorsally from a hypertrophied dorsal annulus fibrosus, laterally by malformed articular facets, and circumferentially by vertebral canal stenosis. Disk herniation may accompany this syndrome.

b. **Diagnosis** is based on the breed and neurologic and radiographic findings.

  (1) **Clinical findings.** The onset of clinical signs is insidious and slowly progressive over months to years. Neurologic signs are consistent with a C1–C5 lesion although the actual site of compression may be slightly caudal.

   (a) Neurologic signs are first noted in the hindlimbs and include ataxia with postural and proprioceptive deficits. Difficultly rising from a sitting or recumbent position may be noted. Spinal reflexes in the hindlimbs are normal to hyperreflexic.

   (b) Mild ataxia progresses to severe ataxia with a wide-based stance and dragging of the paws. The forelimbs are involved, but not as severely as the hind limbs.

   (c) Some chronically affected dogs develop a choppy forelimb gait with rigid flexion of the neck. These dogs may resist manipulation of the neck, but pain does not seem to be present.

  (2) **Laboratory findings.** Analysis of CSF is normal.

  (3) **Radiographic findings**

   (a) **Survey radiographs** may be normal. Visible abnormalities include tipping of the cranial aspect of the vertebra into the spinal canal, collapse of one or more disk spaces, calcification of one or more disks, remodeling of vertebrae resulting in stenosis at the cranial aspect of vertebral bodies, sclerosis of vertebral endplates, and degenerative changes in the articular facets.

   (b) **"Stress" radiography** (i.e., flexion of the neck to demonstrate spinal cord compression) or **"traction" radiography** (i.e., placement of traction on the spine to reduce the compressive lesion) may be required to adequately demonstrate the lesion. However, the results of "stress" procedures may be misinterpreted and these procedures can cause additional injury to the spinal cord.

   (c) **Myelography** is required to determine the extent and location of the spinal cord compression, most often located at the C6–C7 and C5–C6 interspaces.

c. **Treatment.** The presence of concurrent disease (e.g., hypothyroidism, cardiomyopathy), not an uncommon finding in Great Danes and Doberman pinschers, may need to be taken into consideration. Untreated dogs will continue to slowly progress.

  (1) **Medical treatment.** Measures include cage rest, exercise restriction, corticosteroid therapy, use of a neck brace to limit cervical movement, and the use of a harness instead of a collar. **Low-dose corticosteroids** may help some dogs for months to years; however, the underlying compression remains.

  (2) **Surgery** (e.g., dorsal laminectomy, ventral slot decompression, ventral stabilization with lag screw fixation, fusion of adjacent vertebral bodies) may be considered if neurologic signs progress or are initially severe.

d. **Prognosis.** The prognosis depends on the rate of disease progression, the severity of clinical signs on initial presentation, the number of sites of spinal cord compression identified radiographically, and the presence or absence of concurrent disease. The overall prognosis is guarded.

  (1) Some dogs can be maintained in a reasonable state for many months to years with medical therapy.

  (2) Animals that are still ambulatory and have mild to moderately severe clinical signs have a fair prognosis for long-term recovery if treated surgically.

3. **Lumbosacral stenosis** is an acquired or congenital syndrome of spinal canal narrowing at the lumbosacral junction that results in compression of the cauda equina region of the spinal cord. **Congenital lumbosacral stenosis** is rare and recognized most often in small-breed dogs. **Acquired lumbosacral stenosis** is a common degenerative disease that affects large-breed, male dogs, especially German shepherds. It is usually diagnosed in dogs 3–7 years of age. The condition is very rare in cats.

   a. **Diagnosis** is based on the characteristic clinical signs and radiographic demonstration of cauda equina compression at the lumbosacral area.

   (1) **Clinical findings** result from compression of the cauda equina.

   (a) Signs are usually insidious and develop over several months. **Lumbosacral pain** (elicited by deep palpation, dorsoflexion of the tail, or caudal extension of the hindlimbs); a **reluctance to sit, jump,** or **climb stairs; difficulty rising; lameness; proprioceptive deficits; muscle atrophy; weakness** and **flexor hyporeflexia** of the hindlimbs (i.e., depressed withdrawal reflexes due to sciatic nerve paresis); and **paralysis of the tail** may be noted. **Paresthesia** or **hyperesthesia of the perineum and tail** can develop and is associated with self-mutilation of the area. **Urinary** or **fecal incontinence** or both may result from pudendal nerve paresis, but this is rare.

   (b) The term **cauda equina syndrome** refers to the set of clinical and neurologic findings that result from cauda equina dysfunction and is sometimes used synonymously with lumbosacral stenosis; however, lumbosacral stenosis is only one of many causes of cauda equina syndrome. Other causes of cauda equina dysfunction include spina bifida, discospondylitis, neoplasia, and intervertebral disk disease.

   (2) **Radiographic findings**

   (a) **Survey radiographs.** Findings can include spondylosis of the lateral and ventral margins of the L7–S1 interspace, narrowing or collapse of the L7–S1 disk space and ventral displacement of S1 relative to L7. However, these findings can be observed in dogs without significant cauda equina compression.

   (b) **Contrast radiographs** (e.g., an epidurogram, diskogram, or transosseous vertebral sinus venogram) are necessary to detect compressive lesions.

   (c) **Myelography** will not adequately outline structures in this area.

   (3) **Electromyographic findings.** Electromyographic examination of the muscles of the hindlimb and perineum can map out denervated areas and help support the diagnosis of a cauda equina dysfunction.

   (4) **Surgical findings.** Surgical exploration may be required in some animals when diagnostic testing is inconclusive.

   b. **Treatment**

   (1) **Mildly affected dogs** or those with only lumbosacral pain may respond to stringent exercise restriction for 4–6 weeks and the use of analgesics or anti-inflammatory drugs. However, signs usually recur.

   (2) **Moderately** to **severely affected dogs** or those with recurrent signs are candidates for surgical treatment (e.g., dorsal decompressive laminectomy with or without foraminotomy or facetectomy, and techniques to stabilize or fuse the lumbosacral junction).

   c. **Prognosis**

   (1) With mild clinical signs, the prognosis for return to normal function following surgery is good.

   (2) With severe neurologic signs, especially flaccid paralysis of the urethral and anal sphincter, the prognosis is guarded to poor.

4. **Degenerative myelopathy** is characterized by progressive hindlimb ataxia and paresis. It is predominantly a disease of middle-aged to older German shepherd or German shepherd mixed-breed dogs although it can occur in other dog breeds and cats. Affected dogs are usually over 6 years of age and males are affected more frequently.

   a. **Pathogenesis.** Degenerative myelopathy results from demyelination and axonal degeneration, primarily affecting the white matter of the thoracic spinal cord. The etiology is unknown.

    b. Diagnosis. Signs include slowly progressive hindlimb ataxia with proprioceptive and postural deficits (i.e., over the course of 6 months to 2 years) and paresis in the presence of normal to hyperreflexic spinal reflexes. Signs are consistent with a T3–L3 spinal cord lesion and may be asymmetric. Spinal pain is not a feature of this disorder, and cutaneous and deep pain sensation are normal. Disuse atrophy of the hindlimb musculature develops, and affected dogs are eventually unable to stand or walk because of the hindlimb paresis.

        (1) Diagnosis is based on the breed, neurologic findings consistent with a T3–L3 lesion, a slowly progressive clinical course, lack of apparent spinal pain, and no radiographic, myelographic, or CSF abnormalities (although some dogs have a mild elevation in protein).

        (2) Degenerative myelopathy is a diagnosis of exclusion. Other diseases such as intervertebral disk disease, neoplasia, and severe musculoskeletal disease (e.g., severe hip dysplasia) must be ruled out.

    c. Treatment. There is no effective treatment. Corticosteroids are not beneficial. Some clinicians advocate the use of vitamin E, aminocaproic acid (an anti-inflammatory agent), or moderate exercise.

    d. Prognosis. The prognosis is poor. Most animals become unable to walk within 1 year of diagnosis.

5. Spondylosis deformans involves the development of osteophytes (bony spurs) around the lateral and ventral margins of multiple vertebral end-plates. Bony proliferation may be so severe that it may appear to bridge the intervertebral space and fuse adjacent vertebrae. Degenerative changes in intervertebral disks may be related to the development of spondylosis deformans. In dogs, vertebrae of the caudal thoracic, lumbar, and lumbosacral region are most commonly affected. In cats, the T7–T8 junction is most commonly affected.

    a. Diagnosis. In most animals, no clinical signs result from the bony proliferation. However in rare instances, a bony spur may result in spinal cord or nerve root compression. If clinical signs are apparent, then other diseases that can cause similar signs must be ruled out before spondylosis is held accountable for the signs. Diagnosis is made by survey radiographs of the spine.

    b. Treatment is not required unless clinical signs are attributed to the bony changes. Decompressive surgery may be required in those rare cases with spinal cord or nerve root compression.

C. | **Anomalous disorders**

1. Spina bifida results when vertebral arches fail to fuse dorsally during embryonic development, leaving an open dorsal cleft in the vertebral column. The defect occurs most commonly over the lumbosacral and sacrococcygeal regions of the spinal cord, and English bulldogs and Manx cats are most commonly affected. Spina bifida may be accompanied by protrusion or dysgenesis of the meninges or spinal cord.

    a. Diagnosis is based on radiographic findings.

        (1) Clinical findings. Spina bifida can be clinically silent if there are no concurrent spinal cord defects. However, if spinal cord defects occur, neurologic signs will be consistent with a lesion in the L4–S3 region. Signs can include paresis, paralysis, proprioceptive deficits, and depressed spinal reflexes in the hind limbs. Fecal and urinary incontinence may occur because of flaccid paralysis of the urethral and anal sphincter.

        (2) Radiographic findings. Survey radiographs are sufficient to visualize the defect in the dorsal vertebral arches.

    b. Treatment. There is none.

2. Atlantoaxial subluxation. Congenital malformation or absence of the dens or traumatic rupture of the ligaments attaching the atlas to the axis can result in instability and subluxation of the axis (C2) relative to the atlas (C1), causing cervical spinal cord compression. Congenital disease occurs most often in young, toy-breed dogs (6–18 months of age).

a. **Diagnosis** is based on radiographic findings.
   (1) **Clinical findings.** Neurologic signs are consistent with a C1–C5 lesion. Cervical pain may or may not develop. The head may be held in a tilted or turned position.
      (a) In dogs with congenital disease, signs often develop slowly and progressively as the ligamentous support of the dens deteriorates.
      (b) Minor trauma in dogs with congenital disease may precipitate acute neurologic signs.
      (c) Severe trauma and fracture of the axis in normal dogs can also result in acute signs.
   (2) **Radiographic findings** are best detected on a lateral radiograph with the neck in a slightly ventroflexed position. The body of the axis is displaced dorsally and cranially relative to the atlas, or the axis may be tilted ventrally (to an excessive degree) relative to the atlas. Lateral and lateral oblique views may demonstrate deformity or absence of the dens.
      (a) Initial radiographs should be taken in an awake animal because sedation or general anesthesia increases the risk of overflexing the head and inducing severe spinal cord injury.
      (b) If initial radiographs are inconclusive, additional radiographs taken under general anesthesia with the head slightly flexed ventrally can be considered. Great caution should be exercised.
b. **Treatment**
   (1) **Splinting** of the head and neck and strict **cage rest** for at least 6 weeks may help animals with only cervical pain or mild neurologic deficits, but clinical signs can recur.
   (2) **Surgical stabilization** or **decompression** is indicated in dogs with recurrent neck pain or moderate to severe neurologic deficits.
c. **Prognosis.** The prognosis is fair to good for those dogs with mild to moderate neurologic deficits. The prognosis is guarded for dogs with an acute onset of tetraplegia.

3. **Congenital vertebral abnormalities** are common and most are not associated with clinical signs. The vertebral anomalies observed most often include **transitional vertebrae, hemivertebrae, butterfly vertebrae, block vertebrae, altered location of the anticlinal vertebra, abnormal number of vertebrae,** and **nonfusion of sacral vertebrae.**
   a. **Diagnosis**
      (1) **Clinical findings.** Hemivertebrae is most likely to result in clinical signs. It may result in spinal cord compression (usually in the T3–L3 region) and UMN signs to the hindlimbs. It usually is diagnosed in animals younger than 1 year.
      (2) **Radiographic findings.** Diagnosis is based on survey radiography. Myelography is required if a compressive lesion is suspected.
   b. **Treatment. Surgery** (decompression or stabilization) may be indicated in animals with clinical signs related to vertebral abnormalities.

4. **Sacrococcygeal dysgenesis in Manx cats** is associated with varying degrees of sacral and coccygeal vertebral abnormalities. In cats with dysgenesis or agenesis of sacral or coccygeal vertebrae, spina bifida and malformation of the terminal spinal cord and cauda equina can occur. Sacrococcygeal dysgenesis is inherited in an autosomal dominant fashion and may occur in other breeds of cats.
   a. **Diagnosis**
      (1) **Clinical findings** vary, depending on the degree of spinal cord malformation. Many cats have no clinical signs. If present, signs are observed soon after birth, may be progressive or nonprogressive, and are compatible with a lesion in the L4–Cd5 region. Paresis, paralysis, depressed spinal reflexes, a "bunny hop" gait, and a plantigrade stance can occur in the hindlimbs. Urinary and fecal incontinence can result from flaccid paralysis of the urethral and anal sphincter. Constipation due to megacolon can also occur. A meningocele and draining tract may form over the sacral region.

(2) Radiographic findings. Dysgenesis or agenesis of sacral or caudal vertebrae on survey radiographs of the sacrococcygeal area in combination with the breed and appropriate clinical signs are usually sufficient for diagnosis.

b. **Treatment.** There is no treatment for the neurologic deficits. Recurrent urinary tract infection (UTI) and constipation can be managed with antimicrobial therapy and fecal softening agents or enemas.

c. **Prognosis.** In severely affected cats, the prognosis is very poor. Signs may be progressive. However, many Manx cats are clinically normal.

D. **Nutritional disorders. Hypervitaminosis A in cats** results from excess dietary vitamin A, usually from feeding a diet composed largely of liver. Multiple and extensive bony exostoses form along the cervical and thoracic spine. The disease is slow to develop, and the lesions are usually extensive before clinical signs result. Cervical pain and rigidity and forelimb lameness or paresis can be observed, usually in cats older than 2 years. Diagnosis is based on radiographs and dietary history. Treatment consists of dietary modification. The bony lesions are not reversible, but correcting the dietary imbalance will prevent further development of exostoses.

E. **Neoplastic disorders**

1. **Types.** Tumors may be primary or metastatic and involve the spinal cord or the surrounding structures (i.e., meninges, bone).

   a. In dogs, tumors of the vertebral body, extradural lymphosarcoma, metastatic tumors, and intradural, extramedullary tumors such as meningiomas and nerve sheath tumors (e.g., neurofibroma) are common causes of spinal cord neoplasia. Intramedullary tumors (e.g., gliomas, ependymoma, intramedullary lymphosarcoma) are rare.

   b. In cats, extradural lymphosarcoma is the most common tumor.

2. **Predisposition.** Dogs or cats of any age can be affected, but most spinal tumors are diagnosed in large-breed dogs older than 5 years of age. Lymphosarcoma, however, has a wide age range and in cats, it usually occurs in young adults. Neuroepithelioma (an intradural, extramedullary tumor) usually affects young German shepherd dogs and has a predilection for the T10–L1 region.

3. **Diagnosis.** Definitive diagnosis usually requires CSF analysis, myelography, histopathology, and possibly exploratory surgery and biopsy.

   a. **Clinical findings.** Neoplasms affecting the spinal cord usually result in chronic, slowly progressive signs of spinal cord dysfunction. Signs associated with spinal tumors may mimic those of several other spinal cord conditions (e.g., intervertebral disk disease, degenerative myelopathy, discospondylitis). Signs depend on the region of the spinal cord most affected and may include:

   (1) Pain (common with nerve sheath tumors, bone tumors of the vertebral bodies, or tumors involving or compressing the meninges)

   (2) Lameness

   (3) Acute neurologic signs resulting from tumor-associated hemorrhage into the spinal cord such as may occur with metastatic hemangiosarcoma

   (4) Pathologic fracture of a diseased vertebral body

   (5) Horner's syndrome, resulting from thoracic nerve root tumors

   (6) Paresis or paralysis

   b. **Laboratory findings**

   (1) CSF analysis may reveal a mild to moderate increase in protein concentration and cell count (primarily mononuclear). Occasionally, neutrophils predominate if meningeal inflammation and necrosis have occurred. In general, neoplastic cells are rarely observed in the CSF; however, if lymphosarcoma is located intradurally, neoplastic lymphocytes may be observed.

   (2) Serology. FeLV test results will be positive in most cats with spinal lymphosarcoma.

   c. **Radiographic findings**

   (1) Survey radiography. Radiographs may be normal; however, tumor-associated bony reaction, destruction, or lysis in the vertebral bodies may be observed. Radiographs of the chest or abdomen may detect a primary tumor if the spinal cord tumor is metastatic.

(2) **Myelography** is the most reliable method to demonstrate compressive spinal cord tumors. Various patterns may be observed, depending on the location of the tumor (see Figure 47-2).

4. Treatment

a. **Lymphosarcoma.** Chemotherapy (with or without radiation) may induce a remission and alleviate clinical signs, at least temporarily.

b. **Most other spinal cord tumors** are usually well advanced by the time a diagnosis is made and few can be surgically excised (especially if the tumor is intramedullary).

(1) **Surgical decompression** or **debulking** may be palliative.

(2) **Radiation therapy** may be considered, but data on effectiveness are not available.

(3) **Corticosteroid therapy** may provide some palliative benefit by decreasing edema and inflammation associated with the tumor.

5. Prognosis. The prognosis is poor for nonresectable tumors.

F. Inflammatory disorders

1. Infectious causes

a. **Diskospondylitis.** Infection of intervertebral disks and vertebral bodies usually results from the hematogenous spread of bacteria (e.g., UTI, bacterial endocarditis, pyoderma, prostatitis, orchitis) or foreign body (i.e., plant awn) migration. Infection rarely extends into the meninges or spinal cord, although spreading of infection may occur more frequently with migrating foreign bodies. Male, young to middle-aged, medium- to large-breed dogs are most commonly affected. Diskospondylitis is rare in cats.

(1) **Etiology.** Organisms commonly isolated include *Staphylococcus, Streptococcus,* and *Brucella canis* (dogs only). Fungal, mycobacterial, and other bacterial organisms may also cause diskospondylitis.

(2) **Diagnosis** is based on radiographic findings and culture (usually blood) results.

(a) **Clinical findings.** Signs of spinal pain (most common), fever, anorexia, and lethargy are often present for several weeks or months. Neurologic deficits occur infrequently but can result from spinal cord compression (usually in the T3–L3 region) caused by bony or fibrous tissue proliferation at the site of infection or subluxation of a diseased vertebral body.

(b) **Laboratory findings**

(i) **Cultures.** Blood cultures are positive in over 50% of the cases. Urine cultures may be beneficial.

(ii) **Serology.** Tests for *B. canis* [e.g., rapid slide agglutination tests (RSAT), tube agglutination tests, agar-gel immunodiffusion tests] should be considered.

(iii) **CSF analysis** and **CBC.** CSF abnormalities and inflammatory leukograms are uncommon.

(c) **Radiographic findings**

(i) **Survey radiographs.** Destruction of vertebral end plates adjacent to the infected disk space, collapse of the disk space, and new bone production are typical. The degree of bony destruction can vary from small lytic areas early in the infection to widespread bone lysis in the vertebral body associated with abundant new bone production. Vertebrae in the mid-thoracic area, C6–C7 and L7–S1 are most commonly affected, and multiple disk spaces may be involved. Radiographic lesions may be absent very early in the infection.

(ii) **Bone scans** using radioisotopes may help detect early infections.

(iii) **Myelography** may confirm spinal cord compression.

    (3) Treatment
        (a) Antimicrobial therapy
            (i) Selection should be based on culture and sensitivity results. Otherwise, treatment should be directed toward the most likely pathogen (i.e., *Staphylococcus*), using a **first-generation cephalosporin** (e.g., cephalexin, cefazolin) or a **β-lactamase–resistant penicillin** (e.g., cloxacillin). Parenteral therapy for 5 days followed by 6 weeks of oral therapy is recommended.
            (ii) Monitoring of vertebral lesion resolution should be done via spinal radiographs taken at 2– to 3–week intervals. Animals that do not respond within 1 week may have *B. canis* infection, infection with a resistant bacterial species, fungal infection, a migrating foreign body, or nonbacterial disease (e.g., neoplasia).
        (b) Surgery. Exploration of the site may be warranted in some animals, especially if the treatment response is poor. **Decompression** and **stabilization** may be required in animals with severe neurologic signs or those with less severe signs that do not respond to medical management.
    (4) Prognosis. The prognosis depends on the ability to eliminate the organism and the presence of neurologic signs. Severe neurologic signs are associated with a poor prognosis.
    b. Other infections that can involve the spinal cord include bacterial or fungal meningitis, protozoal myelitis (e.g., toxoplasmosis), rickettsial infection, FIP, and canine distemper myelitis (see II G2).

  2. Noninfectious causes. Disorders that can affect the spinal cord include GME, feline polioencephalomyelitis, and steroid-responsive meningitis (see II G3).

G. **Traumatic disorders**

  1. Acute spinal cord trauma is common in dogs and cats.
    a. Pathogenesis. Spinal cord dysfunction arises from compressive lesions resulting from vertebral body fracture or subluxation or, less commonly, spinal cord swelling in the absence of bony injuries.
    b. Diagnosis is based on history, neurologic signs, and radiographic findings. Clinical findings relate to the extent and location of the spinal cord trauma. The **Schiff-Sherrington sign** is indicative of severe thoracolumbar spinal injury. It is important to evaluate cutaneous and deep pain sensation. The absence of deep pain sensation indicates severe spinal cord injury proximal to the area assessed.
    c. Treatment
        (1) Supportive treatment (i.e., therapy for shock) may be necessary in an acutely traumatized patient.
        (2) Rapid-acting corticosteroids (e.g., prednisolone sodium succinate) administered intravenously followed by the administration of longer-acting corticosteroids (e.g., dexamethasone) for 3 days is indicated to reduce spinal cord edema and swelling.
        (3) Surgical decompression and **stabilization** are indicated in patients with moderate to severe neurologic deficits, obvious vertebral subluxation or fracture (resulting in cord compression), or progressive deterioration in neurologic signs despite medical therapy. Surgery should be performed as soon after the injury as possible.
    d. Prognosis depends on the location and severity of the injury.
        (1) Animals that retain voluntary motor activity have a good prognosis for return to normal function.
        (2) Animals that are paralyzed but retain deep pain sensation have a fair prognosis and may have residual neurologic deficits.
        (3) The absence of deep pain sensation or the presence of LMN signs is associated with a poor prognosis.

  2. Sacrococcygeal fracture or **luxation** is a common traumatic injury in cats, less so in dogs. It results in damage to the cauda equina and neurologic signs consistent with an L4–Cd5 lesion.

    a. Diagnosis. Depending on the severity of the injury, paralysis of the tail, urine and fecal incontinence, or hindleg weakness may result. Diagnosis is based on a history of trauma and radiographic findings.

    b. Treatment

        (1) Supportive treatment includes frequent emptying of the bladder and fecal softeners.

        (2) Definitive treatment entails **surgery.**

            (a) Tail amputation may be warranted to eliminate constant fecal and urine soiling.

            (b) Decompression may be warranted if the sacrum is fractured.

    c. Prognosis is variable. A return of bladder and bowel function is more likely with coccygeal fractures or luxations than with sacral fractures. Neurologic function may return in some cats.

H. Vascular disorders

  1. Fibrocartilaginous embolism (ischemic myelopathy) primarily occurs in large-breed dogs, 3–7 years of age. It has also been reported in small-breed dogs and cats.

    a. Pathogenesis. Acute paresis or paralysis results from ischemic necrosis of the spinal cord parenchyma. The origin of the fibrocartilaginous embolus is unknown, but it may arise from the nucleus pulposus of intervertebral disks.

    b. Diagnosis is based on history, clinical signs, and the exclusion of other causes of acute neurologic disease. The absence of pain helps to distinguish this disorder from other causes of acute nonprogressive spinal cord disease (e.g., intervertebral disk disease).

        (1) Clinical findings. Signs are acute and nonprogressive, although they may appear progressive in the first few hours after the injury. Neurologic signs reflect the region affected (usually, but not exclusively, the thoracolumbar region) and are commonly asymmetric. UMN, LMN, or both signs occur. The severity of signs can vary from mild paresis to paralysis and loss of deep pain sensation. Spinal pain is not a feature of this disorder.

        (2) Laboratory findings. Analysis of CSF is usually normal, but a mild increase in protein and cell count may occur.

        (3) Radiographic findings. Myelography is normal, but mild cord swelling may be observed.

    c. Treatment. Corticosteroids may help reduce any spinal cord swelling in the first 24–48 hours, but after 48 hours, corticosteroids are not useful. **Supportive** and **nursing care** is required for recumbent, nonambulatory patients.

    d. Prognosis. Approximately 50% of animals will regain sufficient neurologic function to be acceptable pets. Most of the improvement in clinical signs occurs within 7–10 days of the injury, but it may take 6–8 weeks before neurologic signs resolve. If no improvement is observed within 14 days, it is not likely to occur.

        (1) The prognosis is good for animals with strictly UMN signs and intact pain sensation.

        (2) The prognosis is poor if LMN signs are present (C6–T2 or L4–S3 lesions) or deep pain sensation is absent.

  2. Progressive hemorrhagic myelomalacia (PHM)

    a. Pathogenesis. Acute, severe spinal cord injury can cause ascending and/or descending hemorrhagic necrosis of the spinal cord parenchyma. Although uncommon, PHM occurs most frequently after acute (type I) intervertebral disk herniation, but it may also occur after spinal cord trauma.

    b. Diagnosis. Signs of PHM are superimposed on those of the initial spinal cord injury. PHM is suspected when neurologic signs acutely deteriorate in an otherwise stable patient (e.g., a dog with a T3–L3 lesion develops LMN signs to the hindlimbs or anal sphincter indicative of an L4–Cd5 lesion). Signs progress rapidly over hours to 1–2 days.

    c. Treatment. There is no treatment.

    d. Prognosis. The prognosis is very poor. The hemorrhagic necrosis will continue to progress to the medullary respiratory centers and death ensues (usually within 24–48 hours). Those who survive have severe, irreversible spinal cord damage.

3. **Vasculitis** of meningeal vessels around the spinal cord is described under breed-associated meningeal vasculitis (see II G 3 d).

IV. DISORDERS OF THE PERIPHERAL NERVES AND THE NEUROMUSCULAR JUNCTION

A. Localizing signs

1. **Neuropathic syndrome** is a constellation of neurologic abnormalities that result from peripheral nerve dysfunction. Because motor and sensory fibers often travel in the same nerve, diseased peripheral nerves often result in both decreased motor and sensory function. However, signs associated with abnormal motor or sensory function may predominate. Characteristic abnormalities associated with peripheral nerve motor dysfunction appear as **LMN signs.** Chronic neurogenic atrophy can result in fibrosis of involved muscles and limb contracture. Pain sensation may range from normal to completely absent, depending on the nature of the disorder.

   a. Although less common than motor neuropathies, primary sensory neuropathies occur and can result in decreased pain sensation, proprioceptive deficits, abnormal sensation or sensitivity (paresthesia), self-mutilation (resulting from abnormal sensation), and reduced or absent spinal reflexes but without neurogenic muscle atrophy.

   b. Rarely, autonomic neuropathies can occur (e.g., feline dysautonomia) and may result in anisocoria or dilated pupils, reduced tear or saliva production, reduced GI motility (e.g., constipation, megaesophagus), and bradycardia.

2. **Mononeuropathy** involves dysfunction of a single peripheral or CN and results in localized, often acute, dysfunction (e.g., facial or radial nerve paralysis). Trauma is a common cause.

3. **Polyneuropathy** involves multiple nerves. Although polyneuropathies may be acute in onset, many of them have a slow and insidious onset. The resulting signs are usually bilaterally symmetric and often begin in the hindlimbs. The involvement of CNs in polyneuropathies is uncommon but can occur. Abnormal function of the neuromuscular junction (such as results from botulism or tick paralysis) can mimic polyneuropathies.

B. **Trauma.** Traumatic neuropathy is common and may result from bone fractures, iatrogenic damage, (e.g., surgery, injection of irritating substances), deep lacerations, or severe tissue stretching.

1. **Diagnosis** is based on the history and neurologic deficits.
   a. **Clinical findings** reflect the nerves affected (most commonly the radial and sciatic nerve and the brachial plexus) and include flaccid paralysis to the affected muscle groups and reduced cutaneous sensation. Mapping of reduced cutaneous sensation can be used to indicate the nerves affected and return of function.
      (1) **Radial nerve injury**
         (a) **Injuries above the elbow** result in an inability to extend the elbow, carpus, and digits, an inability to support weight, and reduced pain sensation over the dorsal aspect of the paw and craniolateral aspect of the forearm.
         (b) **Injuries below the elbow** will interfere with extension of the carpus and digits only. The animal may walk on the dorsal surface of the paw. Pain sensation is reduced over the dorsal aspect of the paw and craniolateral aspect of the forearm.

(2) Sciatic nerve injury
  (a) If the injury is proximal (i.e., before the nerve branches into the common peroneal and tibial nerve), stifle flexion and the withdrawal reflex are absent.
  (b) If only the common peroneal nerve is damaged, there is an inability to flex the hock and extend the digits. Cutaneous sensation is reduced over the craniodorsal aspect of the paw, hock, and stifle.
  (c) If only the tibial nerve is injured, the hock cannot be extended or the digits flexed. Cutaneous sensation is reduced over the plantar surface of the paw.
(3) Brachial plexus avulsion
  (a) Extreme stretching or abduction of the forelimb can damage the plexus, usually by avulsing the ventral nerve roots (C6–T2) from the spinal cord.
  (b) The extent of the neurologic deficits ranges from weakness of a single muscle group to total paralysis and loss of pain sensation over the entire forelimb.
b. Other findings. Electromyography and nerve conduction velocities can substantiate neurologic findings in equivocal cases.

2. Treatment
  a. Supportive therapy includes bandaging of peripheral limbs or the use of an Elizabethan collar to prevent damage to paws or limbs by dragging or self-mutilation (as nerves begin to regenerate 2–3 weeks after injury).
  b. Physical therapy (e.g., limb manipulation, muscle massage) can help reduce the severity of muscle atrophy and slow fibrotic changes.
  c. Amputation of the affected limb or arthrodesis of an affected joint (when possible) should be considered if improvement is not noted after 1 month.

3. Prognosis is usually guarded to poor.
  a. Nerves can regenerate slowly if the supporting tissue around the axons has not been damaged too severely. The closer the nerve injury is to the innervated muscle, the better the chances are for successful reinnervation.
  b. If no improvement in motor or sensory function has been noted within 1 month of the injury, then improvement is unlikely.

C. **Facial nerve paralysis** is common in dogs and cats.

1. Etiology. Infection (otitis media or interna), inflammation, foreign bodies, nasopharyngeal polyps, or tumors of the middle ear can damage the facial nerve. Facial nerve paralysis can also be idiopathic or associated with hyperadrenocorticism.

2. Diagnosis. If no cause for the facial nerve paralysis is found, then a diagnosis of idiopathic disease is justified. Idiopathic disease accounts for about 75% of the cases of facial nerve paralysis in dogs and 25% in cats.
  a. Clinical findings
    (1) Clinical signs result from the paralysis of facial muscles and include a drooped lip, eyelid, and ear. Drooling may result from the loss of lip tone. Keratoconjunctivitis sicca (dry eye) may result from an inability to close the eyelids. If facial nerve paralysis has resulted from middle ear disease, a head tilt and Horner's syndrome may be present.
    (2) Otoscopic findings may reveal otitis externa. Otitis media or interna is usually an extension of otitis externa.
  b. Laboratory findings. Serum biochemistry may detect changes associated with hyperadrenocorticism (e.g., increased ALP).
  c. Radiographic findings. Radiographs of the tympanic bulla may reveal changes consistent with otitis media or interna (e.g., bony reaction, increased density) or neoplasia. Radiographs of the nasopharynx may reveal a nasopharyngeal polyp.

3. Treatment is focused on the underlying disorder, if one can be identified. There is no specific treatment for idiopathic disease.

   a. Artificial tear supplements may be necessary.
   b. Corticosteroids may be helpful.

4. **Prognosis.** In patients with idiopathic disease, some return of facial nerve function is common over 1–2 months.

D. **Idiopathic trigeminal nerve paralysis** is a rare condition of dogs that results in paralysis of the muscles of mastication. Affected dogs have a dropped jaw and difficulty eating; otherwise, they are clinically and neurologically normal. Affected dogs may need to be fed with their head elevated to improve their ability to eat. No treatment, including corticosteroids, alters the course of the disease. Dogs fully recover within 4–6 weeks.

E. **Peripheral vestibular nerve dysfunction** can be congenital, idiopathic, or caused by otitis media or interna, middle ear tumors or polyps, trauma, or aminoglycoside ototoxicity. Peripheral vestibular disease must be differentiated from central vestibular (i.e., brain stem) disease (see II A 4–5; Table 21-1).

1. **Otitis media– or otitis interna–related peripheral vestibular nerve dysfunction.** Otitis interna may account for as many as 50% of all cases of acute peripheral vestibular disease.
   a. Pathogenesis. Otitis media or interna usually occurs as an extension of otitis externa, which can be caused by bacterial or mycotic infections or ear mites. The involvement of the inner ear gives rise to vestibular signs.
   b. Diagnosis is based on neurologic signs compatible with peripheral vestibular disease, an otoscopic examination, and radiographs of the tympanic bulla.
      (1) Clinical findings
         (a) Otitis media is clinically indistinguishable from otitis externa (ear pain, scratching, rubbing, head shaking). An opaque, cloudy, discolored, bulging, torn or absent tympanic membrane may be associated with middle ear disease. Facial nerve paralysis or Horner's syndrome may occur.
         (b) Otitis interna. Vestibular signs (i.e., head tilt, spontaneous horizontal or rotatory nystagmus, falling or rolling to the affected side) occur with otitis interna, and often lessen in severity over several days.
      (2) Radiographic findings
         (a) Otitis media produces a soft tissue density within the (normally air-filled) tympanic bulla, sclerosis, or thickening of the wall of the tympanic bulla and bony proliferation of the bulla that may extend into the petrous temporal bone and temporomandibular joint. Radiographic changes may not be evident for several weeks in acute cases.
         (b) Otitis interna usually does not produce radiographic changes.
   c. Treatment
      (1) Antibiotic therapy should be based on culture and sensitivity testing. Samples for culture are best obtained directly from the middle ear via myringotomy. If a reliable culture cannot be obtained, a first-generation cephalosporin (e.g., cephalexin, cefadroxil), chloramphenicol, or trimethoprim/sulfadiazine are acceptable choices. Antibiotics should be administered for 3–6 weeks.
      (2) Surgical drainage (i.e., bulla osteotomy) of the tympanic bulla is indicated if there is radiographic (and otoscopic) evidence of infection or if medical therapy alone has failed. Surgical drainage is required in most animals with well-established otitis media or interna.
   d. Prognosis. If otitis media/interna is diagnosed early and treated appropriately, the prognosis for recovery is good. Some animals are left with a residual head tilt and possibly facial nerve paralysis and Horner's syndrome.

2. **Canine idiopathic (geriatric) vestibular disease** is a common cause of acute, unilateral vestibular signs in elderly dogs (mean age, 12.5 years). Head tilt, spontaneous nystagmus (often rotatory), falling, rolling, and ataxia are common. Nausea and vomiting can occur. Diagnosis is based on the elimination of other causes of peripheral vestibular diseases, especially otitis media or interna. Treatment is primarily sup-

portive; most signs resolve within 1–2 weeks. Antihistamines (e.g., diphenhydramine) may help reduce nausea. A few dogs will have a mild residual head tilt. Recurrences can occur but are uncommon.

3. **Feline idiopathic vestibular disease** is very similar to canine idiopathic vestibular disease, but it can occur in cats of any age. Also, there may be an increased incidence in the northeastern United States and a seasonal increase in cases in the summer and early fall. Signs and onset are the same as those of canine idiopathic vestibular disease. Diagnosis is based on the exclusion of other causes of peripheral vestibular disease. Treatment consists of supportive care. Most cats start to improve within a few days, and signs are usually resolved within 2–3 weeks.

4. **Neoplasia-related peripheral vestibular disease.** Tumors can arise from the tympanic bulla or bony labyrinth or extend into the middle or inner ear from the external ear canal (e.g., squamous cell carcinoma, ceruminous gland adenocarcinoma). Although rare, nerve sheath tumors (e.g., neurofibroma, neurofibrosarcoma) may involve the vestibular nerve itself.
   a. **Diagnosis** is based on radiographs of the tympanic bulla and petrous temporal area, surgical exploration and biopsy, or both. Signs are consistent with a peripheral vestibular disorder, and have a slow, progressive course. Facial nerve paralysis, Horner's syndrome, or both may occur.
   b. **Treatment.** Most tumors in this area are not resectable. Chemotherapy and radiation therapy could be considered in some cases.

5. **Congenital vestibular disease** has been recognized in German shepherds, Doberman pinschers, Akitas, English cocker spaniels, and Siamese and Burmese cats. Unilateral peripheral vestibular signs are usually noticed shortly after birth or within the first few weeks of life (almost always by 3 months of age). Deafness may also be present. Diagnosis is based on age of onset and the exclusion of other causes of peripheral vestibular disease. Many animals will compensate sufficiently to be acceptable pets.

6. **Aminoglycoside ototoxicity–related peripheral vestibular disease.** The use of aminoglycoside antibiotics (e.g., gentamicin), usually in prolonged high dosages, can be associated with degeneration of the vestibular and cochlear structures of the ear. Unilateral or bilateral vestibular signs as well as deafness can result. Diagnosis is based on history and clinical signs. The vestibular signs resolve in most dogs if the drug is promptly withdrawn. Deafness may be permanent.

F. **Deafness**

1. **Deafness resulting from CNS disruption of auditory tracts** is rare.

2. **Conductive deafness** can result from middle or external ear disease or obstruction.

3. **Peripheral** (i.e., **cochlear) neural deafness** can have multiple causes.
   a. **Congenital deafness** is usually hereditary and can be unilateral or bilateral. Breeds most commonly (but not exclusively) affected include blue-eyed, white-coated cats, Dalmatians (highest prevalence, 20%–30%), Australian heelers, English setters, Catahoulas, and Australian shepherds. Diagnosis is usually based on age, breed, and an abnormal BAER (especially if unilateral deafness is present).
   b. **Ototoxic agents**
      (1) **Aminoglycoside antibiotics,** systemic or topical (otic), are one of the most common causes of drug-induced degeneration of vestibular or cochlear structures (or both).
         (a) Streptomycin and gentamicin tend to cause more vestibular damage.
         (b) Neomycin, kanamycin, amikacin, and tobramycin are more likely to cause cochlear damage.
      (2) **Other potentially ototoxic agents** include topical polymyxin B and chloramphenicol, many antiseptic solutions, diuretics (e.g., ethacrynic acid, furosemide), and cisplatin. Topical agents such as propylene glycol, ceruminolytic

agents, and detergents can also be ototoxic if the tympanic membrane has been ruptured.

   c. **Aging** is a common cause of deafness in old dogs. The hearing impairment is typically gradual in onset. Diagnosis is based on age and the absence of other ear disease.

G. **Peripheral nerve sheath tumors (schwannomas, neurofibromas, neurilemomas).** Although any nerve or nerve root can be affected, these tumors occur most often in the brachial plexus region. Lymphosarcoma can occasionally involve nerve roots.

   1. Diagnosis

     a. Clinical findings

      (1) Tumors in the brachial plexus usually result in a slowly progressive, unilateral forelimb lameness associated with muscle atrophy. Although pain may be elicited with deep palpation in the axillary region, the tumor is usually not palpable. Early in the course of tumor development, signs may be difficult to distinguish from musculoskeletal or other neurologic causes of forelimb lameness (e.g., intervertebral disk herniation).

      (2) Horner's syndrome may result if the T1–T3 nerve roots are affected.

      (3) Occasionally, these tumors will grow into the spinal canal through the intervertebral foramen and cause spinal cord compression (UMN signs distal and ipsilateral to the lesion may be apparent).

     b. Radiographic findings

      (1) **Survey radiographs** of the spine may reveal bony changes in or widening of the intervertebral foramen due to an expanding tumor.

      (2) **Myelograms** may be useful in detecting spinal cord compression if UMN signs are apparent.

     c. Electromyographic findings. Electromyography can be used to map the distribution of denervation to muscle groups and help localize the nerves affected.

   2. Treatment

     a. Surgical resection is the treatment of choice. However, if many nerve roots are affected, excision may be impossible and resection of the tumor and limb amputation may be indicated. If the spinal canal has been invaded, complete resection is rarely possible.

     b. Corticosteroids may be helpful in reducing nerve edema or inflammation and alleviating clinical signs.

   3. Prognosis varies with the number of nerves or nerve roots involved and the extent of tumor growth. The prognosis may be good with a localized tumor of a single nerve. It is poor if the spinal canal is involved.

H. **Polyneuropathies**

   1. Etiology. Polyneuropathies may be idiopathic. They have also been associated with:

     a. Endocrine diseases (e.g., diabetes mellitus, hypothyroidism)

     b. Toxins or **drugs** (e.g., organophosphates, vincristine, lead)

     c. Immune-mediated diseases [e.g., systemic lupus erythematosus (SLE)]

     d. Breed-associated causes (e.g., Birman cat polyneuropathy, laryngeal paralysis and polyneuropathy in young Dalmatians)

     e. Paraneoplastic syndromes (in dogs with bronchogenic carcinoma, insulinoma, hemangiosarcoma, leiomyosarcoma, undifferentiated sarcoma, adrenal adenocarcinoma, or synovial cell sarcoma)

   2. Diagnosis. Endocrine, toxic, paraneoplastic, or immune-mediated causes must be ruled out. Histopathologic examination of a peripheral nerve biopsy is required for definitive diagnosis.

     a. Clinical findings

      (1) **Motor neuropathies.** Widespread LMN signs of multiple limbs are noted. Signs are usually slowly progressive over several months; however, the hindlimb weakness and plantigrade stance associated with diabetic neuropathy

in cats may develop rapidly (i.e., in less than 1 week). Clinical signs from other diseases may be apparent.

(2) **Sensory neuropathies** have been documented in boxers, long-haired dachshunds, Jack Russell terriers, English pointers, and others. Paresthesia, reduced pain sensation, self-mutilation, proprioceptive deficits, and ataxia are noted.

b. **Other findings.** Electromyography and nerve conduction velocities can help document the presence of a polyneuropathy.

3. **Treatment.** The underlying disorder should be treated, if possible. Corticosteroid treatment in idiopathic disease may or may not be beneficial.

4. **Prognosis** depends on the underlying cause and its reversibility. In some animals, the neuropathy resolves spontaneously; in other animals, their condition slowly deteriorates.

I. **Acute polyradiculoneuritis (coonhound paralysis)** is the most common acute polyneuropathy seen in dogs; it can occur in adult dogs of any breed or sex. It also can occur in cats.

1. **Etiology.** This syndrome has been associated with exposure to raccoon saliva (i.e., bites), but many dogs do not have a history of such exposure. The disorder probably has an immunologic basis.

2. **Diagnosis** is based on clinical and neurologic signs.
   a. **Clinical findings.** Signs usually appear 7–10 days after exposure to raccoons, if documented, and include weakness and hyporeflexia beginning in the hindlimbs, rapidly ascending to the forelimbs, and usually progressing to tetraplegia within 12 hours to 7 days. Neurologic signs are consistent with widespread LMN disease.
      (1) Motor dysfunction is more affected than sensory function. As a result, cutaneous pain sensation is usually normal. Some dogs appear to have increased sensation (hyperesthesia) to painful stimuli.
      (2) Perineal reflexes and CNs are normal.
      (3) In rare cases, bilateral facial nerve paralysis or respiratory muscle paralysis (and death) has been observed.
   b. **Laboratory findings**
      (1) **Histopathologic findings** include widespread demyelination and inflammation, primarily affecting the nerve roots (especially ventral roots) and peripheral spinal nerves.
      (2) **CSF analysis** is normal although a mild increase in protein concentration may be present.
   c. **Electromyographic findings** include denervation (fibrillation) potentials after 5–7 days and reduced nerve conduction velocities.

3. **Treatment** is primarily supportive (e.g., nursing care, physiotherapy) until neurologic signs begin to improve. Recovery usually begins within 1 week, but full recovery may take several weeks to 2–3 months.

4. **Prognosis.** Some dogs do not improve at all or make an incomplete recovery, and recurrences may occur. Occasionally, dogs will die of respiratory muscle paralysis. Overall, however, the prognosis is good.

J. **Botulism** is a rare cause of diffuse LMN disease in dogs.

1. **Pathogenesis.** Ingestion of spoiled food containing a preformed toxin produced by *Clostridium botulinum* results in inhibition of acetylcholine release from neuromuscular junctions. Widespread paralysis develops within hours or days of toxin ingestion.

2. **Diagnosis** is based on neurologic findings and a history of ingestion of spoiled food. Rabies is a differential diagnosis.
   a. **Clinical findings**

      (1) Ascending LMN paralysis starts in the hindlimbs and eventually results in tetraplegia.

      (2) Pain sensation is normal.

      (3) Spinal reflexes are reduced or absent.

      (4) Widespread CN involvement is common and can lead to dysphagia, drooling, regurgitation (due to megaesophagus), and mydriasis. CN involvement usually distinguishes botulism from acute polyradiculoneuritis and tick paralysis.

    b. Electromyographic findings are normal because it is the neuromuscular junction, not the nerve, that is affected. A normal EMG can distinguish botulism and tick paralysis from acute polyradiculoneuritis.

    c. Laboratory findings. Definitive diagnosis requires the detection of botulinum toxin in feces or blood.

  3. Treatment is supportive. Enemas or laxatives can be used to speed the removal of botulinum toxin from the GI tract. Most dogs recover in 1–3 weeks.

K. **Tick paralysis.** Tick infestation with *Dermacentor variabilis* or *Dermacentor andersoni* can cause an ascending LMN paralysis that begins in the hindlimbs. Tick paralysis is attributed to a neurotoxin originating from the tick that blocks transmission across the neuromuscular junction.

  1. Diagnosis is based on clinical signs and documented or suspected tick infestation.

    a. Clinical findings. Signs begin 5–9 days after tick infestation and rapidly progress to tetraplegia over 24–72 hours. They include reduced or absent spinal reflexes without muscle atrophy. The CNs are usually spared, but dysphagia, mild facial or trigeminal nerve paralysis, and an altered bark can occur.

    b. Electromyographic findings are normal (no denervation potentials) because the neuromuscular junction is affected, not the nerves.

  2. Treatment. Tick removal or insecticidal dips result in rapid clinical improvement and recovery within 24–72 hours.

  3. Prognosis. Without treatment, death results from respiratory paralysis within 1–5 days. Recovery following tick removal is usually complete.

L. **Myasthenia gravis** is associated with reduced transmission across the neuromuscular junction.

  1. Etiology. Myasthenia gravis can occur as a congenital disorder, but most myasthenia gravis in dogs is acquired and results from the immune-mediated destruction of acetylcholine receptors in the neuromuscular junction. Myasthenia gravis may also occur in cats.

    a. Congenital myasthenia gravis has been documented in Jack Russell terriers, springer spaniels, and smooth-coated fox terriers.

    b. Acquired myasthenia gravis can occur in any age or breed of dog, but young dogs (between the ages of 2 and 3 years) and old dogs (between the ages of 9 and 10 years) are affected more often. German shepherds may be predisposed. In elderly dogs, myasthenia gravis may also appear as a paraneoplastic syndrome associated with thymomas.

  2. Diagnosis. Myasthenia gravis is diagnosed on the basis of clinical signs and a significant antibody titer to acetylcholine receptors. A presumptive diagnosis can be based on a positive response to edrophonium chloride or a decremental response in muscle action potentials following motor nerve stimulation.

    a. Clinical findings. Hallmark sign is progressive muscle weakness associated with exercise.

      (1) Congenital myasthenia gravis is usually detected when puppies begin to ambulate (3–8 weeks of age).

      (2) Acquired myasthenia gravis. The main clinical sign is progressive muscle weakness with exercise. Apparently normal strength can progress to recumbency and an inability to rise after several minutes of modest exercise. With rest, muscle strength returns. Megaesophagus (associated with regurgitation) may accompany the skeletal muscle weakness, or it may be the only sign. Occasionally, an altered bark and dilated pupils may be present.

b. Radiographic findings can include a mediastinal mass (i.e., thymoma), megaesophagus, or aspiration pneumonia.

c. Other findings. A positive response to edrophonium chloride (a short-acting cholinesterase inhibitor) produces a transient increase in strength in a weak animal. However, interpretation is subjective, and borderline results are difficult to interpret.

3. Treatment

a. Long-acting cholinesterase inhibitors (neostigmine, pyridostigmine) can improve and control clinical signs in many dogs. Both **underdosing (myasthenic crisis)** and **overdosing (cholinergic crisis)** of cholinesterase inhibitors can increase muscle weakness and result in death. An edrophonium response test can differentiate underdosing from overdosing: an underdosed animal will improve, and an overdosed animal will transiently worsen or remain the same. Atropine is indicated to reverse overdose symptoms.

b. Corticosteroids at immunosuppressive doses are indicated in animals with acquired disease that do not respond to cholinesterase inhibitors alone and do not have aspiration pneumonia (a common complication in myasthenic animals).

4. Prognosis. The prognosis is fair to good if there is a good response to cholinesterase inhibitors and aspiration pneumonia is not present. Esophageal function may not return to normal with therapy, and severe megaesophagus is a significant risk factor for the development of aspiration pneumonia.

a. If aspiration pneumonia develops, the prognosis is fair to poor.

b. Some animals undergo spontaneous remission.

V. DISORDERS OF MUSCLE

A. Localizing signs

1. Clinical signs

a. Weakness is the predominant sign of muscle disorders (at least those affecting the limb musculature). The weakness is usually persistent although it may be exacerbated by exercise. As opposed to most, but not all, causes of neurologic weakness, pain sensation is normal with muscle disease.

b. Muscle pain (myalgia), fever, and lethargy are present in some of the inflammatory disorders.

c. Muscle atrophy is common, but hypertrophy can occur (i.e., myotonia).

2. Laboratory findings

a. Serum creatine kinase elevation occurs as a result of leakage from muscle cells and is specific for muscle damage. However, serum creatine kinase concentration may range from normal to markedly elevated in muscle disorders.

b. AST elevation can also occur following muscle injury, but it is less specific for muscle than creatine kinase levels.

3. Electromyographic abnormalities are present with many, but not all, muscle diseases.

a. Inflammatory myopathies tend to be associated with fibrillation potentials (which also occur with denervation) and positive sharp waves.

b. Degenerative myopathies are more often associated with complex repetitive discharges (high-frequency discharges).

4. Muscle biopsy is usually needed to confirm the presence of muscle disease, characterize the pathologic process, and make therapeutic decisions.

B. **Infectious myopathies**

1. **Toxoplasmosis** is discussed in II G 2 d.

2. **Neosporosis** is discussed in II G 2 e.

3. **Bacterial myositis** is uncommon. It is usually focal, and often secondary to bite wounds, lacerations, or surgery. *Staphylococcus intermedius* and *Clostridium perfringens* are the most common pathogens. Antimicrobial therapy should be based on culture and sensitivity results. Surgical debridement and drainage are often required.

C. **Immune-mediated myositis**

1. **Polymyositis** is a rare, diffuse, immune-mediated inflammatory muscle disorder that occurs in dogs and cats. Large-breed, middle-aged dogs are most commonly affected.
   a. **Pathogenesis.** This myositis primarily affects appendicular muscles although laryngeal and esophageal muscles may be affected in some dogs. Polymyositis may occur alone or be associated with SLE, thymoma, or myasthenia gravis.
   b. **Diagnosis**
      (1) **Clinical findings.** Signs may be intermittent early in the disease. Muscles of the head are usually spared, and there are no neurologic abnormalities.
         (a) Muscle weakness exacerbated by exercise is the most common sign. Muscle pain, muscle atrophy, fever, lethargy, and a stilted gait may also be observed.
         (b) Some dogs will have an altered bark (due to laryngeal involvement), dysphagia, drooling, or regurgitation (due to megaesophagus).
      (2) **Laboratory findings. Serum creatine kinase** is mildly to moderately elevated. Serologic tests can help rule out SLE and myasthenia gravis.
      (3) **Electromyographic findings** are nonspecific and consist of fibrillation potentials, positive sharp waves, and prolonged insertional activity.
      (4) **Radiographic findings** may include megaesophagus or aspiration pneumonia. Thoracic radiographs can help rule out thymoma.
      (5) **Muscle biopsy findings.** Results may be negative because of the multifocal nature of the disease, but typically, a lymphocytic–plasmacytic inflammatory response is observed with varying degrees of muscle fiber necrosis and fibrosis. Negative findings should not rule out polymyositis if clinical and laboratory signs are highly suggestive. Muscle biopsies should be examined closely to rule out toxoplasmosis or neosporosis.
   c. **Treatment**
      (1) **Corticosteroids** are indicated in the absence of aspiration pneumonia.
      (2) **Antibiotics** and **supportive care** are indicated in the presence of aspiration pneumonia. Corticosteroid therapy can begin after resolution of the pneumonia.
   d. **Prognosis** is usually good unless severe megaesophagus or aspiration pneumonia is present. Occasionally, dogs require long-term therapy or alternative immunosuppressive medications (e.g., azathioprine).

2. **Masticatory muscle myositis (eosinophilic myositis, atrophic myositis)** is a reasonably common disorder in dogs. Large-breed dogs (especially German shepherds and retriever breeds) are preferentially affected.
   a. **Pathogenesis.** This myositis results from immune-mediated inflammation, involving antibodies to type 2M muscle fibers (found only in masticatory muscles). Although eosinophilic inflammation can occur with masticatory myositis, it is uncommon.
   b. **Diagnosis** is based on histopathologic examination of muscle biopsies or detection of serum antibodies to type 2M muscle fibers.
      (1) **Clinical findings**
         (a) In acute cases, the masticatory muscles may be swollen and painful, and pain is associated with attempts to open the jaw. Anorexia, depres-

sion, fever, and submandibular and prescapular lymphadenopathy may occur.

(b) Atrophy of the masseter muscles is often the first abnormality noted, usually associated with varying degrees of trismus (inability to open the mouth) due to fibrosis of the masticatory muscles. Masseter muscle atrophy is not accompanied by systemic illness and rarely by muscle pain, and may be a sequela to acute episodes of myositis or may develop without previous signs.

(2) **Laboratory findings.** Some dogs with acute signs have inflammatory leukograms (with or without eosinophilia). Serum creatine kinase levels are normal to mildly elevated. Histology reveals mononuclear inflammation with low numbers of eosinophils and varying degrees of muscle fiber necrosis and fibrosis.

(3) **Electromyographic findings** are similar to those of other inflammatory myopathies.

(4) **Differential diagnoses** include other conditions associated with pain on jaw opening (i.e., retrobulbar abscesses, tooth or temporomandibular joint problems) and other causes of masseter muscle atrophy (i.e., idiopathic trigeminal nerve paralysis).

c. **Treatment**

(1) **Corticosteroids** in immunosuppressive doses are indicated. Improvement is usually rapid in dogs with acute signs and slower in dogs with primarily muscle atrophy and trismus. The dose is usually tapered off over a few months. Long-term maintenance therapy or more potent immunosuppressive medications (e.g., azathioprine) may be necessary.

(2) **Supportive measures.** A soft gruel-like food may need to be fed to dogs with severe trismus.

d. **Prognosis** is variable depending on the degree of trismus. Relapses are common. Dogs with severe fibrosis and trismus may not improve to a great extent.

3. **Dermatomyositis** is a rare condition associated with immune-mediated dermatitis and polymyositis. It is primarily recognized as a familial disorder seen in young rough and smooth-coated collies and Shetland sheepdogs.

a. **Diagnosis** is based on breed, age, and skin or muscle biopsy findings.

(1) **Clinical findings**

(a) Skin lesions usually appear by 3 months of age and consist of erythema, crusts, ulcers, and alopecia affecting the inner side of the pinna, head, and skin surfaces subject to friction. Pruritus is absent or mild.

(b) Severely affected dogs also develop polymyositis with generalized muscle atrophy, facial muscle paresis, decreased jaw tone, masticatory muscle atrophy, and a stiff gait.

(c) Dysphagia may result from pharyngeal dysfunction, and regurgitation may result from megaesophagus.

(2) **Histopathologic findings**

(a) **Skin biopsies** reveal hydropic degeneration of the basal cell layer and separation at the dermoepidermal junction (with or without a perivascular mononuclear infiltrate).

(b) **Muscle biopsies** reveal muscle fiber necrosis, atrophy, and regeneration along with a mononuclear cell inflammatory infiltrate and fibrosis.

(3) **Electromyographic findings** are similar to those of other inflammatory myopathies.

b. **Treatment.** Although corticosteroids have been used, the results are variable. In mildly affected dogs, signs may spontaneously resolve. Affected dogs should not be bred.

D. Metabolic myopathies

1. **Hyperadrenocorticism** or **glucocorticoid excess** can, in rare instances, result in a degenerative myopathy. Degenerative myopathy resulting from hyperadrenocorticism

or glucocorticoid excess is noted most often in small-breed, middle-aged, female dogs.

   a. Diagnosis
      (1) Clinical findings. Unilateral hindlimb stiffness progressing to the other hindlimb (and, to a lesser extent, the forelimbs) is usually the initial sign. Generalized muscle atrophy and weakness are common. Signs of glucocorticoid excess (endogenous or exogenous) are present.
      (2) Laboratory findings may include an elevation in serum creatine kinase.
      (3) Electromyographic findings may include complex repetitive discharges.
   b. Treatment involves withdrawal of glucocorticoid therapy or control of the hyperadrenocorticism.
   c. Prognosis. Complete recovery from the myopathy is uncommon.

2. **Hypothyroidism** has been associated with a subclinical myopathy characterized by type 2 muscle fiber atrophy.

3. **Hypokalemic polymyopathy** is frequently recognized in severely hypokalemic cats and, to a lesser extent, dogs.
   a. Pathogenesis. In cats, hypokalemia can develop secondary to prolonged anorexia, aggressive fluid diuresis, polyuria or polydipsia, chronic renal failure, and the administration or consumption of urine-acidifying agents or diets. A reduction in serum potassium is associated with hyperpolarization of muscle membranes, which increases the stimulus required to depolarize muscle membranes (and result in muscle contraction). As a result, generalized muscle weakness results. If the reduction in serum potassium is severe, perfusion to skeletal muscles is decreased (due to vasoconstriction of vessels supplying muscle beds) and can result in ischemia.
   b. Diagnosis is based on clinical signs of muscle weakness associated with hypokalemia.
      (1) Clinical findings include mild to profound generalized muscle weakness (the hallmark sign), ventroflexion of the head (due to weak cervical muscles), and muscle pain.
      (2) Laboratory findings include serum potassium less than 3.0 mEq/L if muscle weakness is apparent and mild to marked serum creatine kinase elevation.
      (3) Electromyographic findings. Abnormalities (i.e., increased spontaneous activity) are generalized.
      (4) Histopathologic findings. Muscle biopsies are usually normal.
   c. Treatment. Oral potassium gluconate therapy is preferred unless life-threatening respiratory muscle weakness is present. Parenteral potassium supplementation is via intravenous lactated Ringer's solution with added potassium chloride. Long-term potassium supplementation is required in some cats to maintain a normal serum potassium concentration.
   d. Prognosis. The prognosis is excellent. Adequate potassium supplementation usually resolves clinical signs within 24–36 hours.

E. Inherited myopathies

1. **X-linked muscular dystrophy** is a group of myopathies in dogs and cats. It is characterized by progressive muscle degeneration inherited in an X-linked fashion. X-linked muscular dystrophy is usually associated with the lack of a membrane-associated protein called dystrophin.
   a. Diagnosis is based on breed, sex, age of onset, and histopathologic (with or without immunocytochemical) examination of muscle biopsies.
      (1) Clinical findings. Signs may appear as early as 6 weeks, progress rapidly between 3 and 6 months, then stabilize.
         (a) Affected dogs (usually golden retrievers, Irish terriers, Samoyeds, Rottweilers, Belgian shepherds, and miniature schnauzers) may develop trismus, a stilted gait, atrophy of truncal and masseter muscles, plantigrade stance, kyphosis (with lordosis later), and exercise intolerance. Muscle fibrosis and contracture can develop.
         (b) Aspiration pneumonia and cardiac failure may also occur.

    (2) **Laboratory findings** always include a marked elevation in serum creatine kinase.

    (3) **Electromyographic findings.** The EMG reveals prominent complex repetitive discharges.

  b. Treatment. There is no specific therapy, but signs may improve with physical therapy and possibly corticosteroid administration.

2. Labrador retriever myopathy is a progressive degenerative myopathy inherited in an autosomal recessive fashion. The disease occurs in both yellow and black Labrador dogs.

  a. Diagnosis is based on age, breed, and characteristic clinical signs.

    (1) **Clinical findings.** Signs include a stilted gait with the advancement of the hindlimbs simultaneously, temporalis muscle atrophy, ventroflexion of the neck, and weakness (which may be exacerbated by exercise, cold, or excitement). Spinal reflexes in the limbs may be depressed. In rare instances, dogs may become recumbent. Clinical signs begin between 6 weeks to 7 months of age and usually do not progress after 6–8 months of age.

    (2) **Laboratory findings.** Serum creatine kinase levels are mildly elevated.

    (3) **Electromyographic findings.** The EMG may reveal spontaneous activity.

    (4) **Histopathologic findings.** Muscle biopsy reveals fibrosis and variation in the size, necrosis, and regeneration of muscle fibers.

  b. Treatment. There is no specific treatment, but diazepam may help some dogs.

  c. Prognosis. The prognosis is fair to good. Most dogs are not severely debilitated.

3. Myotonia is the persistent contraction of muscles following an external stimulus or voluntary contraction. A myotonic syndrome is recognized in chow chows and is believed to be inherited in an autosomal recessive fashion. Myotonia has also been documented sporadically in other breeds. Myotonia is thought to result from a shift in the resting muscle membrane potential closer to the threshold level.

  a. Diagnosis is based on characteristic clinical signs, muscle hypertrophy, breed, and electromyography findings.

    (1) **Clinical findings.** A stiff gait is common, mostly in the hindlimbs. Hypertrophy of most muscles is often present. Severely affected dogs may have difficulty rising or walking, and the joints are difficult to flex. In some dogs, percussion of a muscle results in sustained dimple (from muscle fiber contraction). In some cases, the condition stabilizes, whereas in others, it gradually deteriorates.

    (2) **Laboratory findings.** Serum creatine kinase levels may be mildly elevated.

    (3) **Electromyographic findings.** The EMG may reveal high frequency discharges that wax and wane (i.e., the "dive bomber" sound).

    (4) **Histopathologic findings.** Muscle biopsy findings are nonspecific.

  b. Treatment. Procainamide, and to a lesser extent phenytoin and quinidine, have been beneficial in some dogs.

DIRECTIONS: Each of the numbered items or incomplete statements in this section is followed by answers or by completions of the statement. Select the ONE numbered answer or completion that is BEST in each case.

1. A neurologic examination is performed on a dog with a unilateral right hindlimb lameness. Abnormal findings are restricted to the right hindlimb. There is decreased proprioception and the withdrawal reflex is reduced. Cutaneous pain sensation appears to be decreased over the dorsal aspect of the paw. The patellar and perineal reflexes are normal. These findings are most consistent with:

(1) spinal cord injury (L4–L6 region).
(2) peripheral nerve injury (sciatic nerve).
(3) spinal cord injury (L6–S1 region).
(4) peripheral nerve injury (femoral nerve).
(5) peripheral nerve injury (pudendal nerve).

2. A dog is presented because of drooling. Examination reveals that the left lip appears to droop and the left eyelid is held partially closed. A gentle tap at the medial canthus of the left eye does not elicit a blink or closure of the eyelid. No other abnormalities are noted on a physical or neurologic examination. Which one of the following conditions is the most likely cause of the abnormalities?

(1) Trigeminal nerve paralysis
(2) Hypoglossal nerve paralysis
(3) Facial nerve paralysis
(4) Vestibular nerve dysfunction
(5) Oculomotor nerve paralysis

3. A cerebrospinal fluid (CSF) sample is collected from a 2-year-old male German shepherd with cervical pain. The cell count (> 100 cell/μl) and protein concentration (> 100 mg/dl) are markedly elevated. The cells are predominantly nondegenerate neutrophils. The findings in this dog are most consistent with:

(1) cervical intervertebral disc disease.
(2) trauma.
(3) cervical spondylomyelopathy.
(4) cervical fibrocartilaginous emboli.
(5) steroid-responsive meningitis.

4. A veterinarian is presented with a 4-month-old female Labrador retriever. The owner is concerned because the puppy seems more uncoordinated than expected for a puppy. The puppy is in otherwise good health. The puppy is bright and alert but has a wide-based stance and is visibly ataxic. Muscular strength is normal and the gait appears hypermetric. Intention tremors of the head are obvious when the puppy is offered some food. Which of the following is the most likely diagnosis for this puppy?

(1) Cerebellar disease
(2) Cerebrocortical disease
(3) Cervical spinal cord (C1–C5) disease
(4) Brain stem disease
(5) Cervical spinal cord (C6–T2) disease

5. An 8-year-old female spayed mixed-breed dog is presented because of a head tilt and incoordination. On neurologic examination, mentation is normal and there is a prominent head tilt to the right. Spontaneous nystagmus that changes direction with alterations in the position of the head is present. The right fore- and hindlimb appear weak, and the dog is slow to replace the fore- and hindlimb paws when they are knuckled over on the dorsal surface. No other physical or neurologic abnormalities are noted. The neurologic signs are consistent with which one of the following conditions?

(1) Idiopathic vestibular disease
(2) Otitis media or interna
(3) Cerebellar disease
(4) Central vestibular disease
(5) Cervical intervertebral disc disease (C1–C5)

6. An unvaccinated dog that has bitten a child is examined by a veterinarian. No abnormalities are noted. To rule out the possibility of rabies, quarantine for this dog:

(1) should be a minimum of 10 days.
(2) should be a minimum of 14 days.
(3) should be a minimum of 7 days.
(4) should be a minimum of 21 days.
(5) is not necessary because the dog would be showing clinical signs if it were rabid.

7. A 5-year-old beagle is presented because of the acute onset of hindlimb paresis. The dog is bright and alert, but weak in both hindlimbs. On neurologic examination, the findings include bilateral proprioceptive deficits of the hindlimbs, normal to hyperreflexic patellar reflexes, normal hindlimb withdrawal reflexes, normal perineal reflexes, and an area of hyperpathia over the lumbar spine. The front limbs and the cranial nerves (CNs) are normal. What is the most likely diagnosis?

(1) Fibrocartilaginous embolism at T3–L3
(2) Cervical spondylomyelopathy at C1–C5
(3) Intervertebral disk disease at T3–L3
(4) Meningitis
(5) Intervertebral disk disease at L4–Cd5

8. Of the following dog breeds, which one has a predisposition for the development of cervical spondylomyelopathy (wobbler syndrome)?

(1) Dachshund
(2) Labrador retriever
(3) Irish wolfhound
(4) German shepherd
(5) Doberman pinscher

9. An 8-year-old male German shepherd is presented for incoordination and weakness in the hindlimbs. The owner reports that incoordination and scuffing of the hind paws first started several months ago but now the dog seems worse and has difficulty rising and climbing into the car. The dog has been otherwise healthy with a good appetite and attitude. A neurologic examination reveals bilateral proprioceptive deficits and poor hopping reactions in both hindlimbs. The dog can walk but is weak in the hindlimbs. The patellar and hindlimb withdrawal reflexes are normal to hyperreflexic. The perineal reflex is normal. The front limbs and cranial nerves (CNs) are normal. Other than a moderate degree of muscle atrophy in both hindlimbs, no areas of pain in the hindlimbs or spine are detected. Analysis of cerebrospinal fluid (CSF) and a myelogram are normal. What is the most likely diagnosis?

(1) Cervical spondylomyelopathy
(2) Lumbosacral stenosis
(3) Degenerative myelopathy
(4) Chronic (type II) disk herniation
(5) Spinal cord neoplasia

10. Bacterial organisms commonly isolated from dogs with diskospondylitis include:

(1) *Pasteurella multocida, Escherichia coli,* and *Pseudomonas aeruginosa.*
(2) *Staphylococcus* species, *Streptococcus* species, and *Brucella canis.*
(3) *B. canis, Mycobacterium avium,* and *Proteus mirabilis.*
(4) *Staphylococcus* species, *E. coli,* and *P. aeruginosa.*
(5) *Streptococcus* species, *Klebsiella* species, and *E. coli.*

11. A 10-year-old female spayed mixed-breed dog is presented because of the acute onset of head tilt and falling. The owner first noted the head tilt yesterday, and the dog has been very unsteady on her feet and falling over and rolling. The owner reports that the dog has been healthy up until now. The owner also gave the dog two doses of amoxicillin the day before the head tilt started because the dog was pruritic. On a neurologic examination, the dog has a severe head tilt to the left and rotatory nystagmus. There are no proprioceptive deficits or weakness. No other cranial nerve (CN) abnormalities are noted, and spinal reflexes are normal. An otoscopic examination of the external ear canals is normal. Which one of the following is the most likely diagnosis?

(1) Brain stem neoplasia
(2) Otitis media or otitis interna
(3) Neoplasia of the middle or inner ear
(4) Idiopathic vestibular disease
(5) Adverse drug effect

12. Congenital deafness is most likely in which one of the following breeds?

(1) German shepherds
(2) Dalmatians
(3) Siamese cats
(4) Bichons frisé
(5) Doberman pinschers

13. Which one of the infectious agents listed below might be found on a muscle biopsy from a dog younger than 4 months of age with hindlimb rigidity, hyporeflexia, and muscle atrophy?

(1) *Clostridium perfringens*
(2) *Blastomyces dermatitidis*
(3) *Neospora caninum*
(4) *Cryptococcus neoformans*
(5) *Rickettsia rickettsii*

14. Profound weakness develops in a 16-year-old female spayed cat that is being treated for chronic renal failure. The owner reports that the cat's appetite has been poor for the last 4–5 days but the extreme weakness did not seem to develop until today. On physical examination, the cat is in sternal recumbency and cannot stand. It is holding its head in a ventroflexed position and cannot lift it. What would be the most likely cause of this cat's weakness?

(1) Worsening uremia
(2) Feline ischemic encephalopathy
(3) Acute polyradiculoneuritis
(4) Immune-mediated polymyositis
(5) Hypokalemia

DIRECTIONS: Each of the numbered items or incomplete statements in this section is negatively phrased, as indicated by a capitalized word such as NOT, LEAST, or EXCEPT. Select the ONE numbered answer or completion that is BEST in each case.

15. A 9-year-old male neutered Border collie is presented because of seizures. The owner reports that the seizures began 2 weeks ago and the dog has had three seizures since then. The owner feels the dog is healthy but not as active as before the seizures began. Neurologic and physical examinations are normal. Of the diseases listed below, which one is LEAST likely to be the cause of the seizures in this dog?

(1) Brain neoplasia
(2) Hypoglycemia
(3) Liver failure
(4) Granulomatous meningoencephalitis (GME)
(5) Idiopathic epilepsy

ANSWERS AND EXPLANATIONS

1. The answer is 2 [I C 2 e (1) (b)]. The reduced withdrawal reflex in the right hindlimb suggests either a spinal cord injury in the L6–S1 region or a peripheral nerve injury (i.e., to the sciatic nerve). The strict unilateral nature of the signs would make peripheral nerve injury more likely than spinal cord injury, which is usually associated with bilateral signs (asymmetric or symmetric). The normal patellar reflex rules out a spinal cord lesion in the L4–L6 region or damage to the femoral nerve. Also, a normal patellar reflex would support a diagnosis of peripheral sciatic nerve injury because a spinal cord lesion would rarely be so isolated as to affect only the withdrawal reflex (L6–S1) and not the patellar reflex (L4–L6). The absence of an abnormal perineal reflex would rule out pudendal nerve disease.

2. The answer is 3 [Table 47-2]. The signs are typical of facial nerve paralysis (motor to facial muscles). Loss of the sensory branches of the trigeminal nerve may abolish the palpebral reflex (eye blink) but would not affect the facial muscles (i.e., drooping of the lip). Hypoglossal nerve paralysis is ruled out by the fact that there are no abnormalities associated with the tongue. The lack of head tilt and nystagmus rule out vestibular nerve disease. Oculomotor nerve dysfunction would manifest with pupillary dilation, loss of the pupillary light reflex (PLR), and possibly, ventrolateral strabismus.

3. The answer is 5 [Table 47-3; II G 3 c]. Steroid-responsive meningitis is the only predominantly inflammatory condition listed. It typically results in an intensely inflammatory cerebrospinal fluid (CSF) with mostly neutrophils. Intervertebral disk disease, cervical spondylomyelopathy, and fibrocartilaginous emboli do not cause marked changes in the CSF. Trauma to the neck could be associated with normal CSF or evidence of hemorrhage within the CSF, but a marked inflammation would be absent.

4. The answer is 1 [II A 2]. The neurologic signs of ataxia, normal strength, hypermetria, and intention tremors are typical of cerebellar disease. Cerebrocortical disease is often associated with changes in mentation or seizures.

Cervical spinal cord disease would be associated with proprioceptive deficits or paresis, either upper motor neuron (UMN, C1–C5) or lower motor neuron (LMN, C6–T2) in nature. Brain stem disease can also be associated with proprioceptive deficits or paresis and CN abnormalities or altered mentation.

5. The answer is 4 [II A 5; Table 21-1]. The neurologic abnormalities are most consistent with a central vestibular lesion. Although a head tilt is common to both peripheral and central vestibular disease, nystagmus that changes direction with altered head positions and especially paresis and proprioceptive deficits in the ipsilateral fore- and hindlimbs are suggestive of central or brain stem disease. Head tilt is usually not a feature of cerebellar disease and is never a feature of spinal cord disease (unless multifocal disease is present).

6. The answer is 2 [II G 2 a]. Dogs can shed rabies virus in their saliva up to 13 days before showing clinical signs.

7. The answer is 3 [III A 2 c, B 1 b (1) (a) (i)]. The neurologic signs suggest a T3–L3 lesion. Pain (hyperpathia) is a consistent feature of intervertebral disk disease. Pain is not a feature of fibrocartilaginous embolism. In dogs with meningitis, the pain is usually in the cervical area, and neurologic deficits are not common but can occur.

8. The answer is 5 [III B 2]. Doberman pinschers and Great Danes are two breeds that are predisposed to cervical spondylomyelopathy (wobbler syndrome), but all large-breed dogs may be affected.

9. The answer is 3 [III B 4]. The most likely diagnosis is degenerative myelopathy. The neurologic signs are consistent with a T3–L3 lesion. In addition, degenerative myelopathy occurs primarily in German shepherds and related breeds. Cervical spondylomyelopathy is characterized by neurologic signs of a C1–C5 lesion, and lumbosacral stenosis results from compression in the cauda equina region. The absence of pain also makes lumbosacral stenosis unlikely. Although cerebrospinal fluid (CSF) analysis may be normal with degenerative myelopathy, disk herniation, or spinal cord neoplasia, a normal myelogram would only occur with degenerative myelopathy. Extradural compression should be evident with disk herniation. Variable patterns (e.g., extradural compression, intradural–extramedullary compression, intramedullary compression) may be seen on a myelogram with spinal cord neoplasia.

10. The answer is 2 [III F 1 a (1)]. Although many bacterial organisms and some fungal organisms can cause diskospondylitis, most cases are associated with *Staphylococcus* species, *Streptococcus* species, and *Brucella canis.*

11. The answer is 4 [IV E 2]. Idiopathic vestibular disease produces acute peripheral vestibular signs (as seen in this dog), often in aged dogs. Brain stem neoplasia can be ruled out by the lack of central vestibular signs. Otitis media or otitis interna would be an important differential, but no evidence of either otitis externa or otitis media or interna was observed on otoscopic examination. Although the lack of otoscopic examination findings does not rule out otitis media or otitis interna, it makes it less likely. Neoplasia of the middle or inner ear could produce these signs, but the onset would likely be more gradual. An adverse drug effect resulting in vestibular signs can been associated with aminoglycoside antibiotics (e.g., gentamicin) but not with amoxicillin.

12. The answer is 2 [IV F 3 a]. Congenital deafness (unilateral or bilateral) is common in the Dalmatian breed (prevalence of 20%–30%). It is uncommon in German shepherds, Siamese cats, Bichons frisé, and Doberman pinschers.

13. The answer is 3 [II G 2 e]. *Neosporum caninum* is most likely to be found on a muscle biopsy from a young dog with hindlimb rigidity, hyporeflexia, and muscle atrophy. This clinical presentation has been observed with neosporosis or toxoplasmosis. Both of these organisms may be detected on muscle biopsies. All of the other organisms, except *Clostridium perfringens,* do not primarily infect muscle. The clinical presentation of *C. perfringens* infection is usually one of a focal myositis rather than the clinical syndrome described in the question.

14. The answer is 5 [V D 3]. Hypokalemia is a common cause of muscle weakness. Cats with chronic renal failure, and especially those that are anorectic, are predisposed to the development of hypokalemia. Although worsening uremia may cause weakness, it does not tend to develop rapidly and to such a severe degree. Feline ischemic encephalopathy is usually associated with marked behavioral changes or seizures. Acute polyradiculoneuritis is extremely rare in cats. Immune-mediated polymyositis can cause severe weakness, but it usually has a slow, insidious onset.

15. The answer is 5 [II H 1 b]. Seizures that begin in dogs older than 5 years of age are unlikely to be related to idiopathic epilepsy. In older animals, neoplasia and organ failure are more likely. Inflammatory disease has a broad age range. Hypoglycemia may occur in young or old dogs and is due to many causes.

Chapter 48

Hematologic and Immunologic Diseases

I. TRANSFUSION THERAPY

A. Blood groups

1. **Canine blood groups.** Dogs have eight blood groups, which are designated as dog erythrocyte antigen (DEA) 1.1, 1.2, and 3 to 8.
   a. **Transfusion reactions.** Transfusion to dogs that have preformed antibodies to DEA 1.1 or 1.2 can result in hemolysis and transfusion reactions. However, dogs rarely have performed antibodies to DEA 1.1 or 1.2, so transfusion reactions are rare in dogs that have never had a transfusion.
   b. **Universal donors** are negative for DEA 1.1, 1.2, and 7.

2. **Feline blood groups.** Cats have two major blood groups (A and B) and one rare type (AB).
   a. **Transfusion reactions.** Giving type A blood to a cat with type B blood can cause severe transfusion reactions.
      (1) **Type A.** Most domestic short- and long-haired cats in North America have type A blood and a low level of antibody to type B blood.
      (2) **Type B.** This blood type is most prevalent in purebred Abyssinian, Birman, British shorthair, Devon Rex, Himalayan, Persian, Scottish fold, and Somali cats. It has not been found in Siamese cats. Most cats with type B blood have high levels of antibody to type A blood.
   b. **Universal donors** do not exist in cats.

B. Blood components

1. **Cellular components**
   a. **Whole blood.** Red blood cells (RBCs) and plasma proteins provide both RBC mass and volume support.
      (1) **Fresh whole blood** (transfused within a few hours of collection) contains viable platelets and coagulation factors and is indicated when, in addition to mass and volume support, coagulation support is required [e.g., warfarin intoxication, thrombocytopenia, vonWillebrand's disease (vWD)].
      (2) **Stored whole blood** lacks viable platelets and coagulation factors V, VIII, and vonWillebrand's factor (vWF).
   b. **Packed RBCs** are produced by removing most of the plasma. They can provide RBC mass when volume or coagulation support is not needed.
   c. **Platelet-rich plasma** is used for patients that are thrombocytopenic but not anemic.

2. **Plasma components**
   a. **Fresh frozen plasma** contains coagulation factors and is used most often for patients that have coagulopathies but no anemia.
   b. **Stored frozen plasma** (harvested from stored whole blood) can supply plasma proteins for volume support or albumin for severely hypoalbuminemic patients. Although stored frozen plasma contains minimal factor V, VIII, and vWF, it has adequate concentrations of vitamin K–dependent coagulation factors (II, VII, IX, X).
   c. **Cryoprecipitate,** which is not widely available, contains about 10 times the concentration of coagulation factors of fresh frozen plasma, enabling the administra-

tion of high concentrations of coagulation factors without a large volume of plasma.

C. **Indications for transfusion therapy**

1. **Anemia.** Indications for RBC mass (with or without plasma) include:
   a. A packed cell volume (PCV) of less than 10%
   b. A PCV that has decreased rapidly to less than 20% in dogs or less than 12%–15% in cats
   c. The loss of more than 30% of the blood volume (30 ml/kg in dogs, 20 ml/kg in cats)
   d. Blood loss that is associated with collapse
   e. Poor response to fluid therapy in an animal with acute hemorrhage and shock

2. **Bleeding tendency.** Indications for fresh whole blood or plasma include:
   a. Life-threatening hemorrhage
   b. Surgery in an animal known to have a bleeding disorder

3. **Thrombocytopenia.** Indications for fresh whole blood (if anemia is present), fresh plasma, or platelet-rich plasma include:
   a. Life-threatening hemorrhage due to thrombocytopenia
   b. Surgery in a thrombocytopenic animal

4. **Hypoproteinemia.** Indications for plasma (fresh, fresh frozen, or stored) include:
   a. Plasma albumin concentrations less than 1.5 g/dl
   b. Surgery in a hypoproteinemic animal

5. **Hypovolemia.** Whole blood or plasma may be indicated for volume support if severe hemodilution (i.e., reduced plasma protein concentration and RBC mass) is resulting from aggressive intravenous fluid administration during shock therapy.

D. **Administration of transfusion therapy.** In general, 10 ml/kg of whole blood will raise the packed cell volume (PCV) by 10%. Administration should begin slowly (to observe for adverse effects) and be completed within 4 hours (to decrease the risk of bacterial growth in the administration equipment). If a reaction is suspected (see I E), the transfusion should be stopped, and antihistamines and corticosteroids should be administered. If the reaction is not serious and signs abate, the transfusion can usually be restarted without consequence.

1. **Dogs.** Crossmatching is recommended, but if not possible, blood from a universal donor may be used. The target PCV is 25%–30%.

2. **Cats.** Preformed antibodies to other blood groups do occur in cats; therefore, **crossmatching** or blood typing before transfusion is much more important in cats than in dogs. Purebred cats of the breeds listed in I A 2 a (2), cats that have received blood transfusions in the past, and cats that will require multiple transfusions should be crossmatched. The target PCV is 15%–20%.

E. **Complications of transfusion therapy**

1. Mild effects, which include pyrexia (mostly in cats), nausea (hypersalivation), vomiting (mostly in dogs), urticaria, and chills, are infrequent.

2. Severe, life-threatening reactions (i.e., acute hemolysis, respiratory distress) are very rare.

3. Other adverse effects include disease transmission [e.g., feline leukemia virus (FeLV)], hypothermia (following the administration of cold blood components), hypocalcemia (from overly aggressive administration of citrated blood components), and hyperammonemia (in the presence of reduced liver function or a portosystemic shunt). Ammonia levels increase over time in stored whole blood.

II. DISORDERS OF RED BLOOD CELLS

A. **Anemia** is present if the PCV, hematocrit, or RBC count is less than the reference range for the age and species of animal. (Generally, the PCV is less than 38% in dogs and less than 24% in cats.) Puppies and kittens younger than 4–6 months of age often have a slightly subnormal hematocrit.

1. **General considerations**
   a. **Clinical findings**
      (1) **Specific signs** of anemia include exercise intolerance, lethargy, weakness, pica, pale mucous membranes, tachycardia, and a systolic murmur (if the PCV is less than 20%–25%).
      (2) **Nonspecific signs** that may relate to the underlying cause include icterus, petechiae, ecchymoses, blood in the stool, lymphadenopathy, hepatomegaly, and splenomegaly.
   b. **Diagnostic evaluation.** Anemia is a symptom of underlying disease, so a thorough patient evaluation is required. The first step in identifying the cause of anemia is to categorize the anemia as regenerative or nonregenerative.
      (1) **Regenerative anemias** are due to blood loss (internal or external) or RBC hemolysis. Characteristics that can help distinguish blood loss from RBC hemolysis are presented in Table 48-1.
         (a) In dogs, a regenerative anemia is present if the reticulocyte count is greater than 150,000 cells/μl or the reticulocyte index (RI) or reticulocyte production index (RPI) is greater than 1.0 (Tables 48-2 and 48-3).
         (b) In cats, a regenerative anemia is present if the aggregate reticulocyte count (types II and III) is greater than 50,000 cells/μl or the punctate reticulocyte count is greater than 500,000 cells/μl (see Table 48-2).
      (2) **Nonregenerative anemias** usually develop chronically and are often due to anemia of chronic disease (ACD), bone marrow disease, or renal disease. A nonregenerative anemia is present when the reticulocyte count or the RI is less than the values discussed for regenerative anemias.
2. **Regenerative anemias**
   a. **Blood loss anemia.** Anemia associated with blood loss is influenced by the initiating disease process, the rapidity of blood loss (i.e., peracute, acute, or chronic), and the location of the hemorrhage (i.e., external, internal). A reduc-

TABLE 48-1. Differentiation between Blood Loss and Hemolytic Causes of Regenerative Anemia

	Blood Loss	Hemolysis
Serum protein	Normal to low	Normal to high
Evidence of bleeding	Common	Rare
Icterus	Absent	Common
Hemoglobinemia	Absent	Common
Spherocytosis	Absent to mild	Moderate to marked
Red blood cell (RBC) inclusions (e.g., Heinz bodies, infectious agents)	Absent	Occasional
Autoagglutination	Absent	Occasional
Direct Coomb's test	Negative	Usually positive with IHA
Splenomegaly	Absent	Common
Reticulocyte index (RI)*	1–3	$\geq$3**

IHA = immune-mediated hemolytic anemia.
Modified with permission from Murtaugh R, Kaplan P (eds.): *Veterinary Emergency and Critical Care Medicine,* St. Louis, Mosby-Year Book, 1992, p 361.
* Dogs only.
** May be <3 early in disease.

TABLE 48-2. Degree of Regenerative Response Based on Reticulocyte Percentage and Number

	Dog		Cat		
Degree of Regeneration	Reticulocyte Percentage	Reticulocyte Count (cells/μl)	Reticulocyte Percentage	Aggregate Reticulocyte (II & III) Count (cells/μl)	Punctate Reticulocyte Count (cells/μl)
None	1	60,000	0–0.4	<15,000	<200,000
Slight	1–4	150,000	0.5–2	50,000	500,000
Moderate	5–20	300,000	3–4	100,000	1,000,000
Marked	21–50	>500,000	>5	>200,000	1,500,000

tion in plasma (total) protein is an important clue when trying to distinguish blood loss anemia from hemolytic anemia. However, decreased plasma protein is delayed in peracute blood loss and is usually not present if blood loss is internal.

(1) Peracute blood loss occurs over minutes to hours.

    (a) Laboratory findings

        (i) PCV and **total protein.** The PCV and total protein may not decrease until 12–24 hours after hemorrhage (sooner if intravenous fluids are administered). Blood loss into the peritoneal cavity can result in **autotransfusion** of RBCs via the lymphatics and a rapid restoration of the PCV (e.g., within a few days). Blood loss into tissue does not result in autotransfusion because the RBCs are degraded.

        (ii) Reticulocyte response

        Dogs. The reticulocyte response in dogs is detected in about 72 hours and peaks in 5 days.

        Cats. In cats, aggregate reticulocytes peak in about 4 days and punctate reticulocytes peak in about 7 days. Aggregate reticulocytes usually disappear by 1 week posthemorrhage whereas punctate reticulocytes remain elevated for about 3 weeks.

TABLE 48-3. Calculation of the Reticulocyte Index (RI) or the Reticulocyte Production Index (RPI)*

1. Calculate the corrected reticulocyte percentage (CRP)

$$CRP = \text{reticulocyte \%} \times \frac{\text{patient hematocrit}}{45}$$

2. Calculate the reticulocyte index (RI)

$$RI = \frac{CRP}{\text{reticulocyte life span}}$$

Reticulocyte Life Span (days)	Patient Hematocrit (%)
1.0	45
1.5	35
2.0	25
2.5	15

3. Interpretation of the RI

RI < 1.0: Nonregenerative anemia
RI 1.0–3.0: Regenerative anemia (most consistent with blood loss)
RI ≥ 3.0: Regenerative anemia (most consistent with hemolysis)

* Dogs only.

(iii) White blood cell (WBC) count. A stress leukocytosis is often evident within a few hours of hemorrhage.

(iv) Platelet count. Platelet numbers are usually normal but can be decreased following marked hemorrhage. Thrombocytosis starts the third day posthemorrhage.

(b) Treatment. Objectives include:

(i) Correction of hypovolemia (more important initially than replacing the decreased RBC mass)

(ii) Location and cessation of hemorrhage

(iii) Restoration of circulating volume with intravenous fluid (i.e., crystalloid) therapy or blood transfusion (if the hematocrit declines precipitously following intravenous fluid administration)

(2) Acute blood loss occurs over days. Hypovolemia is usually not severe because of fluid movement into the vascular compartment from extravascular sources, but the anemia can be marked.

(a) Laboratory findings

(i) Total protein. The total protein is reduced.

(ii) Reticulocyte response. The reticulocyte response is moderate to marked.

(b) Treatment. Objectives include:

(i) Location and cessation of the hemorrhage

(ii) Replacement of RBC mass with a blood transfusion if the PCV is significantly decreased

(iii) Correction of the underlying cause

(3) Chronic blood loss occurs over weeks to months. A **regenerative anemia** develops initially, but as iron deficiency develops, a **nonregenerative anemia** becomes established. The vascular volume is usually maintained despite severe anemia.

(a) Etiology. In young animals, **hookworm infestation** and **severe external parasitism** are common causes of chronic blood loss. In adult animals, **bleeding tendencies** and **bleeding from gastrointestinal (GI) ulcers** or **tumors** are more common causes.

(b) Laboratory findings include those of **iron deficiency.** Iron deficiency is determined by the rate and volume of blood loss and the age of the animal. Diagnostic features of iron deficiency include RBC microcytosis and hypochromasia and a reduced serum iron concentration and transferrin saturation. The total iron binding capacity is usually normal and there are no hemosiderin deposits in the bone marrow.

(c) Treatment. Objectives include:

(i) Correction of the low RBC mass (as opposed to correction of hypovolemia)

(ii) Correction of the underlying cause

(iii) Administration of iron salts (e.g., ferrous sulfate, ferrous gluconate) to iron-deficient animals

b. Hemolytic anemia. RBC destruction can be intravascular (i.e., occurring inside the vascular compartment) or extravascular (i.e., occurring outside the vascular compartment). Extravascular hemolysis, which is more common, results from RBC removal by the mononuclear-phagocyte system (mostly in the liver and spleen).

(1) Congenital hemolytic anemia. Congenital causes of hemolytic anemia are rare and include RBC enzyme deficiencies (e.g., pyruvate kinase deficiency in basenjis, beagles, and West Highland white terriers or phosphofructokinase deficiency in English springer spaniels), feline porphyria, and stomatocytosis in chondrodysplastic Alaskan malamutes.

(2) Immune-mediated hemolytic anemia (IHA). Primary IHA, which has no underlying cause and is most common in dogs, is the focus of the discussion. Most frequently affected are young to middle-aged female poodles, cocker spaniels, Irish setters, and Old English sheepdogs. **Secondary IHA** can result from drug administration, infectious agents (e.g., FeLV), and neoplasia, and is more common in cats.

(a) Pathogenesis
    (i) Immunoglobulin G (IgG). The most common mechanism of RBC destruction involves the binding of IgG antibody to the surface of RBCs, resulting in the selective extravascular destruction of antibody-coated RBCs (via phagocytosis by the mononuclear-phagocyte system). In dogs, frequently only portions of the RBC are removed by phagocytic cells, resulting in the formation of **spherocytes** (i.e., RBCs that are smaller and lack a central area of pallor).
    (ii) Immunoglobulin M (IgM). If IgM antibody is the primary antibody involved, intravascular hemolysis is more likely because IgM is more efficient than IgG at activating complement.

(b) Clinical findings include the acute onset of lethargy, depression, weakness, as well as vomiting and abdominal pain (in some animals), mucous membrane pallor, dehydration, petechiation or ecchymoses (if concurrent thrombocytopenia is present), icterus (due to the generation of bilirubin from hemoglobin metabolism at a rate that exceeds the liver's capacity to excrete it), fever, hepatosplenomegaly, and a systolic murmur (due to the anemia).

(c) Laboratory findings
    (i) A moderate to marked regenerative anemia with marked spherocytosis is common. A nonregenerative anemia is present in some dogs resulting from either marrow stem cell damage or peracute hemolysis.
    (ii) Thrombocytopenia due to immune-mediated removal may also be apparent.
    (iii) A neutrophilic leukocytosis with a left shift, monocytosis, and increased numbers of nucleated RBCs may occur.
    (iv) The plasma protein concentration is normal to increased. Plasma may be red-tinged (from intravascular hemolysis) or icteric (from increased serum bilirubin).
    (v) Hemoglobinuria (port wine–colored urine) may be noted. Bilirubinuria is common.
    (vi) Autoagglutination within a blood collection tube or on a microscope slide may be present. When equal volumes of blood and normal saline are mixed together on a microscope slide, normal rouleaux will disperse and autoagglutination will not.

(d) Diagnosis
    (i) A **regenerative anemia with moderate to marked spherocytosis** is a hallmark sign of IHA, although mild spherocytosis may accompany any cause of regenerative anemia or RBC fragmentation. The presence of autoagglutination or a positive Coombs' (antiglobulin) test is supportive for IHA. However, the Coombs' test is negative in 10%–30% of dogs with IHA.
    (ii) Diagnosis of the nonregenerative form, although problematic, can be based on the presence of spherocytosis, a positive Coombs' test, and evidence of an interruption in RBC development on bone marrow examination.

(e) Treatment
    (i) Immunosuppressive therapy with corticosteroids (e.g., prednisone) usually produces improvement within 1–4 days. Corticosteroids act primarily by suppressing RBC phagocytosis by the mononuclear-phagocyte system. Concurrent use of corticosteroids and cyclophosphamide may be necessary in dogs with acute severe anemia, autoagglutination, icterus, or signs of intravascular hemolysis. Immunosuppressive therapy is gradually reduced to the lowest effective dose over several months. Drug therapy may be required for several months only or for the rest of the animal's life.
    (ii) Low-dose heparin administration during initial therapy may minimize the increased risk of thromboembolic disease.
    (iii) Blood transfusions may be required.

   (iv) Other treatments for refractory cases include danazol, cyclosporine, azathioprine, human immunoglobulin (purified polyclonal IgG), plasmapheresis, or splenectomy.
- **(f) Complications** of IHA include drug-induced immunosuppression leading to sepsis, acute renal failure (from hemoglobin nephrotoxicity), pulmonary thromboembolism, and drug-induced vomiting and pancreatitis.
- **(g) Prognosis.** The prognosis is variable. Response to initial therapy and long-term control is achieved in many dogs. However, some dogs with severe disease do not respond to any therapy and die or are euthanized within a few days of admission.
- **(3) Infectious causes of hemolytic anemia**
  - **(a) Hemobartonellosis** is the most common cause of hemolytic anemia in cats. It occurs in cats of all ages, with a peak incidence between the ages of 4 and 6 years. Male cats are affected more often, probably because of increased roaming and fighting.
    - **(i) Etiology** and **pathogenesis.** *Hemobartonella felis* is an epicellular rickettsial parasite of RBCs. Most transmission is thought to occur via blood-sucking arthropods (i.e., fleas) and, to a lesser extent, via bite wounds. Episodes of anemia result from intermittent parasitemia and the removal of infected RBCs by the mononuclear-phagocyte system.
    - **(ii) Clinical signs.** The most common clinical signs are depression, anorexia, weakness, weight loss, pale mucous membranes, and occasionally splenomegaly and icterus.
    - **(iii) Laboratory findings.** A regenerative anemia (with or without monocytosis) varies from mild to severe. During the acute phase of the disease, infected RBCs can be recognized in stained blood smears in about 50% of affected cats. A positive Coombs' test is not unusual, and autoagglutination is sometimes observed.
    - **(iv) Diagnosis** is based on the observation of *H. felis* organisms on RBCs or a positive response to antimicrobial therapy. *H. felis* organisms on RBCs must be differentiated from Howell-Jolly bodies, basophilic stippling, and *Cytauxzoon felis*. Because of the cyclic nature of parasitemia, the absence of visible organisms does not rule out the disease; conversely, the presence of rare organisms does not necessarily indicate that these organisms are inducing disease and anemia.
    - **(v) Treatment.** Cats should be treated with tetracycline or doxycycline for 3 weeks. Prednisone can be added to inhibit RBC destruction if the anemia is severe or progressive. Blood transfusion may be required in severely anemic cats.
    - **(vi) Prognosis.** About one-third of untreated cats will die following experimental infection. Untreated cats that recover often remain infected for months to years. Approximately 40% of cats with hemobartonellosis are infected with feline leukemia virus (FeLV). The immunosuppressive effects of FeLV enable the infection to become established and may exacerbate the clinical signs and slow recovery. The long-term prognosis is good in treated cats free of FeLV.
  - **(b) Babesiosis** is a rare cause of hemolytic anemia.
    - **(i) Etiology.** *Babesia canis* is a protozoan that infects RBCs. It is transmitted by the brown dog tick, *Rhipicephalus sanguineus*.
    - **(ii) Diagnosis.** Clinical signs vary from a mild to moderate anemia, fever, and lethargy to intravascular hemolysis, hemoglobinemia, hemoglobinuria, severe acidosis, dehydration, and weakness. Many dogs have a positive Coombs' test. Diagnosis is based on visualizing the organism within RBCs on a blood smear.
    - **(iii) Treatment.** Fluid therapy, blood transfusions, or bicarbonate administration may be required in severely ill dogs. Effective antiparasitic drugs (e.g., imidocarb) are not available in North America. Although less effective, tetracycline is recommended.

(c) **Cytauxzoonosis** is seen primarily in the southern United States. The infection is caused by *Cytauxzoon felis,* a protozoan that infects tissue macrophages, blood monocytes, and RBCs in cats. Cytauxzoonosis is characterized by fever, dyspnea, hemolytic anemia, thrombocytopenia, icterus, and splenomegaly. Diagnosis is made by visualizing the organisms in RBCs. There is no known successful treatment, and cytauxzoonosis is rapidly fatal.

(4) **Miscellaneous causes of hemolytic anemia** include hypophosphatemia, neonatal isoerythrolysis, microangiopathic hemolytic anemia, oxidant injury (e.g., onion ingestion in dogs, zinc toxicity, acetaminophen toxicity, methylene blue toxicity, benzocaine toxicity, phenothiazine toxicity), and drugs (e.g., sulfas, penicillins, cephalosporins, anticonvulsants, methimazole, propylthiouracil).

3. **Nonregenerative anemias** most often result from primary or secondary bone marrow disease; therefore, bone marrow aspiration or biopsy is frequently required.

   a. **ACD** is the most common cause of nonregenerative anemia in dogs and cats.

   (1) **Etiology.** ACD occurs secondary to many chronic inflammatory, degenerative, or neoplastic diseases. It results from the sequestration of iron within bone marrow mononuclear-phagocyte cells.

   (2) **Laboratory findings**

   (a) The mild to moderate anemia is usually normocytic and normochromic. Serum iron may be mildly reduced and the total iron binding capacity is normal.

   (b) The main differential is iron-deficiency anemia, differentiated by bone marrow examination and serum ferritin concentration.

   (i) **ACD.** Abundant iron stores are usually visible in the marrow. Serum ferritin concentrations are normal.

   (ii) **Iron-deficiency anemia.** Abundant iron stores are not usually visible in the marrow. Serum ferritin concentrations are reduced.

   (3) **Treatment** is focused on reversing the underlying disease.

   b. **Hypoproliferative anemia**

   (1) **Etiology.** Hypoproliferative anemias can result from:

   (a) Bone marrow disease, including maturational abnormalities induced by toxins (e.g., estrogen, chemotherapy) and infection (e.g., FeLV infection, ehrlichiosis)

   (b) The physical crowding out of normal marrow cells by neoplastic cells (e.g., myeloproliferative disorders, lymphosarcoma), fibrous tissue (i.e., myelofibrosis), or bone (i.e., osteosclerosis)

   (2) **Laboratory findings.** In addition to anemia, many of these diseases affect other cell lines and result in thrombocytopenia and neutropenia. Pure red cell aplasia or erythroid hypoplasia or aplasia may be associated with FeLV infection in cats or immune-mediated mechanisms in dogs.

   (3) **Specific disorders**

   (a) **FeLV infection** is the most common cause of anemia of any kind in cats. FeLV may cause a regenerative anemia via immune-mediated RBC destruction; however, in most cats, it results in a nonregenerative anemia caused by pure red cell aplasia (erythroid hypoplasia), myeloaplasia (all cell lines affected), myelodysplasia, myeloproliferative disorders, or myelofibrosis. **Laboratory findings,** in addition to anemia, may include RBC macrocytosis and other cytopenias. **Treatment** of the nonregenerative anemia is primarily supportive (i.e., blood transfusions, good nutrition, treatment of concurrent illness). The anemia usually progresses despite therapy.

   (b) **Estrogen toxicity** can result from repeated high doses of diethylstilbestrol, single injections of estradiol cypionate, estrogen-secreting Sertoli cell tumors in dogs, or prolonged estrus in ferrets. All cell lines are affected, resulting in neutropenia, thrombocytopenia, and a nonregenerative anemia. Paradoxically, leukocytosis develops initially but is soon followed by profound marrow suppression. **Diagnosis** is based on a history of estrogen administration or the detection of an estrogen-secreting tumor. **Treatment** is primarily supportive (i.e., blood transfusions). Many dogs die of sepsis, refractory anemia, or hemorrhage.

- **(c)** **Myelofibrosis** and **osteosclerosis** are considered sequelae to marrow injury or disease and have been associated with myeloproliferative disorders, FeLV infection, and pyruvate kinase deficiency.
- **(d)** **Pure red cell aplasia in dogs** is thought to be caused by the immune-mediated destruction of erythroid precursors in the bone marrow.
  - **(i)** **Diagnosis.** In addition to a moderate to severe nonregenerative anemia, some dogs have a positive Coombs' test. Diagnosis is based on bone marrow examination and response to therapy.
  - **(ii)** **Therapy.** Most dogs respond to immunosuppressive therapy (similar to that used in IHA) and supportive care. Lifelong drug therapy is frequently required.

- **c.** **Anemia of renal disease** results from reduced erythropoietin production in the kidneys.
- **d.** **Anemia of endocrine disorders.** Hypothyroidism and hypoadrenocorticism can be associated with a mild nonregenerative anemia.

B. **Erythrocytosis (polycythemia)** refers to an increase in the RBC mass.

1. **Etiology.** Causes of erythrocytosis are listed in Table 48-4.

2. **Diagnosis**
   - **a.** **Clinical findings.** Signs do not develop until the PCV is greater than 65%–70%. Most signs are related to hyperviscosity and sluggish blood flow. They include central nervous system (CNS) signs (e.g., changes in mentation, seizures) and paroxysmal sneezing (congestion of the nasal mucosa).
   - **b.** **Laboratory findings**
     - **(1)** Concurrent thrombocytosis may occur in dogs with polycythemia vera.
     - **(2)** Microcytosis is common in patients with absolute polycythemia.
     - **(3)** The polycythemia associated with hyperadrenocorticism, hyperthyroidism, and corticosteroid or androgen administration is usually mild.
   - **c.** A **diagnostic approach** is summarized in Figure 48-1.

TABLE 48-4. Causes and Classification of Polycythemia in Dogs and Cats

Relative polycythemia
   Hemoconcentration
Absolute polycythemia
   Primary
      Polycythemia rubra vera
   Secondary
      Appropriate (in the presence of tissue hypoxia)
         Pulmonary disease
         Right-to-left cardiac shunt
         High altitude
         Hemoglobinopathies
      Inappropriate (in the absence of tissue hypoxia)
         Hyperadrenocorticism
         Hyperthyroidism
         Renal masses
         Nonrenal neoplasia

Reprinted with permission from Nelson RW, Couto GC (eds.): *Essentials of Small Animal Internal Medicine,* St. Louis, Mosby-Year Book, 1992, p 909.

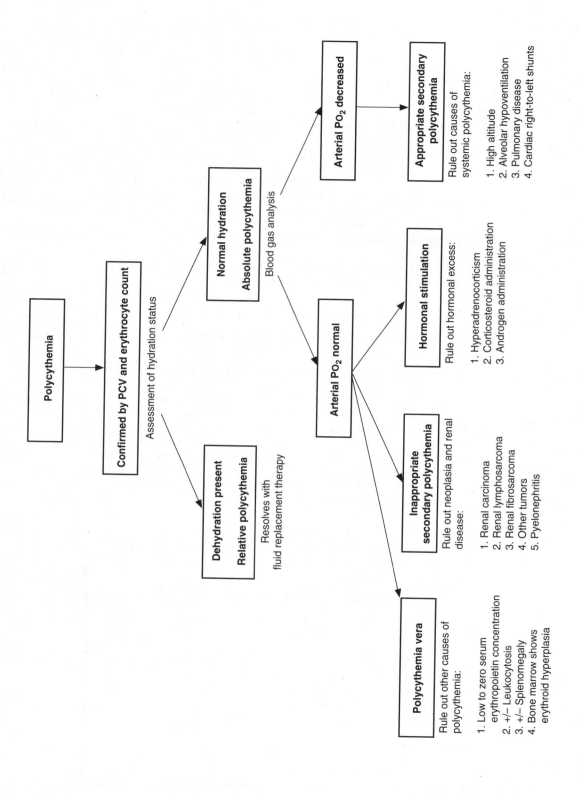

3. Treatment
  a. Relative polycythemia is treated by correcting the dehydration.
  b. Absolute polycythemia. The underlying disorder should be treated, if possible. For polycythemia vera, hydroxyurea may help suppress RBC production. Intermittent phlebotomy may be required to keep the PCV below 65%.

III. DISORDERS OF WHITE BLOOD CELLS

A. Leukocytosis

  1. Neutrophilia. Leukocytosis is almost always accompanied by neutrophilia because neutrophils make up the largest fraction of the blood leukocytes.
    a. Etiology
      (1) Inflammation. Acute suppurative inflammation is a common cause of neutrophilia and may result from:
        (a) Bacterial, fungal, protozoal, or viral infection
        (b) Nonseptic (often immune-mediated) disease processes
        (c) Neoplasia (associated with secondary bacterial infection, tumor necrosis, damage to adjacent tissue, or a paraneoplastic effect)
      (2) Stress or **steroid response.** The stress or steroid response, which results from endogenous or exogenous steroids, is a very common cause of neutrophilia.
      (3) Exercise or **epinephrine response.** The exercise or epinephrine response is associated with a mild transient leukocytosis. Cats tend to have a greater response than dogs.
      (4) Leukemia (see III B) is caused by the neoplastic proliferation and circulation of any one or a combination of blood leukocytes.
    b. Diagnosis. Differentiation between the causes of neutrophilia is based on the number of band and mature neutrophils and the relative changes in the number of other leukocytes (Figure 48-2).
      (1) Inflammation produces a **left shift,** which is an increased number of band (immature) neutrophils.
        (a) A **regenerative left shift** is present when the increased number of band neutrophils does not exceed the number of mature neutrophils. It indicates that the animal is adequately compensating for neutrophil demand.
        (b) A **degenerative left shift** is present when the number of band neutrophils exceeds the number of mature neutrophils. It indicates an aggressive inflammatory process in which the body cannot keep up with neutrophil demand.
        (c) A **leukemoid reaction** is used to describe an extremely elevated neutrophil count accompanied by a severe left shift. It is associated with severe inflammatory disease and can be difficult to distinguish from chronic myelogenous leukemia (CML).
      (2) Stress or **steroid response.** The classic pattern is that of a moderate mature

---

FIGURE 48-1. Diagnostic approach to polycythemia. Relative polycythemia (hemoconcentration) is suggested if an elevated packed cell volume (*PCV*) is accompanied by an increase in total protein and clinical signs of dehydration. Absolute polycythemia requires radiographs and a blood gas analysis to rule hypoxia due to cardiovascular or pulmonary disease in or out. If hypoxia is absent, serum erythropoietin levels should be measured. If serum erythropoietin is low, then polycythemia vera is likely present. If the serum erythropoietin level is high, then abdominal radiographs (with or without renal ultrasound) should be performed to detect renal masses or other neoplasia, which may be secreting erythropoietin. Pao_2 = arterial oxygen tension. (Redrawn and modified with permission from Morrison WB: Polycythemia. In *Textbook of Veterinary Internal Medicine,* 4th ed. Edited by Ettinger SJ and Feldman EC. Philadelphia, WB Saunders, 1995, p 198.)

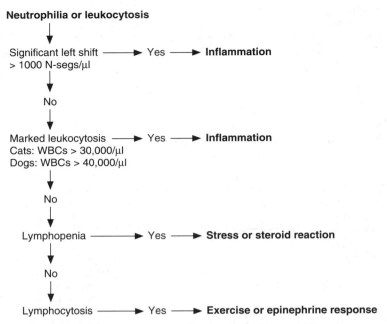

Neutrophilia or leukocytosis

Significant left shift ⟶ Yes ⟶ **Inflammation**
> 1000 N-segs/µl

No

Marked leukocytosis ⟶ Yes ⟶ **Inflammation**
Cats: WBCs > 30,000/µl
Dogs: WBCs > 40,000/µl

No

Lymphopenia ⟶ Yes ⟶ **Stress or steroid reaction**

No

Lymphocytosis ⟶ Yes ⟶ **Exercise or epinephrine response**

FIGURE 48-2. Diagnostic approach for determining the cause of neutrophilia or leukocytosis. This diagram does not consider myeloid or lymphoid leukemia, which could be associated with marked leukocytosis and circulating abnormal cells. *WBCs* = white blood cells. (Redrawn and modified with permission from Willard MD, Tvedten H, Turnwald GH (eds): *Small Animal Clinical Diagnosis by Laboratory Methods*, 2nd ed. Philadelphia, WB Saunders, 1994, p 57.)

neutrophilia (i.e., no band neutrophils are present), lymphopenia, eosinopenia, and monocytosis.

(3) **Exercise** or **epinephrine response.** In contrast to a stress response, lymphocytosis is often present.

(4) **Leukemia** is characterized by a marked leukocytosis or abnormal (i.e., immature or blast-like cells) circulating leukocytes.

c. **Treatment** is focused on the underlying disorder.

2. **Lymphocytosis** can be associated with the exercise or epinephrine response in cats, or prolonged antigenic stimulation, leukemia, or hypoadrenocorticism in dogs. Antigenic stimulation can result from chronic infection (e.g., ehrlichiosis) or vaccination. In dogs with persistent marked lymphocytosis (with normal cell morphology), ehrlichiosis or chronic lymphocytic leukemia (CLL) should be suspected.

3. **Eosinophilia** is usually associated with parasitism or allergic reactions. Less commonly, it can be associated with hemopoietic and nonhemopoietic neoplasms, infectious diseases, or estrus (in dogs). It may also be idiopathic (e.g., hypereosinophilic syndromes). Diagnostic approaches to eosinophilia in cats and dogs are given in Figure 48-3.

4. **Monocytosis** can be caused by a stress or steroid response, chronic inflammatory disease, or any disease process involved in cell destruction and removal. Pyogranulomatous or granulomatous diseases are likely to be associated with monocytosis. Chronic bacterial infections, systemic fungal infections, IHA, and lymphosarcoma are relatively common causes. If a stress or steroid pattern is absent, then an inflammatory cause should be sought.

5. **Basophilia** results from the same disease processes that cause eosinophilia. Basophilia in the absence of eosinophilia may be associated with altered lipid metabolism and lipemia.

B. **Leukemia** should be suspected in the presence of marked leukocytosis and/or circulating abnormal leukocytes (e.g., immature, blast-like cells).

1. **General considerations.** Leukemias are broadly classified (Table 48-5) according to time course and cell type [i.e., myeloid (nonlymphoid) and lymphoid].

   a. **Acute** versus **chronic disease** can often be differentiated with routine laboratory examination.

      (1) **Acute leukemia** is usually associated with aggressive biologic behavior, circulating blast cells, and short survival times.

      (2) **Chronic leukemia** often has a slow, insidious onset, well-differentiated circulating cells, and is associated with a longer survival time.

   b. **Myeloid** versus **lymphoid disease.** Differentiation of myeloid and lymphoid disease requires special cytochemical staining in most cases.

2. **Acute leukemia**

   a. **Canine.** In dogs, acute myeloid leukemias are more common than acute lymphoid leukemias.

      (1) **Diagnosis** is based on physical findings and the complete blood count (CBC).

         (a) **Clinical findings** are vague and nonspecific. They commonly include lethargy, anorexia, weight loss, splenomegaly (often marked), hepatomegaly, and lymphadenopathy (mild). Shifting-leg lameness, persistent fever, vomiting, diarrhea, pale mucous membranes, and petechial hemorrhages can also occur.

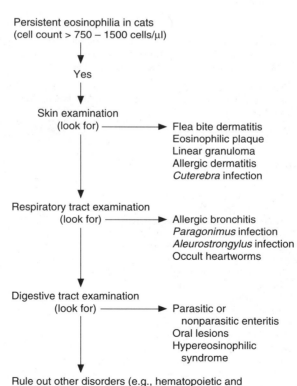

FIGURE 48-3. (*A*) Diagnostic approach to eosinophilia in cats. (Redrawn and modified with permission from Williard MD, Tvedten H, Turnwald GH (eds): *Small Animal Clinic Diagnosis by Laboratory Methods*, 2nd ed. Philadelphia, WB Saunders, 1994, p 65.)

B.

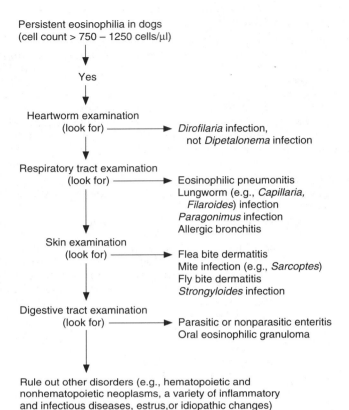

Persistent eosinophilia in dogs
(cell count > 750 – 1250 cells/μl)

↓

Yes

↓

Heartworm examination
(look for) ——————→ *Dirofilaria* infection,
                                    not *Dipetalonema* infection

↓

Respiratory tract examination
(look for) ——————→ Eosinophilic pneumonitis
                                    Lungworm (e.g., *Capillaria,
                                    Filaroides*) infection
                                    Paragonimus infection
                                    Allergic bronchitis

↓

Skin examination
(look for) ——————→ Flea bite dermatitis
                                    Mite infection (e.g., *Sarcoptes*)
                                    Fly bite dermatitis
                                    Strongyloides infection

↓

Digestive tract examination
(look for) ——————→ Parasitic or nonparasitic enteritis
                                    Oral eosinophilic granuloma

↓

Rule out other disorders (e.g., hematopoietic and
nonhematopoietic neoplasms, a variety of inflammatory
and infectious diseases, estrus, or idiopathic changes)

FIGURE 48-3. (*B*) Diagnostic approach to eosinophilia in dogs. (Redrawn and modified with permission from Willard MD, Tvedten H, Turnwald GH (eds): *Small Animal Clinical Diagnosis by Laboratory Methods,* 2nd ed. Philadelphia, WB Saunders, 1994, p 65.)

TABLE 48-5. Classification of Leukemias in Dogs and Cats

Acute leukemia
  Acute myeloid (myelogenous) leukemia (AML)
    Undifferentiated myeloid leukemia
    Acute myelocytic leukemia
    Acute progranulocytic leukemia
    Acute myelomonocytic leukemia
    Acute monoblastic/monocytic leukemia
    Acute erythroleukemia
    Acute megakaryoblastic leukemia
  Acute lymphoid leukemia (ALL)
    Acute lymphoblastic leukemia
    Acute leukemia of large granular lymphocytes
Chronic leukemia
  Chronic myeloid (myelogenous) leukemia (CML)
  Chronic myelomonocytic leukemia
  Chronic lymphoid leukemia (CLL)
  Chronic lymphoid leukemia (large granular lymphocyte variant)
  Subacute myelomonocytic leukemia

Modified with permission from Nelson RW, Couto GC (eds.): *Essentials of Small Animal Internal Medicine,* St. Louis, Mosby-Year Book, 1992, p 872.

(b) Laboratory findings
    (i) A marked leukocytosis with large numbers of abnormal blast-like cells is usually present. Occasionally, aleukemic leukemia is present (i.e., neoplastic cells are seen only in the bone marrow).
    (ii) Anemia and thrombocytopenia are present in many dogs.

(c) Bone marrow examination and **fine needle aspirate** of an enlarged liver, spleen, or lymph nodes is indicated to ascertain the extent of disease.

(d) Differential diagnoses. Acute leukemia may be difficult to differentiate from lymphosarcoma with circulating blast lymphocytes.
    (i) Lymphosarcoma is more likely if the lymphadenopathy is marked, there are no systemic signs of illness, and hypercalcemia is present.
    (ii) Acute leukemia is more likely if there are systemic signs of illness, thrombocytopenia or anemia, and more than 40%–50% of the cells in bone marrow samples are blast cells.

(2) Treatment. Most dogs with acute leukemia respond to chemotherapy poorly and have short remission times. Dogs with acute lymphoblastic leukemia are more responsive to chemotherapy than dogs with acute myelogenous leukemia, but survival times are still short (1–3 months).

(3) Prognosis. The prognosis is very poor.

b. Feline. Approximately two-thirds of acute leukemias in cats are myeloid [acute myeloid leukemia (AML)], and one-third are lymphoid [acute lymphoid leukemia (ALL)].

(1) Diagnosis is based on a CBC and bone marrow examination. Tests for FeLV and FIV should be performed.

(a) Clinical findings are similar to those of dogs and include lethargy, weight loss, anorexia, hepatosplenomegaly, lymphadenopathy, mucous membrane pallor, and fever.

(b) Laboratory findings
    (i) CBC. In addition to leukocytosis and abnormal circulating (blast-like) cells, most cats have concurrent thrombocytopenia or anemia. During the course of AML in cats, the cell type may shift from one to another (i.e., granulocytes to monocytes).
    (ii) Serology. Approximately 90% of cats with acute leukemia are FeLV-positive.

(2) Treatment

(a) ALL. Multiple-drug combination chemotherapy has resulted in survival times of 1–7 months.

(b) AML. Many chemotherapeutic agents have been tried, but responses have been poor and survival times short (2–10 weeks).

3. Chronic leukemia

a. Canine. CLL is more common than chronic myeloid leukemia (CML) and may be the most common leukemia in dogs.

(1) Diagnosis

(a) Clinical findings. In approximately 50% of cases, clinical signs are nonspecific and may include lethargy, anorexia, weight loss, fever, polyuria, polydipsia, intermittent lameness, generalized lymphadenopathy, mucous membrane pallor, intermittent vomiting and diarrhea, and hepatosplenomegaly. In the other 50%, clinical signs are absent and the leukemia is discovered during routine blood testing. Dogs with CLL may develop marked generalized lymphadenopathy and hepatosplenomegaly due to a large cell lymphoma as a terminal event.

(b) Laboratory findings
    (i) CLL. The presence of marked lymphocytosis (greater than 20,000 cells/μl) comprised of well-differentiated lymphocytes is almost pathognomonic. A monoclonal gammopathy, and rarely, IHA, immune-mediated thrombocytopenia, or neutropenia may also accompany CLL. Anemia (80% of cases) and thrombocytopenia (50% of cases) may be present. An increase in the number of well-differentiated lymphocytes is observed on a bone marrow examination.

        (ii) CML. Anemia and leukocytosis characterized by the presence of myelocytes occurs. Some dogs will develop a blast crisis (immature cells in circulation and bone marrow) after having CML for several months or years.

     (c) Differential diagnosis

        (i) CLL. Less marked lymphocytosis can be associated with chronic antigenic stimulation (e.g., ehrlichiosis) or CLL; the two disorders may be difficult to distinguish.

        (ii) CML can be especially difficult to distinguish from a leukemoid reaction. The diagnosis is based on ruling out all other causes of neutrophilia (e.g., inflammation). Infiltration of solid organs such as the liver and spleen may occur with CML and can help distinguish it from other causes of marked neutrophilia or monocytosis.

   (2) Treatment

     (a) CLL. Asymptomatic dogs may not require treatment. Treatment with chlorambucil or a combination of chlorambucil and prednisone is recommended if clinical signs or organomegaly are present. The response to therapy may be slow and it may take 1–6 months before cell counts begin to decline.

     (b) CML can be treated with hydroxyurea. The treatment of a blast crisis is often unrewarding.

   (3) Prognosis

     (a) CLL. Survival times of untreated and treated dogs can be prolonged (over 2 years).

     (b) CML. Survival times of treated dogs average 4–15 months.

 b. Feline. Chronic leukemias in cats are extremely rare. CLL has been described and appears to have a clinical course similar to that in dogs.

4. Myelodysplastic (preleukemic) syndromes

 a. Diagnosis

   (1) Clinical findings. In dogs, myelodysplastic syndromes can be associated with lethargy, anorexia, hepatosplenomegaly, fever, and mucous membrane pallor. Most affected cats are FeLV-positive and have signs similar to dogs.

   (2) Laboratory findings. Hematologic findings consist of anemia, leukopenia, and thrombocytopenia, alone or in combination. Macrocytosis, the absence of circulating blast cells, reticulocytopenia, and the presence of macrothrombocytes are also common.

   (3) Bone marrow examination reveals normal to increased cellularity. Blast cells comprise less than 30% of marrow cells, and there are maturational abnormalities affecting all cell lines. Megaloblastic RBC precursors are common.

 b. Treatment consists of supportive care (e.g., fluids, blood transfusion, antibiotics) and the administration of low-dose cytosine arabinoside and anabolic steroids (e.g., nandrolone decanoate).

 c. Prognosis. Some dogs and many cats eventually develop ALL.

C. **Leukopenia**

 1. Neutropenia

  a. Etiology. Causes of neutropenia include:

   (1) Severe inflammation. Overwhelming bacterial sepsis (e.g., diffuse peritonitis, pyothorax, septicemia) can cause neutropenia.

   (2) Bone marrow disease. Common causes of bone marrow disease resulting in neutropenia include myeloproliferative and lymphoproliferative disorders, anticancer chemotherapy, griseofulvin administration (in cats), parvovirus infection, and FIV and FeLV infections.

   (3) Peripheral immune-mediated destruction is an uncommon cause of neutropenia.

  b. Diagnosis

   (1) Severe inflammation. A degenerative left shift accompanied by toxic changes in the neutrophils is usually present and should prompt an immediate and aggressive search for a septic focus.

(2) **Bone marrow disease.** Neutropenia associated with bone marrow disease is usually not associated with a marked band response or toxic change. Neutropenia from bone marrow disease is often associated with decreases in other cell lines (e.g., thrombocytopenia, anemia). Bone marrow examination is indicated if primary bone marrow disease is suspected.

  c. **Treatment** is focused on the underlying disorder.

    (1) **Severe sepsis** may require thoracic or abdominal cavity lavage and drainage, surgical debridement of infected tissue, therapy to counteract shock, and aggressive antimicrobial therapy.

    (2) **Bone marrow disease.** If bone marrow disease is present, prophylactic antibiotic therapy is indicated if the neutropenia is marked.

2. Lymphopenia may be associated with a stress or steroid response or anticancer chemotherapy.

3. Combined cytopenias. Cytopenias of either two (bicytopenia) or all (pancytopenia) cell lines can result from bone marrow disease or peripheral destruction.

  a. **Etiology**

    (1) **Bone marrow diseases** that can result in pancytopenia include drug-induced damage (e.g., estrogen), infectious disease (e.g., chronic ehrlichiosis, FeLV), neoplastic infiltration, and myelofibrosis.

    (2) **Peripheral destruction** of two or more cell lines can be caused by combined IHA with immune-mediated thrombocytopenia, sepsis, disseminated intravascular coagulation (DIC), and splenomegaly (e.g., hypersplenism, hemolymphatic neoplasia).

  b. **Diagnosis.** The combination of historical information, physical findings, abdominal radiographs, laboratory testing (e.g., CBC, serology), and a bone marrow examination should provide a specific diagnosis.

IV. DISORDERS OF HEMOSTASIS

A. General considerations

1. Normal hemostasis. A delicate balance exists between those forces that initiate coagulation (i.e., platelets, coagulation factors) and those that inhibit coagulation (i.e., the fibrinolytic system, antithrombin III, and others). This balance prevents excessive hemorrhage or thrombosis.

  a. **Platelet adhesion** occurs rapidly following exposure of subendothelial collagen. Adequate amounts of vWF are necessary for platelet adhesion. Following adhesion, platelets release a variety of potent mediators (e.g., thromboxane A_2), which recruit more platelets into the vessel wall defect to form a temporary platelet (primary hemostatic) plug.

  b. **Coagulation cascade.** The coagulation cascade is activated concurrently. Its main purpose is to generate fibrin strands that are interspersed within the platelet plug to strengthen the closure of the defect (secondary hemostatic plug).

  c. **Fibrinolytic system.** The fibrinolytic system (i.e., plasmin) removes the fibrin plug after the endothelial surface has healed.

2. Etiology and **pathogenesis of disorders of hemostasis.** Breed, age, gender, previous bleeding episodes, affected littermates, and concurrent drug therapy may all provide clues as to the cause of a bleeding tendency (characterized by spontaneous hemorrhage or excessive bleeding following minor trauma or in the absence of trauma). Bleeding disorders are caused by one or a combination of four basic abnormalities.

  a. **Vascular abnormalities** in small blood vessels and capillaries can result in spontaneous bleeding, but these conditions (e.g., Ehlers-Danlos syndrome, vasculitis) are rare.

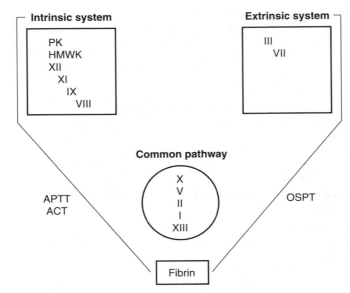

FIGURE 48-4. Diagram of the intrinsic, extrinsic, and common pathways of the coagulation cascade. *ACT* = activated clotting time; *APTT* = activated partial thromboplastin time; *HMWK* = high–molecular-weight kininogen; *OSPT* = one-stage prothrombin time; *PK* = prekallikrein. (Modified and redrawn with permission from Nelson RW, Couto CG (eds): *Essentials of Small Animal Internal Medicine*, St. Louis, Mosby-Year Book, 1992, p 927.)

  b. **Platelet abnormalities** are one of the most common causes of bleeding disorders in dogs. They result from either a decreased number of platelets (i.e., thrombocytopenia) or abnormal platelet function. Immune-mediated thrombocytopenia and vWD are two common examples.
  c. **Coagulation factor abnormalities** result from a single or multiple factor deficiency. The coagulation cascade is comprised of three enzymatic cascades (Figure 48-4): the intrinsic system (factors XII, XI, IX, and VIII), the extrinsic system [factors III (tissue thromboplastin) and VII], and the common pathway (factors X, V, II, I, XIII, and fibrin).
  d. **Fibrinolytic abnormalities.** Excessive fibrinolytic activity can result in spontaneous bleeding but its occurrence as a sole abnormality is rare. It is usually associated with other hemostatic defects, such as DIC. The excessive degradation of fibrin by plasmin generates fibrin degradation products.

 3. **Diagnosis of disorders of hemostasis**

TABLE 48-6. Hemorrhage Patterns Associated with Platelet and Coagulation Factor Abnormalities

Clinical Sign	Thrombocytopenia or Platelet Dysfunction	Coagulation Factor Deficiency
Petechia	Common	Rare
Large hematomas	Rare	Common
Bleeding into body cavities	Rare	Common
Hemarthrosis	Rare	Common
Renewed bleeding after initial clot	Rare	Common
Ocular hemorrhage	Small, retinal hemorrhages	Hyphema, scleral hemorrhage

TABLE 48-7. Laboratory Test Results in Various Disorders of Hemostasis

Disorder	Platelet Count	MBT	PT	APTT	ACT	FDPs
Thrombocytopenia	↓	↑	N	N	N*	N
Platelet dysfunction (e.g., vWD)	N	↑	N	N†	N†	N
Hemophilia A (factor VIII deficiency) or B (factor IX deficiency)	N	N	N	↑	↑	N
Anticoagulant rodenticide toxicity (e.g., warfarin)	N‡	N	↑	↑	↑	N
DIC	↓	↑	↑	↑	↑	↑

ACT = activated clotting time; APTT = activated partial thromboplastin time; DIC = disseminated intravascular coagulation; FDPs = fibrin degradation products; MBT = mucosal bleeding time; N = normal; PT = prothrombin time; vWD = vonWillebrand's disease.
* May be prolonged with severe thrombocytopenia.
† Usually normal, but may be prolonged in vWD if there is concurrent factor VIII deficiency.
‡ Mild to moderate thrombocytopenia may accompany acute hemorrhage.

    a. Vascular abnormalities. A prolonged buccal mucosal bleeding time or vasculitis documented on a skin biopsy are supportive.

    b. Platelet abnormalities

        (1) Clinical findings. The character of the hemorrhage is highly variable, but there are consistent differences between platelet-associated hemorrhages and those caused by coagulation factor deficiency (Table 48-6).

        (2) Laboratory findings. A platelet count will reveal thrombocytopenia. *In vitro* platelet aggregation testing can also be performed to assess platelet function, but this test is not widely available. The mucosal bleeding time is prolonged (primarily with abnormal platelet function, but also if thrombocytopenia is severe). Laboratory test results in various disorders of hemostasis are summarized in Table 48-7.

    c. Coagulation factor abnormalities

        (1) Clinical findings. Characteristics of the hemorrhage associated with coagulation factor abnormalities are summarized in Table 48-6.

        (2) Laboratory findings

            (a) Prothrombin time (PT). The PT, which evaluates the extrinsic and common pathways, may be prolonged.

            (b) Activated partial thromboplastin time (APTT) and **activated clotting time (ACT).** The APTT and ACT, which evaluate the intrinsic and common pathways, may be prolonged. The ACT is less sensitive than the APTT and can also be prolonged with severe thrombocytopenia; however, it is an inexpensive, quick, and easy test to perform.

            (c) Specific factor assays can also be performed to identify a single (usually congenital) factor deficiency.

    d. Fibrinolytic system abnormalities (i.e., excessive fibrinolysis) will result in elevated serum levels of fibrin degradation products.

B. **Platelet abnormalities**

    1. Thrombocytopenia

        a. Etiology. Thrombocytopenia is caused by decreased production in the bone marrow or increased peripheral utilization, destruction, or sequestration of platelets (Table 48-8).

        (1) Dogs. In dogs, idiopathic immune-mediated thrombocytopenia (IMT) and *Ehrlichia canis* infection are the most common causes.

        (2) Cats. Decreased platelet production from viral infection (e.g., FeLV, FIV) or bone marrow neoplasia is the most common cause.

TABLE 48-8. Causes of Thrombocytopenia

Decreased platelet production
  Megakaryocytic hypoplasia (immune-mediated)
  Idiopathic bone marrow aplasia
  Drug-induced marrow injury (e.g., estrogen toxicity)
  Infectious agents [e.g., feline leukemia virus (FeLV) infection, *Ehrlichia canis* infection]
  Bone marrow neoplasia
  Myelofibrosis
Increased peripheral utilization, sequestration, or destruction
  Immune-mediated destruction
    Idiopathic immune-mediated thrombocytopenia
    Adverse drug effect
    Infectious agents (e.g., cyclic thrombocytopenia caused by *Ehrlichia platys* infection)
  Live-virus vaccination
  Microangiopathy
  Disseminated intravascular coagulation (DIC)
  Vasculitis [e.g., *Rickettsia rickettsii* infection (Rocky Mountain spotted fever)]
  Splenomegaly
  Splenic torsion
  Endotoxemia or sepsis
  Acute hepatic necrosis
  Neoplasia (immune-mediated, microangiopathy)

---

   b. Diagnosis
      (1) Clinical findings are summarized in Table 48-6. The platelet count must usually fall below 20,000 platelets/μl before spontaneous hemorrhage occurs (the reference range = 200,000–500,000 platelets/μl).
      (2) Laboratory findings
         (a) An **automated platelet count** is the most reliable method of assessing platelet numbers. A subjective estimate may be obtained from a blood smear (reference range = 8–30 platelets/oil immersion field).
         (b) Bone marrow examination is indicated in all animals with a persistent platelet count of less than 30,000 platelets/μl.
            (i) Megakaryocytic hyperplasia is suggestive of peripheral utilization or destruction of platelets.
            (ii) Few or no megakaryocytes is suggestive of decreased production resulting from bone marrow disease.
      (3) Other findings. A thorough patient evaluation to detect underlying disease may include coagulation tests to detect other hemostatic defects (e.g., DIC), serologic tests for infectious diseases (e.g., FeLV, *Ehrlichia canis*), and radiographic or ultrasound examination to detect neoplasia or splenomegaly.

   2. IMT is common in dogs and rare in cats. Female dogs, toy breeds, and Old English sheepdogs are affected most frequently.
      a. Diagnosis is based on the presence of thrombocytopenia, adequate numbers of megakaryocytes, and the exclusion of underlying diseases (i.e., no identifiable neoplasia, negative serology for infectious agents, no other hemostatic defects).
         (1) Clinical findings. Signs are usually acute. The pattern of hemorrhage is typically that of a platelet abnormality and can include skin and mucous membrane petechial hemorrhages, epistaxis, mucosal bleeding, hematuria, and melena. Splenomegaly may occur. If significant hemorrhage has occurred, lethargy, weakness, and mucous membrane pallor may be observed. If blood loss is minimal, the animal may be asymptomatic.
         (2) Laboratory findings
            (a) CBC. Platelet numbers are usually very low (i.e., less than 20,000/μl). A regenerative anemia of variable severity may be present if blood loss

has occurred. IHA can occur simultaneously. Concurrent IHA (especially in a Coombs'-positive patient) would support a diagnosis of IMT.

(b) Bone marrow examination reveals megakaryocytic hyperplasia. No other marrow abnormalities are present.

(c) Serology. Although developed, no tests to detect antiplatelet antibody in serum are commercially available.

b. Treatment

(1) Acute therapy

(a) Administration of **corticosteroids** (e.g., prednisone) at immunosuppressive doses usually results in an increase in platelet numbers within 2–4 days. The dose of prednisone is gradually reduced over 1–2 months to the lowest effective dose that will maintain platelet numbers in an acceptable range (i.e., greater than 100,000/μl).

(b) Cyclophosphamide or **azathioprine** may be added if there is no response to prednisone.

(c) Transfusion of blood components (e.g., whole blood, packed RBCs, platelet-rich plasma) may be required in animals that become severely anemic or have marked ongoing hemorrhage.

(d) Vincristine, danazol, or **splenectomy** can be considered in animals refractory to other attempts at therapy.

(2) Maintenance therapy. If required in addition to prednisone, azathioprine rather than cyclophosphamide is preferred for maintenance therapy.

c. Prognosis. In general, the prognosis is good. Most animals can be controlled with drug therapy; however, treatment is often lifelong. Death, if it occurs, is usually caused by GI hemorrhage.

3. Platelet dysfunction

a. Congenital defects in platelet function are rare with the exception of **vWD.** In dogs, vWD is the most common congenital bleeding disorder. The highest prevalence is in Doberman pinschers. Pembroke Welsh corgis, Scottish terriers, German shepherds, miniature schnauzers, golden retrievers, standard poodles, and Shetland sheepdogs are also commonly affected. In cats, vWD is extremely rare.

(1) Etiology

(a) Autosomal dominant inheritance with incomplete penetrance occurs in most breeds (e.g., Doberman pinschers). Heterozygotes or carriers may be clinically normal or have a severe bleeding disorder. Homozygote dominant dogs all have a severe bleeding disorder.

(b) Autosomal recessive inheritance occurs less commonly, usually in Scottish terriers and Chesapeake Bay retrievers. Heterozygotes are clinically normal, and all homozygote recessives have a severe bleeding disorder.

(2) Pathogenesis. vWD results from a deficiency of vWF, which is produced in endothelial cells and megakaryocytes and circulates in the blood in a complex with factor VIII. Occasionally, dogs may also have reduced factor VIII levels. vWF is composed of a group of variously sized molecules (multimers) made up of repeating identical polypeptide subunits.

(a) Type I vWD. The concentration of all vWF multimers is low. Type I vWD occurs in Doberman pinschers as well as other breeds.

(b) Type II vWD. The concentration of high–molecular-weight vWF multimers is low. Type II vWD occurs most commonly in German short-haired pointers.

(c) Type III vWD is characterized by the complete absence of all vWF multimers. Type III vWD occurs most commonly in Scottish terriers and Chesapeake Bay retrievers.

(3) Diagnosis

(a) Clinical findings. Dogs may be asymptomatic or have a severe bleeding disorder. Some dogs will be several years old before a bleeding episode occurs. Because vWF is necessary for platelet adhesion, a deficiency results in signs consistent with platelet dysfunction.

(i) When hemorrhage occurs, it has a pattern typical of platelet dysfunction. Signs can include petechial hemorrhages, epistaxis, gingival bleeding, hematuria, melena, prolonged bleeding following surgery or trauma, and lameness.

    (ii) If factor VIII levels are low, hemorrhage typical of a factor deficiency can occur (e.g., hematomas, bleeding into body cavities).

  (b) Laboratory findings

    (i) Diagnosis is based on documenting reduced concentrations of vWF in the plasma. This is referred to as **vWF:Ag (antigen)** and is expressed as a percentage of normal (normal = 60%–172%). Values of 50%–60% are equivocal, but values **less than 50%** are diagnostic. Factors that may elevate plasma vWF:Ag include pregnancy, elevated body temperature, exercise, and medication with thyroid hormone or desmopressin.

    (ii) Although not specific for vWD, the **mucosal bleeding time** is a reliable and rapid screening test and is usually prolonged in dogs with vWD.

  (4) Treatment. There is no long-term specific factor replacement therapy available for dogs.

    (a) Desmopressin (a vasopressin analogue) can be considered in dogs with type I vWD that have significant bleeding.

      (i) Desmopressin increases the release of vWF from endothelial stores and can shorten the mucosal bleeding time in most dogs with vWD.

      (ii) Presurgical administration of desmopressin or transfusion of fresh or fresh frozen plasma can temporarily (for a few hours) increase plasma vWF levels and normalize hemostasis.

    (b) Thyroid hormone supplementation may help raise vWF levels and decrease the risk of hemorrhage. Hypothyroidism can aggravate the severity of vWD.

    (c) Transfusion with fresh whole blood may be required in dogs with severe life-threatening hemorrhage.

  (5) Breeding recommendations

    (a) All breeding animals should have normal levels of vWF.

    (b) In breeds with a high prevalence of the disease, asymptomatic carriers should be bred to normal animals if it is necessary to breed the asymptomatic carrier.

    (c) Carriers should not be bred together.

    (d) No animal that has a clinical bleeding tendency should be bred.

  b. Acquired defects in platelet function can result from **drugs** [e.g., aspirin and other nonsteroidal anti-inflammatory drugs (NSAIDs), some antibiotics, phenothiazines] or **diseases** (e.g., uremia, liver failure, myeloproliferative disorders, dysproteinemias).

C. | **Coagulation factor abnormalities**

  1. Congenital factor deficiencies are uncommon in dogs and very rare in cats. **Hemophilia A (factor VIII deficiency)** and **hemophilia B (factor IX deficiency)** are the most common disorders.

    a. Diagnosis. Most congenital factor deficiencies are diagnosed in animals younger than 1 year. The severity of the bleeding tendency is proportional to the degree of factor deficiency. Many animals are asymptomatic but have prolonged coagulation times. The pattern of hemorrhage (i.e., hematomas, hemarthrosis, body cavity bleeds, delayed bleeding after trauma or surgery) suggests coagulation factor deficiency. A congenital factor deficiency is likely if a factor deficiency pattern of hemorrhage occurs in a young animal and only the PT or APTT is prolonged (suggesting a single rather than a multiple factor deficiency). Definitive diagnosis requires a specific factor assay.

    b. Treatment is supportive.

  2. Acquired factor deficiencies

a. **Liver failure** can lead to reduced production of factors.
b. **Vitamin K deficiency.** Vitamin K is required for the activation of factors II, VII, IX, and X. Vitamin K deficiency can be caused by malabsorption or anticoagulant rodenticide intoxication.
   (1) **Malabsorption** due to intestinal disease is a rare cause of vitamin K deficiency.
   (2) **Anticoagulant rodenticide intoxication** is the most common cause of vitamin K deficiency.
      (a) **Pathogenesis.** All agents work by inhibiting the enzyme vitamin K epoxide reductase, which results in the rapid depletion of vitamin K. Many agents are available and differ primarily in their length of action.
         (i) Short-acting agents (e.g., warfarin). Multiple exposures or a single large exposure are usually required to cause toxicity. Clinical signs are apparent within 3–5 days of ingestion.
         (ii) Longer-acting agents (e.g., diphacinone, brodifacoum, bromadoline) are more potent, and a single exposure often produces clinical signs within 1–3 days.
      (b) **Diagnosis** is based on suspected rodenticide ingestion, the acute onset of factor-like hemorrhage, and appropriate laboratory findings.
         (i) **Clinical findings.** Signs only become apparent once hemorrhage occurs. The bleeding is typical of a factor deficiency and can include hematomas and bleeding into body cavities (very common), muscle, or fascial planes. Hemorrhage is often acute and may not be readily apparent if the blood loss is internal. An acute onset of weakness, mucous membrane pallor, dyspnea (from hemothorax), or abdominal enlargement (hemoabdomen) may be observed. Death may occur from hypovolemic shock, acute cardiac tamponade (hemorrhage into pericardial sac), or CNS dysfunction (resulting from CNS hemorrhage).
         (ii) **Laboratory findings.** Prolongation of the PT and APTT or ACT suggests a multiple-factor deficiency. The mucosal bleeding time and platelet count are usually normal. Because factor VII has the shortest half-life of the vitamin K–dependent factors, prolongation of the PT may precede prolongation of the APTT.
      (c) **Treatment.** Vitamin K_1 is the treatment of choice. It takes 6–12 hours before enough factors are replenished to stop hemorrhage.
         —For short-acting agents, vitamin K_1 therapy is administered for 1 week. The PT should be assessed 2–3 days after stopping therapy (or the ACT 3–4 days later) to confirm that all the rodenticide has been metabolized. If the PT is prolonged, treatment is repeated for another week and the PT is again rechecked.
         —For long-acting agents, vitamin K_1 therapy should be administered for a minimum of 3 weeks and rechecked as described above. Animals that are in hypovolemic shock or have severe ongoing hemorrhage require intravenous fluid administration and the transfusion of fresh whole blood (which will immediately provide sufficient factors to stop hemorrhage and replenish the RBC mass and blood volume). If the rodenticide has been recently ingested (within a few hours), emesis can be induced followed by activated charcoal administration and prophylactic vitamin K_1 therapy for 1 week.

D. **Fibrinolytic abnormalities.** DIC is relatively common in dogs but rare in cats. DIC is a secondary phenomenon that develops from one or a combination of the following factors: a marked release of tissue thromboplastin, widespread exposure of subendothelial collagen, or the release of enzymes or procoagulant substances into the circulation. Conditions associated with DIC in relative order of frequency (high to low) include hemangiosarcoma, sepsis, IHA, pancreatitis, electrocution, heat stroke, heartworm disease, and other malignancies.

1. **Pathogenesis.** DIC results from the widespread and simultaneous activation of platelets, the coagulation cascades, and the fibrinolytic system. This activation leads to diffuse microvascular thrombosis; depletion of platelets, coagulation factors, and anticoagulant factors (e.g., antithrombin III); and the generation of fibrin degradation products, leading to the paradoxical development of spontaneous bleeding and thrombosis. DIC results in hemorrhage and organ ischemia and damage (e.g., acute renal failure) due to thrombosis.

2. **Diagnosis**
   a. **Clinical findings.** The severity of DIC can vary from being clinically silent (only evident on laboratory tests) to acute and fulminant, resulting in multiple organ failure and death. Signs of the underlying disease are usually readily apparent.
      (1) Absence of clinical signs is more common with malignancy-associated DIC.
      (2) With acute DIC, signs of hemorrhage (platelet or factor deficiency pattern), lethargy, weakness, shock, and signs associated with organ failure (e.g., vomiting, diarrhea, dyspnea) may occur.
   b. **Laboratory findings.** Diagnosis is based on the presence of thrombocytopenia, prolongation of the PT and APTT, and increased fibrin degradation products. Reduced blood antithrombin III concentration is an additional and sensitive indicator of DIC. Animals with acute DIC usually have all of the laboratory abnormalities; patients with less severe DIC may have fewer abnormalities.

3. **Treatment.** The underlying cause should be corrected, if possible. The patient should be monitored to detect and prevent complications (e.g., sepsis, acid–base and electrolyte abnormalities). A positive response to therapy is indicated by improved patient status, an increased platelet count, a reduced PT and APTT, and increased antithrombin III concentrations.
   a. **Intravenous fluid therapy** should be administered to maintain tissue perfusion and oxygenation.
   b. **Transfusion of fresh whole blood** or **plasma** controls intravascular coagulation by replenishing platelets, coagulation factors, and antithrombin III.
   c. **Heparin** helps prevent further coagulation, although its use and correct dose is somewhat controversial. The dosage of heparin can be proportional to the severity of the DIC or can be based on the amount required to prolong the APTT to 1.5–2 times normal.

4. **Prognosis**
   a. **Clinically silent DIC.** The prognosis depends on the nature of the underlying disease.
   b. **Acute, severe DIC.** The prognosis is grave. Most animals die despite aggressive therapy.

V. DISORDERS OF THE LYMPH NODES AND SPLEEN

A. **Lymphadenopathy.** The term "lymphadenopathy" (i.e., disease of the lymph nodes) is also used to refer to lymph node enlargement (lymphadenomegaly). Reactive and infiltrative lymphadenopathies are the most common causes of lymph node enlargement in dogs and cats.

1. **Etiology**
   a. **Reactive lymphadenopathy** (proliferation of normal lymph node cell populations) is associated with many infectious and noninfectious inflammatory diseases.
   b. **Infiltrative lymphadenopathy** (infiltration of neoplastic cells, less commonly inflammatory cells such as eosinophils) is most frequently caused by lymphoma and metastatic neoplasia.
   c. **Lymphadenitis** (predominance of neutrophils or macrophages in the lymph node) is usually caused by infection of the lymph node.

    d. Idiopathic lymphadenopathy can also occur.

2. Diagnosis

    a. Patient history. A history of travel may suggest infectious diseases with a geographic distribution (e.g., rickettsial diseases, deep mycoses).

    b. Clinical findings. The submandibular, prescapular, and popliteal lymph nodes are the only ones that can be routinely palpated; however, if marked generalized lymphadenopathy occurs, other lymph nodes (e.g., axillary, inguinal nodes) may become palpable.

        (1) If regional lymphadenopathy is present, the area drained by the lymph nodes should be carefully evaluated.

        (2) Marked generalized lymphadenopathy is usually due to lymphoma or, less commonly, lymphadenitis.

    c. Diagnostic imaging findings. Radiography or ultrasonography may detect intraabdominal or intrathoracic lymphadenopathy.

    d. Laboratory findings. Fine-needle aspirates of enlarged lymph nodes and cytologic examination usually enables categorization of enlargement as reactive, neoplastic, or lymphadenitis.

        (1) The presence of reactive lymphadenopathy may necessitate an extensive workup (e.g., routine laboratory work, serology, radiography, ultrasonography) to detect underlying inflammatory disorders.

        (2) A diagnosis of lymphoma can usually be made on the basis of lymph node cytology. If lymph node cytology is equivocal, an excisional or needle biopsy of superficial or deep lymph nodes can be performed for histopathologic examination.

B. **Lymphosarcoma (lymphoma)**

    1. Feline. Lymphosarcoma (lymphoma) accounts for 60%–90% of all hemolymphatic tumors in cats. Feline lymphoma can take several anatomic forms (in order from most to least common): mediastinal, alimentary, multicentric, leukemic, and miscellaneous; however, the prevalence of one form over another may vary with the geographic area.

    a. General considerations

        (1) Etiology. In cats, lymphosarcoma is usually induced by **FeLV infection.**

        (2) Treatment

            (a) Chemotherapy. Lymphosarcoma is one of the most responsive tumors to chemotherapy. Multiple-drug combinations are recommended over single agents. The COAP [cyclophosphamide, Oncovin (vincristine), cytosine arabinoside, prednisone] and CHOP [cyclophosphamide, hydroxydaunorubicin (doxorubicin), Oncovin (vincristine), prednisone] drug protocols are commonly used.

            (b) Radiation therapy can be considered for focal lymphosarcoma or for masses that are compressing important structures (e.g., mediastinal, epidural masses).

            (c) Surgery

                (i) Resection can be successful in cases of focal GI involvement.

                (ii) Enucleation may be considered in localized ocular involvement.

            (d) Prednisone alone can be used for short-term palliation of clinical signs if chemotherapy is not an option.

        (3) Prognosis. Complete remission (defined as a greater than 75% reduction in lymph node or tumor size) is induced with chemotherapy in 16%–79% of cases, depending on the anatomic form. In general, there is a 60%–70% complete remission rate with a median survival of 5–7 months.

            (a) Animals with mediastinal or multicentric lymphosarcoma respond better and have the longest survival times (median survival, 2–18 months or longer).

            (b) Animals with alimentary and renal lymphosarcoma are associated with fewer complete remissions and shorter survival times (median survival, 5–10 months).

(c) Survival time is shorter for cats that only partially respond or are FeLV-positive.

b. **Mediastinal lymphosarcoma.** Typically, young cats (age 2–3 years) are affected.

    (1) **Clinical findings.** Signs reflect the presence of a space-occupying mass and pleural effusion and include dyspnea, regurgitation, cyanosis, a noncompressible cranial thorax, and dorsocaudal displacement of cardiac sounds.

    (2) **Diagnostic imaging findings.** Pleural effusion is often present and can obscure visualization of the cranial mediastinal mass on thoracic radiographs. Radiographic signs include tracheal elevation and pleural effusion.

    (3) **Laboratory findings**

        (a) Diagnosis can usually be reached by cytologic evaluation of pleural fluid. The pleural fluid tends to be moderately to highly cellular and lymphoblastic cells are often present.

        (b) Occasionally, fine-needle aspiration of the mass is necessary. Ultrasound guidance can help reduce the risk of vessel damage.

        (c) Approximately 80% of cats with mediastinal lymphoma are FeLV-positive.

c. **Alimentary lymphosarcoma** tends to affect older cats (mean age, 8 years). GI involvement may be diffuse or focal, and regional lymph nodes and the liver may also be affected. The most common sites are the small intestine (50% of cases), stomach (25% of cases), and the ileocecocolic junction and colon.

    (1) **Clinical findings.** Signs include vomiting, diarrhea, weight loss, and anorexia. Malabsorption can occur and may result in signs of a protein-losing enteropathy (PLE) and hypoalbuminemia.

    (2) **Diagnostic imaging findings.** Radiography may reveal evidence of bowel obstruction, diffuse bowel wall thickening, and mesenteric lymphadenopathy.

    (3) **Laboratory findings**

        (a) Diagnosis can be obtained by needle aspiration of an enlarged mesenteric lymph node or bowel segment or by biopsy of the intestinal mucosa (via endoscopy) or bowel wall (via laparotomy).

        (b) Only approximately 30% of affected cats are FeLV-positive, possibly because alimentary lymphosarcoma is of B lymphocyte origin whereas most FeLV-induced lymphosarcoma is of T lymphocyte origin.

    (4) **Treatment.** Diffuse GI involvement can be treated with chemotherapy.

d. **Multicentric lymphosarcoma.** Solid hemolymphatic organs are involved, including the deep and superficial lymph nodes, the liver, the spleen, or bone marrow (secondary involvement). Extranodal involvement is common (i.e., eyes, kidneys, CNS).

    (1) **Clinical findings.** Signs vary with the degree of organ involvement and dysfunction. Some cats may be asymptomatic except for enlarged lymph nodes, which are usually markedly enlarged. Hepatosplenomegaly and tonsillar enlargement are common findings.

    (2) **Laboratory findings**

        (a) The diagnosis can often be established by the cytologic examination of lymph node aspirates; however, histopathology may be required.

        (b) Eighty percent of cats with the multicentric form of lymphosarcoma are FeLV-positive.

e. **Miscellaneous forms of lymphosarcoma**

    (1) **Ocular lymphosarcoma.** Primary or secondary ocular involvement is observed in about 10% of cats with lymphosarcoma. Lesions can occur in any area of the eye, but anterior uveal and chorioretinal lesions are most common. Most cats are FeLV-positive.

    (2) **Renal lymphosarcoma.** Renal involvement can be primary or secondary, and one or both kidneys can be affected. The kidneys are enlarged and irregular. Clinical findings are usually a result of renal failure and uremia. More than 50% of cats are FeLV-positive.

    (3) **Neural lymphosarcoma.** Primary neural involvement is rare, but involvement secondary to renal or multicentric lymphosarcoma is reasonably common. The mean age of affected cats is 3–4 years, and males may be predis-

posed. Eighty percent of cats are FeLV-positive. The CNS is involved more frequently than peripheral nerves.

(a) **Epidural lymphosarcoma.** Lymphosarcoma is the second most common CNS tumor in cats (following meningioma). The tumor is often epidural in the thoracolumbar region and results in spinal cord compression with subsequent hindlimb paresis or paralysis. Cerebrospinal fluid (CSF) analysis usually fails to reveal abnormalities in epidural lymphosarcoma. Definitive diagnosis is usually obtained by surgical biopsy.

(b) **Leptomeningeal lymphosarcoma** is rare and tends to affect intracranial structures in a diffuse pattern. CSF abnormalities are usually present (increased protein, increased cell count, presence of neoplastic lymphocytes). Most cats are FeLV-positive.

(4) **Cutaneous lymphosarcoma** is rare in cats. The mean age of affected cats is 8–10 years. Most cats with cutaneous lymphosarcoma are FeLV-negative. Lesions may consist of papules, nodules, tumors, erythematous plaques, crusts, ulcers, and alopecia. Pruritus may be present. Diagnosis is based on skin biopsy.

2. Canine. Lymphosarcoma (lymphoma) is one of the most common malignant neoplasms in dogs. Breeds that may be at increased risk include boxers, basset hounds, St. Bernards, Scottish terriers, Airedales, and bulldogs. Dachshunds and Pomeranians are at a lower risk. The average age at onset is 6–7 years with a range from 6 months to 15 years. The most common anatomic forms are multicentric, mediastinal, alimentary, and cutaneous. Less common are the ocular and CNS forms.

a. General considerations

(1) **Laboratory findings.** In addition to the diagnostic findings specific to the anatomic form of lymphoma, the following may be noted:

(a) Total blood leukocyte counts are often normal.

(b) Lymphoblastic cells in the circulation are occasionally observed and are an indicator of bone marrow involvement and advanced disease.

(c) A mild to moderate nonregenerative anemia resulting from chronic disease is observed in some animals. Occasionally, the anemia may be secondary to immune-mediated hemolysis, blood loss, or bone marrow destruction and replacement by neoplastic cells.

(d) Thrombocytopenia can also be observed.

(e) A monoclonal gammopathy is detected in some dogs.

(f) Hypercalcemia is present in approximately 10% of cases. Lymphosarcoma is the most common cause of persistent moderate to marked hypercalcemia in dogs.

(2) **Treatment**

(a) **Multiple-drug combination chemotherapy** similar to that used in cats can achieve partial remission (i.e., 50% reduction in lymph node or tumor size) in 90% of patients and complete remission in 75% of patients.

(i) Alimentary and cutaneous lymphosarcoma are not as responsive to chemotherapy as other forms.

(ii) Prior treatment with corticosteroids may decrease the response to chemotherapy.

(b) **Prednisone** alone can be considered for short-term palliation of clinical signs if chemotherapy is not an option.

(3) **Prognosis.** Relapses are common and usually occur within the first 6 months of therapy. With effective chemotherapy and owner compliance, median survival times range from 6–12 months, and are occasionally as long as 2–3 years. Percent 1-year survival ranges from 10%–50%.

b. Multicentric lymphosarcoma accounts for approximately 80% of cases of lymphosarcoma in dogs. Many organs, including the lungs, spleen, liver, bone marrow, and peripheral blood, can be involved. The extent of organ involvement can be established by thoracic and abdominal radiographs, ultrasonography (with or without fine-needle aspirate of the liver or spleen), and a bone marrow examination.

    (1) Clinical findings. Multicentric lymphosarcoma is characterized by generalized marked lymphadenopathy. Weight loss and inappetence may be present, although many dogs have no systemic signs of illness. Hepatosplenomegaly may be detected.

    (2) Diagnostic imaging findings

        (a) Thoracic radiographs can reveal sternal and tracheobronchial lymphadenopathy, or nodular, focal, alveolar, or interstitial pulmonary densities.

        (b) Abdominal radiographs may reveal hepatomegaly, splenomegaly, or sublumbar and mesenteric lymphadenopathy.

    (3) Laboratory findings. The diagnosis is usually established by fine-needle aspiration of enlarged lymph nodes. In some cases, lymph node biopsy may be required.

  c. Mediastinal lymphosarcoma. Cranial mediastinal lymphoma results in a large space-occupying mass that can compress the trachea, large vessels, and esophagus. Pleural effusion is often present.

    (1) Clinical findings can include coughing, dyspnea, regurgitation, and edema of the head and neck.

    (2) Diagnostic imaging findings. Widening of the cranial mediastinum and elevation and compression of the trachea may be identified on thoracic radiographs.

    (3) Laboratory findings. Definitive diagnosis can usually be obtained by examination of the pleural fluid or, if necessary, ultrasound-guided fine-needle aspiration of the mass.

  d. Alimentary lymphosarcoma is usually associated with malabsorptive disease and results from bowel wall infiltration.

    (1) Clinical findings often include weight loss, vomiting, chronic diarrhea, and (occasionally) melena.

    (2) Laboratory findings. Histologically, the disease is characterized by focal or diffuse neoplastic infiltrates in the bowel wall. The liver, spleen, and mediastinal lymph nodes can also be affected. Mucosal biopsies obtained with an endoscope are relatively superficial and may not detect the tumor if it is deeper within the bowel wall. Diagnosis requires GI biopsy (endoscopically or surgically).

  e. Cutaneous lymphosarcoma. Tumors can appear as solitary or generalized lesions in the form of nodules, plaques, or ulcerations. The lesions have been characterized as erythematous plaques that eventually ulcerate. Over 50% affected dogs have involvement of other sites such as the liver, spleen, and lymph nodes. Diagnosis is based on skin biopsy examination.

  f. Ocular lymphosarcoma. The eye may be involved as a primary single site or as an extension of another form. Conjunctival, corneal, uveal, and retinal involvement can occur.

  g. Neural lymphosarcoma. The CNS can be a primary or secondary site. Peripheral nerve involvement is less common. Signs can be attributable to multifocal CNS disease, focal spinal cord involvement, or peripheral nerve dysfunction. Diagnosis is based on the observation of neoplastic lymphocytes in the CSF or surgical biopsy.

C. Splenomegaly

  1. Etiology

    a. Inflammatory (e.g., **suppurative, eosinophilic, granulomatous) splenomegaly** is caused by many infectious agents.

    b. Hyperplastic splenomegaly is caused by chronic inflammatory diseases (e.g., IHA).

    c. Congestive splenomegaly is caused by portal hypertension, splenic torsion, and tranquilizers.

d. Infiltrative splenomegaly is caused by neoplasia (e.g., lymphoma, plus many others), extramedullary hematopoiesis, or amyloidosis.

e. Splenic infarction from thrombosis of splenic vessels can also result in splenomegaly.

2. **Diagnosis**
   a. **Clinical findings.** Clinical signs of the underlying disease usually predominate. The spleen is usually not easily palpable unless it is enlarged. The spleen may be smooth and diffusely enlarged or nodular. When splenomegaly or splenic disease is the primary abnormality (e.g., splenic torsion), signs may include anorexia, depression, weakness, vomiting, diarrhea, polyuria, polydipsia, and abdominal distention.
   b. **Diagnostic imaging findings.** Abdominal radiographs, and especially ultrasonograms, can aid in the assessment of splenic size and determination of whether the disease process is diffuse or focal. Mass lesions can be characterized (e.g., as solid or cavitary).
   c. **Laboratory findings**
      (1) **Hematology**
         (a) **Hypersplenism** (increased function) can be associated with the accelerated removal of RBCs, platelets, and leukocytes. Hypersplenism can result in a regenerative anemia, thrombocytopenia, or neutropenia (or a combination thereof).
         (b) **Hyposplenism** (reduced function or splenectomy) can be associated with an increased number of target cells, acanthocytes, Howell-Jolly bodies in RBCs, reticulocytes, and platelets.
      (2) **Other tests.** Percutaneous fine-needle aspiration of the spleen is a noninvasive and easy method of characterizing the disease process. A laparotomy to visualize and biopsy the spleen may be necessary.

3. **Treatment.** Splenectomy is indicated if there is splenic torsion, splenic rupture, symptomatic splenomegaly, or splenic masses.

D. **Splenic masses** are common in dogs, less so in cats. Splenic masses may be neoplastic (e.g., hemangiosarcoma, hemangioma) or nonneoplastic (e.g., hematoma, abscess, regenerative hyperplasia). **Hemangiosarcoma** is the most common splenic tumor in dogs, and is seen most often in male German shepherds (and related crosses) and golden retrievers. It is rare in cats.

1. **Pathology.** Hemangiosarcoma has an aggressive biologic behavior, and about 50% of dogs have metastatic disease at the time of diagnosis. Metastatic lesions are commonly found in the liver, omentum, right atrium of the heart, peritoneum, kidneys, and lungs.

2. **Diagnosis** is usually based on a combination of clinical signs of hemorrhage, the presence of a splenic mass and hemoabdomen, laboratory findings, and metastatic disease (in some patients). Splenic hematoma, the main differential for hemangiosarcoma, is not accompanied by intraabdominal hemorrhage, metastatic lesions, or laboratory abnormalities.
   a. **Clinical findings.** Rupture of this very vascular tumor often causes signs reflective of intraabdominal hemorrhage (e.g., anorexia, lethargy, weakness, mucous membrane pallor, abdominal distention). Signs associated with metastatic lesions may predominate in some dogs.
   b. **Laboratory findings.** Many hematologic abnormalities result from hemorrhage, reduced splenic function, microangiopathic damage to RBCs, and DIC (approximately 50% of dogs have laboratory abnormalities consistent with DIC). Anemia (usually regenerative), nucleated RBCs, poikilocytes, acanthocytes, schistocytes, Howell-Jolly bodies, thrombocytopenia, and neutrophilia are common; the presence of acanthocytes and hemangiosarcoma has been correlated.

3. **Treatment**
   a. **Splenectomy** is the main treatment for dogs without metastatic disease. How-

ever, microscopic or undetectable metastasis is frequently present, resulting in short survival times.

    b. Adjuvant immunotherapy using a mixed bacterial vaccine and multiple-drug chemotherapy has been used in conjunction with splenectomy but has only prolonged survival to a modest degree.

4. Prognosis. The prognosis is usually poor.

    a. With splenectomy alone, median survival times have been reported to range from 19 to 83 days.

    b. With splenectomy plus aggressive chemotherapy, median survival times have been reported to range from 141 to 179 days. With the addition of immunotherapy (i.e., liposome encapsulated muramyl tripeptide-phosphatidylethanolamine), the median survival time has increased to 273 days.

VI. DISORDERS OF THE IMMUNE SYSTEM

A. Immune deficiency may be **congenital** or **acquired** (Table 48-9). Congenital immune deficiency is rare.

1. Pathogenesis. Immune deficiency may primarily affect either humoral (antibody-mediated) or cell-mediated immune function, or both may be affected. The main signs of immune deficiency relate to increased susceptibility to infection and include infections that are recurrent, difficult to resolve, or caused by normally nonpathogenic organisms.

    a. Defects in humoral immunity are commonly associated with bacterial infection.

    b. Poor cell-mediated immunity is usually associated with recurrent fungal, protozoal, or viral infection.

2. Diagnosis can be difficult, but immune deficiency is suggested by the identification of a disease known to cause immune deficiency (e.g., FeLV or FIV infection), decreased neutrophil and lymphocyte counts, reduced serum immunoglobulin levels,

TABLE 48-9. Diseases Associated with Immune Deficiency

Congenital

    Canine cyclic hematopoiesis (grey collies)

    Canine granulocytopathy syndrome (Irish setters)

    Leukocyte surface glycoprotein deficiency

    Pelger-Huët anomaly (domestic shorthair cats)

    Chediak-Higashi syndrome (Persian cats)

    C3 deficiency

    Combined immunodeficiency (basset hounds)

    Selective IgA deficiency (German shepherds, Shar peis, beagles)

    Failure of passive (immunoglobulin) transfer in neonates

Acquired

    Infections [e.g., feline leukemia virus (FeLV) infection, feline immunodeficiency virus (FIV) infection, feline panleukopenia virus infection, canine parvovirus infection, canine distemper virus (CDV) infection, systemic fungal infections, demodicosis, ehrlichiosis]

    Drug therapy (e.g., with corticosteroids, many cancer chemotherapeutic drugs)

    Hyperadrenocorticism

    Diabetes mellitus

    Malignant neoplasia

and abnormal macrophage or B and T lymphocyte function (assessed with specialized in vitro tests).

B. **Immune-mediated diseases**

1. **Hypersensitivity reactions**
   a. **Type I hypersensitivity reactions** involve immunoglobulin E (IgE), mast cells or basophils, and the release of pharmacologically active mediators (e.g., histamine).
      (1) **Pathogenesis.** IgE that is produced in response to antigen exposure (often epidermal) binds to the surface of local mast cells or basophils; if excess IgE is produced, it will enter the circulation and bind to these cells in other body tissues, priming the body for local and systemic reactions. When antigen reenters the body, it binds to IgE molecules on the surface of local mast cells, resulting in degranulation and the release of a variety of preformed and secondary mediators such as histamine, serotonin, proteases, heparin, cytokines, and lipid mediators (e.g., prostaglandins, leukotrienes). An acute local inflammatory reaction (e.g., wheals, urticaria, edema) or systemic inflammatory reaction (e.g., anaphylactic shock) results.
      (2) **Etiology.** Diseases associated with type I reactions include local and systemic anaphylaxis, atopy, and flea allergy dermatitis.
   b. **Type II hypersensitivity reactions** result from **antibody-dependent cytotoxicity.**
      (1) **Pathogenesis.** Antibodies are formed to "self" (endogenous) antigens or foreign (exogenous) antigens that become associated with a cell surface or basement membrane. Damage occurs in response to any of the following:
         (a) Bound antibody interacts with cytotoxic effector cells, resulting in destruction or damage to target cells or basement membranes.
         (b) Bound antibody activates complement, resulting in cellular destruction.
         (c) Circulating cells that have antibody bound to their surface are removed from the circulation by the mononuclear phagocyte system.
      (2) **Examples** of type II reactions include IHA and IMT.
   c. **Type III hypersensitivity (immune-complex) reactions** involve immune complexes that are deposited in various tissues and incite tissue or organ damage. Deposited immune complexes trigger a variety of inflammatory responses (e.g., complement activation, mast cell degranulation, platelet activation or aggregation). Type III reactions are associated with systemic lupus erythematosus (SLE), rheumatoid arthritis, and various chronic inflammatory or infectious diseases.
   d. **Type IV hypersensitivity (cell-mediated) reactions** involve a sensitized population of T cells that upon subsequent reexposure to an antigen initiate a cellular inflammatory response. Examples of type IV reactions include contact hypersensitivity or allergy and some infectious diseases that result in chronic granulomatous inflammation (e.g., tuberculosis).

2. **Systemic anaphylaxis** is an acute, life-threatening event that results from the widespread activation and degranulation of mast cells following exposure to an antigen (e.g., drugs, hormones, vaccines, iodinated contrast media, snake venom).
   a. **Pathogenesis.** Most, but not all, anaphylactic reactions involve IgE-mediated mast cell degranulation. Certain drugs and complement fragments (C3a and C5a) can interact directly with mast cells and cause degranulation and anaphylaxis (anaphylactoid reactions). Mast cell degranulation results in the release of primary mediators (e.g., histamine, chemotactic factors) followed by the generation of secondary mediators (prostaglandins, leukotrienes, thromboxane A_2, platelet-activating factor). The combined action of these mediators results in a vasogenic shock, bronchoconstriction, excess airway mucous production, dyspnea, and hypoxemia.
   b. **Diagnosis** is based on a history of exposure to a potential antigen and on clinical signs. The clinical signs of anaphylaxis can be local or systemic. Local signs may precede a systemic reaction.
      (1) **Localized anaphylaxis** usually results in urticaria, wheals, pruritus, and erythema close to the site of antigen exposure.

    (2) **Systemic anaphylaxis** involves multiple organs and begins at a site distant from the location of antigen exposure. Systemic signs are different between dogs and cats and are related to the predominant shock organ.

        (a) In dogs, the shock organs are the liver and GI tract. Initial signs may include excitement, vomiting, defecation, and urination, followed by respiratory depression and collapse. Death can occur within 1 hour if untreated.

        (b) In cats, the shock organ is the lung. Initial signs can include extreme pruritus of the head and neck followed by dyspnea, profuse salivation, vomiting, incoordination, and collapse.

  c. Treatment

    (1) **Localized anaphylaxis** can usually be successfully treated with antihistamines and corticosteroids. Epinephrine injected at the site of antigen exposure (e.g., bee sting) may be helpful. Animals should be monitored closely for 12–24 hours to detect the development of systemic signs.

    (2) **Systemic anaphylaxis.** Prompt and aggressive treatment is essential.

        (a) **Epinephrine** should be administered intramuscularly or subcutaneously and repeated every 15–20 minutes as needed.

        (b) **Therapy for shock** (i.e., intravenous fluids, corticosteroids with or without positive inotropic therapy, and atropine) and **respiratory support** (i.e., supplemental oxygen, possible endotracheal intubation or tracheostomy, bronchodilators) should follow.

3. Pemphigus diseases are a group of autoimmune skin diseases characterized by the formation and deposition of antibodies in epidermal intercellular spaces (a type II hypersensitivity reaction). Autoimmune skin disease may also result from bullous pemphigoid, SLE, and discoid (cutaneous) lupus erythematosus.

  a. Types. The four forms of pemphigus differ in the distribution pattern of skin lesions and where in the epidermis the antibodies are deposited.

    (1) **Pemphigus foliaceous** is one of the more common autoimmune skin diseases. It is a progressive disorder recognized in dogs 3–7 years of age. Newfoundlands, bearded collies, Akitas, and schipperkes may be at increased risk. Pemphigus foliaceous usually begins as crusty lesions around the face; crusting, scaling, and alopecia are the most common lesions. Patchy or generalized lesions can develop, and pruritus is variable.

    (2) **Pemphigus erythematosus** may be an initial stage or a less severe form of pemphigus foliaceous. Skin lesions are usually confined to the face and include erythema, crusting, oozing, and alopecia.

    (3) **Pemphigus vulgaris** typically causes ulceration of the epidermis with a predilection for mucocutaneous junctions and oral mucous membranes. Ninety percent of affected animals have oral lesions (e.g., ulcerative stomatitis, gingivitis, glossitis). Pain and pruritus may occur. The onset may be slow or rapid, and systemic signs of illness may develop.

    (4) **Pemphigus vegetans** is rare and is thought to represent a less severe form of pemphigus vulgaris. During healing of the ulcerative skin lesions, verrucous vegetations and papillomatous proliferations develop.

  b. Diagnosis is based on skin biopsy and immunologic staining (immunoperoxidase, immunofluorescence) to document the deposition of antibodies.

  c. Treatment. Immunosuppressive doses of **corticosteroids** (e.g., prednisone) are used initially.

    (1) If a positive response is observed, the dosage of corticosteroid is gradually reduced over a 1- to 2-month period to administration every other day.

    (2) If no response occurs, azathioprine, cyclophosphamide, or gold salts (aurothioglucose) can be added to the treatment regimen.

  d. Prognosis

    (1) **Pemphigus foliaceous.** Approximately 75% of affected dogs can be managed successfully without significant drug side effects.

    (2) **Pemphigus erythematosus.** Most dogs can be treated successfully.

(3) **Pemphigus vulgaris.** Affected dogs have a poor prognosis, and most die of sepsis or progressive debilitation.

(4) **Pemphigus vegetans.** Little is known regarding the prognosis for animals with this disorder.

4. **SLE** is a rare disease of dogs and cats. It has been reported in dogs from 8 months to 14 years of age. Breeds that may be predisposed include poodles, German shepherds, collies, Shetland sheepdogs, Irish setters, and Afghans.

  a. **Pathogenesis.** SLE results from the formation of autoantibodies to many "self" antigens (e.g., deoxyribonucleic acid, RBCs, neutrophils, platelets). Organ and tissue damage occurs via type II, type III, and type IV hypersensitivity reactions.

  b. **Diagnosis** can be difficult because of the multisystemic manifestations. A combination of joint, skin, renal, or hematologic disease is suggestive of SLE.

    (1) **Clinical findings**

      (a) **Joint disease** (an immune-mediated nonerosive polyarthritis) is the most common manifestation of SLE in dogs.

      (b) **Skin disease** is the second most common manifestation of SLE. Skin lesions observed include pruritic seborrheic dermatitis (most severe around the face, ears, and limbs), mucocutaneous ulcerations, ulcerative or hyperkeratotic footpads, and subcutaneous nodules (with or without fistulae).

      (c) **Fever** (constant or intermittent) is present in more than 50% of affected dogs.

      (d) **Renal disease** is manifested as an immune complex (membranoproliferative) glomerulonephritis.

      (e) **Other signs** include CNS signs, polymyositis, and pleuritis.

    (2) **Laboratory findings**

      (a) **Hematology**

        (i) **Anemia** occurs in about 35% of dogs and can be either nonregenerative (ACD) or regenerative (IHA or blood loss caused by immune-mediated thrombocytopenia). Most animals with IHA will be Coombs'-positive and have spherocytosis.

        (ii) **Thrombocytopenia** occurs in about 10% of SLE patients and is immune-mediated due to the generation of antiplatelet antibodies. If thrombocytopenia is severe (i.e., the platelet count is less than $20,000/\mu l$), petechial hemorrhages, retinal hemorrhage, hematuria, and melena may occur.

        (iii) **Neutropenia** may be observed.

      (b) **Antinuclear antibody (ANA) titer.** A significant ANA titer is a key supportive finding. Normal animals and animals with inflammatory disease not related to SLE may have low ANA titers.

      (c) **LE cell preparation.** This is an *in vitro* test to detect ANAs in blood. An LE cell preparation is considered to be more specific but less sensitive than an ANA titer. However, some consider the LE cell preparation to be of marginal value due to the frequency of false-negative and false-positive reactions.

      (d) **Cytology.** SLE joint disease is characterized by the presence of large numbers of nondegenerate neutrophils in the joint fluid. The presence of spontaneously occurring LE cells (cells that have phagocytosed nuclear material) in joint fluid, peripheral blood, or bone marrow is highly suggestive of SLE.

      (e) **Skin biopsy** primarily reveals an interface dermatitis (i.e., hydropic degeneration and/or lichenoid cell infiltration at the dermoepidermal junction). Immunofluorescent staining reveals immunoglobulin deposition along the dermoepidermal junction (an LE band).

      (f) **Urinalysis.** Proteinuria due to glomerulonephritis occurs in approximately 50% of patients with SLE.

    (3) **Diagnostic criteria** include the major and minor signs. A definitive diagnosis of SLE requires a significant ANA titer and one of the following: two major

signs, or one major and two minor signs. A diagnosis of probable SLE requires a significant ANA titer and one major sign or two minor signs.

(a) **Major signs** include polyarthritis, skin disease, Coombs'-positive anemia, significant thrombocytopenia or neutropenia, and polymyositis.

(b) **Minor signs** include fever, CNS signs, and pleuritis.

c. **Treatment.** Immunosuppressive doses of **prednisone** are used initially and are tapered to the lowest effective dose. **Azathioprine** is added to the regimen for animals that are refractory to prednisone alone.

d. **Prognosis** depends on the extent of organ involvement (especially if renal failure is present) and the severity of hematologic abnormalities.

(1) Approximately 40% of dogs die within the first year of therapy because of bronchopneumonia, sepsis, or steroid-induced pancreatitis.

(2) Disease in animals with primarily joint and skin involvement may be controlled better and these animals may survive longer.

5. **Paraproteinemia (monoclonal gammopathy)** develops from the production of immunoglobulin from a single, expanded clonal population of plasma cells.

a. **Etiology.** Causes include multiple myeloma, CLL, lymphosarcoma, plasma cell leukemia, primary macroglobulinemia, amyloidosis, and idiopathic (benign) monoclonal gammopathy. Occasionally, chronic inflammatory or infectious diseases (e.g., ehrlichiosis) may be the cause.

b. **Diagnosis.** Monoclonal gammopathies may be associated with a bleeding tendency (primarily caused by platelet dysfunction) and hyperviscosity syndrome. Hyperviscosity can result in heart failure (from chronic volume overload), CNS signs resulting form sluggish blood flow and hypoxia (e.g., depression, coma, ataxia, dementia), and renal damage resulting from tubular toxicity caused by filtered protein.

6. **Plasma cell tumors (multiple myeloma).** Plasma cell tumors are rare in dogs and very rare in cats.

a. **Pathogenesis.** Most plasma cell tumors occur in bone and cause a diffuse increase in plasma cell numbers in the bone marrow. Occasionally, solitary bone tumors (without diffuse marrow involvement) and extramedullary tumors (which do not involve bone or bone marrow) occur. Solitary bone tumors may actually be an early stage before diffuse marrow involvement occurs. Animals with multiple myeloma are immunocompromised and susceptible to bacterial infection.

b. **Diagnosis**

(1) **Clinical findings.** Signs result from a direct effect of the tumor (i.e., osteolytic lesions, bone pain, pathologic fractures, hypercalcemia) or from increased serum concentrations of immunoglobulin (i.e., hyperviscosity, renal disease). **Hypercalcemia** (resulting from increased bone absorption), **renal disease,** and **hyperviscosity** are common manifestations of multiple myeloma.

(a) Hyperviscosity and increased immunoglobulin concentrations may result in petechiation, epistaxis, retinal hemorrhages, or signs of congestive heart failure. Hyperviscosity is most common with IgM gammopathies.

(b) Hypercalcemia or renal failure may cause polyuria and polydipsia.

(c) Lameness, bone pain, weakness, pale mucous membranes, fever, lethargy, and hepatosplenomegaly may also be detected.

(2) **Laboratory findings**

(a) **Hematology.** Mild leukopenia and anemia are relatively common secondary to marrow replacement by plasma cells. About 25% of dogs have leukopenia and 70% have a nonregenerative anemia. Severe thrombocytopenia occurs in about 16% of cases.

(b) **Serum biochemical profile.** Hypercalcemia is present in about 15%–20% of affected animals. Serum biochemistry may reveal renal failure, which occurs in about 30% of patients with plasma cell tumors.

(c) **Serum protein electrophoresis.** The globulin concentration is usually markedly increased due to monoclonal gammopathy. A serum protein electrophoresis is required to document the presence of a monoclonal versus a polyclonal gammopathy (caused by chronic inflammation).

(d) **Immunoglobulin electrophoresis** can be considered to identify the immunoglobulin class.

(i) In dogs, plasma cell tumors secrete IgG and IgA with equal frequency.

(ii) In cats, most tumors secrete IgG.

(3) **Diagnostic imaging findings.** Bony lesions are present in about 50% of patients. Increased bone resorption can lead to either generalized osteoporosis or localized, osteolytic "punched-out" lesions with no evidence of bone repair at the margins. Osteolytic lesions are more common than diffuse osteoporosis. The long bones, vertebral bodies, and pelvis are most frequently affected.

(4) **Diagnostic criteria.** Diagnosis is based on the presence of:

(a) Bone marrow plasmacytosis (more than 20% plasma cells)

(b) Osteolytic bone lesions [in the absence of bone lesions, the combination of bone marrow plasmacytosis and a progressive increase in serum myeloma protein (monoclonal gammopathy) is diagnostic]

(c) Monoclonal gammopathy

(d) Urine myeloma protein (Bence-Jones proteinuria)

c. **Treatment**

(1) **Chemotherapy.** A combination of **melphalan** (an alkylating agent) and **prednisone** will reduce the population of tumor cells but will not eradicate the tumor. Response to drug therapy can be assessed by monitoring laboratory changes and bony lesions. The monoclonal gammopathy usually decreases by 50% in 8–12 weeks and will frequently disappear with prolonged therapy.

(2) **Phlebotomy** and replacement with normal saline can be performed if hyperviscosity is present.

(3) **Intravenous fluid diuresis, furosemide administration,** and **corticosteroid therapy** may be used to treat hypercalcemia. Fluid diuresis will also help decrease the level of azotemia associated with renal failure and correct dehydration (if present).

(4) **Blood transfusion** should be considered if the anemia is severe.

(5) **Antimicrobial therapy.** Prompt and aggressive antimicrobial therapy is indicated if signs of infection develop.

d. **Prognosis**

(1) **Solitary plasma cell tumors.** The prognosis for animals with solitary plasma cell tumors (e.g., of the skin or GI tract) is good if complete surgical excision is possible.

(2) **Diffuse plasma cell tumors**

(a) **Dogs.** Despite the lack of tumor cell eradication with chemotherapy, a significant prolongation and an enhanced quality of life can be expected in most animals who undergo chemotherapy for diffuse plasma cell tumors. A median survival time of 540 days has been reported in dogs treated with melphalan (with or without prednisone). The median survival in dogs treated with prednisone alone was 220 days.

(i) The presence of renal failure, severe hyperviscosity, hypercalcemia, or extensive bony lysis is associated with a poorer prognosis.

(ii) Many patients with sepsis, renal failure, hemorrhage, or intractable spinal or bone pain either die or are euthanized.

(b) **Cats.** The prognosis in cats is poorer than in dogs and most do not survive longer than 2–3 months following diagnosis.

DIRECTIONS: Each of the numbered items or incomplete statements in this section is followed by answers or by completions of the statement. Select the ONE numbered answer or completion that is BEST in each case. See Appendix for normal laboratory reference ranges.

1. A complete blood count (CBC) from a dog reveals a packed cell volume (PCV) of 20% with a reticulocyte percentage of 8% and a reticulocyte count of 180,000/μl. Total protein is 4.5 g/dl (SI units = 45 g/L. There are no other abnormalities noted. These data would be most consistent with:

(1) zinc toxicity.
(2) warfarin poisoning (with hemorrhage).
(3) immune-mediated hemolytic anemia (IHA).
(4) anemia of chronic disease (ACD).
(5) estrogen toxicity.

2. Which one of the following criteria would be most supportive of a diagnosis of immune-mediated hemolytic anemia (IHA)?

(1) Acanthocytosis
(2) Strongly regenerative anemia
(3) Howell-Jolly bodies
(4) Marked spherocytosis
(5) Marked polychromasia

3. Which of the following transfusions presents the highest risk of a severe transfusion reaction?

(1) Blood from a purebred cat is transfused into a nonpurebred cat.
(2) Blood from a purebred dog is transfused into a mixed-breed dog.
(3) Blood from a mixed-breed dog is transfused into a purebred dog.
(4) Blood from a nonpurebred cat is transfused into a purebred cat.
(5) Blood from a mixed-breed dog is transfused into another mixed-breed dog.

4. Which one of the following diseases would most likely be associated with a degenerative left shift?

(1) Septic peritonitis
(2) Immune-mediated polyarthritis
(3) Sarcoptic mange
(4) Lower urinary tract infection (UTI)
(5) Bone marrow neoplasia

5. A 7-month-old male golden retriever experiences prolonged bleeding from the incision site following castration. The oral mucosal bleeding time is prolonged. A platelet count, prothrombin time (PT), and activated partial thromboplastin time (APTT) are normal. Which one of the following diseases would be consistent with the abnormalities in this dog?

(1) Anticoagulant rodenticide poisoning
(2) Hemophilia A
(3) Hemophilia B
(4) vonWillebrand's disease (vWD)
(5) Liver failure

6. Which one of the following statements regarding feline lymphosarcoma is true?

(1) Neoplastic lymphoblasts are commonly observed in the blood.
(2) Mediastinal lymphoma is a disease of middle-aged to older cats.
(3) Alimentary lymphoma is a disease of middle-aged to older cats.
(4) Hypercalcemia is common.
(5) Multicentric lymphoma is the most common form of lymphosarcoma in cats.

7. Which combination of clinical signs would be most consistent with systemic anaphylaxis in a cat?

(1) Seizures, pale mucous membranes, shock
(2) Vocalization, acute collapse, shock
(3) Extreme pruritus of the head and neck, dyspnea, profuse salivation
(4) Urination, defecation, vomiting
(5) Urination, defecation, excitement, shock, collapse

ANSWERS AND EXPLANATIONS

1. The answer is 2 [II A 1 b (1) (a), 2 a]. The data are most consistent with a regenerative anemia resulting from blood loss [i.e., increased reticulocyte response, a reticulocyte index (RI) greater than 1.0 (i.e., 1.6), reduced total protein]. The only disorder listed associated with blood loss is warfarin poisoning. Anemia of chronic disease (ACD) and estrogen toxicity result in a nonregenerative anemia. Hemolytic anemia (which could be immune-mediated or caused by zinc toxicity) is usually associated with normal total protein and a higher reticulocyte response (i.e., the RI is often greater than 3.0).

2. The answer is 4 [II A 2 b (2) (c) (d)]. Marked spherocytosis is a strong indicator of immune-mediated damage to red blood cells (RBCs). Acanthocytes are usually associated with hemangiosarcoma and liver disease but not immune-mediated hemolytic anemia (IHA). Although a strong regenerative anemia is common with IHA, it is not as specific as marked spherocytosis. Howell-Jolly bodies are associated with hyposplenism and regeneration. Marked polychromasia indicates the presence of many reticulocytes and is consistent with a regenerative response, but it is not specific for IHA.

3. The answer is 4 [I A 2 a]. Many purebred cats have a high prevalence of type B blood and have a high level of naturally occurring antibodies to type A blood. Most nonpurebred cats (i.e., domestic long- or shorthair cats) have type A blood and low levels of antibody to type B blood. Therefore, severe transfusion reactions are more likely to occur when type A blood (most prevalent in nonpurebred cats) is transfused into cats with type B blood (most prevalent in purebred cats). Dogs usually do not have naturally occurring antibodies to other canine blood groups; therefore, severe transfusion reactions are unlikely following a first-time transfusion.

4. The answer is 1 [III A 1 b (1) (b)]. A degenerative left shift is usually associated with marked inflammation, often caused by severe, overwhelming bacterial infection (e.g., septic peritonitis). Immune-mediated disease, sarcoptic mange, or lower urinary tract infection (UTI) rarely result in this degree of inflammation. Bone marrow neoplasia would be more likely to result in neutropenia (with or without other cytopenias) without a band response.

5. The answer is 4 [IV B 3 a, Table 48-7]. The coagulation test results are consistent with platelet dysfunction. The only disease listed that causes platelet dysfunction is von Willebrand's disease (vWD). Although liver failure can result in abnormal platelet function, the predominant abnormality is usually reduced production of coagulation factors. A normal prothrombin time (PT) and activated partial thromboplastin time (APTT) would make anticoagulant rodenticide poisoning, hemophilia A or B, and liver failure unlikely. All of these disorders are associated with multiple- or single-factor deficiencies and would prolong the PT, the APTT, or both. Also, the mucosal bleeding time is unaffected in factor deficiencies.

6. The answer is 3 [V B 1 c]. Alimentary lymphosarcoma is more common in middle-aged to older cats and is an important differential for chronic gastrointestinal (GI) signs in cats in this age range. Circulating neoplastic lymphoblasts are uncommon. Mediastinal lymphoma is typically seen in cats 2–3 years of age. Hypercalcemia is rare in cats with lymphoma. It is more common in dogs. In cats, mediastinal and alimentary lymphoma are more common than multicentric lymphoma.

7. The answer is 3 [VI B 2 b (2) (b)]. Clinical signs of systemic anaphylaxis in cats include extreme pruritus of the head and neck followed by dyspnea, profuse salivation, vomiting, incoordination, and collapse. The lung is the shock organ in cats [as opposed to the gastrointestinal (GI) tract and liver, the primary shock organs in dogs], and dyspnea is a prominent feature. Excitement, urination, defecation, vomiting, respiratory depression, and collapse are common signs of systemic anaphylaxis in dogs.

Chapter 49

Infectious Diseases

I. BACTERIAL DISEASES

A. **Abscesses.** In cats, most abscesses occur as a result of a cat bite. Anaerobic bacteria and *Pasteurella* species are the most common causative organisms. In addition to the abscess itself, fever, anorexia, and regional lymphadenopathy may be seen. Treatment requires lancing and draining unruptured abscesses. Antibiotic treatment with penicillin, amoxicillin, ampicillin, or metronidazole may be necessary; the prognosis is generally good.

B. **Actinomycosis**

1. **Etiology.** Actinomycosis is caused by branching, filamentous, Gram-positive bacteria found in the oral cavity of dogs and cats. Infection usually results from wound infection.

2. **Diagnosis**
   a. **Clinical findings** may include fever, lymphadenopathy, tachypnea or dyspnea, lameness, abdominal distention, or an abscess or draining tract. Infection is usually localized to one body cavity or one tissue site.
   b. **Laboratory findings**
      (1) **Complete blood count (CBC).** A CBC will usually show a leukocytosis with a shift toward immaturity.
      (2) **Examination of exudate.** Grossly, fluid obtained from the infection site may contain yellow "sulfur granules." Cytologically, pyogranulomatous inflammation is found along with non–acid-fast, branching filamentous organisms.
      (3) **Culture** of the organism is necessary for diagnosis.
   c. **Radiographic findings** will vary with the tissue involved. For example:
      (1) Pleural effusion may be seen with pleural infection.
      (2) Lysis and periosteal reaction may be seen with bony infection.
      (3) Ascites may be seen with peritoneal infection.

3. **Treatment** and **prognosis.** Treatment requires drainage and debridement of the infection site along with systemic antibiotic treatment. Penicillin is the antibiotic of choice. The prognosis is generally good with appropriate treatment.

C. **Borreliosis (Lyme disease)** is discussed in Chapter 46 III B 1.

D. **Botulism** is rare in dogs and does not occur in cats.

1. **Etiology.** Botulism is caused by ingestion of spoiled food or dead animals that contain the *Clostridium botulinum* toxin.

2. **Diagnosis.** Presumptive diagnosis is often based on the history and the clinical findings. The diagnosis can be confirmed by electromyography or by finding the bacterial toxin in serum, vomitus, feces, or food.
   a. **Clinical findings** are those of lower motor neuron (LMN) disease and parasympathetic dysfunction because the toxin blocks acetylcholine release. Signs may include weakness, lack of spinal reflexes, drooling, dysphagia, and mydriasis. Pain sensation is normal. With severe disease, respiratory paralysis may occur.
   b. **Electromyography** will show subnormal amplitude of evoked motor potentials and no denervation potentials.

3. **Treatment** and **prognosis.** The treatment is nonspecific and mainly entails supportive care. Laxatives and enemas may be used to remove any toxin still remaining in

the gastrointestinal (GI) tract. The prognosis is generally good unless severe disease causes respiratory paralysis.

E. **Brucellosis.** Cats are not susceptible.

1. **Etiology.** Brucellosis is caused by the Gram-negative coccobacillus *Brucella canis.*

2. **Pathogenesis.** Infection occurs following the exposure of mucous membranes (e.g., oral, nasal, conjunctival, vaginal membranes) to secretions from another infected dog. The organism is then carried by macrophages to genital and lymphatic tissues.

3. **Diagnosis**
   a. **Clinical findings** may include infertility, testicular enlargement (orchitis) and epididymal enlargement (epididymitis), lymphadenopathy, late-gestation abortion, uveitis, fever, back pain (discospondylitis), and lameness (osteomyelitis).
   b. **Laboratory findings**
      (1) **Serology**
         (a) **Rapid slide agglutination tests (RSAT)** are used most often because of their high sensitivity. They have a low specificity, however, so a positive result requires further testing to determine if the animal is truly infected.
         (b) **Tube agglutination tests** are used by many laboratories for confirmation of RSAT test results. False–positive results can still be seen with this test.
         (c) **Agar-gel immunodiffusion** is the best method for confirming positive agglutination test results because of better test sensitivity.
      (2) **Culture** of fluid (e.g., blood, vaginal discharge, semen) or tissue from a site of infection (e.g., a lymph node) may isolate the organism.
      (3) **Other tests.** Nonspecific diagnostic test results may include leukocytosis, monocytosis, hyperglobulinemia, proteinuria, and semen abnormalities.

4. **Treatment** and **prognosis.** Treatment is difficult because *Brucella* is an intracellular organism. Optimal antibiotic treatment is with a combination of minocycline and dihydrostreptomycin, but these drugs can be expensive. Repeated courses of tetracycline and dihydrostreptomycin treatment may also be tried. The prognosis for cure is guarded.

5. **Prevention** requires testing and elimination of infected animals from all breeding programs. Infected bitches should be spayed and treated with antibiotics.

6. **Zoonotic potential.** Humans can become infected with *B. canis* by coming in contact with fluids or tissues from an aborting bitch or urine from an infected male dog.

F. **Campylobacteriosis** is discussed in Chapter 41 IV B 4 b.

G. **Clostridial disease (intestinal)** is discussed in Chapter 41.

H. **Leptospirosis** is rare in cats. Disease is more common in the summer and early fall.

1. **Etiology.** Leptospirosis in dogs is usually caused by the spirochetes *Leptospira icterohaemorrhagiae* or *Leptospira canicola.*

2. **Pathogenesis**
   a. The organism may be acquired through direct contact with an infected animal (wild or domestic) or from contact with contaminated soil, water, or other items. Urine from an infected animal is a concentrated source of infection.
   b. The organisms penetrate mucous membranes and replicate in the circulation. They may then cause vasculitis, renal tubular damage, hepatic damage (more likely with *L. icterohaemorrhagiae*), meningitis, and uveitis.

3. **Diagnosis**
   a. **Clinical findings** vary with the type of infection, immune response of the patient, and the organs or body systems affected. Fever, anorexia, muscle pain, vomiting, petechiae and ecchymoses, cough, oculonasal discharge, dyspnea, and oliguria or anuria may be seen. Icterus may be seen with *L. icterohaemorrhagiae* infection.

    b. Laboratory findings. Definitive diagnosis requires culture of the organism, demonstration of organisms on dark-field microscopy, or demonstration of a fourfold increase in serum antibody titer.

        (1) CBC. A CBC may reveal leukopenia early in the course of the disease, leukocytosis with a shift toward immaturity later in the course of the disease, and thrombocytopenia.

        (2) Serum biochemical profile. A serum biochemical profile usually shows azotemia, hyperphosphatemia, hyponatremia, hypokalemia, hypochloremia, and hypoalbuminemia. Other findings may include increased hepatic enzyme concentrations, hyperbilirubinemia, and increased creatine kinase concentration.

        (3) Urinalysis often shows isosthenuria, proteinuria, hyperbilirubinuria, and inflammatory sediment.

4. Treatment and **prognosis.** Supportive care entails intravenous fluid therapy and treatment for acute renal failure and disseminated intravascular coagulation (DIC), if present. Antibiotic therapy should include penicillin initially, followed by dihydrostreptomycin or tetracycline therapy when renal function has returned to normal. Prognosis varies with the severity of infection and the degree of renal damage.

5. Prevention. Bacterins containing *L. canicola* and *L. icterohaemorrhagiae* are available but are not 100% effective.

6. Zoonotic potential. Humans are susceptible to leptospirosis, so contact with infected urine should be avoided and contaminated areas should be disinfected.

I. **L-form (cell–wall-deficient) bacteria** can cause fever, cellulitis, and synovitis in cats. Infection is caused by contamination of a wound. Treatment is with tetracycline.

J. **Mycobacterial infections**

1. Tuberculous infection

    a. Etiology. Tuberculous infection is caused by *Mycobacterium tuberculosis* (from humans), *Mycobacterium bovis* (from meat products), or less commonly, *Mycobacterium avium* (usually from poultry).

    b. Diagnosis

        (1) Clinical findings. Granulomas may form in the respiratory tract (more common in dogs), GI tract (more common in cats), or lymph nodes. Fever, cough, weight loss, vomiting, diarrhea, dysphagia, lymphadenopathy, or other signs may be noted. Some animals are asymptomatic.

        (2) Laboratory findings. Diagnosis is based on biopsy or culture of one of the granulomatous lesions.

    c. Treatment. Most infected pets are euthanized because of the severity of the disease, poor response to treatment, and the zoonotic potential of the infection (especially with *M. tuberculosis*).

2. Nontuberculous infection

    a. Etiology. Nontuberculous infection can be caused by *Mycobacterium lepraemurium* (feline leprosy), acquired from the bite of an infected rodent, or other atypical mycobacteria acquired as a result of wound contamination.

    b. Diagnosis

        (1) Clinical findings include the presence of cutaneous and subcutaneous nodules.

        (2) Laboratory findings. Diagnosis is by biopsy with demonstration of the presence of acid-fast organisms.

    c. Treatment is usually surgical, although dapsone or rifampin may be used as adjunct treatment.

K. **Nocardiosis**

1. Etiology. Nocardiosis is caused by branching filamentous organisms found in the soil. Infection usually occurs as a result of inhalation or wound infection.

2. **Diagnosis**
   a. **Clinical findings.** Nocardiosis can have several presentations:
      (1) **Subcutaneous nocardiosis** occurs when infection of a wound leads to invasion of deeper tissues. Clinical findings include the wound itself, a draining tract, regional lymphadenopathy, or fever.
      (2) **Infection of a body cavity** with *Nocardia* species may be characterized by fever, dyspnea or tachypnea, and ascites.
      (3) **Disseminated disease.** Clinical signs may include fever, anorexia, lameness, cough, oculonasal discharge, diarrhea, dyspnea and tachypnea, and neurologic abnormalities. *Nocardia* is more likely than *Actinomyces* to cause disseminated disease.
   b. **Laboratory findings**
      (1) **CBC.** A CBC will usually show a leukocytosis with a shift toward immaturity.
      (2) **Cytology.** Cytologic evaluation of fluid from the infection site usually shows pyogranulomatous inflammation and acid-fast, branching, filamentous organisms.
      (3) **Culture.** Diagnosis is based on culture of the organism.
   c. **Radiographic findings** will vary with the tissue involved. For example, pleural effusion may be seen with pleural infection, lysis and periosteal reaction may be seen with bony infection, and ascites may be seen with peritoneal infection.

3. **Treatment** and **prognosis.** Treatment requires drainage and debridement of the infection site along with systemic antibiotic treatment. Sulfonamides are the antibiotics of choice. The prognosis is fair to good with local disease but poor for disseminated disease.

L. **Plague** is caused by *Yersinia pestis*. Wild rodents serve as the main reservoir for the disease, and infection usually occurs as the result of the bite of a flea from an infected rodent or ingestion of the rodent. The disease can be transmitted to humans through the common vector (fleas) or through a bite or scratch from the infected animal. Cats may become septicemic, but dogs usually just show mild lymphadenopathy. Treatment is with sulfonamides, tetracycline, or chloramphenicol, but the prognosis is guarded in cats and the zoonotic potential must be considered.

M. **Salmonellosis** (see also Chapter 41)

1. **Etiology** and **pathogenesis.** Many species of *Salmonella* can infect dogs and cats. Infection usually occurs from contact with infected animals or through ingestion of contaminated food. The organism can also be isolated from clinically normal dogs and cats. The bacteria invade and multiply in the intestinal mucosa.

2. **Diagnosis**
   a. **Clinical findings.** In dogs, fever, diarrhea, vomiting, and weight loss are most common, but in cats, diarrhea is uncommon. Shock, neurologic abnormalities, pneumonia, and other signs may be seen if septicemia occurs. Some animals are asymptomatic carriers.
   b. **Laboratory findings.** Diagnosis is based on fecal or blood culture and the presence of appropriate clinical signs.

3. **Treatment**
   a. GI disease alone often resolves with supportive care. Antibiotic treatment in animals who only have signs of GI disease is controversial because of the risk of increasing resistance and possibly promoting a carrier state.
   b. Septicemic animals should be treated with ampicillin, enrofloxacin, trimethoprim/sulfa, or cephalothin while awaiting results of sensitivity testing. Supportive care should also be instituted.

4. **Prognosis** is good with GI disease but poor with septicemia.

5. **Zoonotic potential.** Salmonellosis can be transmitted to humans, so good hygiene should be used and all contaminated areas should be disinfected.

N. **Streptococcal infection**

1. **Etiology.** Streptococci are Gram-positive facultatively anaerobic coccal bacteria. Nonhemolytic streptococci can be part of the normal flora in dogs and cats, whereas β-hemolytic streptococci are more commonly pathogenic.

2. **Diagnosis**
    (1) **Clinical findings** vary with the organ or tissue affected and may include fever, pollakiuria and dysuria [in the case of urinary tract infection (UTI)], cervical lymphadenopathy (in the case of strangles), cough (with bronchitis or pneumonia), dyspnea and tachypnea (with pneumonia or pleural effusion), a cardiac murmur (with endocarditis), or back pain (with discospondylitis).
    (2) **Laboratory findings.** Diagnosis is based on culture. Other diagnostic test results vary with the organ or tissue affected.

3. **Treatment** and **prognosis.** Treatment is with penicillin, ampicillin, or a cephalosporin. Ampicillin or trimethoprim/sulfa is recommended for β-hemolytic streptococcal UTI. The prognosis varies with the severity of the infection.

4. **Zoonotic potential.** Group A streptococci (e.g., *Streptococcus pyogenes*) can be acquired by pets from humans. Infected pets, which may be asymptomatic, can serve as a source of reinfection for humans.

O. **Tetanus**

1. **Etiology.** Tetanus is caused by wound contamination with *Clostridium tetani,* a Gram-positive, spore-forming anaerobic bacillus found in the soil.

2. **Pathogenesis.** Under anaerobic conditions, the bacterium changes to a vegetative form and produces toxins that travel via peripheral nerves to the spinal cord, where the toxin blocks neurotransmitter release from inhibitory interneurons (Renshaw cells).

3. **Diagnosis** is usually based on the clinical findings and the history of a recent wound. Clinical findings result from loss of neural inhibition and may include trismus (lockjaw), pain, a stiff gait, elevated third eyelids, erect ears and tail, contraction of the facial muscles, and tetany. Death can result from respiratory failure.

4. **Treatment**
    a. Antibiotic therapy with penicillin or metronidazole should be instituted, and the wound should be debrided. Equine origin tetanus antitoxin can be administered to neutralize the toxin, but a test dose should always be given first.
    b. Supportive care often includes intravenous fluid therapy, nutritional support, a quiet environment, and medication to decrease the tetany (e.g., acepromazine, chlorpromazine, diazepam, phenobarbital, pentobarbital).

5. **Prognosis**
    a. With mild to moderate disease, the prognosis is usually good, but recovery may take several weeks.
    b. With severe, rapidly progressive disease, the prognosis is guarded because respiratory failure can occur.

P. **Tularemia,** a rare disorder of cats and dogs, is caused by *Francisella tularensis.* Rabbits and wild rodents serve as the reservoir for the infection, and the bacterium is thought to be transmitted by blood-sucking insects or ingestion of infected meat. Infected cats may transmit the infection to humans through a scratch or bite. Both dogs and cats may serve as hosts for the insect vector. Clinical findings may include fever, cough, dyspnea, lymphadenopathy, icterus, and other signs.

Q. **Yersiniosis** (intestinal) is discussed in Chapter 41.

II. FUNGAL DISEASES

A. Aspergillosis

1. **Etiology** and **pathogenesis.** Aspergillosis is most commonly caused by *Aspergilla fumigatis,* but other species can also be pathogenic and may be more likely to cause disseminated disease. The organisms are present in the environment. Infection usually occurs by inhalation and is facilitated by underlying disease, trauma, or defective immune mechanisms. Infection is rare in cats.

2. **Diagnosis**
   a. **Clinical findings**
      (1) **Nasal infection** is seen most commonly in young to middle-aged male dogs. Clinical findings usually include chronic nasal discharge, sneezing, and stertor. The discharge may initially be unilateral, progressing to bilateral.
      (2) **Disseminated aspergillosis.** Anorexia, fever, weight loss, depression, lameness, back pain, or neurologic abnormalities may be seen.
      (3) **Focal aspergillosis** is rare but may cause coughing (in the case of pulmonary infection) or lameness (in the case of osteomyelitis).
   b. **Laboratory findings.** In disseminated disease, a CBC, serum biochemical profile, and urinalysis will often show neutrophilia, azotemia, an increased serum alkaline phosphatase (SAP) concentration, hyperproteinemia, and other abnormalities, depending on the tissues involved. Diagnosis is based on cytology or fungal culture. Serologic testing can support a diagnosis if other test results are appropriate but should not be used alone for diagnosis.
   c. **Radiographic findings**
      (1) **Nasal aspergillosis.** Nasal radiographs often show lysis of the turbinates and an increased soft tissue density in the nasal cavity and possibly in the sinuses. Rhinoscopy may allow visualization of fungal plaques.
      (2) **Disseminated disease.** Thoracic radiographs may show a diffuse interstitial pulmonary pattern, and radiographs of an affected limb may show bony lysis and mild periosteal reaction.

3. **Treatment**
   a. **Nasal infection** best responds to introduction of enilconazole into the nasal cavity and frontal sinuses (via indwelling catheters). Other treatments that have been used alone or in combination include dilute povidone iodine flushes, intranasal clotrimazole, oral ketoconazole, and oral itraconazole.
   b. **Disseminated infection** is very difficult to treat. Itraconazole has produced remission in some patients, but continuous therapy has been required. New imidazole compounds may prove to be more efficacious.

4. **Prognosis** is fair to good with treatment of nasal aspergillosis but poor with disseminated disease.

B. Blastomycosis.
In the United States, blastomycosis is most common in the Mississippi River Valley. Young, large-breed, male dogs are most often affected. Blastomycosis is rare in cats.

1. **Etiology.** Blastomycosis is caused by *Blastomyces dermatitidis,* a saprophytic, dimorphic fungus. The organism is found in the soil, and infection usually occurs via inhalation.

2. **Diagnosis**
   a. **Clinical findings** are quite variable.
      (1) **Pulmonary infection** may result in fever, chronic cough, mucopurulent nasal discharge, exercise intolerance, dyspnea, anorexia, and weight loss.
      (2) **Cutaneous disease** may produce skin lesions, draining tracts, and localized lymphadenopathy.
      (3) **Disseminated disease** may produce generalized lymphadenopathy, lameness, draining tracts, blindness, testicular swelling, and neurologic abnormal-

ities. On physical examination, fever, lymphadenopathy, pulmonary crackles and tachypnea, bone or joint pain, conjunctivitis, uveitis, and retinal lesions may be noted.

b. Laboratory findings

  (1) CBC. A CBC may show a nonregenerative anemia and a leukocytosis characterized by a neutrophilia and monocytosis.

  (2) Serum biochemical profile. Findings may include hyperglobulinemia and mild hypercalcemia.

  (3) Cytology. Identification of the organisms in cytologic samples from the lungs, lymph nodes, draining skin lesion, or a bony lesion is the optimal method of diagnosis.

  (4) Serology, especially agar gel immunodiffusion, can support the diagnosis but should not be used as the primary diagnostic test.

c. Radiographic findings. Thoracic radiographs commonly show a nodular interstitial pulmonary pattern, and radiographs of affected bones may show lysis and periosteal proliferation.

3. Treatment. Amphotericin B, ketoconazole, itraconazole, or a combination of some of these drugs have been effective. Treatment can be expensive and may be associated with complications:

a. Nephrotoxicity can result from amphotericin B, so close monitoring of blood urea nitrogen (BUN) levels is required.

b. Anorexia and vomiting may be caused by ketoconazole.

c. Acute respiratory distress syndrome or a hypersensitivity to the organism in the lungs may also occur with treatment and can result in rapidly progressive dyspnea and pulmonary compromise.

4. Prognosis is fair with all but central nervous system (CNS) disease, for which the prognosis is grave.

5. Zoonotic potential. Blastomycosis is unlikely to be transmitted from a dog or cat to humans unless contamination of an open wound occurs. However, humans can acquire the infection from the environment in the same manner as their pets.

C. **Coccidioidomycosis** is seen primarily in semi-arid areas. Young, large-breed dogs are most commonly infected; cats are resistant.

1. Etiology and **pathogenesis.** Coccidioidomycosis is caused by the saprophytic dimorphic fungus *Coccidiodes immitis.* Arthrospores of the organism are inhaled from the environment. Once inhaled, they produce endospores, which then spread throughout the body.

2. Diagnosis

a. Clinical fndings

  (1) Pulmonary disease. Acute pulmonary disease may result in fever, cough, dyspnea, inappetence, and weight loss.

  (2) Cutaneous disease may produce skin lesions, draining tracts, and regional lymphadenopathy.

  (3) Disseminated disease may result in lameness, bone pain or swelling, peripheral lymphadenopathy, neurologic abnormalities, or other signs.

b. Laboratory findings

  (1) CBC. A CBC may show a mild nonregenerative anemia and a leukocytosis characterized by a neutrophilia.

  (2) Serum biochemical profile. Findings may include hyperglobulinemia and mild hypoalbuminemia.

  (3) Cytology. Identification of the organism in cytologic samples from the lungs, skin lesions, lymph nodes, bony lesions, or other affected tissues is the optimal method of diagnosis.

  (4) Serology can support the diagnosis but may also produce false-negative results.

c. Radiographic findings. Thoracic radiographs may show a mixed or interstitial pulmonary pattern. Radiographs of any bony lesions may show periosteal reaction.

3. **Treatment** and **prognosis.** Ketoconazole or itraconazole is the current treatment of choice. The prognosis is good with treated pulmonary disease but poor with disseminated disease.

4. **Zoonotic potential.** Direct transmission from dogs to humans has not been reported.

D. **Cryptococcosis** is the most common systemic fungal infection in cats. It is uncommon in dogs.

1. **Etiology** and **pathogenesis.** Cryptococcosis is caused by *Cryptococcus neoformans,* an encapsulated, saprophytic, yeast-like fungus. The organisms are found in soil, especially soil containing droppings from pigeons and other birds. Infection occurs via inhalation.

2. **Diagnosis**
   a. **Clinical findings.** Presentations vary from localized cutaneous disease to nasal disease to disseminated disease. Clinical disease usually only occurs in animals with a deficient immune system.
      (1) **Cutaneous disease.** Skin lesions, draining tracts, and regional lymphadenopathy may be seen in infected cats.
      (2) **Nasal disease.** Stertor, chronic nasal discharge, sneezing, and a nasal mass may be present in infected cats.
      (3) **Disseminated disease.** Fever, depression, anorexia, weight loss, neurologic abnormalities, ocular discharge, and uveitis may be seen. Ocular examination may also reveal optic neuritis and retinal lesions. In dogs, CNS and ocular disease are most common and may be manifested as depression, amaurosis (loss of sight without an apparent eye lesion), ataxia, circling, seizures, paresis, and other abnormalities.
   b. **Laboratory findings**
      (1) **CBC.** A CBC may show a leukocytosis characterized by a neutrophilia.
      (2) **Serum biochemical profile.** Findings may be normal or may show a hyperglobulinemia or changes consistent with organ dysfunction (disseminated disease).
      (3) **Cytology.** Identification of the organism in cytologic samples obtained from a cutaneous or nasal swab, cerebrospinal fluid (CSF), or other tissue or fluid sample is the optimal method of diagnosis. The organisms may be in macrophages or extracellular.
         (a) Organisms are best demonstrated with India ink, new methylene blue, or Gram staining.
         (b) In an animal with neurologic signs, **CSF analysis** may show hypercellularity in addition to *Cryptococcus* organisms.
      (4) **Serology** should only be used for diagnosis if appropriate clinical findings and other test results are present and the organism cannot be found directly. The latex agglutination capsular antigen test (LCAT) is more useful for monitoring therapy than for making a diagnosis.
   c. **Radiographic findings.** Nasal radiographs may show lysis of turbinates or a soft tissue density in the nasal cavities and sinuses.

3. **Treatment**
   a. In cats, nasal cryptococcosis has been successfully treated with amphotericin B and flucytosine, ketoconazole and flucytosine, ketoconazole alone, itraconazole, and fluconazole.
   b. In dogs, amphotericin and ketoconazole have been used unsuccessfully to try to treat CNS cryptococcosis.

4. **Prognosis.** In cats with nasal or cutaneous disease who undergo treatment, the prognosis is fair to good. CNS disease in dogs carries a grave prognosis.

E. **Dermatomycosis** affects only the skin in dogs and cats and does not cause systemic disease. It can be transmitted to humans.

F. **Histoplasmosis.** In the United States, the disease is seen primarily in the Mississippi and Ohio River Valleys. Infection is most common in young hounds and sporting-breed dogs.

1. **Etiology** and **pathogenesis.** Histoplasmosis is caused by *Histoplasma capsulatum*, a saprophytic, dimorphic fungus. The organisms are found in the soil, especially that which contains bird or bat droppings. Infection occurs via inhalation or ingestion.

2. **Diagnosis**
   a. **Clinical findings.** Some animals will show only a transient fever and cough and will then clear the infection.
      (1) In dogs, GI disease is most common. Fever, vomiting, diarrhea, weight loss, and anorexia will often be seen. Coughing, dyspnea, tachypnea, and icterus may also be seen with more disseminated disease. Skin lesions, chorioretinitis, lameness, and neurologic abnormalities are rare.
      (2) In cats, fever, dyspnea, cough, weight loss, anorexia, pale mucous membranes, and lymphadenopathy are most common. Other signs may include ocular lesions (conjunctivitis, uveitis, retinal lesions), lameness, and skin lesions.
   b. **Laboratory findings**
      (1) **CBC.** A CBC may show a mild nonregenerative anemia and a leukocytosis characterized by a neutrophilia.
      (2) **Serum biochemical profile.** Findings may include panhypoproteinemia, increased hepatic enzyme concentrations, hyperbilirubinemia, electrolyte abnormalities, and other changes depending on the organs or tissues affected.
      (3) **Cytology.** Identification of the organism in samples from the GI tract, lungs, lymph nodes, liver, bone, bone marrow, or other sites is the optimal method of diagnosis. Organisms will sometimes also be seen on a buffy coat smear.
      (4) **Serology** can support the diagnosis if appropriate clinical signs and other test results are compatible, but serology alone is not reliable.
   c. **Radiographic findings**
      (1) **Survey radiographs.** Thoracic radiographs may show a nodular interstitial pattern and hilar lymphadenopathy. Abdominal radiographs may show hepatomegaly and lymphadenopathy.
      (2) **Contrast radiographs** of the GI tract may show intestinal wall thickening.
   d. **Upper GI endoscopy** or **colonoscopy** may reveal gross mucosal lesions and will allow biopsies to be obtained for histopathology.

3. **Treatment** and **prognosis.** Amphotericin B and ketoconazole, amphotericin B alone, ketoconazole alone, and itraconazole have been used successfully. The prognosis is usually fair to good if the disease is not advanced at the time of diagnosis.

4. **Zoonotic potential.** The disease is not transmitted from pets to humans; however, humans may acquire the infection from the environment in the same manner as the pet.

G. **Phycomycosis** is discussed in Chapter 41 III B 7.

H. **Protothecosis** is discussed in Chapter 41 IV C 5 c.

I. **Sporotrichosis**

1. **Etiology** and **pathogenesis.** Sporotrichosis is caused by *Sporothrix schenckii*. The organisms are found in the soil, and transmission usually occurs via wound contamination. Disseminated disease is rare.

2. **Diagnosis.** Clinical findings most commonly include an ulcerated skin nodule/papule and possible regional lymphadenopathy. Diagnosis is by culture of a biopsy or cytology specimen.

3. **Treatment** and **prognosis.** Ketoconazole, itraconazole, and iodides have successfully been used in the treatment of cutaneous disease. Disseminated disease may require treatment with amphotericin B and ketoconazole or itraconazole. Localized infection carries a good prognosis if treated, but the prognosis with disseminated disease is guarded.

4. **Zoonotic potential.** Humans can contract sporotrichosis from animals if contamination of a wound occurs.

III. PARASITIC DISEASES

A. **Amebiasis** is discussed in Chapter 41 IV C 2 e.

B. **Babesiosis.** In the United States, the disease has not been seen in cats and is rare in dogs.

1. **Etiology.** Babesiosis is caused by *Babesia canis* and *Babesis gibsoni* in dogs and *Babesia felis, Babesia cati,* and other organisms in cats. The organisms are intracellular erythrocytic parasites transmitted by the tick *Rhipicephalus sanguineous.*

2. **Diagnosis**
    a. **Clinical findings.** Three clinical syndromes may be seen.
       (1) **Peracute disease** causes shock and sudden death.
       (2) **Acute disease** causes intravascular hemolysis; icterus, pale mucous membranes, anorexia, lethargy, and vomiting may be seen.
       (3) **Chronic disease** may cause fever, inappetence, and weight loss. Various other signs have been reported.
    b. **Laboratory findings**
       (1) **CBC.** A CBC may show a regenerative anemia, leukocytosis, and thrombocytopenia.
       (2) **Serum biochemical profile** and **urinalysis.** Findings may include hyperbilirubinemia, azotemia, hyperbilirubinuria, and proteinuria.
       (3) **Blood smear.** Definitive diagnosis is made by observation of the organisms in erythrocytes.
       (4) A **Coombs' test** may be positive.
       (5) **Serology** can be used to detect occult infection.

3. **Treatment** and **prognosis.** Treatment is with imidocarb, if available, in addition to supportive care. The prognosis varies with the form and severity of the disease.

C. **Balantidiosis** is discussed in Chapter 41 IV C 2 f.

D. **Coccidiosis** is discussed in Chapter 41 IV B 2 d.

E. **Cytauxzoonosis.** In the United States, cytauxzoonosis is seen primarily in the southeastern and south central areas of the country but is rare. Cytauxzoonosis is caused by the protozoan *Cytauxzoon felis.* The organism is thought to be transmitted by ticks or other arthropods, with wild felines serving as the disease reservoir. Clinical findings include fever, icterus, depression, pale mucous membranes, and dyspnea as a result of hemolytic anemia. Diagnosis is based on observation of the organisms in erythrocytes or tissues. There is no treatment; hence, the prognosis is grave.

F. **Encephalitazoonosis** is a rare disease caused by the microsporidian *Encephalitozoon cuniculi.* Infection occurs via oronasal contact with infected urine. The zoonotic potential remains in question. Clinical findings may include pale mucous membranes, hematuria, pollakiuria or polyuria, neurologic abnormalities, or poor growth in puppies. Cats often show muscle spasms and paralysis. Diagnosis is by observation of spores in the urine or serology, although serology will not be positive for several weeks in the cat. There is no treatment.

G. **Giardiasis** is discussed in Chapter 41 IV B 2 c.

H. **Hepatozoonosis.** In the United States, hepatozoonosis has been found near the coast of Texas.

1. **Etiology** and **pathogenesis.** Hepatozoonosis is caused by *Hepatozoon canis* in the dog. Infection occurs via ingestion of an infected tick (*Rhipicephalus sanguineous*). Released sporozoites penetrate the intestinal wall and spread to other tissues.

2. **Diagnosis**
   a. **Clinical findings** may include fever, anorexia, weight loss, pain, oculonasal discharge, diarrhea, cough, hyperesthesia, and other signs. The signs may wax and wane.
   b. **Laboratory findings**
      (1) **CBC.** A CBC may show mild anemia and marked leukocytosis characterized by neutrophilia, lymphocytosis, and monocytosis.
      (2) **Serum biochemical profile.** Serum biochemistry may show an increase in the SAP concentration and mild hypoglycemia.
      (3) **Urinalysis** may reveal proteinuria.
      (4) **Cytology** or **histopathology** is necessary for definitive diagnosis.
   c. **Radiographic findings.** Periosteal reaction may be seen near the origins and insertions of muscles.

3. **Treatment.** There is no specific treatment. Some animals will clear the infection. Symptomatic treatment, including nonsteroidal anti-inflammatory drugs (NSAIDs), may be useful during clinical episodes.

I. **Leishmaniasis**

1. **Etiology** and **pathogenesis.** Leishmaniasis is primarily caused by the protozoan *Leishmania donovani* in the dog, but other *Leishmania* species can be pathogenic. Transmission occurs via sandfly bite. Dogs and rodents are primary vertebrate hosts. Infection of cats is incidental.

2. **Diagnosis**
   a. **Clinical findings** are variable but may include skin lesions (e.g., ulcers, pustules, nodules, erythema, plaques), lymphadenopathy, lethargy, weight loss, joint pain, petechiae and ecchymoses, muscle pain, and pale mucous membranes.
   b. **Laboratory findings**
      (1) **CBC** and **urinalysis.** Nonspecific findings include anemia, leukocytosis characterized by a neutrophilia with a shift toward immaturity, leukopenia, hyperglobulinemia, azotemia, proteinuria, and hematuria.
      (2) **Cytology.** Definitive diagnosis is by observation of the organisms in samples (e.g., blood, lymphatic tissue, splenic tissue, or bone marrow).
      (3) **Serology** can support the diagnosis in the presence of appropriate clinical signs and test results.

3. **Treatment** and **prevention.** Meglumine antimonate, if available, can be used, although retreatment is often needed. Supportive care should also be instituted. Prevention is aimed at avoidance of sandflies (e.g., confinement in a sandfly-free kennel during the evening and night).

4. **Zoonotic potential.** Transmission from animals to humans is rare but can occur as a result of accidental inoculation with infected blood or tissues. Human infection can also occur via the common vector.

J. **Neosporum infection**

1. **Etiology** and **pathogenesis.** Neosporum infection is caused by the protozoan *Neospora caninum.* Infection is thought to occur as a result of ingestion of tachyzoites and tissue cysts. Transplacental infection can also occur.

2. Diagnosis

a. **Clinical findings** are primarily those of neuromuscular disease and may include LMN paralysis, muscle pain, weakness, muscle atrophy, and other neurologic abnormalities. Rigidity of the rear limbs is common as the disease progresses. Other clinical signs similar to those of toxoplasmosis (see III L 2 a) may also be seen but are less common.

b. **Laboratory findings.** Diagnosis is by demonstration of a fourfold increase in serum titers or by immunochemical staining of a muscle biopsy if muscular signs are present.

3. Treatment and prognosis. There is no treatment. Treatment as discussed for toxoplasmosis (see III L 3) can be tried, but the prognosis is grave.

K. *Pneumocystis* infection is rare but may cause pneumonia in immunosuppressed patients.

L. Toxoplasmosis

1. **Etiology** and **pathogenesis.** Toxoplasmosis is caused by the protozoan *Toxoplasma gondii*. Cats are the definitive hosts. Infection occurs when the cat ingests sporulated oocysts, tachyzoites, or bradyzoites encysted in an intermediate host (e.g., fish, amphibians, reptiles, mammals). The organisms encyst in body tissues, and when the cysts rupture, released bradyzoites cause a hypersensitivity reaction and tissue damage. Cats later shed unsporulated oocysts, which sporulate and become infective 1–3 days later. The enteroepithelial cycle occurs only in cats.

a. Herbivores become infected by ingestion of sporulated oocysts shed by cats.

b. Transplacental infection can also occur.

2. **Diagnosis**

a. **Clinical findings.** Clinical disease is more common in young or immunosuppressed cats. Most infections are asymptomatic.

(1) In cats, clinical signs are quite variable and may include fever, lymphadenopathy, icterus, vomiting, cough, dyspnea and tachypnea, weakness, muscle swelling and pain, neurologic abnormalities, and anterior uveitis. Chorioretinitis may also be detected with an ophthalmologic examination.

(2) In dogs, acute fever, vomiting, diarrhea, icterus, dyspnea, anorexia, lymphadenopathy, and weight loss may be seen with generalized disease. Primary CNS infection (e.g., weakness, tremors, paresis, paralysis, seizures) can also occur.

b. **Laboratory findings**

(1) **CBC.** A CBC may reveal leukopenia.

(2) **Serum biochemical profile.** Findings may include hypoproteinemia, hyperbilirubinemia, increased hepatic enzyme concentrations, and an increased creatine kinase concentration.

(3) **Urinalysis** may reveal hyperbilirubinuria.

(4) **CSF analysis.** In animals with CNS signs, CSF analysis may reveal increased protein concentration and increased lymphocytes.

(5) **Serology.** Definitive diagnosis is usually made by serology. Immunoglobulin M (IgM) titers are more indicative of a recent or active infection than are immunoglobulin G (IgG) titers. Paired titers are needed with IgG. Titers may also be negative with primary CNS infection.

(6) **Biopsy** of affected tissues or organs may yield a diagnosis.

c. **Radiographic findings** may include a mixed interstitial–alveolar pulmonary pattern.

3. **Treatment** and **prognosis.** Clindamycin or a combination of trimethoprim/sulfa, pyrimethamine, and folinic acid should be combined with supportive care. The prognosis is poor with CNS disease but fair to good with other forms of infection.

4. **Zoonotic potential.** In pregnant women, infection during pregnancy can result in harm to the fetus and abortion, stillbirth, or congenital defects. Neonates and immunosuppressed individuals are susceptible to generalized infection. Susceptible individuals should avoid undercooked meat, gardening (i.e., to minimize the potential

of coming into contact with contaminated soil), and cleaning the litter box (i.e., to minimize contact with cat feces).

M. Trichomoniasis is discussed in Chapter 41 IV C 2 d.

N. Trypanosomiasis

1. **Etiology** and **pathogenesis.** Trypanosomiasis is a rare disorder caused by the protozoans *Trypanosoma brucei* (in cats) and *Trypanosoma cruzi* (in dogs). The organism is carried by blood-sucking insects of the family *Reduviidae*. Infection occurs when an infected insect defecates on a wound or exposed mucous membranes. The amastigotes later can cause an inflammatory myocarditis.

2. **Diagnosis**
   a. **Clinical findings**
      (1) Acute signs may include anorexia, lymphadenopathy, hepatomegaly, ascites, tachycardia, weak pulses, and diarrhea.
      (2) Chronic signs are usually those of cardiomyopathy (e.g., lethargy, exercise intolerance, dyspnea and tachypnea). Sudden death can occur.
   b. **Laboratory findings.** The organism may be present in cytology samples (e.g., lymph node aspirates) or a capillary blood sample, but animals can also be positive without clinical signs of the disease.
   c. **Diagnostic imaging findings.** Results of thoracic radiographs, an electrocardiogram(ECG), and cardiac ultrasonography are often consistent with cardiomyopathy with or without heart failure.

3. **Treatment** is not currently available in the United States.

4. **Zoonotic potential.** Human infection can occur via common insect vectors.

IV. RICKETTSIAL DISEASES

A. *Coxiella burnetii* **infection** rarely causes clinical signs in dogs or cats, but is the causative agent of Q fever in humans. Human infection is usually acquired from livestock but can be acquired from contact with periparturient fluids and tissues from an infected cat or dog.

B. Ehrlichiosis

1. **Etiology**
   a. *Ehrlichia canis* is the most common causative organism of ehrlichiosis; it is the focus of this discussion.
   b. *Ehrlichia platys* can cause a cyclic thrombocytopenia.
   c. *Ehrlichia equi* affects neutrophils of immunosuppressed patients.
   d. *Ehrlichia risticii* may cause a transient fever, diarrhea, and lymphadenopathy in cats.

2. **Pathogenesis.** The organisms multiply and infect mononuclear cells and then spread to mononuclear phagocytic cells throughout the body, resulting in cytopenia and vasculitis. Ehrlichiosis is transmitted by *Rhipicephalus sanguineous,* the brown dog tick.

3. **Diagnosis**
   a. **Clinical findings** vary with the stage of the disease and the organs and tissues affected.
      (1) In the acute phase, fever, anorexia, weight loss, epistaxis and other types of hemorrhage, cough, oculonasal discharge, lameness, and neurologic signs may be seen. These signs may resolve without treatment. In some animals, the disease then becomes asymptomatic, although laboratory abnormalities may still be present.

(2) In the chronic stage, pale mucous membranes, ocular lesions (e.g., anterior uveitis, hyphema, retinal hemorrhage), peripheral edema, and neurologic signs may be seen.

b. Laboratory findings

(1) **CBC.** A CBC usually shows a thrombocytopenia during the acute stage and a bicytopenia [a decrease in two cell lines (e.g., decreased leukocyte and platelet levels)] or pancytopenia during the chronic stage.

(2) **Serum biochemical profile** and **urinalysis** may reveal hyperglobulinemia (monoclonal or polyclonal gammopathy), hypoalbuminemia, increased hepatic enzyme concentrations, and proteinuria.

(3) **CSF analysis** may reveal increased lymphocyte numbers when neurologic signs are present.

(4) **Arthrocentesis** may confirm a polyarthritis.

(5) **Serology** or **cytology** are necessary for definitive diagnosis.

4. Treatment

a. Treatment with tetracycline, doxycycline, or chloramphenicol will readily resolve acute or subclinical infections.

b. Severe chronic infections require prolonged antibiotic treatment and may also require transfusions (for severe anemia) or concurrent glucocorticoid therapy (for secondary immune-mediated cell destruction).

5. Prognosis. Acute or subclinical infection carries a good prognosis if treated. Chronic infection carries a guarded to fair prognosis.

6. Prevention is primarily aimed at tick control. Prophylactic antibiotic therapy may be used during tick season in endemic areas.

C. **Hemobartonellosis** is discussed in Chapter 48 II A 2 b (3) (a) .

D. *Rochalimaea henselae* infection rarely causes clinical disease in cats but can cause "cat scratch disease" in humans. It may also cause bacillary angiomatosis and pleosis hepatitis in immunocompromised people.

E. **Rocky Mountain spotted fever**

1. Etiology and **pathogenesis.** *Rickettsia rickettsii* is the causative organism. Rabbits and rodents are the main reservoirs for the disease, and the infection is primarily transmitted through the bite of an infected tick.

a. *Dermacentor variabilis* is the vector in the midwestern United States and on the eastern coast.

b. *Dermacentor andersoni* is the vector in the western United States.

2. Diagnosis

a. Clinical findings. Infection causes a vasculitis and variable clinical signs. In the United States, the disease is seen predominately in the spring and summer.

(1) Common signs include fever, anorexia, vomiting, diarrhea, depression, lymphadenopathy, lethargy, and petechiae and ecchymoses. Other signs may include cough, dyspnea, peripheral edema, oculonasal discharge, joint pain, muscle pain, neurologic signs (e.g., ataxia, hyperesthesia, seizures), anterior uveitis, and decreased vision.

(2) On physical examination, petechiae, peripheral edema, arrhythmias, retinal hemorrhage or edema, joint swelling, splenomegaly, and neurologic abnormalities may be found.

b. Laboratory findings

(1) **CBC.** A CBC often shows a thrombocytopenia and a leukopenia (early) or a leukocytosis (later) characterized by a shift toward immaturity and a monocytosis.

(2) **Serum biochemical profile.** The serum biochemical profile may show increased hepatic enzyme concentrations, azotemia, hypoalbuminemia, hyperglobulinemia, and electrolyte abnormalities.

(3) CSF analysis. Increased neutrophils may be present, or there may be no abnormal findings.

(4) Serology. Diagnosis is based on serologic testing (with acute or acute and convalescent serum samples, depending on the test utilized) or immunofluorescent staining of a biopsy specimen.

3. **Treatment** and **prognosis.** Treatment is with tetracycline, doxycycline, or chloramphenicol in addition to supportive care. The prognosis is good with prompt treatment, with most animals showing notable improvement in 2–3 days.

4. **Prevention** is aimed at tick control.

F. **Salmon poisoning (rickettsial enteritis)** is discussed in Chapter 41 IV B 5.

V. VIRAL DISEASES

A. **Coronaviral enteritis.** Canine coronaviral enteritis and feline coronaviral enteritis are discussed in Chapter 41 IV B 3 b and f.

B. **Distemper**

1. **Etiology** and **pathogenesis.** The canine distemper virus (CDV) is a morbillivirus. Infection can occur when droplets of infected secretions are inhaled. Dogs are most susceptible at 3--6 months of age because maternal antibodies wane during that time. Spread of the infection in the body initially occurs via tissue macrophages and later via circulating virus. The extent of clinical disease is partially dependent on the animal's immune status.

2. **Diagnosis.** A presumptive diagnosis of acute or subacute disease is often made based on the history and clinical findings.
   a. **Clinical findings**
      (1) Non-neurologic signs. Anorexia, nasal discharge, ocular discharge, fever, cough, vomiting, diarrhea, and a skin rash may be noted. Chorioretinitis may be found with acute disease; retinal hyperreflectivity may be found with chronic disease.
      (2) Neurologic signs are quite variable, depending on the severity and chronicity of the infection. Some dogs show no neurologic signs.
         (a) Acute disease. "Chewing gum" or other seizures, circling, myoclonus, and blindness may be seen.
         (b) Subacute disease. Myoclonus or other neurologic abnormalities occur weeks to months after the non-neurologic signs.
         (c) Chronic disease
            (i) A multifocal encephalitis can occur with chronic infection of young dogs. Progressive rear limb ataxia and weakness, head tremors, head tilt, and cranial nerve deficits may be seen.
            (ii) "Old dog encephalitis" can occur with chronic infection in older dogs. Depression, behavior changes, circling and decreased vision may be seen.
   b. **Laboratory findings**
      (1) CBC. Findings may include lymphopenia.
      (2) CSF analysis may reveal increased protein and cell numbers when neurologic signs are present. Antidistemper antibody in CSF can confirm CDV infection (either acute or chronic).
      (3) Serology. Fluorescent antibody testing of conjunctival or respiratory epithelial smears or a buffy coat smear may confirm the diagnosis. A negative test result, however, does not rule out distemper.

3. **Treatment.** There is no definitive treatment. Supportive care and control of secondary bacterial infections should be instituted.

4. **Prognosis.** Mild disease carries a fair prognosis, although neurologic signs may develop at a later time. In the case of acute disease with progressive neurologic signs, the prognosis is grave. Anticonvulsant medications and glucocorticoid therapy may help control neurologic signs or slow the progression of the signs in those dogs with milder or nonprogressive signs.

5. **Prevention.** Efficacious vaccines are available and are usually administered at 4-week intervals beginning when the puppy is 6–8 weeks of age. Because the virus that causes human measles is antigenically related to CDV, the human measles vaccine can be used for puppies younger than 6 weeks.

C. **Feline immunodeficiency virus (FIV) infection**

1. **Etiology** and **pathogenesis**
   a. Feline immunodeficiency virus (FIV) infection is caused by a lentivirus. Infection usually occurs as a result of a bite wound from an infected cat; therefore, outdoor male cats are at greatest risk. Placental and colostral transmission may also occur but is rare.
   b. The virus ultimately causes a decrease in number and activity of T lymphocytes, especially T helper cells, and also infects macrophages. Once infected, the cat will not clear the virus. FIV infection may slightly increase the risk of neoplasia.

2. **Diagnosis**
   a. **Clinical findings** are highly variable but are primarily related to secondary infections as a result of the immunosuppression. Fever, weight loss, lymphadenopathy, diarrhea, chronic oculonasal discharge or cough, gingivitis, oral ulceration, pale mucous membranes, neurologic disease, and many other signs may be seen. An infected cat may be asymptomatic for months to years or may first show a transient fever, lymphadenopathy, or diarrhea before a long asymptomatic period.
   b. **Laboratory findings**
      (1) **CBC.** A CBC may show a nonregenerative anemia, a neutropenia, or a leukocytosis.
      (2) **Serum biochemical profile, urinalysis,** and **radiographic findings** vary according to the type of secondary disease present.
      (3) **Serology.** Definitive diagnosis is based on the detection of antibodies to FIV using ELISA.

3. **Treatment.** There is no specific treatment. Supportive care and appropriate treatment of any secondary disorders should be instituted.

4. **Prognosis.** The long-term prognosis is grave because most infected cats ultimately die of a secondary or opportunistic infection. However, infected cats may also remain asymptomatic for months to years, and treatment of secondary disorders may prolong life once signs do occur.

5. **Prevention.** There is no vaccine; therefore, the only prevention available is avoidance of exposure to infected cats.

D. **Feline infectious peritonitis (FIP)**

1. **Etiology** and **pathogenesis.** FIP is caused by a coronavirus that is antigenically very similar to the coronavirus that causes feline coronaviral enteritis.
   a. Infection occurs via the oronasal route with subsequent viral replication in epithelial cells. The virus then circulates in mononuclear cells and triggers a type III hypersensitivity reaction. Immune complex deposition and pyogranuloma formation near small vessels are responsible for clinical disease.
   b. Most cats are fairly resistant to the development of clinical disease. Cats younger than 2–3 years and older cats are most susceptible.

2. **Diagnosis**
   a. **Clinical findings** are quite variable and may include fever, anorexia, depression, weight loss, vomiting, diarrhea, icterus, seizures or other neurologic signs, abor-

tion, uveitis, granulomatous retinal lesions, and other signs. In the "wet" form of the disease, abdominal distention (caused by ascites) and tachypnea and dyspnea (caused by pleural effusion or pericardial effusion) may also be seen.

b. **Laboratory findings**

    (1) **CBC.** Findings may include a mild nonregenerative anemia and a leukopenia or a leukocytosis with a shift toward immaturity.

    (2) **Serum biochemical profile.** Findings often include hyperglobulinemia. Azotemia or increased hepatic enzyme concentrations may be seen if the kidneys or liver, respectively, are affected. Protein electrophoresis results are consistent with a polyclonal gammopathy.

    (3) **Fluid analysis** ("wet" form of the disease). Fluid obtained from one of the body cavities is usually yellow and viscous and has a high protein concentration and a low to moderate number of nucleated cells.

    (4) **CSF analysis.** Analysis of CSF samples taken from an infected cat showing neurologic signs often reveals an increase in protein concentration and an increase in neutrophils, lymphocytes, and macrophages.

    (5) **Biopsy** is the only antemortem way to confirm the diagnosis of FIP.

    (6) **Serology** alone will not establish the diagnosis because of the cross reactivity of feline enteric coronavirus with serologic tests for FIP. A very high titer or a fourfold increase in the antibody titer in the face of appropriate clinical signs supports a diagnosis of FIP but does not confirm it. Also, some cats that are very ill with FIP may have negative titers.

c. **Diagnostic imaging findings.** Radiographs may confirm the presence of peritoneal, pleural, or pericardial fluid. Ultrasonography is useful for confirming pericardial effusion and for ruling out other causes of fluid accumulation.

3. **Treatment.** There is no specific therapy. Prednisone, cyclophosphamide, or both may slow the progression of the disease if treatment is initiated when only mild clinical signs are present.

4. **Prognosis.** The disease is usually fatal.

5. **Prevention.** A vaccine has recently become available, but the efficacy is less than 100%.

E. | **Feline leukemia virus (FeLV) infection**

1. **Etiology.** FeLV infection is caused by an oncovirus. Three subgroups of FeLV have been found: A, B, and C. Subgroup A is most common. Subgroups B and C occur as a coinfection with subgroup A.

2. **Pathogenesis.** Infection occurs through contact with secretions, especially saliva, from an infected cat.

a. The gp70 envelope protein allows the virus to bind to feline cells. The virus replicates in the oropharyngeal lymphatic tissue and then infects lymphocytes and macrophages, which enter the circulation. The virus replicates in systemic lymphatic tissues and the bone marrow, and infected neutrophils enter the circulation. Finally, epithelial and glandular tissues are infected. This entire process usually takes 2–4 weeks.

b. Only some cats that are exposed to the virus become persistently infected and develop clinical signs related to FeLV infection within 2–3 years. The majority of cats exposed to the virus will clear the infection before the virus-infected cells are released from the bone marrow.

3. **Diagnosis**

a. **Clinical findings** are highly variable. Pale mucous membranes, weakness, depression, anorexia, vomiting, weight loss, icterus, fever, lymphadenopathy, oral ulceration, neurologic signs, or signs of secondary infection or neoplasia (especially lymphosarcoma, leukemia, and myelodysplasia) may be seen. The p15e envelope protein is responsible for the immunosuppression and anemia found in many infected cats.

b. **Laboratory findings**

(1) **CBC.** Findings may include a nonregenerative anemia, macrocytosis, leuko-penia, thrombocytopenia, or leukemia.

(2) **Serum biochemical profile** and **urinalysis.** Findings vary depending on the organ systems affected.

(3) **Serology** is the basis for definitive diagnosis. The p27 core antigen is the antigen detected by the two most commonly used diagnostic tests [i.e., ELISA and immunofluorescent antibody].

    (a) ELISA

        (i) An ELISA test performed on a blood sample will detect viral antigen in the circulation. If the result is positive, especially in a clinically normal cat or one with minimal clinical signs of disease, an immunofluorescent antibody test should be performed or the cat should be isolated from other cats and another ELISA test performed in 1–2 months. If test results are still positive at that time, it is unlikely the cat will clear the infection.

        (ii) The ELISA test can also be performed on tears and saliva. A positive ELISA from one of these secretions means that the virus reached the epithelial and glandular tissues and the cat is unlikely to clear the virus. This test is usually reserved for cattery situations because there is a higher incidence of false–positive and false–negative results as compared to ELISA tests on blood.

    (b) Immunofluorescent antibody. The immunofluorescent antibody test detects viral antigen within circulating cells. If it is positive, the cat is unlikely to clear the virus. Because leukopenia may cause a false–negative test result, a bone marrow aspirate may be a better specimen for the immunofluorescent antibody test in a leukopenic cat.

(4) **Virus isolation** and **feline oncornavirus-associated cell membrane antigen (FOCMA) testing** are usually only performed on a research basis. FOCMA is not a portion of the virus; rather, it is an antigen that may be found in infected cat cells.

   c. Radiographic findings may include lymphadenopathy, a mass, ascites, pleural effusion, or organomegaly if a secondary infection or lymphosarcoma (see Chapter 48 V B) is present.

4. Treatment. There is no specific treatment. Any secondary infection or neoplasia should be treated appropriately.

5. Prognosis. The long-term prognosis is grave for persistently infected cats. Most die of an FeLV-related disorder within 3 years of diagnosis.

6. Prevention. Several FeLV vaccines are available. Although none provides 100% protection from infection, they may decrease the chance of infection in high-risk (i.e., outdoor or indoor-outdoor) cats. Preventing contact with infected cats is optimal.

F. | **Infectious hepatitis** is rare in dogs and cats.

1. Etiology and **pathogenesis.** Canine infectious hepatitis is caused by canine adenovirus type 1. Infection occurs via the oronasal route. The virus replicates regionally and then causes viremia and dysfunction of parenchymal and reticuloendothelial cells.

2. Diagnosis

   a. Clinical findings. Most animals have few or no clinical signs. With severe disease, anorexia, fever, lymphadenopathy, vomiting, diarrhea, ascites, and petechiae and ecchymoses may be seen. Corneal edema may be seen during recovery as a result of the immune response.

   b. Laboratory findings

      (1) **CBC.** Early in the infection, neutropenia and a possible thrombocytopenia may be seen.

      (2) **Serum biochemical profile.** Serum alanine aminotransferase (SALT) concentrations are increased with clinical disease.

      (3) **Serology.** A fourfold increase in the serum titer confirms the diagnosis.

3. **Treatment** and **prognosis.** Treatment is supportive only. The prognosis is good with mild or subclinical infection but poor with severe disease.

4. **Prevention.** A vaccine is available based on cross-reactivity of canine adenovirus 1 and canine adenovirus 2.

G. **Herpesvirus infection**

1. **Etiology.** Herpesvirus infections usually result from oronasal contact with secretions from an infected animal. Venereal and transplacental infection can also occur.

2. **Diagnosis.** A presumptive diagnosis is often made based on the history and clinical signs.
   a. **Clinical findings**
      (1) Infected newborns may show weakness, diarrhea, nasal discharge, petechiation, or acute death. Cerebellar signs may also be seen at birth.
      (2) Infected adult cats may have fever and nasal and ocular discharge. Infertility can also occur.
      (3) Infected adult dogs may be infertile or may experience abortion, vaginitis, or balanoposthitis. Herpesvirus also plays a role in kennel cough.
   b. **Laboratory findings.** Definitive diagnosis in adult animals is based on virus isolation, observation of intranuclear inclusion bodies on an epithelial swab or scraping, or a positive serological titer, but a negative result does not rule out the diagnosis.

3. **Treatment** is symptomatic only.
   a. Antibiotic therapy (e.g., with ampicillin or trimethoprim/sulfa) may be used to treat secondary bacterial infection if the disease is chronic.
   b. Humidification and decongestants may also help lessen the clinical signs in cats with chronic upper respiratory infection.

4. **Prognosis.** For neonates, the prognosis is grave. For adult animals, the disease will rarely cause death but the infection may persist and cause chronic or chronic intermittent clinical signs.

5. **Prevention.** A feline vaccine is available but is not 100% efficacious.

H. **Panleukopenia** is discussed in Chapter 41 IV B 3 e.

I. **Parvovirus infection** is discussed in Chapter 41 IV B 3 a.

J. **Pseudorabies** is caused by a swine herpesvirus that can also affect other mammals. Infection occurs through ingestion of infected material. Clinical findings include behavioral changes followed by intense pruritus of the head and rapidly progressive neurologic signs (usually seizures). There is no treatment, and death commonly occurs within 48 hours of the onset of signs. Diagnosis is made at postmortem through histology of the brain or virus isolation.

K. **Rabies**

1. **Etiology.** Rabies is caused by a rhabdovirus. Bats, skunks, raccoons, and other wild animals serve as the reservoir for the disease. All warm-blooded animals are susceptible.

2. **Pathogenesis.** Infection occurs when saliva from an infected animal enters a wound (often a bite wound) or contacts conjunctival or nasal mucosa. The virus travels to the CNS along nerve fibers.

3. **Diagnosis.** Rabies should always be suspected if an animal from an endemic area has rapidly progressive neurologic signs. Definitive diagnosis requires postmortem evaluation of brain tissue.
   a. **Clinical findings**
      (1) An initial **prodromal phase,** characterized by a behavioral change, may be seen.

    (2) Next, an **excitative phase** may be seen. The excitative stage may be characterized by drooling, dysphagia, marked behavioral changes (e.g., the animal may appear "furious" or "dumb"), ataxia, seizures, and various other neurologic abnormalities.

    (3) The final phase, the **paralytic phase,** is characterized by rapidly progressive paresis and paralysis; death results from respiratory arrest. The time from the onset of clinical signs until the time of death is less than 10 days.

  b. Laboratory studies. Fluorescent antibody testing of a mucosal smear or a biopsy of a sensory vibrissae may yield a positive result, but a negative result does not rule out rabies. Other test results are nonspecific (e.g., CSF analysis will show only an increase in mononuclear cells and protein concentration).

4. Treatment and **prognosis.** There is no treatment, and the prognosis is grave.

5. Prevention. An efficacious vaccine is available, although it does not always prevent infection. Avoiding contact with wild animals is recommended.

6. Zoonotic potential

  a. Rabies can be transmitted from an infected dog or cat to humans; therefore, gloves and masks should be worn when working with an animal suspected of having rabies. High-risk individuals (e.g., veterinarians, laboratory workers) should receive pre-exposure immunizations. A bite from the infected animal poses the greatest risk.

  b. When a human is bitten by a suspect animal:

    (1) If the animal is showing neurologic signs, the animal should be euthanized and the brain tissue tested.

    (2) If the animal has an owner, the animal should be isolated and observed for 10 days. If the animal does not have an owner, the animal should be euthanized and the brain tissue tested.

    (3) The case should be reported to the appropriate public health authorities so that postexposure immunization of any exposed humans can be initiated.

L. **Feline upper respiratory tract infection** is discussed in Chapter 40 I C 1.

DIRECTIONS: Each of the numbered items or incomplete statements in this section is followed by answers or by completions of the statement. Select the ONE numbered answer or completion that is BEST in each case.

1. Active blastomycosis and histoplasmosis infections are most accurately diagnosed by:

(1) thoracic radiographs.
(2) intradermal skin testing.
(3) serology.
(4) cytology.

2. Monoclonal gammopathy on a serum protein electrophoresis may be seen with:

(1) feline infectious peritonitis (FIP).
(2) ehrlichiosis.
(3) chronic antigenic stimulation.
(4) blastomycosis.

3. An enzyme-linked immunosorbent assay (ELISA) test for feline leukemia virus (FeLV) is performed on a blood sample from a cat who has been adopted from an animal shelter, and the cat tests positive. What conclusions can the veterinarian draw from this test result?

(1) The cat has been exposed to the virus and may be currently infected.
(2) The cat has been exposed to the virus but probably is not currently infected.
(3) The cat should be euthanized, because it will inevitably die from FeLV-related disease.
(4) The cat has lymphosarcoma.

4. A cat tests positive for feline immunodeficiency virus (FIV) on an enzyme-linked immunosorbent assay (ELISA) test. What conclusions can be drawn from this test result?

(1) The cat has been exposed to the virus and is currently infected.
(2) The cat has been exposed to the virus but probably is not currently infected.
(3) The cat is protected from FIV-related disease because it has been exposed previously.
(4) The cat has FIV-related disease.

5. Which antibiotics are the treatment of choice for actinomycosis and nocardiosis, respectively?

(1) Sulfonamide, cephalosporin
(2) Enrofloxacin, clindamycin
(3) Penicillin, sulfonamide
(4) Gentamicin, cephalosporin
(5) Enrofloxacin, amoxicillin-clavulanic acid

6. A Gram stain of a nasal swab from a cat with chronic mucopurulent nasal discharge shows the presence of multiple yeast-like organisms. The most likely diagnosis is:

(1) aspergillosis.
(2) cryptococcosis.
(3) chronic bacterial rhinitis secondary to a foreign body.
(4) coccidioidomycosis.
(5) chronic herpesvirus infection.

7. A 6-year-old spayed female golden retriever is presented with rapidly progressive weakness. On physical examination, you find mydriasis and hyporeflexia of all 4 limbs. Mentation and pain sensation are normal. The most likely diagnosis is:

(1) tetanus.
(2) botulism.
(3) cryptococcosis.
(4) rabies.

8. A 3-year-old neutered male Irish setter is presented with a 6-week history of mucopurulent nasal discharge and sneezing. Other than the nasal discharge, the physical examination is normal. Nasal radiographs show an increased soft tissue density in the nasal cavity and some turbinate lysis. On rhinoscopy, multiple yellowish plaques are seen. The most likely diagnosis is:

(1) cryptococcosis.
(2) blastomycosis.
(3) coccidiomycosis.
(4) aspergillosis.

DIRECTIONS: Each of the numbered items or incomplete statements in this section is negatively phrased, as indicated by a capitalized word such as NOT, LEAST, or EXCEPT. Select the ONE numbered answer or completion that is BEST in each case.

9. Which one of the following diseases is NOT a zoonotic disease?

(1) Brucellosis
(2) Leptospirosis
(3) Toxoplasmosis
(4) Salmonellosis
(5) Ehrlichiosis

1. The answer is 4 [II B 2 b (3), F 2 b (3)]. A diagnosis of blastomycosis or histoplasmosis should be based on observation of the organism in a cytologic sample (e.g., lymph node aspirate, bronchial washing, or an impression smear from a skin lesion). Thoracic radiographs may show a miliary nodular pattern suggestive of mycotic infection, but such changes are not pathognomonic. Serologic titers can also support the diagnosis but may be elevated because of a previous infection.

2. The answer is 2 [IV B 3 b (2)]. Hyperglobulinemia is relatively common with ehrlichiosis; the gammopathy may be monoclonal or polyclonal. In contrast, feline infectious peritonitis (FIP) virus infection and chronic antigenic stimulation both cause only a polyclonal gammopathy.

3. The answer is 1 [V D 3 b (3) (a)]. A single positive enzyme-linked immunosorbent assay (ELISA) test for feline leukemia virus (FeLV) indicates viral exposure and possible infection, but it is possible the cat may still clear the virus. An immunofluorescent antibody test should be performed or the cat should be isolated and another ELISA test should be performed 1–2 months later. If the immunofluorescent antibody test or a second ELISA test is positive, then the infection will probably persist and FeLV-related disease will develop in the future. The ELISA test and the immunofluorescent antibody test indicate nothing about the presence or absence of lymphosarcoma.

4. The answer is 1 [V C]. A positive result on an enzyme-linked immunosorbent assay (ELISA) test for feline immunodeficiency virus (FIV) indicates that the cat has acquired the virus and developed FIV antibodies. These antibodies do not clear the virus, however, and the cat will remain persistently infected. The antibodies also do not protect against FIV-related diseases, and a secondary infection or other secondary disease months to years later will usually cause the cat's death.

5. The answer is 3 [I B 3, J 3]. Penicillins are the antibiotic of choice for the treatment of actinomycosis, and sulfonamides are most effective in the treatment of nocardiosis.

6. The answer is 2 [II D 2 b (3)]. Cryptococcal infection typically causes signs of nasal disease in cats, and the causative organisms are encapsulated yeast-like organisms. Aspergillosis is rare in cats, and the organisms are not encapsulated. Cats are resistant to coccidioidomycosis. Both chronic bacterial rhinitis and chronic viral rhinitis can cause chronic nasal discharge, but yeast-like organisms should not be seen on cytology.

7. The answer is 2 [I D, I O, II D, V K]. Mydriasis and lower motor neuron (LMN) weakness are typical signs of botulism because the bacterial toxin blocks acetylcholine release. In contrast, with tetanus, neurotransmitter release from inhibitory neurons is blocked, so the loss of inhibition results in a stiff gait, trismus, erect ears and tail, and tetany. Cryptococcosis can cause neurologic disease in the dog, but central nervous system (CNS) signs such as depression, ataxia, circling, seizures, or paresis with hyperflexia are more common. With rabies, the neurologic signs are also central in origin and would not include hyporeflexia and normal mentation.

8. The answer is 4 [II A, II B, II C, II D]. Aspergillosis is the most likely diagnosis based on the signs of mucopurulent nasal discharge and sneezing, the radiographic findings of both an increased soft tissue density and turbinate lysis in the nasal cavity, and the visualization of multiple plaques with rhinoscopy; a biopsy or culture would be needed to confirm the diagnosis. Cryptococcosis is the most common fungal infection because of the nasal cavity in cats, but in dogs, central nervous system (CNS) and ocular disease are far more common. Blastomycosis and coccidiomycosis do not commonly cause nasal disease, especially in the absence of any systemic signs of illness.

9. The answer is 5 [I E 6, G 6, L 5; III L 4; IV B]. Ehrlichiosis is not transmitted from dogs or cats to humans, but brucellosis, leptospirosis, toxoplasmosis, and salmonellosis may be. Care should be taken to avoid contact with infected body fluids and secretions when handling infected animals, and appropriate disinfection measures should be carried out.

Chapter 50

Oncologic Diseases

I. GENERAL PRINCIPLES

A. **Etiology.** The cause of most tumors is not known. Genetic factors, infectious agents, exposure to carcinogens or radiation, trauma, and implants of foreign materials (e.g., orthopedic implants) may all play a role in certain types of neoplasia.

B. **Pathogenesis.** Tumors can adversely affect the host in a variety of ways:

1. **Primary tumors** can alter tissue or organ function or create a mass effect.

2. **Metastatic lesions** occur when malignant cells spread via the circulation or the lymphatic system.

3. **Paraneoplastic syndromes** are effects of the tumor that occur away from the primary tumor or metastatic lesions.

   a. **Anemia** is common in animals with cancer and may result from chronic disease, blood loss, secondary immune-mediated disease, malnutrition, microangiopathic disease, myelophthisis, chemotherapy, or other mechanisms.

   (1) **Anemia of chronic disease (ACD)** is most common. Resolution requires treatment of the neoplasia.

   (2) **Blood loss anemia** may occur with gastrointestinal (GI) neoplasia, mast cell tumors (and secondary GI ulceration), secondary coagulopathies, and other mechanisms. Treatment requires resolution of the hemorrhage and supplementation with ferrous sulfate.

   (3) **Microangiopathic hemolytic anemia** occurs most commonly with disseminated intravascular hemolysis (DIC) and with hemangiosarcoma. Treatment requires supportive care (e.g., intravenous fluids), possibly heparin therapy for DIC, and treatment of the neoplasia.

   (4) **Immune-mediated hemolytic anemia (IHA)** can occur secondary to various neoplasms. Treatment includes supportive care, prednisone and other immunosuppressive medications, and treatment of the neoplasia.

   (5) **Anemia caused by chemotherapeutic suppression of the bone marrow** is rare. Myelosuppression is usually seen much sooner, leading to the limitation of chemotherapy before the erythrocytes are significantly affected.

   b. **Cancer cachexia** is weight loss that occurs despite adequate nutritional intake in a patient with a malignant neoplasm. Relative insulin resistance, hyperlactasemia, and abnormal protein and fat metabolism all contribute to this syndrome. Nutritional support and removal or minimization of the neoplasia are needed to control the weight loss.

   c. **Erythrocytosis** is uncommon but can result from increased erythropoietin production by a tumor, tumor production of a factor that stimulates erythropoietin production or release, or physiologic erythropoietin production in response to tumor-induced hypoxia. Clinical signs, differential diagnoses, and treatment are discussed in Chapter 48 II B. Definitive treatment of the neoplasm will resolve the erythrocytosis.

   d. **Fever** often results from secondary infection but can also be induced by the tumor itself. Treatment requires therapy for the primary neoplasm. Nonsteroidal anti-inflammatory drugs (NSAIDs) or antipyretic drugs may be used for symptomatic relief.

    e. Hypercalcemia (see also Chapter 43 Part II:III C). Malignancy is the most common cause of hypercalcemia in dogs and cats and is caused by local osteolysis (such as occurs with multiple myeloma, lymphosarcoma, and mammary adenocarcinoma) and systemic release of a parathyroid hormone (PTH)-related protein (such as occurs with anal sac adenocarcinoma or lymphosarcoma). Definitive treatment of the neoplasia will resolve the hypercalcemia.

    f. Hyperglobulinemia is most common with multiple myeloma but may also be seen with lymphosarcoma, some leukemias, and primary macroglobulinemia. Clinical signs are those of hyperviscosity and include hemorrhage, decreased vision, and neurologic abnormalities. Renal failure, congestive heart failure, and retinal detachment may also occur. Treatment is aimed at the primary neoplasm. Plasmapheresis may also be useful but is not always available.

    g. Hypertrophic osteopathy occurs most commonly with metastatic pulmonary lesions; the cause is unknown. Clinical findings include lameness, pain, and swelling of the long bones. Radiographically, periosteal proliferation is seen along the bone shafts, beginning with the distal bones (i.e., the digits) and progressing proximally. Treatment includes resolution or removal of the pulmonary tumors in addition to symptomatic treatment with glucocorticoids.

    h. Hypocalcemia is uncommon but may occur with hypomagnesemia caused by cisplatin treatment and with tumor lysis syndrome.

    i. Hypoglycemia is most common with an insulinoma (see Chapter 44 IV B), but it may also be seen with other tumors (e.g., hepatoma, hepatocellular adenocarcinoma, lymphosarcoma, hemangiosarcoma) as a result of increased tumor utilization of glucose, tumor production of an insulin-like substance, or tumor-induced alterations in glucose metabolism. Definitive treatment of the neoplasia will resolve the hypoglycemia.

    j. Neurologic dysfunction is uncommon as a paraneoplastic syndrome, but peripheral neuropathies have been seen in association with some tumors, and myasthenia gravis can occur in association with thymoma. Treatment is aimed at the primary tumor.

    k. Thrombocytopenia can occur as a result of decreased platelet production, platelet sequestration, increased platelet consumption (if DIC is present) or increased platelet destruction (i.e., immune-mediated thrombocytopenia). Regardless of the underlying mechanism, treatment of the underlying neoplasm is needed for resolution of the thrombocytopenia. Supportive care and heparin therapy (if DIC is present) may be helpful. Prednisone or other immunosuppressive treatment may be useful with immune-mediated platelet destruction.

C. **Diagnosis**

    1. History and **physical examination**
      a. Signalment. Breed, age, sex, and coloration will predispose certain dogs and cats to development of some types of tumors. Specific risk factors are discussed in the sections on individual neoplasms.
      b. Clinical findings vary widely, depending on the site of the primary tumor and the presence of metastatic disease or paraneoplastic syndromes.

    2. Diagnostic tests
      a. Cytology. Cytologic evaluation of a fine-needle aspirate should be performed before other more invasive or costly tests. This approach is effective for skin and subcutaneous masses as well as masses in many internal organs or tissues (e.g., lymph nodes, liver, spleen, kidneys, prostate, thyroid, lung, mediastinum, intra-abdominal masses).
        (1) Cytology may show changes consistent with inflammation, hyperplasia, and malignancy, or it may be normal.
          (a) Criteria of malignancy may include a decrease in the nuclear:cytoplasmic ratio, the presence of multiple nucleoli, pleomorphism, multiple nuclei, and other changes.
          (b) Special caution must be used in evaluation of samples from the respira-

tory tract, bladder, and prostate because hyperplasia and dysplasia can look similar to neoplasia.

    (2) Cytology may also allow differentiation of carcinomas, sarcomas, and round cell tumors.

        (a) Carcinomas arise from epithelial tissues. Cytology often shows the presence of clumps of round or polygonal cells. The cytoplasm is often dark blue, and vacuolization is common. Large nuclei and nucleoli may be seen.

        (b) Sarcomas arise from mesenchymal tissues. Cytology often shows the presence of spindle-shaped to oval cells, which often form "tails" and have nuclei that distend the central part of the cell. The cytoplasm is usually reddish-blue, and the nuclei may be irregular. Few cells are seen on cytology samples because these tumors do not exfoliate well.

        (c) Round cell tumors. Cytology often shows individual round cells. Other cytologic characteristics are discussed in the sections on the individual neoplasms (e.g., lymphosarcoma, histiocytomas, mast cell tumors, melanomas, and transmissible venereal tumors).

  b. Biopsy. Histologic evaluation is recommended if cytology is not diagnostic. Depending on the location and size of the mass, a needle biopsy, incisional biopsy, or excisional biopsy may be obtained.

  c. Diagnostic imaging techniques. Malignant masses require further evaluation to determine the extent of the primary disease and the presence or absence of metastasis, paraneoplastic disease, or concurrent but unrelated disease.

    (1) Thoracic radiographs (ventrodorsal and right and left lateral views) should be obtained to look for evidence of pulmonary metastasis. Even if no radiographic abnormalities are seen, micrometastasis may be present. With some types of neoplasia, intrathoracic lymphadenopathy or metastatic bone lesions may also be seen.

    (2) Abdominal radiographs and **abdominal ultrasonograms** should be considered for an animal with a mass that may spread to the abdominal cavity or for an animal with clinical signs or laboratory test results that suggest abdominal organ dysfunction. Lymphadenopathy, organomegaly, irregular contour of an abdominal organ, or potential metastatic lesions (especially in the liver) may be visible.

  d. Laboratory studies

    (1) Complete blood count (CBC). A CBC may show anemia, leukocytosis, leukopenia, or hyperproteinemia.

    (2) Serum biochemical profile and **urinalysis.** These studies may reveal hypercalcemia, hypoglycemia, or hyperglobulinemia as a paraneoplastic syndrome. Other abnormalities vary with the organ systems affected by the neoplasia or concurrent disease.

3. Staging. In addition to providing an index of the extent of the neoplastic disease, staging can help determine the best treatment options and the prognosis. Staging usually follows the World Health Organization's tumor/node/metastasis (TNM) guidelines. Although the specific guidelines vary with the type of neoplasia, the same general format is used.

  a. T designates the **tumor** size or extent and levels usually range from T_1 to T_4.

  b. N designates the number and characteristics of regional lymph **nodes** affected by the neoplasm and ranges from N_1 to N_3. A concurrent a or b designation is used for some neoplasms.

  c. M designates the presence or absence of **metastasis** (i.e., M_0 or M_1).

D. Treatment

1. Surgery

  a. Indications

    (1) Surgery is most commonly used to treat localized neoplastic disease. If a tumor is malignant, the tumor should be excised along with at least a 2- to 3-cm wide margin of normal tissue, if possible.

(2) Surgery may also be used as a diagnostic tool to obtain biopsies and to help stage the disease, or to treat urinary or GI obstruction or perforation caused by neoplasia.

b. Complications. Potential complications of surgery include hemorrhage, altered organ or tissue function, and altered appearance.

2. Radiation therapy may be used for treatment of localized or regional neoplasia or as palliative therapy in patients with terminal disease. Because radiation therapy is most effective against a small tumor volume, it may be used in conjunction with surgery or chemotherapy.

a. Indications. Radiation therapy has been shown to have some effect in the treatment of lymphoid neoplasia, thymomas, mast cell tumors, nasal adenocarcinoma, squamous cell carcinoma, basal cell carcinomas, transitional cell carcinomas, and pituitary tumors. Radioactive iodine therapy is also effective against functional thyroid tumors.

b. Complications. Potential side effects or complications of radiation therapy vary with the tumor site and may include moist desquamation of the overlying skin, tissue necrosis, fistula formation, permanent local alopecia, keratoconjunctivitis sicca, and later stricture formation or cataract development.

c. Technique. Radiation therapy is administered as frequent small doses in order to maximize the therapeutic effects while minimizing adverse effects. Orthovoltage radiation is used to treat superficial tumors, but cobalt-60 or a linear accelerator is needed to treat deeper tumors. The full effects of treatment may not be seen for weeks to months.

3. Chemotherapy is not usually curative. Rather, it is used for systemic or metastatic tumors, those that cannot be surgically removed, or in conjunction with surgery for suspected micrometastasis.

a. Cell cycle. Neoplastic and other dividing cells follow a set cell cycle (Figure 50-1). The timing of this cycle influences tumor and tissue growth as well as the efficacy and potential side effects of chemotherapy (and radiation therapy).

(1) The **mitotic index** is the percentage of cells in mitosis.

(2) The **growth fraction** is the proportion of growing or dividing cells. Chemotherapy kills a **constant proportion,** rather than a constant number, of cells. In general, rapidly dividing cells are more susceptible to chemotherapy.

(3) Chemotherapeutic agents may be **cell cycle phase-nonspecific** or **cell cycle phase-specific.**

(a) Cell cycle phase-nonspecific drugs work against cells in various stages of the cell cycle. These agents will also kill resting cells.

(b) Cell cycle phase-specific drugs work against cells in a specific stage of the cell cycle.

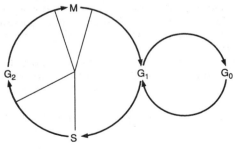

FIGURE 50-1. Cell cycle. The G_1 (gap 1) phase is a presynthetic phase during which RNA and enzymes are synthesized for later DNA production. DNA synthesis occurs during the S (synthesis) phase, and the mitotic spindle apparatus is synthesized during the G_2 (gap 2) phase. Mitosis occurs during the M phase. The G_0 (gap 0) phase is a true resting phase. Cells may go into G_0 from G_1 and can then later return to the G_1 phase. (Reprinted with permission from Ahrens FA: *NVMS Pharmacology.* Baltimore, Williams & Wilkins, 1996, p 230.)

b. Combination chemotherapy is used most often.
   (1) Each drug used in the treatment protocol should have some efficacy against the tumor when used as a single agent.
   (2) The drugs should work through different mechanisms.
   (3) Ideally, the toxicities should differ.
c. Chemotherapeutic drugs
   (1) Alkylating agents (e.g., chlorambucil, cisplatin, cyclophosphamide, melphalan) are cell cycle phase-nonspecific drugs. They work to prevent cell replication by cross-linking DNA. Myelosuppression and GI toxicity are the most common side effects.
   (2) Antimetabolites (e.g., cytosine arabinoside, 5-fluorouracil, methotrexate) are cell cycle phase-specific drugs. The drugs work during the S phase of mitosis to prevent replication by mimicking normal cell metabolites. Myelosuppression and gastroenteritis are the most common side effects.
   (3) Antineoplastic antibiotics (e.g., doxorubicin, mitoxantrone) are cell cycle phase-nonspecific drugs. They damage cellular DNA and prevent replication. Myelosuppression is the most common side effect.
   (4) Plant alkaloids (e.g., vinblastine, vincristine) are cell cycle phase-specific drugs. The drugs are active during the M phase; they disrupt the mitotic spindle. Myelosuppression, gastroenteritis, and necrosis (if given perivascularly) are the most common side effects.
   (5) Hormones (e.g., prednisone) do not usually cause cell death but may be useful in treatment of several types of neoplasia.
   (6) Miscellaneous chemotherapeutic agents include L-asparaginase.
d. Complications. In addition to killing neoplastic cells, chemotherapy will also kill some rapidly dividing non-neoplastic cells (e.g., bone marrow cells, intestinal villi). Most chemotherapeutic agents have a low therapeutic index, but host factors also affect toxicity. For example, cats are more susceptible to anorexia, vomiting, and bone marrow suppression, whereas collies, Old English sheepdogs, and West Highland white terriers are more susceptible to myelosuppression and gastroenteritis.
   (1) Cardiotoxicity can result from doxorubicin treatment. Echocardiographic evaluation is recommended prior to initiation of doxorubicin treatment and prior to every third treatment (i.e., every 9 weeks).
      (a) Acute cardiotoxicity is manifested as cardiac arrhythmias during or shortly after treatment. Pretreatment antihistamine administration may prevent this complication.
      (b) Chronic cumulative cardiotoxicity is more common and can be seen when the total dose of doxorubicin approaches or exceeds 240 mg/m^2 in dogs. Clinical signs and echocardiographic findings are consistent with dilated cardiomyopathy. Doxorubicin cardiotoxicity is rare in cats but can occur with administration of cumulative doses exceeding 150–170 mg/m^2.
   (2) Dermatologic toxicity
      (a) Local tissue necrosis may result from the perivascular administration of vincristine or doxorubicin. Use of a catheter for administration, careful monitoring of the patency of the catheter, dilution of the drug, and thorough flushing of the catheter after drug administration will minimize this risk.
      (b) Alopecia occurs in some animals, especially woolly-haired dogs because their hair growth is more synchronous. Doxorubicin, cyclophosphamide, and 5-fluorouracil most commonly cause this side effect.
      (c) Delayed hair regrowth. Many animals treated with chemotherapy may have delayed regrowth of clipped hair because hairs in the growth (anagen) phase are also affected by chemotherapy.
   (3) GI toxicity is the second most common side effect of many chemotherapeutic agents in veterinary medicine. Nausea and vomiting occur most often, but diarrhea can also occur.
      (a) Vomiting is minimized by slow administration of intravenous drugs and treatment with metoclopramide or prochlorperazine.

    (b) **Diarrhea** seen following doxorubicin therapy (3–7 days post-treatment) or methotrexate therapy (2 or more weeks post-treatment) will usually respond to supportive care.

    (c) **Pancreatitis** is a rare side effect of chemotherapy but has been reported in a small number of dogs treated with L-asparaginase or combination chemotherapy. Anorexia and vomiting may be seen within 1 week of treatment.

    (d) **Hepatic toxicity** is rare but can occur with cyclophosphamide, methotrexate, or azathioprine administration.

  (4) Hematologic toxicity. Hematologic toxicity is the most common side effect seen with most chemotherapeutic agents because of the bone marrow's rapid rate of division and growth. The nadir of the bone marrow effect is usually 7–10 days following treatment. **Neutropenia** is usually seen first, followed by **thrombocytopenia,** and rarely, **anemia.**

    (a) Neutropenia may necessitate dropping the drug from the therapeutic protocol on a temporary or permanent basis.

    (b) There may be no clinical signs related to the bone marrow suppression, especially if only myelosuppression has occurred. However, these patients are very susceptible to infection and sepsis and should be closely monitored, especially if the neutrophil count is less than 2000 cells/μl. Febrile, neutropenic patients should be promptly and aggressively evaluated for sepsis, and supportive care and antibiotic therapy (e.g., gentamicin or amikacin and cephalothin) should be initiated.

  (5) Hypersensitivity can occur in response to L-asparaginase, doxorubicin, and other drugs. Urticaria, wheals, or anaphylaxis may be seen. Temporary discontinuation of chemotherapy, administration of an antihistamine and possibly a glucocorticoid, and subsequent drug administration at a slower rate will resolve most mild reactions. Anaphylaxis requires discontinuation of chemotherapy and administration of antihistamines, glucocorticoids, and, possibly, epinephrine.

  (6) Neurotoxicity can occur in cats following the administration of 5-fluorouracil; therefore, this agent is contraindicated in cats. Vincristine will also occasionally cause a peripheral neuropathy.

  (7) Pulmonary toxicity is caused by cisplatin in cats. Acute dyspnea and pulmonary edema are followed by death despite aggressive supportive care. For this reason, cisplatin should not be used in this species.

  (8) Urologic and **renal toxicity**

    (a) Cyclophosphamide causes a sterile hemorrhagic cystitis in 5%–25% of treated dogs; this complication is rare in cats. Clinical signs include hematuria, pollakiuria, and dysuria, and the diagnosis is made based on the history and a urinalysis and urine culture to rule out infection. Treatment includes prompt discontinuation of cyclophosphamide treatment, furosemide administration to initiate diuresis, and possibly prednisone and antibiotic treatment. Intravesicular installation of dilute formalin or dimethyl sulfoxide (DMSO) may be helpful in more resistant cases.

    (b) Cisplatin and high-dose methotrexate treatment and doxorubicin treatment can induce renal failure in dogs. With cisplatin therapy, saline diuresis prior to and following drug administration helps minimize this risk.

  (9) Other side effects. Acute tumor lysis syndrome results from the rapid death and lysis of some tumor cells. The syndrome is rare in veterinary medicine but has been reported in a small number of dogs with lymphosarcoma. Hyperphosphatemia, azotemia, and hyperkalemia occur within hours to a few days of treatment and death usually follows despite aggressive supportive care.

4. Hyperthermia is sometimes used in conjunction with chemotherapy or radiation therapy.

5. Immunotherapy may be used in conjunction with chemotherapy, radiation therapy, or surgery for the control of some neoplasms.

6. **Nutritional support** may be needed in addition to treatment of the neoplasia itself. Most cancer patients are malnourished as a result of anorexia, inability to eat, altered metabolism, maldigestion or malabsorption, and the effects of the primary therapy.

II. SPECIFIC NEOPLASMS

A. Multisystemic neoplasms

1. **Hemangiosarcoma** is discussed in Chapter 48 V D.

2. **Leukemia** is discussed in Chapter 48 III B.

3. **Lymphosarcoma** is discussed in Chapter 48 V B.

4. **Mast cell tumors** are the most common type of skin tumor in dogs and are fairly common in cats. Middle-aged to older animals are most commonly affected, and brachycephalic breeds of dogs are at increased risk.

   a. **Etiology.** The exact cause of the tumors is unknown.

   b. **Pathogenesis**

      (1) In addition to their mass effects, mast cell tumors may cause systemic signs of disease following the release of heparin, histamine, and other vasoactive substances.

      (2) Approximately half of all canine mast cell tumors are benign. Lesions in the perineal, preputial, and inguinal areas and on the distal limbs are more likely to spread to other tissues.

   c. **Diagnosis**

      (1) **Clinical findings** vary with the site of disease.

         (a) **Cutaneous lesions**

            (i) In **dogs,** subcutaneous and cutaneous lesions are most common. The lesions may be single or multiple and may appear as a papule, nodule, mass, or diffuse skin thickening. Manipulation of the lesion may cause erythema, swelling, and bruising near the lesion **(Darier's sign)** as a result of release of vasoactive substances from the tumor.

            (ii) In **cats,** most cutaneous mast cell tumors occur as a single lesion on the head of a middle-aged to older cat. A rare form of histiocytic mast cell tumors, in which multiple benign mast cell tumors usually regress without treatment, may be seen in young Siamese cats.

         (b) **Visceral disease.** In cats, a visceral form of the disease may also occur. In the visceral form, systemic mast cell disease (mast cell leukemia) or intestinal involvement occurs. Anorexia, vomiting, and abdominal distention are common, and splenomegaly is usually palpable.

         (c) **Other findings**

            (i) In dogs, spread to the lymph nodes, spleen, and liver can occur and may be manifested as anorexia, vomiting, lethargy, weight loss, pale mucous membranes, and hepatosplenomegaly.

            (ii) GI ulceration may result from tumor release of histamine, and increased surgical hemorrhage may result from tumor release of heparin.

      (2) **Cytology findings.** Cytologic evaluation can be diagnostic. A needle aspirate will usually reveal round cells containing multiple purple granules.

      (3) **Biopsy findings.** Histologic examination of a biopsy sample may be useful because histologic grade has been correlated with prognosis (i.e., grade 1 mast cell tumors generally have a better prognosis).

      (4) **Laboratory findings**

         (a) **CBC.** A CBC often reveals no abnormalities, but eosinophilia, basophilia, and other nonspecific abnormalities (e.g., anemia, leukocytosis) may be seen.

         (b) **Serum biochemical profile.** Serum biochemistry results are usually normal but may include hyperglobulinemia.

        (c) **Fecal occult blood test.** A fecal occult blood test should be considered as a screening test for the presence of GI ulceration secondary to the mast cell tumor.

    (5) **Diagnostic imaging findings.** Thoracic and abdominal radiographs may reveal internal lymphadenopathy or organomegaly if visceral or systemic disease is present.

  d. Treatment

    (1) **Solitary mass.** Surgical excision is recommended if the mass is solitary and adequate margins can be obtained. Radiation therapy can also be used with a solitary superficial mass. A second surgery or radiation therapy can be used to treat local recurrence.

    (2) **Disseminated** or **metastatic disease** is treated with prednisone. If prednisone becomes ineffective, combination therapy with prednisone, cyclophosphamide, and vinblastine can be initiated.

    (3) **GI ulceration** should be treated with a histamine-2 (H_2) antagonist and, if clinical signs of ulceration are present, sucralfate.

B. **Bone neoplasms**

  1. Osteosarcoma is the most common bone tumor in dogs; it is less common in cats. Middle-aged to older, large- and giant-breed dogs are at greatest risk.

    a. Etiology. The inciting cause is unknown.

    b. Pathogenesis. In dogs, the tumor is usually locally aggressive, and early metastasis to the lungs is common. Metastasis to other bones can also occur. In cats, metastasis is rare.

    c. Diagnosis

      (1) **Clinical findings** usually include lameness and a localized painful swelling of the affected limb. The metaphyseal region of the distal radius, distal tibia, and proximal humerus are the most common sites for development of osteosarcoma.

      (2) **Biopsy findings.** Biopsy is usually diagnostic if taken from the center of the lesion.

      (3) **Radiographic findings**

        (a) **Radiographs of the affected limb** usually show an area of lysis and bony proliferation in the metaphyseal region. The lesion does not usually cross the joint.

        (b) **Thoracic radiographs** (three views) should be taken to look for pulmonary metastasis. Even if no radiographic lesions are seen, micrometastasis is still likely to be present.

        (c) **Survey skeletal radiographs** may be useful to look for metastatic bone lesions, especially if pain is detected on physical examination.

    d. Treatment of canine osteosarcoma is **amputation** and **cisplatin** chemotherapy. The addition of chemotherapy has been shown to prolong the survival time. Chemotherapy also alters the biologic behavior of the tumor so that bone metastasis is more common and pulmonary metastasis is less common. In cats, amputation is often curative.

    e. Prognosis

      (1) The long-term prognosis for dogs with osteosarcoma is grave because of the high incidence of micrometastasis at the time of diagnosis.

      (2) The long-term prognosis for cats with osteosarcoma is usually good.

  2. Chondrosarcomas and **fibrosarcomas** of bone are rare. Both are similar to osteosarcoma, although chondrosarcomas may be somewhat slower to metastasize. Treatment is amputation.

  3. Metastatic bone lesions can occur with prostatic adenocarcinoma, transitional cell carcinoma, hemangiosarcoma, and mammary adenocarcinoma in dogs.

C. **Cardiac neoplasia** is discussed in Chapter 39 IX A.

D. **Endocrine neoplasia** is discussed in Chapter 44.

E. **GI neoplasia** is discussed in Chapter 41.

F. **Hepatic neoplasia** is discussed in Chapter 42 I B 12.

G. **Mammary neoplasia** is discussed in Chapter 45 I C 5 e.

H. **Mediastinal neoplasia** is discussed in Chapter 40 V B 6 a.

I. **Neurologic neoplasia** is discussed in Chapter 47 II E, III E, and IV E 4, G.

J. **Oropharyngeal neoplasia** is discussed in Chapter 41 I B 3 g and I D 2 b.

K. **Pancreatic neoplasia** is discussed in Chapter 42 II B 3.

L. **Perineal** and **perianal neoplasia** are discussed in Chapter 41 IV E 6.

M. **Prostatic neoplasia** is discussed in Chapter 43 Part I:XII D.

N. **Renal neoplasia** is discussed in Chapter 43 Part I: XII A.

O. **Reproductive neoplasia** is discussed in Chapter 45 I C 6 f, 7 c–d, and II B 3 f.

P. **Respiratory neoplasia** is discussed in Chapter 40.

Q. **Skin tumors** are the most common tumor in dogs and the second most common tumor in cats. Most types are more common in older animals; but histiocytomas, viral papillomas, and transmissible venereal tumors are more common in young dogs. Basset hounds, boxers, bull mastiffs, Scottish terriers, and weimaraners are at increased risk for development of skin tumors.

   1. Etiology. The exact etiology is not known.

   2. Pathogenesis. Most cutaneous masses are benign in dogs but malignant in cats.

   3. Types
   a. **Basal cell tumors** develop from the basal cells of the epidermis and other skin structures and may be benign or malignant. Basal cell tumors are one of the more common skin tumors in cats.
      (1) **Clinical findings.** The only clinical sign is the presence of a firm, solid or cystic, sessile or pedunculated mass. In cats, the mass may be found on the head, trunk, or limbs. In dogs, masses are most commonly found on the head, neck, or shoulders. The mass is often pigmented and may be ulcerated.
      (2) **Treatment.** No treatment is needed for benign tumors. Basal cell carcinomas should be treated with surgery or radiation therapy.
   b. **Ceruminous gland adenomas** or **adenocarcinomas** develop from the ceruminous glands in the external otic canal. These are the most common tumor of the external ear and are more common in cats.
      (1) **Clinical findings.** The mass is usually brown and pedunculated, produces cerumen, and is located near the tympanic membrane. Adenomas and adenocarcinomas may appear similar upon gross examination, but adenocarcinomas are more invasive.
      (2) **Treatment** entails surgery (tumor resection with an adenoma or total ear ablation with an adenocarcinoma) or radiation therapy.
   c. **Epidermal inclusion cysts** usually occur secondary to obstruction of a hair follicle. Clinically, a cutaneous cyst containing thick white to brown material is seen. **Dermoid cysts** are similar to epidermal inclusion cysts except that dermoid cysts are the result of a developmental abnormality and may contain hair, sebum, and keratinized material in addition to fluid. No treatment is needed, but the mass may be surgically excised if it is causing a problem.

d. Histiocytomas ("button tumors") are benign tumors that develop from monocyte-macrophage cells in the skin. They are most common in young dogs and usually appear as round, reddish-pink, alopecic nodules. Treatment is not usually needed because the lesions commonly spontaneously regress in 1–2 months. Surgical excision may be performed if a mass is causing a problem.

e. Keratoacanthomas (intracutaneous cornifying epitheliomas) are benign tumors of young dogs. They develop from the epithelium between the hair follicles. The only clinical sign is the presence of a soft to firm mass or nodule with a pore on the surface. The mass often contains a thick paste-like material. No treatment is needed, but the mass may be surgically excised if it is causing a problem.

f. Lymphosarcoma. Cutaneous lymphosarcoma is discussed in Chapter 48 V B 1 e (4) and 2 e.

g. Mast cell tumors are discussed in II A 4.

h. Melanomas develop from melanocytes or melanoblasts in the skin. The tumors are most commonly seen as a brownish-black nodule on the face, trunk, feet, scrotum, nailbeds, or mucocutaneous junctions. In dogs, melanomas near mucocutaneous junctions or the nailbeds are more likely to be malignant. Treatment is surgical excision.

i. Papillomas are benign tumors that develop from squamous epithelial cells. These tumors are common in dogs but rare in cats. In puppies, the lesions are caused by a virus, but the cause is unknown in older dogs.
  (1) Clinical findings. The only clinical sign is the presence of one or more wartlike growths, which may be pedunculated and may bleed if irritated.
  (2) Treatment. No treatment is usually needed in young dogs. In older dogs, the masses can be surgically excised if they are causing a problem.

j. Sebaceous gland adenomas and **adenocarcinomas** develop from the epithelium of the sebaceous glands. Sebaceous gland adenomas are common in dogs, especially older dogs, but rare in cats, and sebaceous gland adenocarcinomas are rare. The only clinical sign is the presence of one or more firm, pink, hairless, lobulated, wart-like growths. The masses may ulcerate and bleed if traumatized. No treatment is usually needed, but surgical excision can be performed if the masses are causing a problem.

k. Squamous cell carcinomas are malignant tumors that develop from squamous epithelial cells. The exact etiology is not known, but repeated exposure of hypopigmented skin to ultraviolet radiation increases the risk. Squamous cell carcinomas are more common in older animals.
  (1) Clinical findings. Squamous cell carcinoma usually appears as a nonhealing ulcer or a red proliferative mass. In cats, the nose, lips, ears, and eyelids are the most commonly affected sites. In dogs, the abdomen, limbs, toes, scrotum, lips, and nose are more common sites. The tumor is locally invasive with later spread to lymph nodes and the lungs.
  (2) Treatment is surgical excision or radiation therapy if excision is not possible.

l. Transmissible venereal tumors are discussed in Chapter 45.

R. **Soft tissue tumors**

1. **Etiology.** The exact etiology is not known. Basset hounds, boxers, German shepherd dogs, Great Danes, golden retrievers, and Saint Bernards may be at increased risk.

2. **Types**
   a. Fibromas and **fibrosarcomas** arise from fibrocytes and are relatively common tumors in dogs and cats. The cause is not known in most cases, but infection with feline sarcoma virus can cause multiple benign tumors in young cats. In dogs and in older cats, the tumor occurs most often as a single mass on the trunk or limbs and is usually firm and nodular. Fibrosarcomas rarely metastasize but are locally invasive. Treatment is surgical.
   b. Hemangiopericytomas are benign tumors that develop from pericytes surrounding arterioles. They are common in middle-aged to older dogs. The tumor usually occurs as a slow-growing mass on one of the limbs. Treatment is surgery, radiation therapy, and possibly hyperthermia, but recurrence is common.

c. Hemangiosarcomas are discussed in Chapter 48 V D.

d. Leiomyomas and **leiomyosarcomas** infrequently arise from smooth muscle of the arrector pili muscles and cutaneous blood vessels; more commonly, they arise from the gastrointestinal and genitourinary tract. In superficial tissues, these tumors appear as a solitary, firm, infiltrative mass. Metastasis is possible. Treatment is surgical removal.

e. Lipomas and **liposarcomas** arise from adipocytes.

(1) Pathogenesis

(a) Lipomas are rare in cats but are common in middle-aged to older dogs where the tumor is usually seen as a soft, well-circumscribed, smooth subcutaneous mass on the trunk or proximal extremity. **Infiltrative lipomas** infiltrate adjacent tissues, as the name implies.

(b) Liposarcomas are uncommon but are also infiltrative and poorly circumscribed. Metastasis to the lungs and liver can occur.

(2) Diagnosis. A biopsy may be needed to differentiate an infiltrative lipoma from a liposarcoma because the oily material obtained with a needle aspirate often washes off the slide in the fixative.

(3) Treatment

(a) Lipomas do not require treatment unless the size or location causes a problem.

(b) Liposarcomas should be surgically excised, but complete excision is often difficult.

f. Lymphangiomas and **lymphangiosarcomas** are rare tumors of the lymphatic vessels. The tumor usually appears as a solitary mass and may be locally invasive. Metastasis is rare even with a lymphangiosarcoma. Treatment is surgical removal.

g. Malignant fibrous histiocytomas are uncommon tumors composed of fibroblast-like and histiocyte-like cells. The tumor usually occurs as an invasive subcutaneous mass that may invade bone. Metastasis is rare. Treatment is surgical removal.

h. Myxomas and **myxosarcomas** are rare tumors in dogs and cats. The tumor occurs in older animals, usually as a soft, fluctuant, poorly defined, infiltrative mass. Treatment is surgical removal, but local recurrence is common.

i. Rhabdomyomas and **rhabdomyosarcomas** are uncommon tumors that develop in striated muscle. Bladder, heart, and appendicular muscles are most often involved. These tumors are locally invasive and may metastasize. Treatment of bladder and skeletal muscle tumors is with surgery, although complete excision may be difficult.

j. Synovial cell sarcomas are uncommon in dogs and rare in cats. They arise from periarticular tissue and affect bones on either side of a joint. The tumors are locally aggressive and also metastasize fairly rapidly. Treatment is with amputation if metastasis has not occurred.

DIRECTIONS: Each of the numbered items or incomplete statements in this section is followed by answers or by completions of the statement. Select the ONE numbered answer or completion that is BEST in each case.

1. Gastrointestinal (GI) ulceration is most common secondary to:

(1) leukemia.
(2) hemangiosarcoma.
(3) fibrosarcoma.
(4) multicentric lymphosarcoma.
(5) mast cell tumor.

2. The anemia seen with neoplastic disease is most commonly a result of:

(1) disseminated intravascular coagulation (DIC).
(2) chronic disease.
(3) chemotherapeutic suppression of the bone marrow.
(4) immune-mediated hemolytic anemia.
(5) blood loss.

3. A nonhealing ulcerated mass on the pinna of the ear of a 10-year-old, male, outdoor cat is most likely:

(1) lymphosarcoma.
(2) a melanoma.
(3) a squamous cell carcinoma.
(4) a fibrosarcoma.
(5) a papilloma.

4. At which one of the following sites is a melanoma most likely to be malignant?

(1) Nailbed
(2) Face
(3) Lateral thorax
(4) Dorsal flank
(5) Thigh

5. A 10-year-old neutered male Boston terrier is presented because of a cutaneous inguinal nodule. Several minutes after palpating the nodule, you notice erythematous swelling of the adjacent tissue. This nodule is most likely a:

(1) hemangiosarcoma.
(2) mast cell tumor.
(3) basal cell tumor.
(4) sebaceous gland adenoma.

6. An 8-year-old neutered male domestic shorthair cat is presented with a three-month history of lameness and swelling near the distal radius. Radiographs of the affected limb show a lytic and proliferative lesion of the distal radius; a biopsy confirms the diagnosis of osteosarcoma. No metastatic lesions are seen on thoracic radiographs. You advise the owner that:

(1) there is a good chance for a cure if the affected limb is amputated.
(2) there is a good chance for a cure if the affected limb is amputated and chemotherapy with cisplatin is instituted.
(3) although the cat cannot be cured, amputation of the affected limb will slow the progression of the disease.
(4) although the cat cannot be cured, amputation of the affected limb and cisplatin chemotherapy can extend the cat's life.
(5) despite normal thoracic radiographs, micrometastasis is likely present, so there is no treatment for the cat.

DIRECTIONS: Each of the numbered items or incomplete statements in this section is negatively phrased, as indicated by a capitalized word such as NOT, LEAST, or EXCEPT. Select the ONE numbered answer or completion that is BEST in each case.

7. Which one of the following pairings of chemotherapeutic agent and potential side effect is INCORRECT?

(1) Vincristine— tissue necrosis if given perivascularly
(2) Cyclophosphamide— sterile hemorrhagic cystitis
(3) Cisplatin— cardiotoxicity
(4) L-Asparaginase— hypersensitivity reaction
(5) Doxorubicin— neutropenia

8. Osteosarcoma commonly occurs in all of the following sites in dogs EXCEPT the:

(1) distal radius.
(2) proximal humerus.
(3) distal tibia.
(4) proximal metatarsus.

ANSWERS AND EXPLANATIONS

1. The answer is 5 [II A 4 c (1) (c) (ii)]. Mast cell tumors may cause secondary gastrointestinal (GI) ulceration as a result of tumor release of histamine. Ulceration is uncommon with leukemia, hemangiosarcoma, fibrosarcoma, and multicentric lymphosarcoma. GI hemorrhage can occur with lymphosarcoma if there is gastric or intestinal involvement, but overt ulceration is less common.

2. The answer is 2 [I B 3 a (1)]. Anemia of chronic disease (ACD) is the most common form of anemia in dogs or cats with neoplasia. Disseminated intravascular coagulation (DIC), immune-mediated hemolytic anemia, and blood loss can occur secondary to many neoplastic diseases but are less common. Suppression of erythrocyte production by chemotherapeutic medications is rare.

3. The answer is 3 [II Q 3 I]. Squamous cell carcinoma is most common on the nose, lips, ears, and eyelids of older cats and often appears as a nonhealing ulcer or mass. Because ultraviolet radiation may play a role in the development of squamous cell carcinoma, outdoor cats and those with less pigment in the skin (e.g., white cats) may be at increased risk. Cutaneous lymphosarcoma is less common, and the animal may have multiple lesions. Melanomas are usually pigmented, but not always (amelanotic melanomas). Fibrosarcomas usually appear as firm nodules rather than as ulcerations and are more common on the trunk or a limb. Papillomas are rare in cats.

4. The answer is 1 [II Q 3 I]. Melanomas near the nailbed or mucocutaneous junctions are more likely to be malignant, but histopathology should be done to definitively establish whether the tumor is benign or malignant.

5. The answer is 2 [II A 4]. The occurrence of erythema, swelling, and bruising following palpation of a cutaneous or subcutaneous mass is most consistent with a mast cell tumor; manipulation of the tumor causes release of heparin, histamine, and other vasoactive substances that cause these signs. Hemangiosarcomas, basal cell tumors, and sebaceous gland adenomas all can occur as a cutaneous mass in dogs, but palpation of these tumors does not cause any changes in the adjacent tissues.

6. The answer is 1 [II B 1]. Osteosarcomas are slow to metastasize in cats, so there is a good chance for a cure with amputation of the affected limb. Adjunct cisplatin therapy should **not** be used in cats with any tumor type because it causes fatal pulmonary toxicity. In dogs, the behavior of osteosarcoma is different; optimal treatment includes amputation and adjunct cisplatin chemotherapy, but the long-term prognosis is still grave because of the extremely high incidence of micrometastasis at the time of diagnosis.

7. The answer is 3 [I D 3 d]. Cisplatin can cause renal damage and neutropenia but does not have adverse effects on the heart. Doxorubicin can cause cardiotoxicity but may also cause myelosuppression (i.e., neutropenia). The perivascular administration of vincristine has been associated with tissue necrosis. Cyclophosphamide causes sterile hemorrhagic cystitis in 5%–25% of patients receiving the drug. Hypersensitivity reactions are the major side effect of L-asparaginase therapy.

8. The answer is 4 [II B 1 c (1)]. The distal radius, proximal humerus, and distal tibia are the most common sites of osteosarcoma development in the dog, although the tumor can arise at other locations. A metatarsal osteosarcoma would be rare.

PART III

COMPREHENSIVE EXAM

QUESTIONS

DIRECTIONS: Each of the numbered items or incomplete statements in this section is followed by answers or by completions of the statement. Select the ONE numbered answer or completion that is BEST in each case. See Appendix for normal laboratory reference ranges.

1. A 10-year-old castrated beagle is presented because of incoordination. The dog is ataxic with a head tilt to the right, spontaneous nystagmus is present, and proprioceptive deficits in the right fore- and hindlimb are noted. The most likely cause of the ataxia is:

(1) cerebellar disease.
(2) cervical intervertebral disk disease.
(3) peripheral vestibular disease.
(4) cervical spondylomyelopathy.
(5) brain stem disease.

2. A long-term diabetic patient, a 13-year-old neutered male domestic shorthair cat, is brought to the veterinarian because the clinical signs of diabetes mellitus have recurred despite previous good control of the disease with twice-daily insulin therapy. The owner also comments that the cat's face looks different and that his teeth are no longer normally aligned. Physical examination reveals widened interdental spaces and a facial configuration that does seem different from that seen during previous visits. The owner brings the cat back the following day so that a glucose curve can be obtained; the curve shows persistent hyperglycemia throughout the day. The veterinarian increases the insulin dose, then increases it again, and then increases it again until the cat is receiving 9 units of ultralente insulin twice daily; however, there is a negligible decrease in the blood glucose level. The cat is still very polyuric and polydipsic at home. In addition to the diabetes mellitus, this cat probably also has:

(1) periodontal disease.
(2) hyperadrenocorticism.
(3) renal failure.
(4) acromegaly.
(5) hypercalcemia.

3. Which one of the following congenital defects is usually associated with esophageal dysfunction and regurgitation?

(1) Patent ductus arteriosus (PDA)
(2) Tetralogy of Fallot
(3) Tricuspid valve dysplasia
(4) Persistent right aortic arch (PRAA)
(5) Primary ciliary dyskinesis

4. The best treatment option for a dog affected with mild degenerative joint disease (DJD) or osteoarthritis in several joints would be:

(1) weight control and prednisone therapy.
(2) administration of a nonsteroidal anti-inflammatory drug (NSAID).
(3) weight control and the use of a NSAID as needed.
(4) weight control and strict cage rest.
(5) treatment of the most severely affected joints with intraarticular glucocorticoids

5. Which one of the following factors may contribute to the development of eclampsia in the bitch?

(1) Lack of calcium supplementation during the prepartum period
(2) Large-breed size
(3) Prolonged lactation
(4) Large litter

6. A lesion in which structure would result in altered consciousness?

(1) Pituitary gland
(2) Caudal medulla
(3) Cervical spinal cord
(4) Cerebellum
(5) Rostral brain stem

7. A 9-year-old female cat is brought to the veterinarian because the owner says she has not had much of an appetite. On physical examination, the sclera, inside of the pinnae, and the oral mucous membranes are slightly icteric. This finding would indicate that the serum bilirubin concentration is at least greater than:

(1) 0.5 mg/dl (8.5 μmol/L).
(2) 1.0 mg/dl (17 μmol/L).
(3) 2.0 mg/dl (34 μmol/L).
(4) 3.0 mg/dl (50 μmol/L).
(5) 4.0 mg/dl (67 μmol/L).

8. Dysuria can be associated with:

(1) lower urinary tract infection (UTI).
(2) decreased urethral sphincter tone.
(3) chronic renal failure.
(4) urethral neoplasia.
(5) lower UTI and urethral neoplasia.

9. In cats, which one of the following infectious diseases is most commonly associated with chorioretinitis?

(1) Hemobartonellosis
(2) Calicivirus infection
(3) Toxoplasmosis
(4) Chlamydiosis
(5) Herpesvirus infection

10. A 12-year-old female golden retriever is brought to the veterinarian because of a 3-day history of vomiting and anorexia. Initial laboratory tests and abdominal radiographs show hypercalcemia and enlarged sublumbar lymph nodes. The most likely diagnosis is:

(1) pyometra.
(2) anal sac adenocarcinoma.
(3) anal sac adenoma.
(4) perianal adenoma.
(5) colonic adenocarcinoma.

11. Dyspnea that occurs only on inspiration would most likely be associated with:

(1) lungworm infection.
(2) chronic bronchitis.
(3) pulmonary neoplasia.
(4) laryngeal paralysis.
(5) aspiration pneumonia.

12. Feline infectious peritonitis (FIP) can cause a myriad of clinical signs. The best way to confirm a diagnosis of FIP is:

(1) biopsy of an affected tissue.
(2) demonstration of hypoglobulinemia characterized by a polyclonal gammopathy.
(3) demonstration of characteristic straw-colored, high-protein pleural or peritoneal effusion.
(4) serology.
(5) observation of typical retinal lesions.

13. An 18-month-old male Great Dane is brought to the veterinarian because of incoordination. The owner has noticed slowly worsening incoordination over the last 3 months. The dog is otherwise healthy. A neurologic examination reveals proprioceptive deficits in all four limbs, but the deficit is worse in the hindlimbs. The dog is ataxic and scuffs the dorsal surface of its hind paws. The dog is slow to rise from a sitting position. The patellar reflex is normal to hyperreflexic bilaterally. The fore- and hindlimb withdrawal reflex is normal and cutaneous pain sensation appears normal. No pain is detected in the limbs or over the vertebral column. The cranial nerves are normal. The most likely tentative diagnosis would be:

(1) cerebellar disease.
(2) brain stem disease.
(3) cervical spondylomyelopathy.
(4) degenerative myelopathy.
(5) atlantoaxial subluxation.

14. Passive hepatic congestion most commonly results from:

(1) portosystemic shunts.
(2) right-sided heart failure.
(3) left-sided heart failure.
(4) neoplasms invading the caudal vena cava.
(5) hepatic lipidosis.

15. Bilateral symmetric alopecia that is nonpruritic could be associated with:

(1) hypothyroidism.
(2) scabies.
(3) flea infestation.
(4) atopy.
(5) food allergy.

16. A 5-year-old spayed female mixed-breed dog is brought to the clinic because the owners say she is gaining weight. No other clinical signs have been noted by the owners. The dog is weighed, and she has gained weight since her last visit to the clinic, 10 months ago. Other than the weight gain, the physical examination is unremarkable. The most likely cause of the weight gain is:

(1) hyperinsulinism.
(2) heart failure.
(3) overeating.
(4) hypothyroidism.
(5) hepatic failure.

17. A 4-month-old pug is presented because of difficult and noisy respiration. What collection of upper airway abnormalities is common in this type of dog and may account for the respiratory problem?

(1) Cleft palate, laryngeal stenosis
(2) Tracheal hypoplasia, everted laryngeal saccules, cleft palate
(3) Everted laryngeal saccules, laryngeal collapse, soft palate hypoplasia
(4) Stenotic nares, elongated soft palate, everted laryngeal saccules
(5) Stenotic nares, elongated soft palate, cleft palate

18. The drug of choice for the long-term or chronic control of seizure disorders is:

(1) diazepam.
(2) phenobarbital.
(3) pentobarbital.
(4) acepromazine.
(5) diltiazem.

19. An 8-year-old neutered male Shetland sheepdog is brought to the veterinarian because the owners have noticed that for the past week, the dog has been anorexic and lethargic, with a stilted gait and muscle twitching. A complete blood count (CBC), serum biochemical profile, and urinalysis reveal hypocalcemia and hyperphosphatemia; the remainder of the results are normal. The most likely diagnosis in this dog is:

(1) puerperal tetany.
(2) renal failure.
(3) primary hypoparathyroidism.
(4) malabsorption.
(5) pancreatitis.

20. If a transfusion is required for a dog with hepatic disease, only fresh blood should be used because:

(1) stored blood is deficient in vitamin K.
(2) stored blood increases the risk of thrombosis.
(3) stored blood has a higher concentration of ammonia.
(4) increased free hemoglobin in stored blood will exacerbate the hyperbilirubinemia.
(5) there is an increased risk of a transfusion reaction with the use of stored blood.

21. In which one of the following disease states would aggressive volume expansion using high doses of an intravenous crystalloid solution (e.g., lactated Ringer's solution at 60–90 ml/kg/hr) be contraindicated?

(1) Cardiogenic shock
(2) Severe hemorrhage
(3) Systemic anaphylaxis
(4) Septic shock
(5) Gastric dilatation–volvulus (GDV)

22. On physical examination a 4/6 systolic murmur that is loudest over the heart base is detected in a 3-month-old Newfoundland. Which one of the following conditions is most likely present?

(1) Pulmonic stenosis
(2) Subaortic stenosis (SAS)
(3) Dilated cardiomyopathy
(4) Patent ductus arteriosus (PDA)
(5) Innocent murmur

23. Most abscesses in cats are caused by:

(1) *Staphylococcus*
(2) anaerobic bacteria.
(3) *Pasteurella multocida.*
(4) *Staphylococcus* and anaerobic bacteria.
(5) *Pasteurella multocida* and anaerobic bacteria.

24. A 3-year-old neutered male domestic shorthair cat is brought to the clinic with a 1-day history of vomiting and progressive lethargy. On physical examination, the cat is 6% dehydrated and bunched intestines are felt on abdominal palpation. The most likely diagnosis is:

(1) alimentary lymphosarcoma.
(2) intestinal adenocarcinoma.
(3) inflammatory bowel disease.
(4) a linear foreign body.
(5) salmonellosis.

25. A 4-year-old female Labrador retriever is brought to the veterinarian because she is unable to walk. The dog was fine a couple of hours ago and was loose in a fenced and secure backyard. On neurologic examination, the dog is bright and alert, but she cannot walk or support weight on the hindlimbs. However, the right hindlimb seems to have slightly more strength than the left hindlimb. The patellar reflexes on both legs are normal to hyperreflexic. The hindlimb withdrawal reflexes and anal reflex are normal. No areas of pain can be detected. The front limbs and cranial nerves are normal. Cutaneous pain sensation is reduced but deep pain sensation is present in both hindlimbs. The most likely tentative diagnosis would be:

(1) discospondylitis.
(2) acute intervertebral disk herniation.
(3) degenerative myelopathy.
(4) fibrocartilaginous embolism.
(5) spinal cord trauma.

26. The urine of a polyuric, polydipsic dog has a specific gravity that is greater than 1.030 with water deprivation. What is the most likely diagnosis for this dog?

(1) Primary renal failure
(2) Hyperadrenocorticism
(3) Hypercalcemia
(4) Hypokalemia
(5) Psychogenic polydipsia

27. A 14-year-old spayed female miniature poodle is presented with the complaint of progressive hair loss. Physical examination reveals sparse truncal hair, thin skin, areas of hyperpigmentation, and three areas of thickened skin that feel slightly gritty. The owner reports that the skin problem does not bother the dog. A blood sample for diagnostic testing is obtained, and the dog is sent home. Two hours later, the owner calls and reports that the dog now has a large bruise at the site of the venipuncture; the veterinarian knows that the venipuncture was atraumatic because he drew the blood himself. The most likely diagnosis in this dog is:

(1) hypothyroidism.
(2) estrogen-responsive dermatosis.
(3) hyperadrenocorticism.
(4) Sertoli cell tumor.
(5) growth hormone (GH)–responsive dermatosis.

28. Which one of the following diseases could be associated with a diastolic murmur?

(1) Subaortic stenosis (SAS)
(2) Anemia
(3) Mitral valve insufficiency
(4) Pulmonic stenosis
(5) Aortic valve insufficiency

29. A 7-year-old male St. Bernard is brought to the veterinarian because the dog's urine has been discolored. The dog is bright and alert and has a good appetite. Physical examination is unremarkable. A urinalysis (sample obtained by cystocentesis) reveals the following findings: pH = 6.5, protein = 2+, glucose = negative, bilirubin = 1+. Sediment examination reveals: white blood cells (WBCs) = 30 per high-power field, red blood cells (RBCs) = 20–30 per high-power field, bacteria = 2+, crystals = 1+ (phosphate). The owner cannot afford any more diagnostic tests. The best treatment would be:

(1) gentamicin therapy for 3–4 weeks.
(2) trimethoprim–sulfa therapy for 10–14 days and a calculolytic diet.
(3) trimethoprim–sulfa therapy for 10–14 days.
(4) trimethoprim–sulfa therapy for 3–4 weeks.
(5) enrofloxacin therapy for 10–14 days.

30. An 8-year-old mixed-breed dog is brought to the veterinarian because of an acute onset of dyspnea. No abnormal lung sounds are present and the heart auscults normally. Thoracic radiographs reveal a mild increase in lucency of the lung fields. An arterial blood gas analysis reveals an arterial oxygen tension (Pao_2) of 50 mm Hg and an arterial carbon dioxide tension ($Paco_2$) of 30 mm Hg. The most likely cause of the dyspnea in this dog is:

(1) pulmonary edema.
(2) heart failure.
(3) upper respiratory tract obstruction.
(4) pulmonary arterial thrombus.
(5) allergic bronchitis.

31. Histoplasmosis is most common in dogs from:

(1) the northwest United States.
(2) the southwest United States.
(3) river valleys in the midwestern United States.
(4) southeast Asia, Puerto Rico, and the Caribbean.
(5) California.

32. A 3-year-old mixed-breed dog has a 2-day history of bloody mucoid diarrhea and tenesmus. There are no other clinical signs and a physical examination is normal. Which therapeutic plan is most appropriate?

(1) Withhold food for 24 hours and administer pyrantel pamoate.
(2) Withhold food and water for 24 hours and administer intravenous fluids and antibiotics.
(3) Feed a high-fiber diet and administer antibiotics.
(4) Withhold food and water for 24 hours and administer intravenous fluids and fenbendazole.
(5) Withhold food for 24 hours and administer fenbendazole.

33. Which one of the following diseases can be associated with a hypercoagulable state and spontaneous thrombosis?

(1) Mitral valve insufficiency
(2) Hypothyroidism
(3) Hypoadrenocorticism
(4) Hyperadrenocorticism
(5) Portosystemic shunt

34. Which one of the following is a commonly recognized paraneoplastic syndrome?

(1) Hyperkalemia
(2) Hypernatremia
(3) Hyperchloridemia
(4) Hyperphosphatemia
(5) Hypercalcemia

35. An owner notes that her 4-month-old female Siberian husky's bed always has urine wet spots despite efforts to take the dog outside just before going to bed. She also reports that her dog seems to be continually wet around the vulva and dribbles urine frequently. Physical examination is unremarkable except for a wet vulvar area. A urinalysis is unremarkable. The urine specific gravity is 1.034. The most likely diagnosis is:

(1) urinary incontinence due to urinary tract infection (UTI).
(2) urinary incontinence due to ectopic ureters.
(3) inappropriate urination due to polyuria.
(4) a behavioral problem (i.e., poor house-training).
(5) reproductive hormone—responsive incontinence.

36. A 2-month-old kitten is examined because of incoordination. The kitten is bright and alert and appears to have normal strength. Ataxia, hypermetria, and intention tremors of the head are noted. The most likely cause of this kitten's problems is:

(1) congenital vestibular disease.
(2) hydrocephalus.
(3) lissencephaly.
(4) cerebellar hypoplasia.
(5) spina bifida.

37. Which one of the following statements regarding heartworm disease is true?

(1) Cats are more susceptible to infection than dogs.
(2) Most cats do not have circulating microfilaria.
(3) Neurologic signs due to aberrant larval migration are less common in cats than in dogs.
(4) Pulmonary thromboembolic disease is rare in cats.
(5) Cats typically have large worm burdens.

38. A cat is presented in severe respiratory distress. The cat is open-mouth breathing and the mucous membranes are pink-grey in color. Lung sounds are absent over the ventral aspect of the thoracic cavity bilaterally and are only heard over the dorsal aspects of the chest. The cat is placed in an oxygen cage. What would be the most appropriate next measure to take?

(1) Perform needle thoracocentesis
(2) Anesthetize the cat and place a chest tube
(3) Obtain thoracic radiographs
(4) Order cage rest and diuretic therapy
(5) Blood gas analysis

39. A 10-year-old spayed female mixed-breed dog has mild generalized peripheral edema. The edema may be the result of:

(1) protein-losing nephropathy (PLN).
(2) left-sided heart failure.
(3) oliguric renal failure.
(4) thrombosis.

40. Which organisms are most likely to be associated with bacterial endocarditis?

(1) *Staphylococcus aureus, Escherichia coli, β*-hemolytic streptococci
(2) *Proteus mirabilis, Pseudomonas aeruginosa, S. aureus*
(3) *E. coli, Klebsiella pneumoniae, Enterobacter* species
(4) *β*-Hemolytic streptococci, *P. aeruginosa, K. pneumoniae*
(5) *P. mirabilis, K. pneumoniae, Enterobacter* species

41. An 8-year-old male neutered mixed-breed dog is brought to the veterinarian because over the last 2 months, the owner has noted that the dog has lost weight, vomited occasionally, and passed loose stools. The dog's appetite has been poor and he is thin. Abnormalities noted on a serum biochemical profile include: urea = 42 mg/dl (15 mmol/L), creatinine = 2.1 mg/dl (187 μmol/L), total protein = 4.7 g/dl (47 g/L), and albumin = 2.0 g/dl (20 g/L). Urinalysis (sample obtained by cystocentesis) reveals: pH = 6.0, protein = 1+ (0.1 g/dl), specific gravity = 1.049. Sediment examination reveals: white blood cells (WBCs) = 1 per high-power field, red blood cells (RBCs) = 0 per high-power field, and no casts or crystals. A urine protein:urine creatinine ratio ($U_{Pr}:U_{Cr}$) = 0.1. The best interpretation of these data would be:

(1) glomerular disease and renal failure.
(2) glomerular disease with prerenal azotemia.
(3) prerenal azotemia with urinary tract inflammation.
(4) renal failure and a nonurinary cause of the hypoalbuminemia.
(5) prerenal azotemia and a nonurinary cause of the hypoalbuminemia.

42. If an unvaccinated dog has bitten someone and is showing neurologic signs consistent with intracranial disease, the dog should:

(1) be observed by the owner for 10 days.
(2) be quarantined in a veterinary clinic for 10 days.
(3) be quarantined in a veterinary clinic for 1 month.
(4) be euthanized and the brain submitted for rabies testing.

43. Diabetes insipidus differs from diabetes mellitus in that with diabetes insipidus:

(1) a large quantity of hyposthenuric urine is eliminated.
(2) glucose accumulates in the blood and is eliminated in the urine.
(3) there is no intense thirst.
(4) the appetite is ravenous.
(5) a normal amount of urine is eliminated.

44. An 8-year-old male German shepherd is brought to the veterinarian because he has suddenly become very lethargic. On physical examination, the mucous membranes are pale and the abdomen appears slightly enlarged. A complete blood count (CBC) is normal except for a packed cell volume (PCV) of 19%. Abdominocentesis reveals bloody fluid with a PCV similar to that of peripheral blood. A prothrombin time (PT) and partial thromboplastin time (PTT) are normal. No other physical signs of hemorrhage are apparent. The most likely cause of the intraabdominal hemorrhage would be:

(1) anticoagulant rodenticide poisoning.
(2) ruptured splenic hematoma.
(3) liver failure.
(4) trauma.
(5) splenic hemangiosarcoma.

45. Which one of the following clinical signs commonly results from severe systemic arterial hypertension?

(1) Pleural effusion
(2) Subcutaneous edema
(3) Blindness due to retinal detachment
(4) Ventricular tachycardia
(5) Vomiting

46. Which combination of infectious agents is responsible for 80%–90% of upper respiratory tract infections in cats?

(1) *Mycoplasma* and feline herpesvirus-1
(2) Feline calicivirus (FCV) and *Mycoplasma*
(3) FCV and *Chlamydia psittaci*
(4) FCV and feline rhinotracheitis virus (FRV)
(5) FRV and *Bordetella bronchiseptica*

47. A 3-year-old female German shepherd-cross dog is brought to the veterinarian because of seizures and weakness. The owner reports that the dog started acting strange a few hours ago and had one seizure (approximately 1 minute in duration) approximately 30 minutes before the dog was brought to the veterinarian. The dog also urinated and defecated several times in the house, which is unusual because the dog is well housetrained. On physical examination, the dog is depressed, weak, salivating profusely, and has bilateral epiphora. Moderate dyspnea is present and airway sounds are moist. Muscle fasciculations are noted in the limb muscles. The pupils are miotic bilaterally. The most likely tentative diagnosis would be:

(1) strychnine poisoning.
(2) organophosphate or carbamate poisoning.
(3) idiopathic epilepsy.
(4) warfarin poisoning.
(5) metaldehyde poisoning.

48. A 4-year-old neutered male Boston terrier is brought to the veterinarian because of chronic intermittent vomiting. The vomiting usually occurs 6–10 hours after eating and the vomitus is primarily partially digested food. The dog's appetite is good and no other signs of illness are present. The most likely diagnosis is:

(1) alimentary lymphosarcoma.
(2) hypoadrenocorticism.
(3) pyloric stenosis.
(4) renal failure.
(5) jejunal intussusception.

49. Malignant hyperthermia should be treated with:

(1) dipyrone.
(2) cephalexin.
(3) dantrolene.
(4) external cooling alone.
(5) dexamethasone.

50. A 7-year-old female spayed miniature poodle is presented for a chronic nonproductive cough. The dog has had an intermittent cough for years but it has become more frequent over the last 2 months. The dog is bright and alert. Lung sounds are normal. A 3/6 systolic murmur loudest over the mitral valve area is present. The most likely differential diagnoses to consider at this time would be:

(1) left atrial enlargement, collapsing trachea, and chronic bronchitis.
(2) allergic bronchitis, collapsing trachea, and infectious tracheobronchitis.
(3) collapsing trachea, left atrial enlargement, and allergic bronchitis.
(4) chronic bronchitis, pulmonary neoplasia, and left atrial enlargement.
(5) pulmonary neoplasia, allergic bronchitis, and chronic bronchitis.

51. Which one of the uroliths listed below is most likely to occur in a Dalmatian dog?

(1) Cystine
(2) Struvite
(3) Calcium phosphate
(4) Urate
(5) Calcium oxalate

52. What is the optimal way to confirm a diagnosis of active toxoplasmosis in a cat?

(1) Immunoglobulin G (IgG) titer
(2) Immunoglobulin M (IgM) titer
(3) Observation of typical retinal lesions
(4) Fecal flotation
(5) Therapeutic trial.

53. A 5-year-old male neutered Malamute-cross dog is presented because of an acute onset of weakness. The dog is an outside dog that roams free. The dog seemed normal yesterday afternoon, the last time the dog was observed. On a neurologic examination, the dog is bright and alert but recumbent and unable to move except to lift his head slightly. The patellar reflex is absent on both hindlimbs. The withdrawal reflex is absent on both the fore- and hindlimbs. Pain sensation appears normal. The muscle tone is flaccid. No areas of hyperpathia are detected. The anal reflex and cranial nerves are normal. The most likely diagnosis is:

(1) botulism.
(2) acute cervical disk herniation.
(3) cervical spondylomyelopathy.
(4) cervical spinal cord trauma.
(5) acute polyradiculoneuritis (coonhound paralysis).

54. Pulmonary contusions may not become radiographically detectable until:

(1) 1 hour post-trauma.
(2) 6–12 hours post-trauma.
(3) 30 minutes post-trauma.
(4) 36 hours post-trauma.
(5) 2 hours post-trauma.

55. A 10-year-old male neutered cat is presented for anorexia, lethargy, and vomiting of 2 days' duration. On physical examination, the cat is thin, dehydrated, and depressed. Abdominal palpation is normal, except that both kidneys feel small and slightly irregular. A complete blood count (CBC) reveals a packed cell volume (PCV) of 18% with 0.1% reticulocytes. Abnormalities noted on a serum biochemical profile include: urea = 112 mg/dl (40 mmol/L), creatinine = 6.9 mg/dl (610 μmol/L), phosphorus = 12.4 mg/dl (4.0 mmol/L). Urinalysis is unremarkable and the urine specific gravity is 1.013. What is the most likely diagnosis?

(1) Urinary obstruction
(2) Acute renal failure
(3) Gastrointestinal (GI) disease resulting in vomiting and prerenal azotemia
(4) Chronic renal failure
(5) Hypoadrenocorticism

56. An arterial blood gas analysis is performed on a dog. The results are pH = 7.24, arterial oxygen tension (Pao$_2$) = 65 mm Hg, arterial carbon dioxide tension (Paco$_2$) = 60 mm Hg, and serum bicarbonate concentration = 25 mEq/L. Of the disorders below, which one could result in this acid–base disorder?

(1) Pleural effusion
(2) Urethral obstruction
(3) Hypovolemic shock
(4) Severe and protracted vomiting
(5) Ethylene glycol intoxication

57. A 1-year-old male neutered cat is brought to the veterinarian because of lethargy and anorexia. On physical examination, the cat's respiratory effort is mildly increased and the cranial thorax is firm and noncompressible. These findings suggest:

(1) pleural effusion.
(2) lung lobe consolidation.
(3) heartworm infection.
(4) pulmonary contusions.
(5) cranial mediastinal mass.

58. A 3-year-old female spayed Collie is brought to the veterinarian because of stiffness and inappetence. The dog walks with a stilted gait and is slow to rise from a recumbent position. Pain is elicited when the carpi and hocks are manipulated. There are no other physical abnormalites detected. Radiographs of the right carpus and hock are normal. A complete blood count (CBC), serum biochemical profile, and urinalysis are normal. Synovial fluid is collected from both carpi and hocks and reveals an elevated cell count (estimate = 10,000 cells/μl, 85% nondegenerate neutrophils; normal = <3000 cells/μl). A Lyme titer is negative. The most likely diagnosis is:

(1) *Borrelia burgdorferi* infection.
(2) idiopathic immune-mediated polyarthritis.
(3) polyarthritis associated with systemic lupus erythematosus (SLE).
(4) rheumatoid arthritis.
(5) degenerative joint disease (DJD).

59. A 4-year-old female spayed cocker spaniel is presented because of frequent vomiting and watery diarrhea of 2 days' duration. Physical examination reveals dehydration and lethargy. A complete blood count (CBC) is normal. Abnormalities on a serum biochemical profile include: blood urea nitrogen (BUN) = 42 mg/dl (15 mmol/L), creatinine = 3.1 mg/dl (275 μmol/L). Urinalysis is unremarkable and the urine specific gravity is 1.048. The azotemia is due to:

(1) acute renal failure.
(2) a prerenal cause.
(3) chronic renal failure.
(4) liver failure.
(5) a postrenal cause.

60. Which one of the following would be indicative of conscious perception of pain?

(1) A prick with a needle over the lateral thorax elicits a twitch or ripple in the muscles under the skin in this area.
(2) A toe is pinched and the animal withdraws the limb.
(3) The patellar ligament is tapped with a plexor and the animal extends the stifle joint.
(4) A toe is pinched and the animal turns its head toward the stimulus.
(5) The skin of the perineum is pinched and the animal contracts the anal sphincter.

61. The preferred antimicrobial agent for the treatment of hemobartonellosis in cats is:

(1) tetracycline.
(2) chloramphenicol.
(3) amoxicillin with clavulanic acid.
(4) erythromycin.
(5) trimethoprim/sulfadiazine.

62. The beneficial effects of a reduced-protein diet in dogs and cats with chronic renal failure are:

(1) reduced severity of uremic signs and reduced phosphorus intake.
(2) reduced phosphorus intake and an increase in the glomerular filtration rate (GFR).
(3) reduced severity of uremic signs and reduced potassium intake.
(4) reduced severity of uremic signs and a urine-acidifying effect (leading to a decreased urine pH).
(5) reduced phosphorus and creatinine intake.

63. A 5-year-old female spayed cocker spaniel is brought to the veterinarian because of the acute onset of weakness (over the last day). The dog lives on a farm and roams freely. On physical examination, the dog is weak and depressed. The mucous membranes are pale and icteric. The rectal temperature is normal, but the heart rate and respiratory rate are moderately elevated. No other abnormalities are noted. A complete blood count (CBC) reveals a packed cell volume (PCV) of 15%. The reticulocyte percentage and count are 24% and 530,000/μl, respectively. Marked spherocytosis is present. The platelet count is 10,000/μl. The serum bilirubin concentration is moderately increased and there is marked bilirubinuria. The most likely diagnosis is:

(1) anticoagulant rodenticide poisoning.
(2) acute liver disease.
(3) immune-mediated hemolytic anemia (IHA) and immune-mediated thrombocytopenia (IMT).
(4) blood loss resulting from thrombocytopenia.
(5) blood loss and liver damage due to trauma.

64. A 10-year-old castrated mixed-breed dog is presented because of dysuria of 3 weeks' duration. The dog was castrated at 1 year of age. Rectal examination of the prostate gland reveals asymmetric, firm, nodular enlargement. The most likely prostatic disease in this dog would be:

(1) chronic bacterial prostatitis.
(2) prostatic abscess.
(3) prostatic neoplasia.
(4) acute bacterial prostatitis.
(5) benign prostatic hyperplasia.

65. Which one of the following could be a contraindication for cerebrospinal fluid (CSF) collection?

(1) High-risk candidate for general anesthesia
(2) Cervical pain
(3) Mental depression
(4) Inflammatory central nervous system (CNS) disease
(5) Suspected brain neoplasia

66. A 6-year-old male neutered dachshund is brought to the veterinarian because of the acute onset of hindlimb weakness. The dog was fine the night before, but early this morning, he could not use his hindlimbs. A neurologic examination reveals normal mentation and an inability to stand or voluntarily move the hindlimbs. The patellar and hindlimb withdrawal reflexes are normal to hyperreflexic. Cutaneous pain sensation in the hindlimbs is reduced but deep pain sensation appears to be present. Hyperpathia is detected when the spine is palpated over the thoracolumbar junction. The front limbs and cranial nerves are normal. What is the most likely tentative diagnosis and best treatment plan?

(1) Acute intervertebral disk herniation— surgical decompression as soon as possible
(2) Fibrocartilaginous embolism— supportive care
(3) Acute intervertebral disk herniation— strict cage rest for 1–2 weeks
(4) Spinal cord tumor— surgical decompression or excision as soon as possible
(5) Acute intervertebral disk herniation— strict cage rest and corticosteroid therapy

67. A urethrocystogram obtained from an 8-year-old female dachshund reveals an irregular mass lesion on the ventral wall of the bladder in the trigone area. What is the most likely cause of the lesion?

(1) Squamous cell carcinoma
(2) Adenoma
(3) Granuloma
(4) Transitional cell carcinoma
(5) Adenocarcinoma

68. Moderate to marked masticatory muscle atrophy associated with trismus (i.e., the inability to fully open the mouth) is often associated with:

(1) immune-mediated polymyositis.
(2) idiopathic trigeminal nerve paralysis.
(3) masticatory muscle myositis.
(4) myotonia.
(5) idiopathic facial nerve paralysis.

69. Which one of the following conditions would most likely be associated with eosinophilia?

(1) Septic arthritis
(2) Allergic bronchitis
(3) Corticosteroid administration
(4) Cryptococcosis
(5) Feline leukemia virus (FeLV) infection

70. A 2-year-old cat is presented with a 2-week history of small bowel diarrhea and polyphagia. The most likely diagnosis is:

(1) hyperthyroidism.
(2) an intestinal foreign body.
(3) salmonellosis.
(4) alimentary lymphosarcoma.
(5) cryptosporidiosis.

71. Which set of laboratory findings is most consistent with posthepatic icterus?

(1) increased unconjugated bilirubin, increased serum alkaline phosphatase (ALP), markedly increased serum alanine transferase (ALT)
(2) increased conjugated bilirubin, increased ALP, markedly increased ALT
(3) increased unconjugated bilirubin, markedly increased ALP, increased ALT
(4) increased conjugated bilirubin, markedly increased ALP, increased ALT

72. What is the most common cause of hypothyroidism in dogs?

(1) Thyroid-stimulating hormone (TSH) deficiency
(2) Thyroid agenesis
(3) Lymphocytic thyroiditis
(4) Thyrotropin-releasing hormone (TRH) deficiency
(5) Surgical thyroidectomy

73. A 5-year-old male neutered golden retriever is brought to the veterinarian because the dog tires to the point of an inability to rise after about 2 minutes of exercise. After resting, the dog is able to exercise for a short time again. This problem has been gradually getting worse over the last month. Physical and neurologic examinations are normal. A complete blood count (CBC), serum biochemistry profile, and urinalysis are normal. What is the most likely tentative diagnosis, and how can this diagnosis best be confirmed?

(1) Myasthenia gravis— edrophonium response
(2) Myasthenia gravis— serum acetylcholine receptor antibody titer
(3) Polymyositis— muscle biopsy
(4) Myasthenia gravis— electromyography
(5) Polyneuropathy— nerve conduction velocities

74. A 4-year-old male neutered miniature schnauzer is presented because of weakness and dyspnea. The dog has never been ill until yesterday, when the owner noticed the dog was less active. The dog's condition has deteriorated over the last 24 hours. On physical examination, the dog is depressed, dyspneic, and has pale mucous membranes with diminished lung sounds over the ventral thorax. A complete blood count (CBC) reveals a packed cell volume (PCV) of 19% with 0.1% reticulocytes and a platelet count of 150,000/μl. A thoracic radiograph reveals a moderate degree of pleural effusion. A sample of pleural fluid is obtained. It is extremely bloody with a PCV similar to that of the peripheral blood. The activated clotting time (ACT) is prolonged. The most likely diagnosis is:

(1) acute hemorrhage from trauma.
(2) vonWillebrand's disease (vWD).
(3) immune-mediated thrombocytopenia (IMT).
(4) anticoagulant rodenticide poisoning.
(5) hemophilia A.

75. Normal water consumption for the dog is:

(1) 30–50 ml/kg/day.
(2) 30–50 ml/lb/day.
(3) 50–70 ml/kg/day.
(4) 50–70 ml/lb/day.

76. A monoclonal gammopathy and "punched out" osteolytic lesions seen on radiographs of the pelvis of a dog would be most consistent with:

(1) multiple myeloma.
(2) lymphosarcoma.
(3) chronic lymphocytic leukemia (CLL).
(4) ehrlichiosis.
(5) osteosarcoma.

77. Enzyme-linked immunosorbent assay (ELISA) and immunofluorescent antibody (IFA), the two most common tests for feline leukemia virus (FeLV), detect:

(1) antibodies to the virus.
(2) viral gp70 envelope protein.
(3) viral p15e envelope protein.
(4) viral p27 core antigen.
(5) feline oncornavirus-associated cell membrane antigen (FOCMA).

78. What type of urinary calculi can be seen in association with hepatic dysfunction in dogs and cats?

(1) Struvite
(2) Urate
(3) Cystine
(4) Calcium oxalate
(5) Silica

79. The insulin regimen of choice for initial regulation of nonketotic diabetes mellitus in cats is:

(1) NPH insulin subcutaneously once daily.
(2) crystalline insulin intramuscularly once daily.
(3) ultralente insulin subcutaneously once daily.
(4) lente insulin subcutaneously once daily.
(5) crystalline insulin subcutaneously twice daily.

80. Which of the following are common signs of hypoadrenocorticism in cats?

(1) Anorexia, diarrhea, and weakness
(2) Anorexia, vomiting, and bradycardia
(3) Anorexia, vomiting, and weakness
(4) Polyphagia, diarrhea, and bradycardia
(5) Polyphagia, vomiting, and polyuria

81. What is the best way to confirm a diagnosis of brucellosis?

(1) Tube agglutination test
(2) Rapid slide agglutination test (RSAT)
(3) Agar-gel immunodiffusion test
(4) Uterine biopsy
(5) Testicular biopsy

DIRECTIONS: Each of the numbered items or incomplete statements in this section is negatively phrased, as indicated by a capitalized word such as NOT, LEAST, or EXCEPT. Select the ONE numbered answer or completion that is BEST in each case.

82. An increased body temperature may be seen in association with all of the following disorders EXCEPT:

(1) bacterial endocarditis.
(2) infectious tracheobronchitis ("kennel cough").
(3) toxoplasmosis.
(4) feline infectious peritonitis (FIP).
(5) puerperal tetany.

83. A 9-year-old neutered male mixed-breed dog is brought to the veterinary clinic because the owners have noticed that the dog's abdomen is distended. On physical examination, fluid can be balloted in the abdomen. Which one of the following disorders is NOT likely to be the cause of this dog's abdominal distention?

(1) Hyperadrenocorticism
(2) Intraabdominal neoplasia
(3) Protein-losing nephropathy (PLN)
(4) Right-sided heart failure
(5) Hepatic cirrhosis

84. Which one of the following statements concerning radiation therapy in dogs and cats is FALSE?

(1) Potential side effects include tissue necrosis and permanent localized alopecia.
(2) To minimize the adverse effects of treatment, multiple small doses are administered.
(3) Prior surgery or chemotherapy may increase the effectiveness of radiation therapy by decreasing the tumor volume.
(4) It may take weeks or months to see the full effects of radiation therapy.
(5) Orthovoltage radiation is needed to treat deeper tumors.

85. Which one of the following is NOT a mechanism involved in vomiting?

(1) Irritation of the vomiting center by uremic toxins
(2) Stimulation of the chemoreceptor trigger zone by medications
(3) Stimulation of the vomiting center following neural input from the colon
(4) Stimulation of the chemoreceptor trigger zone following neural input from the cerebrum
(5) Stimulation of the chemoreceptor trigger zone by ammonia

86. Which one of the following condition—breed or phenotype associations is INCORRECT?

(1) Retained deciduous teeth— toy breeds
(2) Cleft palate— brachycephalic breeds
(3) Gingival hyperplasia— boxers
(4) Brachygnathism— brachycephalic breeds
(5) Craniomandibular osteopathy— terriers

87. In dogs, what is the minimum urine specific gravity that suggests that the dog is NOT polyuric?

(1) Less than 1.008
(2) Greater than 1.012
(3) Greater than 1.025
(4) Greater than 1.040

88. A breeder brings a bitch to the veterinarian because the dog is failing to cycle. Which one of the following problems would NOT be a consideration?

(1) Functional ovarian cyst
(2) Hypothyroidism
(3) "Silent" heat
(4) Premature ovarian failure
(5) Hyperadrenocorticism

89. Regurgitation at the time of weaning is a common clinical sign of all of the following disorders EXCEPT

(1) persistent right aortic arch (PRAA).
(2) congenital diverticulum.
(3) congenital esophageal fistula.
(4) inherited megaesophagus.

90. Which one of the following disorders is NOT characterized by weight loss despite polyphagia?

(1) Hyperthyroidism
(2) Diabetes mellitus
(3) Exocrine pancreatic insufficiency (EPI)
(4) Protein-losing enteropathy (PLE)
(5) Protein-losing nephropathy (PLN)

91. All of the following are potential complications of esophageal disease EXCEPT:

(1) perforation.
(2) stricture.
(3) malnutrition.
(4) stomatitis.
(5) chronic respiratory disease.

92. Which one of the following disorders is NOT a common cause of polyuria and polydipsia in an older cat?

(1) Hyperadrenocorticism
(2) Diabetes mellitus
(3) Hyperthyroidism
(4) Renal failure

93. Which one of the following will NOT exacerbate clinical signs of hepatic encephalopathy?

(1) Gastrointestinal (GI) hemorrhage
(2) Acidosis
(3) Constipation
(4) Uremia
(5) A high-protein diet

94. A 2-year-old spayed female Labrador retriever is brought to a veterinary clinic during the peak of summer with severe hyperthermia; the rectal temperature is 106.5°F (41.4°C). Intravenous fluids and nasal oxygen are administered, and the dog is cooled with cool water and a fan. Potential complications that may occur as a result of the severe hyperthermia include all of the following EXCEPT:

(1) disseminated intravascular coagulation (DIC).
(2) congestive heart failure.
(3) hepatic failure.
(4) renal failure.
(5) gastrointestinal (GI) hemorrhage.

95. Gastroesophageal reflux can result in esophagitis. In a dog with reflux-induced esophagitis, all of the following treatments may be helpful EXCEPT:

(1) antibiotics.
(2) histamine-2 (H₂) antagonists.
(3) calcium channel blockers.
(4) metoclopramide.
(5) feeding a low-fat, high-protein diet.

96. Surgical management of gastric dilatation–volvulus (GDV) can encompass more than one surgical maneuver, depending on the individual case. Which procedure would NOT likely be performed in a dog with GDV?

(1) Gastrotomy
(2) Gastrectomy
(3) Pyloroplasty
(4) Gastropexy
(5) Splenectomy

97. Which one of the following is NOT a cause of acquired nephrogenic diabetes insipidus?

(1) Hyperadrenocorticism
(2) Pyelonephritis
(3) Diabetes mellitus
(4) Hypercalcemia
(5) Pyometra

98. Which one of the following is NOT a common pathogen in pyometra?

(1) *Staphylococcus*
(2) *Escherichia coli*
(3) *Pseudomonas*
(4) *Streptococcus*

99. Which one of the following disorders is NOT a potential cause of secondary megaesophagus?

(1) Pneumonia
(2) Myasthenia gravis
(3) Pyloric stenosis
(4) Hypoadrenocorticism
(5) Viral encephalitis

100. Which one of the following is NOT a potential side effect of the use of megestrol acetate for suppression of estrus?

(1) Pyometra
(2) Mammary development
(3) Acromegaly
(4) Clitoral enlargement
(5) Diabetes mellitus

101. A young dog is presented with a 1-day history of pain on opening the mouth. Which one of the following would NOT be a possible cause of the problem?

(1) Masticatory myositis
(2) Sialocele
(3) Retrobulbar abscess
(4) Craniomandibular osteopathy
(5) Oral foreign body

ANSWERS AND EXPLANATIONS

1. The answer is 5 [Chapter 21, Table 21-1]. The presence of a head tilt and spontaneous nystagmus support vestibular dysfunction. The presence of proprioceptive deficits in the right fore- and hindlimb would indicate brain stem disease on the right side (i.e., central vestibular disease). If proprioceptive deficits were absent, peripheral vestibular disease would have been most likely. Cervical spinal cord disease is not accompanied by a head tilt or spontaneous nystagmus unless multifocal disease is present. A head tilt and proprioceptive deficits are typically absent with cerebellar disease.

2. The answer is 4 [Chapter 44 I E 1 b; IV A 6 b (5)]. The lack of response to high doses of exogenous insulin in this cat is consistent with insulin resistance; of the listed disorders, only hyperadrenocorticism and acromegaly would cause such resistance. Although hyperadrenocorticism is slightly more common, albeit still somewhat rare, acromegaly should be suspected in this cat because of the altered facial configuration and the development of widened interdental spaces. Both of these findings are fairly characteristic of acromegaly.

3. The answer is 4 [Chapter 39 V J 3]. Persistent right aortic arch (PRAA) is one of several vascular ring anomalies that may entrap the esophagus dorsal to the heart, resulting in constriction and regurgitation. The esophagus is not affected by patent ductus arteriosus (PDA), tetralogy of Fallot, or tricuspid valve dysplasia. Primary ciliary dyskinesia predominantly affects the ciliated epithelium of the respiratory tract and does not affect esophageal function.

4. The answer is 3 [Chapter 46 III A 1 e]. Weight control is an important facet of treatment in all dogs with degenerative joint disease (DJD). When dogs have mild signs, the use of a nonsteroidal anti-inflammatory drug (NSAID) on an as-needed basis is usually satisfactory. The use of NSAIDs alone without weight control would be less ideal. Exercise limited to an appropriate level aids in maintaining muscle and ligament tone, and therefore, strict cage rest would not be indicated in a dog with mild disease. The use of prednisone (a glucocorticoid) administered into the

joint or orally would not be indicated in a dog with mild signs. Because of the deleterious effect of glucocorticoids on articular cartilage, these agents are usually reserved for those patients with advanced joint disease that are not responsive to other treatments.

5. The answer is 4 [Chapter 45 I C 4 b]. A large litter may result in increased lactation demands and may contribute to the development of eclampsia. Other possible predisposing factors include prepartum calcium supplementation and small-breed size. Because eclampsia occurs most commonly during early lactation, the duration of lactation does not appear to play a role in the development of eclampsia.

6. The answer is 5 [Chapter 22 II]. Any lesion that affects the reticular activating system in the rostral brain stem (midbrain) or its connections to the cerebral cortex will alter the level of consciousness. The pituitary gland, caudal medulla, cervical spinal cord, and cerebellum are not directly involved and lesions in these areas would produce different neurologic signs.

7. The answer is 3 [Chapter 9 III A 2]. Tissue icterus cannot be detected until serum bilirubin concentrations are greater than 2.0–3.0 mg/dl (34–50 μmol/L). Plasma icterus can be detected when the serum bilirubin concentration is greater than 1.5 mg/dl (25 μmol/L).

8. The answer is 5 [Table 32-1]. Dysuria (as well as stranguria and pollakiuria) is indicative of lower urinary (or genital) tract inflammation [such as would occur with a urinary tract infection (UTI)] or obstruction (e.g., urethral neoplasia). Renal failure results in polyuria but not dysuria. Decreased urethral sphincter tone would result in urinary incontinence manifested as involuntary dribbling, not the painful or difficult urination associated with dysuria.

9. The answer is 3 [Chapter 38 II A 1 b]. Toxoplasmosis in cats is commonly associated with a multifocal chorioretinitis, which may or may not be associated with retinal detachment. Anterior uveitis is also common. Although calicivirus infection, herpesvirus infection, and chlamydiosis can result in ocular disease (conjunctivitis; conjunctivitis and corneal ulceration; and conjunctivitis, respectively), the retina is rarely affected. Hemobartonellosis does not usually cause ocular lesions.

10. The answer is 2 [Chapter 41 IV E 6 c]. The most likely diagnosis is anal sac adenocarcinoma. Pyometra can cause vomiting and anorexia, but vaginal discharge (open pyometra) and/or radiographic signs of an enlarged uterus should be seen. Serum calcium is also normal with pyometra. Perianal adenomas and anal sac adenomas cause no systemic signs of illness and would not spread to the sublumbar lymph nodes. Colonic adenocarcinoma could cause sublumbar lymphadenopathy if metastasis had occurred, but hypercalcemia would be uncommon and diarrhea, tenesmus, and constipation are more common findings than vomiting in dogs with colonic adenocarcinoma. In contrast, anal sac adenocarcinomas usually cause no clinical signs directly referable to the primary tumor but instead cause problems through early metastasis and hypercalcemia of malignancy.

11. The answer is 4 [Chapter 28 III A]. Inspiratory dyspnea is most likely to occur with laryngeal paralysis. During inspiration, negative intra-airway pressure is generated in the upper airways, which aggravates obstructive diseases in the upper airway, especially unfixed obstructions such as the paralyzed vocal folds of laryngeal paralysis. Lungworm infection, chronic bronchitis, pulmonary neoplasia, and aspiration pneumonia are predominantly lower airway or pulmonary parenchymal disorders and are associated with expiratory dyspnea or a mixture of inspiratory and expiratory dyspnea.

12. The answer is 1 [Chapter 49 V D 2 b (5)]. The only way to definitively diagnoses feline infectious peritonitis (FIP) is by biopsy and histopathology. Serology can support a tentative diagnosis but cannot confirm the diagnosis because feline enteric coronavirus crossreacts with the FIP assay. Identification of a hypergammaglobulinemia characterized by a polyclonal gammopathy, demonstration of the presence of a straw-colored, high-protein pleural or peritoneal effusion, or identification of retinal lesions can also support a tentative diagnosis but are not pathognomonic for FIP.

13. The answer is 3 [Chapter 47 III A 2 a, B 2]. The neurologic signs are consistent with a C1–C5 lesion; therefore, cerebellar disease, brain stem disease, and degenerative myelopathy can be ruled out. Although atlantoaxial subluxation results in C1–C5 signs, it is usually associated with a congenital malformation of this joint in toy-breed dogs. Acquired atlantoaxial subluxation can occur, but is associated with major trauma to the neck. Great Danes have a predisposition to cervical spondylomyelopathy and in the absence of a history of trauma, this would be the most likely tentative diagnosis.

14. The answer is 2 [Chapter 42 I B 11 d]. Right-sided heart failure resulting from dilated cardiomyopathy, pericardial disease, some congenital cardiac defects, and some cardiac neoplasms is the most common cause of passive hepatic congestion. Portosystemic shunts reduce blood flow through the liver, and hypoxia, but not congestion, is associated with left-sided heart failure. Neoplasms invading the caudal vena cava can cause passive congestion, but such neoplasms are rare. Hepatic neoplasms may cause hepatocellular leakage or alter bile flow, but they rarely affect hepatic blood flow.

15. The answer is 1 [Chapter 36 III A 4 c, 5 c]. Endocrine imbalances (e.g., hypothyroidism) commonly result in nonpruritic bilateral symmetric alopecia. Scabies, flea infestation, atopy, and food allergy may result in symmetric alopecia, but all are very pruritic.

16. The answer is 3 [Chapter 12 II A]. Overeating and overfeeding are the most common causes of weight gain in dogs and cats. Hyperinsulinism and hypothyroidism can cause an increase in body fat, but other clinical signs (e.g., episodic weakness, seizures with hypoglycemia due to hyperinsulinism, alopecia or other dermatopathies associated with hypothyroidism) are usually also present. If a detailed dietary history seems to rule out overeating or overfeeding, then these diagnoses should be considered. With heart failure and hepatic failure, any significant weight gain is usually due to increased fluid retention (e.g., ascites); on physical examination, abdominal fluid may be balloted or abdominal distention may be noted in conjunction with a more generalized loss of body mass.

17. The answer is 4 [Chapter 40 II C 2]. Brachycephalic dogs (e.g., pugs, Boston terriers, Pekingese) are commonly affected with varying combinations of stenotic nares, elongated soft palates, and everted laryngeal saccules (brachycephalic syndrome). Laryngeal collapse can occur in long-standing untreated cases. Tracheal hypoplasia occurs most often as a congenital abnormality in bulldogs. Cleft palate and laryngeal stenosis are not features of brachycephalic syndrome.

18. The answer is 2 [Chapter 24 VI B]. Phenobarbital is the drug of choice for long-term seizure control because it can be administered orally, is inexpensive, has a long half-life, and does not cause significant side effects in most animals. Diazepam is relatively short-acting and although it can be very useful in the acute management of seizuring animals, it is less suited for long-term administration, especially as a single agent. Pentobarbital is an injectable agent used to induce general anesthesia and is not suited for long-term use. Acepromazine is a sedative that can actually lower the seizure threshold and increase the risk of seizure activity. Diltiazem is a calcium channel blocker; it does not have anticonvulsant activity.

19. The answer is 3 [Chapter 44 II A 3 a–b]. Puerperal tetany, renal failure, primary hypoparathyroidism, malabsorption, and pancreatitis can all cause hypocalcemia, but only puerperal tetany and primary hypoparathyroidism will result in the clinical signs of hypocalcemia observed in this dog. Because the dog is a neutered male, puerperal tetany is not a consideration; puerperal tetany also usually results in more acute progressive clinical signs.

20. The answer is 3 [Chapter 48 I B 1 c (7) (b)]. Stored blood has a higher ammonia concentration and therefore should not be used in animals with hepatic disease because the increased blood ammonia may exacerbate signs of hepatic encephalopathy.

21. The answer is 1 [Chapter 31 V A 2 a (3)]. Animals in cardiogenic shock usually have congestive heart failure, a state of sodium and water retention and pulmonary venous congestion and edema. These animals are sensitive to water and sodium loads, which can exacerbate pulmonary congestion and edema. Therefore, intravenous fluid therapy with high-sodium fluids (e.g., lactated Ringer's solution,

normal saline) is administered with caution (or not at all) and at low doses, not at high (shock) doses. Aggressive intravenous fluid therapy is indicated for severe hemorrhage, systemic anaphylaxis, septic shock, and gastric dilatation–volvulus.

22. The answer is 2 [Chapter 39 V C 3 b]. The Newfoundland puppy most likely has sub-aortic stenosis (SAS). The young age of the dog would suggest a congenital cardiac defect and make dilated cardiomyopathy very unlikely. The intensity of the murmur is greater than is usually detected with innocent murmurs and is more consistent with a pathologic murmur. Of the three congenital defects listed [pulmonic stenosis, SAS, and patent ductus arteriosus (PDA)], PDA is usually associated with a continuous murmur and pulmonic stenosis is not as common as SAS (which is inherited in Newfoundlands).

23. The answer is 5 [Chapter 49 I A]. *Pasteurella multocida* and anaerobic bacteria are the most common causes of abscesses in cats.

24. The answer is 4 [Chapter 41 IV B 8 b]. A linear foreign body should be suspected and investigated if bunched intestines are found in a young cat with vomiting and systemic signs of illness. A mass lesion or thickened intestinal walls may be palpable with alimentary lymphosarcoma, but the intestines are usually distributed normally throughout the abdominal cavity. Intestinal adenocarcinomas are more common in older cats and abdominal palpation is often normal or may reveal a mass. The intestines may also feel normal with inflammatory bowel disease or they may be thickened. Salmonellosis may result in fluid-filled bowel loops, but the loops are distributed normally throughout the abdomen.

25. The answer is 4 [Chapter 47 III I 1]. The acute onset of hindlimb paresis due to a T3–L3 lesion with no spinal cord pain and asymmetric neurologic signs in a large-breed dog is suggestive of fibrocartilaginous embolism. Spinal pain is usually a feature of discospondylitis and acute disk herniation and its absence would make these disorders less likely. Degenerative myelopathy is nonpainful and it has a slowly progressive, not an acute, clinical course. Spinal cord trauma can result in acute neurologic deficits (with or without pain), but spinal cord trauma would seem unlikely in a dog in a secure backyard that has been well observed. In addition, there were no other physical signs (e.g., scrapes, bruises, shock) that might be associated with trauma.

26. The answer is 5 [Chapter 44 I B 2 b (4) (b) (vi)]. An animal with psychogenic polydipsia will often concentrate its urine like a normal animal in response to water deprivation. Animals with renal failure, hyperadrenocorticism, hypercalcemia, or hypokalemia are usually unable to concentrate their urine, as the result of either intrinsic renal disease or interference with the action of antidiuretic hormone (ADH) on the kidneys. When undergoing a water deprivation test, these animals will become dehydrated and/or azotemic before a urine specific gravity greater than 1.030 is reached.

27. The answer is 3 [Chapter 37 III B 6]. Truncal alopecia, thin skin, hyperpigmentation, and frequent bruising can all be seen with hyperadrenocorticism. The gritty-feeling areas of thickened skin suggest that calcinosis cutis is also present. Hypothyroidism and growth hormone (GH)–responsive dermatosis can also cause truncal alopecia and hyperpigmentation, but bruising and calcinosis cutis are unlikely. Estrogen-responsive alopecia more typically begins as a perineal alopecia. Sertoli cell tumors occur only in male dogs.

28. The answer is 5 [Chapter 39 I A 3 g (2) (b)]. Diastolic murmurs result from semilunar valve insufficiency (i.e., aortic or pulmonic valve insufficiency) or atrioventricular (AV) valve stenosis. Subaortic stenosis (SAS), anemia, mitral valve insufficiency, and pulmonic stenosis result in a systolic murmur.

29. The answer is 4 [Chapter 43 Part I:VII C 2 a (2); IX B 2 b (2) (a)]. The abnormalities observed on a urinalysis are consistent with a urinary tract infection (UTI). All UTIs in male dogs are potentially complicated by prostatic infection. As a result, antimicrobial therapy should be administered for 3–4 weeks. Both trimethoprim–sulfa and enrofloxacin would be good choices. These agents are effective against most urinary pathogens and would penetrate the prostate gland as well. Gentamicin would be an inappropriate choice because of the high risk of nephrotoxicity with a treatment duration of 3–4 weeks. Furthermore, gentamicin can only be given by injection, which is impractical in this setting. Phosphate crystalluria can be a normal finding and

is not indicative of urolithiasis. Hence, a calculolytic diet would not be indicated.

30. The answer is 4 [Chapter 40 IV H 3]. The combination of dyspnea, minimal thoracic radiographic abnormalities, and hypoxemia is very suggestive of a pulmonary arterial thrombus or pulmonary thromboembolism. The radiographic findings do not support pulmonary edema, heart failure, or allergic bronchitis. The physical examination and radiographic findings are not suggestive of upper respiratory tract obstruction (e.g., inspiratory stridor, radiographically detectable masses or foreign bodies).

31. The answer is 3 [Chapter 49 II F]. Histoplasmosis is acquired through ingestion or inhalation of soil contaminated with bird or bat droppings; in the United States this contamination is most common in and near the midwestern river valleys.

32. The answer is 5 [Chapter 4 VI A]. It is appropriate to withhold food for 24 hours in any dog or cat with vomiting and diarrhea, but it is not necessary to withhold water if there is no vomiting. The dog also does not require intravenous fluid therapy because it is not dehydrated, is not vomiting, and is still drinking water on its own. Intestinal parasites are one of the most common causes of simple enteritis or colitis in dogs, so deworming is appropriate. Whipworms should be suspected because the diarrhea is large bowel in origin (as suggested by the tenesmus and the presence of blood and mucus); fenbendazole is the dewormer of choice. A high-fiber diet is helpful in the management of some cases of colitis but would typically be used after withholding food and after deworming. Antibiotics are not indicated unless bacterial colitis is suspected based on concurrent systemic signs of illness (e.g., decreased appetite, mild lethargy) or the finding of leukocytes and sporulated bacteria on a fecal smear or unless the diagnosis is confirmed by a positive fecal culture.

33. The answer is 4 [Table 39-9]. The increased endogenous glucocorticoid production associated with hyperadrenocorticism can result in a hypercoagulable state. Exogenous glucocorticoid administration may also induce a hypercoagulable state. Mitral valve insufficiency, hypothyroidism, hypoadrenocorticism, and portosystemic shunts are not associated with a tendency for thrombosis.

34. The answer is 5 [Chapter 50 I B 3 e]. Although hyperkalemia, hypernatremia, hyperchloridemia, hyperphosphatemia, and hypercalcemia all may occur in individual patients with neoplasia, only hypercalcemia of malignancy is a recognized paraneoplastic syndrome in dogs and cats. Other paraneoplastic syndromes in veterinary medicine include anemia, cancer cachexia, erythrocytosis, fever, hyperglobulinemia, hypertrophic osteopathy, hypocalcemia, hypoglycemia, and thrombocytopenia.

35. The answer is 2 [Chapter 43:Part I X B 2 b (1) (d)]. The most common cause of urinary incontinence in an immature dog is ectopic ureters, especially in the Siberian husky breed. The urinalysis rules out urinary tract infection (UTI) and polyuria would be very unlikely with a urine specific gravity of 1.034. (If polyuria were present, the urine specific gravity would be less than 1.020.) One cannot absolutely rule out a behavioral problem but the constant dribbling is more indicative of urinary incontinence. Reproductive hormone–responsive incontinence occurs most often in older, spayed, female (usually large-breed) dogs.

36. The answer is 4 [Chapter 47 II A 2, C 2]. The clinical signs are typical for cerebellar disease. Cerebellar hypoplasia (usually caused by *in utero* panleukopenia virus infection) is common in kittens. Congenital vestibular disease (suggested by head tilt and ataxia), hydrocephalus (suggested by mentation changes, seizures, and a domed skull), lissencephaly (suggested by mentation changes and seizures), and spina bifida (suggested by hindlimb paresis) would not be consistent with the neurologic signs observed in this kitten.

37. The answer is 2 [Chapter 39 VI B 3 b (3) (e)]. Most cats do not have circulating microfilaria. Cats are more resistant to heartworm infection and have smaller worm burdens than dogs. Pulmonary thromboembolic disease is common in cats and acute neurologic signs from aberrant larval migration are more common in cats than in dogs.

38. The answer is 1 [Chapter 40 V B 1 c (2)]. The physical examination findings (i.e., decreased lung sounds in the ventral thorax) suggest pleural effusion as the cause of the dyspnea. In cats with severe respiratory distress, needle thoracocentesis is usually less stressful than obtaining thoracic radiographs and it can be life-saving if a significant volume of pleural fluid can be removed. Patient handling for thoracic radiographs may result in death in severely dyspneic animals. Anesthesia would be contraindicated until pleural fluid could be removed and chest tube placement would be premature until the cause of the effusion is determined. Cage rest and diuretic therapy may improve the respiratory signs over the next few days, but more aggressive therapy is indicated in this case. Blood gas analysis would not significantly contribute to patient management at this time. Hypoxemia would be present on the blood gas analysis but this finding could be predicted based on the state of the animal.

39. The answer is 1 [Table 17-1]. With protein-losing nephropathy (PLN), hypoalbuminemia can result in generalized peripheral edema. Thrombosis can also cause peripheral edema as a result of venous obstruction, but the edema is usually localized rather than generalized. Left-sided heart failure alone will not cause generalized edema, although right-sided heart failure can. Oliguric renal failure will not result in generalized peripheral edema unless intravenous fluid administration is overzealous.

40. The answer is 1 [Chapter 39 III B 2]. *Staphylococcus aureus, Escherichia coli*, and β-hemolytic streptococci account for approximately 70% of the cases of bacterial endocarditis in dogs. Although *Proteus mirabilis, Pseudomonas aeruginosa, Klebsiella pneumoniae*, and *Enterobacter* species could cause endocarditis, they are infrequently implicated.

41. The answer is 5 [Chapter 43 Part I:I A 2 a, 4 a]. This dog most likely has prerenal azotemia and a nonurinary cause of hypoalbuminemia. The azotemia is prerenal in origin based on the fact that the urine specific gravity is greater than 1.030. There is no urinary tract inflammation [(as evidenced by the fact that the white blood cell (WBC) count is within normal limits] and the urine protein: urine creatinine ratio (U_{Pr}:U_{Cr}) is less than 1.0; therefore, the protein in the urine could be considered normal or not significant. This would indicate that the hypoalbuminemia is not due to urinary losses and other causes should be sought [e.g., decreased hepatic production, gastrointestinal (GI) losses]. The loose stools noted in this dog would suggest that GI protein losses may be the cause of the hypoalbuminemia.

42. The answer is 4 [Chapter 49 V K 6 (b) (1)]. If a dog has bitten someone and is showing neurologic signs, the dog should be euthanized and the brain submitted for rabies testing because of the zoonotic potential of rabies. If a pet dog has bitten someone but is not showing neurologic signs, it should be quarantined and observed for 10 days. An unowned dog that has bitten someone but is not showing neurologic signs should be euthanized and the brain tested.

43. The answer is 1 [Chapter 44 I B; IV A]. Diabetes insipidus is characterized by the production of large quantities of dilute urine (i.e., with a urine specific gravity that is usually less than 1.010). In both disorders, urine volume is increased, thirst is increased (a compensatory polydipsia), and the appetite is good; the appetite may even be increased with diabetes mellitus. Hyperglycemia and glucosuria are hallmarks of diabetes mellitus, not diabetes insipidus.

44. The answer is 5 [Chapter 48 V D]. The most common clinical presentation for splenic hemangiosarcomas is acute intraabdominal hemorrhage in a German shepherd or a German shepherd crossbred dog. Although the anemia is nonregenerative, it is too soon after the hemorrhage for a reticulocyte response to occur. Coagulation factor deficiency due to anticoagulant rodenticide toxicity or liver failure can be ruled out based on the normal prothrombin time (PT) and partial thromboplastin time (PTT). Thrombocytopenia was not detected on the complete blood count (CBC). Trauma cannot be ruled out but there is no historic or physical evidence to support this diagnosis.

45. The answer is 3 [Chapter 39 XII B 3 a (1)]. Ocular abnormalities, especially blindness following retinal detachment, are the most common signs resulting from arterial hypertension. Although pleural effusion and subcutaneous edema could theoretically result from arterial hypertension, they are more apt to be associated with an underlying disorder (e.g., hypoalbuminemia in nephrotic syndrome). Hypertension can result in left ventricular hypertrophy but ventricular tachycardia is rare. Vomiting is not caused by hypertension but could be related to an underlying disorder associated with hypertension (e.g., hyperthyroidism).

46. The answer is 4 [Chapter 40 I C 1]. Feline calicivirus (FCV) and feline rhinotracheitis virus (FRV, feline herpesvirus-1) account for 80%–90% of upper respiratory tract infections in cats. *Chlamydia psittaci* accounts for most of the remaining infections. *Mycoplasma* and *Bordetella bronchiseptica* infections are rare.

47. The answer is 2 [Chapter 47 II J 4]. The signs are suggestive of organophosphate or carbamate toxicity. The SLUD signs (i.e., salivation, lacrimation, urination, and defecation) are present, as well as other parasympathetic effects (e.g., miosis, muscle fasciculations, bronchoconstriction, increased respiratory secretions). Seizures can occur with strychnine poisoning, idiopathic epilepsy, and metaldehyde poisoning, but the parasympathetic signs would be absent. Warfarin toxicity will only cause seizures if intracranial hemorrhage occurred.

48. The answer is 3 [Chapter 41 III B 8]. Vomiting food 8 or more hours after eating is usually a result of a gastric outflow obstruction such as pyloric stenosis. This diagnosis is also supported by the signalment (a young, male, brachycephalic dog) and the lack of systemic signs of illness. Alimentary lymphosarcoma, hypoadrenocorticism, intussusception, and renal failure are unlikely because anorexia and weight loss are often seen with these disorders. Diarrhea would also likely be seen with lymphosarcoma, hypoadrenocorticism, or an intussusception.

49. The answer is 3 [Chapter 16 V D]. Dantrolene is the appropriate treatment for malignant hyperthermia. External cooling should also be used, but is insufficient on its own to arrest the hyperthermia.

50. The answer is 1 [Chapter 40 III C 4]. Left atrial enlargement (due to mitral valve insufficiency), collapsing trachea, and chronic bronchitis are all common in small-breed dogs. The history and physical examination findings could be present with one or all three conditions existing together. Additional diagnostic testing would be required to differentiate the three disorders. Pulmonary neoplasia and allergic bronchitis are not common in middle-aged small-breed dogs. Infectious tracheobronchitis would be characterized by a more acute history.

51. The answer is 4 [Chapter 43 Part I:VI D; VIII E 3]. In Dalmatian dogs, urate is not metabolized to allantoin as it is in other dogs. As a result, serum and urine urate levels are higher than normal, predisposing Dalmatians to the development of urate urolithiasis.

52. The answer is 2 [Chapter 49 III L 2 b (5)]. An immunoglobulin M (IgM) titer is the best way to confirm the diagnosis of toxoplasmosis. Immunoglobulin G (IgG) titers will also be increased with infection, but paired titers are needed to confirm an active infection. The presence of typical retinal lesions can be supportive of a tentative diagnosis but is not pathognomonic. Response to therapy can also support a tentative diagnosis, but other infections can also respond to the same treatment. Fecal flotation is not a reliable means of diagnosis because the oocysts are only shed periodically.

53. The answer is 5 [Chapter 47 IV I]. The dog most likely has acute polyradiculoneuritis (coonhound paralysis). The presence of diffuse lower motor neuron (LMN) signs (e.g., hypo- or areflexia, flaccid muscle tone) rules out a cervical (C1–C5) lesion. Acute polyradiculoneuritis would be more likely than botulism because botulism is usually characterized by widespread cranial nerve involvement, causing dysphagia, laryngeal paralysis, and megaesophagus. Tick paralysis would be another differential and a thorough examination for ticks and treatment with an insecticidal dip would be indicated.

54. The answer is 2 [Chapter 40 IV I 3]. Pulmonary contusions may not be visible until 6–12 hours post-trauma and in some cases, not until 24 hours later.

55. The answer is 4 [Chapter 43 Part I:IV C]. Renal failure is present based on the presence of azotemia and a urine specific gravity of less than 1.035. The weight loss (as evidenced by the thin body condition) and the nonregenerative anemia suggest that the renal failure is chronic. In addition, no other signs of acute renal failure are present (e.g., hyperkalemia, large numbers of casts in the urine, calcium oxalate crystalluria). Prerenal azotemia may be contributing to the azotemia, but is not the main abnormality because the urine specific gravity is less than 1.035. Hypoadrenocorticism is extremely rare in cats.

56. The answer is 1 [Chapter 43 Part II: V D 1; Table 43-9]. The acid–base disorder present is respiratory acidosis. Of the disorders listed (pleural effusion, urethral obstruction, hypovolemic shock, severe and protracted vomiting, and ethylene glycol intoxication), only pleural effusion could cause a respiratory acidosis. Urethral obstruction, hypovolemic shock, and ethylene glycol poisoning would be expected to be associated with metabolic acidosis. Severe vomiting may be associated with metabolic alkalosis or acidosis.

57. The answer is 5 [Chapter 40 V B 6 a (2) (a)]. A noncompressible cranial thorax in a young cat is suggestive of a cranial mediastinal mass. Pleural effusion, lung lobe consolidation, heartworm infection, and pulmonary contusions will not cause a noncompressible cranial thorax, although they may be associated with increased respiratory effort.

58. The answer is 2 [Chapter 46 III C 1]. Idiopathic immune-mediated polyarthritis is the most likely cause of this dog's stilted gait. A negative Lyme titer would make infection with *Borrelia burgdorferi* very unlikely. The synovial fluid findings are not consistent with degenerative joint disease (DJD). The lack of erosive changes on radiographs makes rheumatoid arthritis less likely. Although an antinuclear antibody (ANA) test or lupus erythematosus (LE) cell preparation were not performed, there are no other clinical or laboratory signs to suggest systemic lupus erythematosus (SLE), such as skin disease, immune-mediated hemolytic anemia (IHA), immune-mediated thrombocytopenia (IMT), or proteinuria.

59. The answer is 2 [Chapter 43 Part I:I A 2 a]. Azotemia in the face of a urine specific gravity greater than 1.030 in a dog is consistent with a prerenal cause because tubular function is intact. Dehydration is a very common cause of prerenal azotemia. A specific gravity greater than 1.030 rules out acute or chronic renal failure (in most cases). There were no physical examination findings that would suggest a postrenal cause (e.g., urinary obstruction, rupture of the urinary tract). Liver failure is often associated with a normal or low blood urea nitrogen (BUN) concentration.

60. The answer is 4 [Chapter 47 I C 2 e]. Conscious perception of pain requires a behavioral response from the animal (e.g., turning its head toward the stimulus, yelping, struggling to get away). All of the other reactions described are spinal reflexes that do not require the conscious perception of pain for the reflex to occur.

61. The answer is 1 [Chapter 48 II A 2 b (3) (a) (v)]. Tetracycline or a tetracycline derivative (e.g., doxycycline) is the best agent for the treatment of hemobartonellosis. In general, rickettsial organisms, such as *Hemobartonella felis,* are responsive to tetracyclines. Although chloramphenicol can be effective, its side effects (anorexia, bone marrow suppression) make it a less desirable option. Amoxicillin with clavulanic acid, erythromycin, and trimethoprim/sulfadiazine would have little or no effect.

62. The answer is 1 [Chapter 43 Part I:IV D 2]. A reduced-protein diet reduces the severity of uremic signs in animals with chronic renal failure. Most of the signs of uremia arise from products of protein metabolism. Because protein contains significant amounts of phosphorus, reduced-protein diets are, by definition, also reduced in phosphorus, which may help ameliorate signs associated with renal secondary hyperparathyroidism. A reduced-protein diet will not increase the glomerular filtration rate (GFR). Because patients with chronic renal failure are already acidotic and have a tendency to develop hypokalemia, reduced-protein diets are not formulated to exacerbate these problems. Creatinine is a product of muscle metabolism, not a dietary constituent.

63. The answer is 3 [Chapter 48 II A 1 b, 2 b (2) (c) (i); IV B 2 a (2) (a); Table 48-3]. The hematologic abnormalities indicate a strongly regenerative anemia. The first thing to do would be to calculate the reticulocyte index (RI) as follows: The corrected reticulocyte percentage (CRP) equals the reticulocyte percentage (24) multiplied by the patient hematocrit (15) divided by 45, or 8. The RI then equals the CRP (8) divided by the reticulocyte life span, which, with a patient hematocrit of 15%, is 2.5 days. Therefore, the RI is 3.2, a value that supports a regenerative anemia and suggests hemolysis as the cause. The marked spherocytosis indicates immune-mediated erythrocyte damage. As a result, a diagnosis of immune-mediated hemolytic anemia (IHA) is justified. Although there are many causes of thrombocytopenia, its occurrence with IHA would suggest that it is also immune-mediated. A strongly regenerative anemia can occur with blood loss from anticoagulant rodenticide poisoning, thrombocytopenia, or trauma, but marked spherocytosis and an RI greater than or equal to 3.0 would favor immune-mediated hemolysis. The icterus and bilirubinuria result from the excessive erythrocyte breakdown and metabolism of hemoglobin. Primary liver disease is unlikely.

64. The answer is 3 [Chapter 43 Part I:XII D 2]. This dog most likely has prostatic neoplasia. A neutered male dog is at low risk for developing bacterial infection of the prostate gland or benign prostatic hyperplasia. However, the risk of neoplasia remains. Therefore, a nodular, asymmetric prostate gland in a neutered male dog would suggest neoplasia as the cause of the enlargement (unless the dog had just been neutered within the last few days to weeks).

65. The answer is 1 [Chapter 47 I D 1 d (2)]. Because cerebrospinal fluid (CSF) collection requires general anesthesia, any condition (neurologic or otherwise) that significantly increases the risk associated with general anesthesia may be a contraindication to CSF collection. Cervical pain, mental depression, inflammatory central nervous system (CNS) disease, and suspected brain neoplasia could be indications for CSF collection.

66. The answer is 1 [Chapter 47 III A 2 c, B 1]. The neurologic examination is consistent with a lesion in the T3–L3 region. The breed, acute onset of signs, and the neurologic findings are all suggestive of an acute intervertebral disk herniation. The presence of severe neurologic signs (i.e., complete paralysis of the hindlimbs) is a strong indication for surgical decompression as soon as possible. Mild or absent neurologic deficits would not necessitate immediate surgery or surgery at all. Fibrocartilaginous embolism can have an acute history but it is usually not painful, neurologic signs are often asymmetric, and large-breed dogs are more commonly affected. Spinal cord tumors are not usually characterized by an acute history and are much less common than disk herniations. However, pain may be present and surgical decompression or excision may be justified.

67. The answer is 4 [Chapter 43 Part I:XII B 3 c (2)]. The trigone area is a common site for bladder neoplasia. Eighty-seven percent of bladder tumors in dogs are transitional cell carcinomas.

68. The answer is 3 [Chapter 47 V C 2]. Masticatory muscle atrophy with trismus is common with masticatory muscle myositis and may be the first manifestation of this disease. Trigeminal nerve paralysis may result in masticatory muscle atrophy but would be associated with a dropped jaw and an inability to close the mouth (if the paralysis was bilateral). Immune-mediated polymyositis usually spares the masticatory muscles. Myotonia is associated with muscle hypertrophy, not atrophy.

69. The answer is 2 [Chapter 48 III A 3]. Eosinophilia often (but not always) accompanies allergic disease or parasitic infection. Corticosteroid administration usually results in eosinopenia rather than eosinophilia. Bacterial, fungal, and viral infections are not associated with eosinophilia.

70. The answer is 4 [Chapter 41 IV B 14 a]. This cat most likely has alimentary lymphosarcoma. Cats with early alimentary lymphosarcoma may have small bowel diarrhea and are polyphagic; with time, however, anorexia occurs. Hyperthyroidism often causes small bowel diarrhea and polyphagia, but the disorder occurs in middle-aged to older cats. Cats with an intestinal foreign body or salmonellosis are usually systemically ill and anorexic, not polyphagic. Cryptosporidiosis may cause diarrhea, but the diarrhea is often bloody and systemic signs of illness are usually present as a result of the coccidial infection or an underlying disease that predisposed the cat to the infection.

71. The answer is 4 [Chapter 9 IV B 1 a (3); Chapter 42 I A 4 b (7)]. The conjugated bilirubin level is usually increased with posthepatic icterus because the bile is unable to flow freely into the small intestine; the bile is mostly conjugated because it has passed through the liver. Serum alkaline phosphatase (ALP) is also usually greatly increased because ALP levels increase with cholestasis. Serum alanine aminotransferase (ALT) levels increase with hepatocellular damage. Some hepatocellular damage can occur secondary to posthepatic obstruction, but the increase in ALT is usually much less significant than the increase in SAP in animals with posthepatic icterus.

72. The answer is 3 [Chapter 44 III A 1]. Lymphocytic thyroiditis is one of the most common causes of hypothyroidism in dogs.

Thyroid-stimulating hormone (TSH) deficiency (i.e., secondary hypothyroidism) and thyrotropin-releasing hormone (TRH) deficiency (i.e., tertiary hypothyroidism) can occur but are rare, as is thyroid agenesis. Surgical thyroidectomy, the most common cause of hypothyroidism in cats, is rarely performed in the dog.

73. The answer is 2 [Chapter 47 IV L]. The clinical sign of weakness following exertion is typical of myasthenia gravis. The definitive diagnosis is made on the basis of finding a significant antibody titer to the acetylcholine receptor. Edrophonium administration can aid in a presumptive diagnosis, but this test provides only a subjective assessment. The clinical signs would not be consistent with polyneuropathy [which is characterized by diffuse lower motor neuron (LMN) signs] or polymyositis (which is characterized by muscle atrophy or pain and increased serum creatine kinase).

74. The answer is 4 [Chapter 48 IV C 2 b (2) (b)]. Anticoagulant rodenticide poisoning is most likely in this miniature schnauzer because of the dog's age, the acute onset of signs, the presence of hemorrhage into a body cavity, and the prolonged activated clotting time (ACT). Trauma would not be associated with a prolonged ACT. vonWillebrand's disease (vWD) cannot be ruled out based on the information provided, but platelet dysfunction is not usually associated with bleeding into body cavities and the ACT is usually unaffected. Although thrombocytopenia is present, it is not significant enough to be associated with spontaneous hemorrhage, which is usually associated with platelet counts below $20,000/\mu$l. Mild to moderate thrombocytopenia is not uncommon with acute hemorrhage. Hemophilia A cannot be ruled out but this disorder would be less likely because of the age of the animal and the lack of prior reports of bleeding (the dog had been neutered).

75. The answer is 3 [Chapter 14 I B]. Normal water consumption for a dog is 50–70 ml/kg/ day. The daily fluid requirement for smaller dogs is near the upper end of this range, whereas larger dogs have daily fluid requirements near the lower end of this range.

76. The answer is 1 [Chapter 48 VI B 6]. Although multiple myeloma, lymphosarcoma, chronic lymphocytic leukemia (CLL), and ehrlichiosis can all be associated with a monoclonal gammopathy, only multiple myeloma is associated with "punched out" osteolytic lesions. Osteosarcoma is not associated with a monoclonal gammopathy and "punched out" osteolytic lesions are uncommon with this tumor.

77. The answer is 4 [Chapter 49 V E 3 b (3)]. Both enzyme-linked immunosorbent assay (ELISA) and immunofluorescent antibody (IFA) detect the p27 core antigen. The IFA test detects only viral antigen associated with infected cells, whereas ELISA will detect any p27 antigen in the circulation.

78. The answer is 2 [Chapter 43 Part I:VIII E 3]. Urate crystals or calculi are sometimes found in dogs and cats with hepatic dysfunction. Because of this, if urate crystals or calculi are seen in a cat or a dog other than a Dalmatian, hepatic function should be evaluated even if no other signs of hepatic disease are present.

79. The answer is 3 [Chapter 44 IV A 5 a (1) (a) (ii)]. Ultralente insulin administered subcutaneously once daily is the insulin regimen of choice for the initial regulation of a nonketotic diabetic cat. The duration of action of NPH and lente insulins in cats tends to be less than 24 hours, so once-daily administration is usually ineffective. Crystalline insulin has an even shorter duration of action and therefore is usually reserved for the treatment of diabetic ketoacidosis.

80. The answer is 3 [Chapter 44 V B 1]. Anorexia, vomiting, and weakness are common in cats with primary hypoadrenocorticism. Although common in dogs with hypoadrenocorticism, diarrhea and bradycardia are uncommon in affected cats. Polyphagia is not characteristic of hypoadrenocorticism in either species.

81. The answer is 3 [Chapter 49 I E 3 b (1) (c)]. An agar-gel immunodiffusion test is the best way to confirm a diagnosis of brucellosis. The tube agglutination test and rapid slide agglutination test (RSAT) have a high sensitivity but lower specificity and therefore may yield false–positive results. Culture of a uterine biopsy or testicular biopsy may also confirm the diagnosis, but these tests are more invasive and costly.

82. The answer is 2 [Chapter 40 III C 1]. Dogs with infectious tracheobronchitis ("kennel cough") do not have a fever or other signs of systemic illness. Animals with bacterial endocarditis, toxoplasmosis, or feline infectious peritonitis (FIP) may have a fever, and hyperthermia can occur with puerperal tetany as a result of increased muscular activity.

83. The answer is 1 [Table 10-2]. The abdominal distention commonly seen in dogs with hyperadrenocorticism is the result of abdominal muscle weakness and hepatomegaly, rather than ascites. Intraabdominal neoplasia, protein-losing nephropathy (PLN), right-sided heart failure, and hepatic cirrhosis can all result in ascites; additional historical information, other physical examination findings, and diagnostic test results will help differentiate these disorders.

84. The answer is 5 [Chapter 50 I D 2 c]. Orthovoltage radiation can be used for superficial tumors but cannot be used to treat deeper tumors without severely damaging the overlying tissues. Cobalt-60 or a linear accelerator is needed for radiation treatment of deeper tumors (e.g., pituitary macroadenomas). Potential side effects of radiation therapy include tissue necrosis and permanent localized alopecia. To minimize the adverse effects of treatment, multiple small doses are administered. Surgery or chemotherapy prior to radiation therapy may increase the effectiveness of the radiation therapy by reducing the tumor volume. It may take weeks or months to see the full effects of radiation therapy.

85. The answer is 4 [Chapter 3 I A]. Drugs, exogenous toxins, and endogenous toxins (e.g., uremic toxins, ammonia) can cause vomiting by stimulating the chemoreceptor trigger zone and/or the vomiting center. Neural input from the colon and other viscera can also stimulate the vomiting center. Cerebral stimulation can cause psychosomatic vomiting, but this is mediated through the vomiting center and not the chemoreceptor trigger zone— the chemoreceptor trigger zone is sensitive to blood-borne toxins.

86. The answer is 4 [Chapter 41 I B 1 a, 3 e, C 1 a–c, 3 a]. Prognathism, not brachygnathism, is commonly seen in brachycephalic breeds. Cleft palates are also more common in brachycephalic breeds. Gingival hyperplasia can be seen in many breeds, but is most common in collies, boxers, and other large-breed dogs. Craniomandibular osteopathy is most common in various terrier breeds. Retained deciduous teeth can be seen in any breed but are far more common in small dogs.

87. The answer is 3 [Chapter 14 IV A 1]. A urine specific gravity that is greater than 1.025 in a nondehydrated, nonglucosuric dog suggests that the dog is not polyuric. An exception to this guideline can occur if large amounts of solutes are present in the urine; these solutes will increase the measured specific gravity even if the kidneys are incapable of concentrating urine adequately.

88. The answer is 1 [Chapter 45 I C 1]. A functional ovarian cyst will usually cause a prolongation of proestrus or estrus rather than a prolonged interestrous interval. With "silent" heat, cycling is normal but clinical signs of estrus are not seen; this is actually an apparent failure to cycle. Hypothyroidism, premature ovarian failure, hyperadrenocorticism, and a nonfunctional ovarian cyst can all cause a prolonged interestrous period.

89. The answer is 3 [Chapter 41 II B 7]. Regurgitation is not a common clinical sign with esophageal fistula unless a foreign body, neoplasia, or infection/inflammation was responsible for the development of the fistulous tract. With congenital esophageal fistula, the problem is a developmental defect and the clinical symptoms are usually referable to the tissue with which the esophagus is connected (e.g., respiratory symptoms with a bronchoesophageal fistula, pleural fluid or adhesions with a pleuroesophageal fistula, soft tissue swelling and an external draining tract with a cutaneous–esophageal fistula). Regurgitation is common with persistent right aortic arch (PRAA), congenital diverticula, and inherited megaesophagus. Clinical symptoms are usually first seen at the time of weaning because liquids are often more easily passed to the stomach than are solid foods.

90. The answer is 5 [Table 11-1]. Most animals with protein-losing nephropathy (PLN) have anorexia rather than polyphagia in addition to their weight loss. With hyperthyroidism, diabetes mellitus, exocrine pancreatic insufficiency (EPI), and some cases of protein-losing enteropathy (PLE), weight loss occurs despite concurrent polyphagia; this weight loss is a result of increased nutrient use, increased nutrient loss, maldigestion, and a combination of increased nutrient loss and malassimilation, respectively.

91. The answer is 4 [Chapter 41 II A 2 b (2)–(3), B 2 d]. Stomatitis does not occur as a complication of esophageal disease, although pharyngeal irritation can occur secondary to repeated regurgitation. Perforation can occur secondary to an esophageal laceration, deep ulceration, pressure necrosis, or deep inflammation. Strictures can occur secondary to any esophageal damage. Malnutrition can result if regurgitation is so severe that inadequate nutrients reach the stomach and intestinal tract or if inappetence or anorexia is present. Recurrent or chronic respiratory disease as a result of aspiration is common.

92. The answer is 1 [Table 14-1]. Diabetes mellitus, hyperthyroidism, and renal failure are the most common causes of polyuria and polydipsia in an older cat. Hyperadrenocorticism does occur in older cats but is rare. In middle-aged and older dogs, hyperadrenocorticism is a common cause of polyuria and polydipsia.

93. The answer is 2 [Chapter 42 I A 3 a]. Gastrointestinal (GI) hemorrhage, alkalosis, constipation, uremia, and consumption of a high-protein diet can all contribute to the clinical signs of hepatic encephalopathy. Acidosis, however, will not exacerbate clinical signs of hepatic encephalopathy.

94. The answer is 2 [Chapter 16 VI B]. Congestive heart failure does not occur as a result of severe hyperthermia, but disseminated intravascular coagulation (DIC), hepatic and renal failure, gastrointestinal (GI) hemorrhage and mucosal sloughing, cerebral edema, rhabdomyolysis, hyperkalemia, and metabolic acidosis can occur.

95. The answer is 3 [Chapter 41 II B 4 c]. Calcium channel blockers have no effect on gastroesophageal reflux. Feeding a low-fat, high-protein diet will increase the lower esophageal sphincter tone, as will administering metoclopramide. Metoclopramide will also promote gastric emptying. Histamine-2 (H_2) antagonists (e.g., cimetidine) decrease gastric acidity (acid in the reflux is one of the compounds responsible for the esophageal irritation). Although reflux esophagitis is not caused by infection, initial antibiotic therapy may help patients by preventing secondary infection of the inflamed mucosa.

96. The answer is 3 [Chapter 41 III B 3 c]. A pyloroplasty (i.e., a transverse incision into the pylorus that is sutured longitudinally) is not commonly performed as treatment for gastric dilatation–volvulus (GDV); a pyloroplasty is most commonly performed in animals with gastric outflow obstruction caused by pyloric hypertrophy. A gastrotomy (i.e., incision into the stomach to remove a large amount of food) is commonly needed to empty the stomach of any remaining gas, liquid, or food so that the stomach can be more easily repositioned; this procedure will also allow visual examination of the gastric mucosa for viability. Discolored areas with poor vascularity or poor contractility are usually resected (i.e., via a gastrectomy). The spleen should also be removed if the vascular supply has been compromised. A gastropexy is usually the final procedure performed; this procedure fixes the stomach in place so that GDV cannot recur.

97. The answer is 3 [Chapter 44 I B 1 b]. Hyperadrenocorticism, pyelonephritis, hypercalcemia, and pyometra all can cause polyuria and polydipsia by interfering with the action of antidiuretic hormone (ADH) on the renal tubules and collecting ducts. Because nephrogenic diabetes insipidus is a disorder characterized by a lack of renal response to ADH, these disorders in effect cause an acquired nephrogenic diabetes insipidus. In contrast, diabetes mellitus causes polyuria through an osmotic diuresis.

98. The answer is 3 [Chapter 45 I C 7 b (1) (b)]. Although many types of bacteria can

cause pyometra, *Escherichia coli*, *Staphylococcus*, and *Streptococcus* are the most common pathogens. *Pseudomonas* is not a common cause of pyometra.

99. The answer is 1 [Table 41-2]. Pneumonia can be a complication of megaesophagus but is not a cause of megaesophagus. Myasthenia gravis and hypoadrenocorticism result in decreased neuromuscular function. Viral encephalitis is believed to disrupt the normal swallowing reflex. The mechanism behind the development of megaesophagus in cats with pyloric stenosis is not known.

100. The answer is 4 [Chapter 45 I C 8 a (2) (a)]. Behavioral changes, pyometra, mammary development, lactation, diabetes mellitus, acromegaly, and an increased risk of mammary neoplasia are all potential side effects of the use of megestrol acetate. Clitoral hypertrophy is not seen with megesterol acetate administration but can occur as a side effect of mibolerone administration for suppression of estrus.

101. The answer is 2 [Chapter 41 I E]. A sialocele may cause drooping and dysphagia if the pharyngeal region is affected, but pain is not usually present. A fluctuant swelling may also be seen with sialocele. Masticatory myositis, retrobulbar abscess, craniomandibular osteopathy, and an oral foreign body would all be possible in this patient. Concurrent clinical signs (e.g., muscle swelling with myositis, exophthalmus with a retrobulbar abscess, mandibular enlargement with craniomandibular osteopathy, drooling with an oral foreign body) may help differentiate these disorders based on the history and physical examination, but these other signs may not be present, especially with only a 1-day history of disease.

APPENDIX—Tables of Normal Reference Values

TABLE A. Normal Reference Values for a Complete Blood Count (CBC)

	Canine		Feline	
	Traditional Units	**SI Units**	**Traditional Units**	**SI Units**
Hemoglobin	13.2–19.2 g/dl	132–193 g/L	8.0–15.0 g/dl	80–150 g/L
Hematocrit	38%–57%	0.38–0.57 L/L	24%–45%	0.24–0.45 L/L
Erythrocytes	$5.6–8.5 \times 10^6/\mu l$	$5.6–8.5 \times 10^{12}/L$	$5.0–10 \times 10^6/\mu l$	$5.0–10 \times 10^{12}/L$
MCV	62–71 mm^3	62–71 fl	39–50 mm^3	39–50 fl
MCH	22–25 pg	22–25 pg	13–17 pg	13–17 pg
MCHC	33.7%–36.5%	337–365 g/L	32%–36%	320–360 g/L
Reticulocytes	0%–1.5%	0%–1.5%	0%–1.5%	0%–1.5%
Platelets	$145–440 \times 10^3/\mu l$	$145–440 \times 10^9/L$	$190–400 \times 10^3/\mu l$	$190–400 \times 10^9/L$
Total nucleated cell count	$6.1–17.4 \times 10^3/\mu l$	$6.1–17.4 \times 10^9/L$	$5.5–15.4 \times 10^3/\mu l$	$5.5–15.4 \times 10^9/L$
Neutrophils	$3.9–12 \times 10^9/\mu l$	$3.9–12 \times 10^9/L$	$2.5–12.5 \times 10^3/\mu l$	$2.5–12.5 \times 10^9/L$
Band neutrophils	$0–1.0 \times 10^3/\mu l$	$0–1.0 \times 10^9/L$	$0–0.3 \times 10^3/\mu l$	$0–0.3 \times 10^9/L$
Lymphocytes	$0.8–3.6 \times 10^3/\mu l$	$0.8–3.6 \times 10^9/L$	$1.5–7.0 \times 10^3/\mu l$	$1.5–7.0 \times 10^9/L$
Monocytes	$0–1.8 \times 10^3/\mu l$	$0–1.8 \times 10^9/L$	$0–0.85 \times 10^3/\mu l$	$0–0.85 \times 10^9/L$
Eosinophils	$0–1.9 \times 10^3/\mu l$	$0–1.9 \times 10^9/L$	$0–0.75 \times 10^3/\mu l$	$0–0.75 \times 10^9/L$
Basophils	$0–0.2 \times 10^3/\mu l$	$0–0.2 \times 10^9/L$	$0–0.2 \times 10^3/\mu l$	$0–0.2 \times 10^9/L$

MCH = mean corpuscular hemoglobin, MCHC = mean corpuscular hemoglobin concentration, MCV = mean corpuscular volume, SI = Système International.

Values derived from Jacobs RM, Lumsden JH. Canine and feline reference values. In *Current Veterinary Therapy XII*. Edited by Bonagura JD, Kirk RW. Philadelphia, WB Saunders, 1995, pp 1395–1417.

TABLE B. Normal Reference Values for Serum Biochemical Analyses

	Canine		Feline	
	Traditional Units	**SI Units**	**Traditional Units**	**SI Units**
Sodium	145–158 mEq/L	145–158 mmol/L	150–165 mEq/L	150–165 mmol/L
Potassium	3.6–5.8 mEq/L	3.6–5.8 mmol/L	3.7–5.8 mEq/L	3.7–5.8 mmol/L
Chloride	105–122 mEq/L	105–122 mmol/L	112–129 mEq/L	112–129 mmol/L
Calcium	9.0–11.8 mEq/L	2.24–2.95 mmol/L	8.9–11.6 mEq/L	2.23–2.9 mmol/L
Phosphorous	1.55–8.05 mEq/L	0.5–2.6 mmol/L	3.2–8.7 mEq/L	1.03–2.82 mmol/L
Urea	5.9–27.2 mg/dl	2.1–9.7 mmol/L	14–28 mg/dl	5–10 mmol/L
Creatinine	0.62–1.64 mg/dl	55–145 μmol/L	0.84–2.04 mg/dl	75–180 μmol/L
Glucose	60–158 mg/dl	3.3–8.7 mmol/L	63–162 mg/dl	3.5–9.0 mmol/L
Cholesterol	106–367 mg/dl	2.74–9.5 mmol/L	58–232 mg/dl	1.5–6.0 mmol/L
Total bilirubin	0–0.41 mg/dl	0–7 mmol/L	0–0.23 mg/dl	0–4 mmol/L
Amylase	400–1800 IU/L	400–1800 U/L	700–2000 IU/L	700–2000 U/L
ALP	0–200 IU/L	0–200 U/L	0–90 IU/L	0–90 U/L
AST	10–50 IU/L	10–50 U/L	10–59 IU/L	10–59 U/L
ALT	0–130 IU/L	0–130 U/L	10–75 IU/L	10–75 U/L
GGT	0–6 IU/L	0–6 U/L	0–2 IU/L	0–2 U/L
Creatine kinase	0–460 IU/L	0–460 U/L	0–580 IU/L	0–580 U/L
Total protein	5.0–7.5 g/dl	50–75 g/L	6.0–8.2 g/dl	60–82 g/L
Albumin	2.2–3.5 g/dl	22–35 g/L	2.5–3.9 g/dl	25–39 g/L
Globulins	2.2–4.5 g/dl	22–45 g/L	2.6–5.0 g/dl	26–50 g/L

ALT = alanine aminotransferase, ALP = alkaline phosphatase, AST = aspartate aminotransferase, GGT = γ-glutamyl transferase, SI = Système International.

Values derived from Jacobs RM, Lumsden JH. Canine and feline reference values. In *Current Veterinary Therapy XII.* Edited by Bonagura JD, Kirk RW. Philadelphia, WB Saunders, 1995, pp 1395–1417.

TABLE C. Normal Reference Values for Urinalysis

	Canine	Feline
Color/turbidity	Yellow/clear	Yellow/clear
Specific gravity	1.001–1.065	1.001–1.080
pH	4.5–8.5	4.5–8.5
Glucose	Negative	Negative
Ketones	Negative	Negative
Bilirubin	Trace to 1+	Negative
Occult blood	Negative	Negative
Protein	Negative to trace	Negative to trace
RBCs per high-power field	0–5	0–5
WBCs per high-power field	0–5	0–5
Casts per low-power field	Occasional hyaline	Occasional hyaline
Epithelial cells per high-power field	Occasional	Occasional
Bacteria per high-power field*	None	None
Crystals per high-power field	Variable	Variable
Urine protein:creatinine ratio	<1.0	<1.0

RBCs = red blood cells, WBCs = white blood cells.
* In samples collected by cystocentisis or catheterization.

TABLE D. Normal Reference Values for Arterial Blood Gases

	Canine	Feline
pH	7.407 (7.351–7.463)	7.386 (7.310–7.462)
P_{CO_2} (mmHg)	36.8 (30.8–42.8)	31.0 (25.2–36.8)
HCO_3^- (mEq/L)	22.2 (18.8–25.6)	18.0 (14.4–21.6)
P_{O_2} (mmHg)	92.1 (80.9–103.3)	106.8 (95.4–118.2)

Values derived from Haskins SC. Blood gases and acid–base balance: clinical interpretation and therapeutic implications. In *Current Veterinary Therapy VIII.* Edited by Kirk RW. Philadelphia, WB Saunders, 1983, pp 201–215.

Index

Italic page number indicates a figure, italic t indicates a table, Q indicates a question, and E indicates an explanation.